W9-AVY-996

Humane Managed Care?

Humane Managed Care?

EDITED BY

GERALD **SCHAMESS**

ANITA **LIGHTBURN**

NASW PRESS
National Association of Social Workers
Washington, DC

Josephine A.V. Allen, PhD, ACSW, President
Josephine Nieves, MSW, PhD, Executive Director

Jane Browning, *Director of Member Services and Publications*
Paula Delo, *Executive Editor*
Christina A. Davis, *Senior Editor*
Christine Cotting, UpperCase Publication Services, *Project Manager*
Caroline Polk, *Proofreader*
Bernice Eisen, *Indexer*
Chanté Lampton, *Acquisitions Associate*
Heather Peters, *Editorial Secretary*

© 1998 by the NASW Press

All rights reserved. No part of this book may be reproduced or transmitted in any form or by any means, electronic or mechanical, including photocopying, recording, or by any information storage and retrieval system, without permission in writing from the publisher.

Library of Congress Cataloging-in-Publication Data

Humane managed care? / edited by Gerald Schamess, Anita Lightburn.
p. cm.
Includes bibliographical references and index.
ISBN 0-87101-294-4 (alk. paper)
1. Managed care plans (Medical care). 2. Managed mental health care. 3. Health maintenance organizations. I. Schamess, Gerald. II. Lightburn, Anita.
RA413.H79 1998
362.1'04258—dc21 98-8336
CIP

Printed in the United States of America

DEDICATION

For our families

and your children,

that you will experience

humane care

Contents

Foreword

Five years ago a new administration stepped forward to design a comprehensive health care reform initiative. At the time, the administration suggested that the federal government build on prototypical "managed care" models, creating an efficient yet equitable public health care system. Congress subsequently fumbled its opportunity to guide the evolution of the new system. Thus, managed care swept with unprecedented speed through our institutions, our medical community, and our work places. A radical, historic shift in society's health care process took place before our astonished eyes, driven totally by market forces and entirely outside regulatory management.

Deep within the maelstrom, America's social workers have been riding the tide of overpowering change. In every setting—hospitals, research institutions, nursing homes, community mental health centers, clinics, schools, private practices, managed care companies—social workers are on the front lines of health care delivery as the nation's largest groups of mental health care providers. Like the canary in the coal mine, the social work profession's fate is a telling indicator of our nation's well-being in the face of the massive conversion to managed care.

Social workers historically have been at the forefront of social change. For 100 years, professional social workers have been addressing the needs of the poor and advocating for improved social conditions. Consequently, it is not surprising that they are once again in the vanguard, assessing the impact of managed care.

Humane Managed Care?—a collaborative effort of Smith College School for Social Work and the National Association of Social Workers—is a compendium of up-to-date research, analysis, experience, and evaluation of this impact on social workers and their clients.

We are confident that our multidisciplinary, wide-ranging review of this phenomenon not only will inform, but also will stimulate an ongoing public policy debate on a crucial topic. By replacing the spiraling costs of a flawed health care system with what appear to be spiraling profits at the expense of quality, what exactly has managed care brought us? How can social workers and other health care professionals "thrive with honor" as they adjust their practices and practice education in response to its demands? This book gives us a framework and the knowledge for examining complex issues and provides a basis for finding a solution.

Those who embrace the responsibility for being change agents will discover effective and ethical responses to managed care. The market-driven care system must be required to adhere to fundamental principles that provide for consumer voice, consumer choice, and service to America's most vulnerable populations. Passage and implementation of a consumers' bill of rights will be a beginning. Regulatory legislation and administrative procedures may be next. But one thing is essential—the continued vigilance and involvement of those committed to equitable social welfare.

JOSEPHINE NIEVES, MSW, PHD
Executive Director
National Association of Social Workers
Washington, DC

Preface

Questions, Concerns, and Opportunities

Is humane care the hallmark of service provision in the managed care revolution? This question dominates conversation among human services professionals as well as consumers. It is a conversation grounded in experience and propelled by the need to grapple with dramatic changes in the provision of care. It is one of the most important questions we must address to remain true to our commitment to healing, protection, and nurturance. We have assembled this volume as an ongoing part of the conversation as it has taken place in a variety of contexts among and by practitioners, managed care providers, educators, and students. The information and perspectives are provided to encourage active participation in the conversation for all who work in or are preparing to work in the human services.

The quality of mental health and health care depends on our unabated efforts to answer questions repeatedly raised about managed care. We need to know what has happened in the conversion of the caregiving relationships previously offered by physicians, social workers, nurses, and psychologists into care that is largely influenced by the dominant term "managed." What outcomes have resulted from the forceful takeover of health and mental health care? Have the long-practiced traditions of humane services provision also been honored and retained as intrinsic to managed care services? As resources have been redistributed, has there been greater access to care within new continua of services? Has better-quality care based on increased accountability been achieved? Have we realized the vision that if preventive care becomes the foundation for health and mental health it will be the most effective means for cost reduction in the long term? Or has the essence and tradition of humane services provision been sacrificed through management systems that embody corporate principles, systems, language, and values. Is humane managed care an oxymoron?

As educators and professionals, we take seriously our responsibility, embodied in our codes of ethics, to uphold the provision of humane services. In a system in which service is designed to be efficient in the short term and profit driven, are we holding on to, incorporating, and advancing principles, ethics, and best practices that are truly humane? Professionals across the human services are grappling with a practice context for which most were never prepared. Major assumptions about humane and effective ways to practice have been called into question as professionals struggle to be "providers" in agencies and institutions where they were trained to be healers, scientists, helpers, and advocates. The consumer language of the marketplace has eclipsed the familiar relational language of therapy. Does the concept of managed care and all related terminology limit the vision and potential for care? The fiscal bottom line is now the standard set by gatekeepers, the interpreters of managed care. It ensures accountability for scarce resources. In lieu of a national health care policy, the marketplace has instituted competition as a mechanism that promises quality care through quality control. Has managed care advanced the quality of care, and is it by definition also humane?

What recalibration has occurred since the management of care has become the dominant way of providing equitable service to the majority of people? Can corporate means and language be transcended and transfigured by the people who are caregivers, the professionals who do not define themselves simply as providers? Can the human beings who offer knowledge, skills, and resources through relationships that require time, respect, and decency turn a managed care provider system into healing and nurturing experiences that meet common human needs, rather than a system offering care that recipients may experience as a semblance of packaged consumer products?

The vigor of management systems has taken hold with the declared intent of improving the performance of service providers. Accountability and demonstration of effective practice are promoted as procedures that ensure quality care. In this new era, complex information systems transport people's lives across unprotected zones to augment efficiency and accountability while potentially violating the established confidence of caretaking relationships. Ethical issues and concerns are mushrooming. Legal and ethical complaints are being brought before courts, accreditation bodies, and state and federal regulatory bodies in an effort to define "humane managed care." And although the new system of accountability and management has solved some of our health care system's problems, it also has created new problems that need to be addressed.

Many contend that managed care does not serve everyone and that it serves unevenly. It has become increasingly evident that humane care in the managed care system is conditional, depending on diagnosis, payer categories, service unit allowances, and available networks that are well resourced. Cost shifting, one of the most notable strategies managed care has used to reduce costs, can disadvantage those who are not fortunate enough to have a support network of family or friends who can provide care when institutions will not. However, the shift from overly expensive inpatient services to outpatient and community-based care can work only if we invest in these new service systems. The promise of comprehensive community-based systems of care must be effectively implemented in the current environment of cost containment and profit making. There is a serious contradiction between comprehensive service delivery, which has been the central commitment of many professionals, and the provider system's primary commitment to "sufficient" service and profitability. Conflicts of interest are inherent as the philosophy of service and care clashes with the philosophy of profit.

Health, mental health, and child care have become "industries," and like other industries are transformed by takeovers and mergers. As conglomerates increase, individual choice becomes more limited. The managed care market system has a track record of reducing costs and saving money over the open-ended fee-for-service approach at a time when health care costs were threatening to spiral out of control. Economically, the potential exists to make a broader range of services available.

In this new order of "providing care" so much depends on whether the "market" will deliver care that men, women, children, and families need and can afford. With government protection receding, market forces may not be moderated fairly for the vulnerable populations—children, elderly men and women, and people who are chronically ill or disabled. In response to reduced benefits structures, limitations have been challenged through legislation promoted to protect individuals from the abuses of the health care market.

Can we all hope that as profit-based managed care systems are being fashioned in the marketplace they will be modified by professionals and consumers? Is it and will it continue to be their advocacy that defines rights and entitlement and ensures that new service continua will be developed in place of more expensive institutional care? Will poor people, disenfranchised nondominant cultural and racial groups, and people with chronic illness or developmental disabilities be able to obtain services in the marketplace? Who will make the decisions about rationing Medicaid resources in the year 2010?

We also are very concerned about the preparation of the upcoming generation of professionals who will not only provide service but will also advocate for humane service provision. Where and how will these professionals be trained when supports for professional training through internships, supervision, and continuing education are being drastically reduced or eliminated? Training programs for "behavioral health care" providers abound, sponsored by newly formed consultant groups and insurers. However, the narrow focus on behavioral health limits professional development. The tradition of shared responsibility for training has been lost in the frenzy of cost cutting accomplished by paring student internships that have been valuable resources and catalysts for learning in health and mental health settings. This dramatic change will transform fieldwork training and the preparation of future practitioners.

In this volume we address these fundamental questions. It has been rewarding for us to see various conversations over the past three years come together to present the complexity we have encountered in trying to answer the questions posed. We have valued the many opportunities that have provoked and stretched our thinking. Two forums that have informed this work are of special note. The first was a special issue of the *Smith Studies—The Human and Corporate Faces of Managed Care—* that was published in June 1996 and included presentations that had been delivered the previous summer in seminars and lectures at the Smith School for Social Work. The second forum was "The First Managed Behavioral Health Care Invitational Conference for New England Graduate Social Work Faculty," held at Boston University School of Social Work in October 1997. This conference was the first of its kind, with 13 schools participating. Support from the Robert Wood Johnson Foundation, the National Institute of Mental Health, obtained by Dean Wilma Peebles-Wilkins, Boston University, in her capacity as chair of the New England Association of Deans and Directors of Schools of Social Work, and with additional support from the Alcohol and Drug Institute at Boston University, brought together leading administrators, policy analysts, and educators to consider the implications of managed care for social work curricula and research. Our inquiry as social work educators was fueled by a host of questions that articulate concern for humane managed care. The keynote presentations from that faculty development conference are included here. New colleagues were also discovered at the conference, and they have become important contributors to this volume.

Geography of This Volume

We are pleased to bring together an unusual collection of scholarly articles and research, as well as case studies from the field. We have gathered a breadth of perspectives provided by a range of health professionals—social workers, psychiatrists, and psychologists as well as administrators, policy analysts, case managers, professional educators, and researchers. The challenge of and for "humane" managed care is presented here as both a public and a private issue affecting health care, mental health care, and related services that support children and families at risk. Those most centrally involved—those responsible for providing care—have presented their experiences and perspectives based on long tenure in human services. State mental health systems, local hospital care, mental health clinics, health maintenance organizations, and network systems of care are described and examined. In the tradition of field studies that bring cases forward for examination, clinicians' and clients' stories are told as "notes from the field." Administrators provide detailed strategic plans that convert fee-for-service and government-funded services to managed care contracts.

Policy issues are considered from the perspectives of health, mental health, and services for children and families. The economics of care, "managed, mismanaged, or unmanaged," is juxtaposed with political decisions that maintain the disadvantaged population in the social system. Educators and researchers also offer meta-analyses, adding another perspective that describes and examines complex outcomes ranging from the type and quality of care given to the state of and future directions for professional social work education.

Part one of this volume sets the stage through policy and program analyses. Part two provides a major case study of one state's "privatization" of its mental health services, beginning with the commissioner's management journal describing the shift to private managed care. In contrast, a longtime professional caregiver who is also an experienced administrator at a psychiatric hospital describes how he and his facility experienced the implementation of the commissioner's strategic re-engineering of mental health. Complementing these two different perspectives are two major research studies that report on the services delivery reconfiguration and utilization outcomes that have resulted. Reports of casualties of this change, including loss of life, are excerpted from a state legislative report. Such tragic outcomes are a sobering postscript to this case study. Overall, the varied and complex documentation of different outcomes provides a unique opportunity for assessing the cost and benefits of privatization in terms of its effects on humane managed care and on mental health services in one state.

Parts three and four present agency and practice perspectives as well as focused discussions of the challenges facing professional social work. Productive evolutions of service are reviewed, with emphasis on accountability, quality assurance, equitable distribution and cost shifting, as well as community-board management. In stark contrast, disturbing practice with adolescents with serious disturbances and with people with mental illness in major hospital and community settings is illustrated with case examples that document practitioners' worst fears. These case studies show how the bottom-line mentality of gatekeepers and administrators combined with employment practices that sacrifice experience and competence in favor of the least-expensive practitioners result in the "dumbing down" of the professions. Best practice, based on skill, knowledge, and the implementation of assessment-based intervention plans, is lost when the corporate value of cost reduction ranks first in determining who will provide services and how they will be provided. It is very difficult to make sense of increased suffering when there is clear potential for help, as well as knowledge and skill that could have been used for healing.

Practice perspectives demonstrate clinicians' resourcefulness and show how humane care still happens. Short-term work, clinical case management, and psychodynamic approaches are explored within the managed care context. One chapter, "Losing Innocents," can be taken as a metaphor for the experience of many managed care practitioners. The author's practice experience raises, both specifically and generally, the most troubling questions concerning the extraordinary challenges faced by those who are very sick and disabled. People who are alone and seriously ill fail to receive care because they are unable to actively shape the managed care they receive as well as need. From these case studies an alarming picture of inhumane care emerges where cost reduction results in care rationing that will not save money in the long term because of the very nature of chronic conditions that will worsen without care, requiring more-involved services at another time. These questions are replayed in the chapter "Notes from a Sinking Ship," a case study of a mental health center's practices of cutting costs to ensure institutional survival but seriously impairing the care of clients with chronic mental illness. In the end, the center may still be lost, along with its tradition of helping a population in great need—an institutional casualty of the managed care revolution.

Part four presents perspectives from the National Association for Social Workers, the Clinical Social Work Federation, and a national study of hospital social work, focusing on the challenges for social work and our allied professions. Obstacles and barriers, such as the deprofessionalization of social work and the takeover of social work roles, are discussed, as are strategies to optimize opportunities for services provision. Important clarifiers of the most salient issues that require new knowledge and approaches make clear how the context of care continues to change substantially. Leaders of professional organizations chronicle the move toward unionization, lobbying, and support for managed care alternatives. The critical path for preserving choice and the fight to maintain the right to elect psychotherapy is charted. Advocacy efforts are detailed for clients and professionals, with collective action and unionization promoted as ways of influencing the corporate giants that now control health and mental health care. Authors also study ethical and legal issues specific to managed care practice and abuse. Special attention is given to confidentiality, professional autonomy, and the reality of managing cost frequently taking precedence over managing care.

The landscape of new opportunities is surveyed in part five, which examines primary care, social work's role in working with state Medicaid contractors, multidisciplinary work in community clinics, clinical case management, and professional affiliation groups. These options describe the frontier for social work practice. With each option, new challenges and opportunities are evident for graduate and continuing education that will enable social workers to move forward toward carving out new ways of providing service.

The challenges for professional education are introduced in part six as sobering realities that are "forcing social work to make choices." Wide-ranging concerns about managed care have acted as catalysts for social work educators who are committed to providing the new "right" direction for curriculum development. With fieldwork training in serious jeopardy, it is important that we all more closely examine what is happening in practice. This also is a time to consider innovative training initiatives, recognizing that collaborative options to support fieldwork can markedly advance learning. Options range from attention to short-term models of treatment to introducing students to postmodern approaches that expand the ways we use helping relationships. Part six is important as an initial effort to chart the future direction of social work education.

Finally, part seven offers direction and resources for the important work of researching managed care. Research is designed to answer questions and to provide information so better decisions can be made about how to use health and child care resources. The two contributions here ably introduce options, possibilities, and directions that research should take. The state of managed care research is broadly reviewed, indicating the value of current studies and the potential of large-scale projects now in progress to answer many of the questions we have asked. Building on the available knowledge and expertise and asking critical questions, these researchers provide direction and resources for future studies.

We believe practitioners, policymakers, managed care providers, educators, researchers, and students should evaluate the human and corporate faces of managed care depicted in this volume. It is our hope that the volume will be a valuable resource in assisting many to address and answer questions posed by the revolution in services delivery. Humane managed care depends on informed professionals who are prepared to grapple with issues involving the relationship between care and fiscal responsibility. This involves grappling with corporate language, systems, and values, as well as the ideology that pushes the frontier of health and mental health care toward preventive community-based care. As professional social workers we are rooted in a tradition of activism that grew to maturity through our work in the Industrial Revolution. In the new market revolution that has enveloped health care and now services for children and families to the extent that they are considered industries, we encounter familiar challenges to social justice and humane practice. We hope that you will examine managed care through the perspectives and experiences of the collected authors in this volume and join with them and other concerned professionals in working for humane managed care.

Acknowledgments

This project has gone through many phases, and we are grateful to the people who have contributed along the way. Our particular thanks to all of the authors. We want to acknowledge those who have given extra time to updating their original work and to those who have written especially for this volume. It has been a pleasure to work with such a committed and able group of professionals. We value the vitality of their thinking and their ongoing work in this area.

We are particularly pleased to have collaborated with Jane Browning, Paula Delo, Christina Davis, and the production staff at NASW. They are a great team, and we have valued their investment in this project. Their vision, enthusiasm, encouragement, and patient attention to details are greatly appreciated. Thanks also to Linda Beebe, who initially shared the vision of Smith's collaboration with NASW to advance social work knowledge of managed care by combining our recent publications in this area.

On the home front, we are indebted to Marjorie Postal, our research analyst at the Smith College School for Social Work, who has been indispensable in coordinating and processing manuscripts. The sheer volume of details has been daunting, and we appreciate her patience, expertise, good humor, and skill. We also want to recognize the expert team who assisted in the production of the special issue of *Smith Studies* from which this volume grew: Joyce Leamy, Louise Krieger, Idene Rodriguez Martin, and Samantha Armour.

We appreciate permission for reprints from the following publishers: American Psychiatric Press, Inc., for work from *Psychiatric Services Journal;* Harwood Academic Publishers for work from *Crisis Intervention and Time Limited Treatment;* Haworth Press for work from the *Journal of Psychoanalytic Social Work, Social Work in Administration,* and *Social*

Work in Health Care; Manticore Publishers for work from *Families in Society;* Mosby-Year Book, Inc., for the use of material from the *Harvard Review of Psychiatry;* NASW Press for reprints from *Health & Social Work* and *Social Work; Open Minds;* the People-to-People Health Foundation for work from *Health Affairs.* The Annie E. Casey Foundation also supported an excellent report (*Managed Care: Challenges for Children and Family Services,* edited by Leslie Scallet, Cindy Brach, and Elizabeth Steele) under the direction of Patrick McCarthy on managed care for children and family services, and that report was the source of the policy chapters in that area.

The support of the New England Association of Deans and Directors of Schools of Social Work in developing the first faculty development conference on managed care provided an important venue for dialogue and learning. We are grateful to the Robert Wood Johnson Foundation, the National Institute of Mental Health, and the Alcohol and Drug Institute at the Boston University School of Social Work for providing support for that conference.

For interest, support, and lively debate, we thank our colleagues and students at Smith College School for Social Work. We are looking forward to continued collaboration and collective action for humane care, however it is managed.

Our clinical mentors, who have taught us about the meaning and value of relationship-based care that addresses the unique feelings and needs that clients bring to clinical encounters, have more than earned our deep appreciation. They taught us about a framework for humane care that has informed all of our work on this volume.

A special vote of thanks goes to our families for generously providing us with good quality managed care as we stretched the envelope to put this volume together. We are committed to working for humane managed care for you and for your children.

GERALD SCHAMESS, MSS
Professor of Social Work

ANITA LIGHTBURN, MSS, MED, EDD
Dean and Elizabeth Marting Truehaft Professor

Smith College School for Social Work
Northampton, MA

PART ONE

Policy Issues

CHAPTER 1

Social Work in a Health and Mental Health Managed Care Environment

Gary Rosenberg

Managed care and the changes in the health care marketplace provide social workers with a challenge and opportunity to enhance services to needy and vulnerable populations, those who are at risk for disability, and those who are chronically ill; to provide prevention and health maintenance services; to critically analyze health policies and practices; to advocate for an equitable system of allocation and access; and to rework the curriculum of schools of social work to prepare practitioners and researchers to enter the health care field of practice.

I will describe the emerging health marketplace—where it is and where it may be heading—and provide an overview of the production, distribution, and financing issues and their effects so far on the delivery of health care services. In selecting some issues and describing their implications for social work practice and education, I hope that these ideas will serve as a foundation for further discussion, analysis, and debate.

Evolving Health Care Marketplace

The process of market-driven health care is still evolving, but some trends are clear. Health care costs are being constrained by reduced lengths of hospital stays; increased ambulatory and community-based care; and reductions in home care benefits available through insurance, managed care organizations, and public programs. Families are, and will be, under increasing pressures to pay more direct costs; provide more hands-on, often technologically complex care; undertake greater burdens for longer times; and forgo more educational, career, and social opportunities (Levine, 1997).

Across the country there are emerging health systems, growth of managed care products, experimental attitudes in state government toward health coverage for poor people, increasing cost sensitivity among businesses, hospital cost-reduction efforts and process redesign, and the formation of physician group practices.

Although American health care policy lags behind that of Western Europe, particularly in access, American health policy has worked well when we deal with real

NOTE: An earlier version of this work was presented at "The First Managed Care Behavioral Health Care Invitational Conference for New England Graduate Social Work Faculty," funded by the Robert Wood Johnson Foundation, the National Institute of Mental Health, and the Alcohol and Drug Institute at the Boston University School of Social Work, October 1997, Boston.

FIGURE **1-1**

Spectrum of Health Services: The System out of Balance

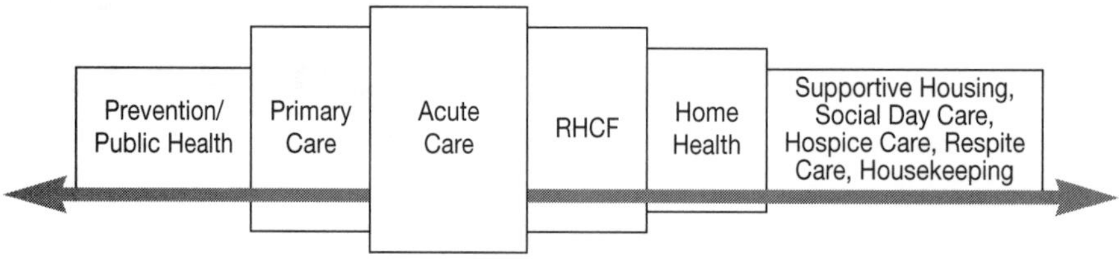

and visible shortages—or as Richmond and Fein (1995) noted, we operate best on the basis of a deficit model: When there was a deficit of hospital and nursing home beds and of physicians and other health professions, we dealt effectively with these deficits. During the same period legislation abounded, including Medicare and Medicaid, regional medical programs, comprehensive health-planning assistance, health professional educational assistance amendments, maternal and infant care under Title V, and neighborhood health care centers and Head Start as part of the Economic Security Act. However, these actions and other pieces of legislation have led to a health system out of balance (Figure 1-1). Hospitals often were built without regard to community needs for other health services. Too much of the health care dollar went into bricks and mortar and not into prevention and primary care on one end of the continuum and into home supports and long-term care on the other end. Community-based organizations were separated from health care organizations and filled in the gaps in care that resulted from the overemphasis on hospital building. Three consequences of this deficit model emerged:

1. A for-profit delivery system materialized and grew rapidly.
2. Health care expenditures increased rapidly without controls.
3. Increased dollars available to hospitals were used for further growth and increased debt service rather than to meet community need.

Yet, no matter what you may think of managed care, it has shifted provider priorities and focused the health delivery system on elements the system neglected in the past (Kotelchuck, 1994; Rosenberg & Holden, 1997). We are moving to a health system whose delivery system is more in balance (Figure 1-2). Managed care has provided incentives for increasing the resources for health education and for long-term care while at the same time halting the growth of hospital-based care. It has created a system that emphasizes efficiency, ambulatory and home care, and cost reduction.

However, access and equity are continuing problems. According to Richmond and Fein (1995), social work will be part of a system that will try to resolve questions such as

- How do we fulfill our commitment to equity—that all are ensured access to quality services?
- How do we ensure that health expenditures are constrained at levels that society judges to be reasonable?

FIGURE **1-2**

Spectrum of Health Services: The System in Balance

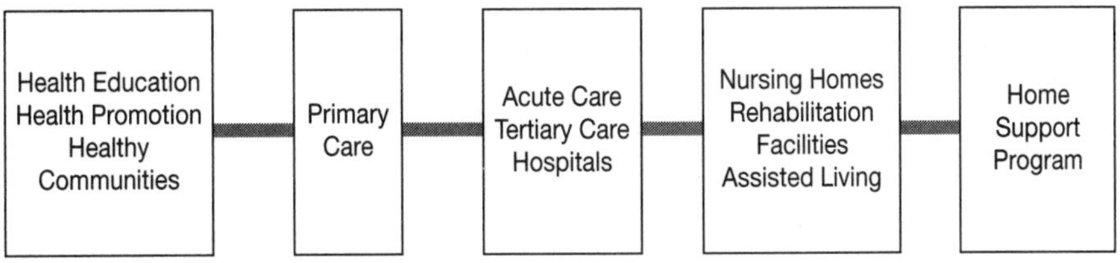

- How do we increase resources for and emphasis on health promotion and disease prevention?
- How do we support the continuation of biomedical and psychosocial research in health?

Policy solutions must focus on the person, his or her social support systems, communities, and the health care delivery systems resources required to meet those needs in a responsible, effective, and efficient manner. Until those issues are successfully addressed, the market forces of managed care will provide solutions to some problems and create and exacerbate other problems.

Access and Cost

The trends in health care provide potential benefits to the consumer by extending the traditional concepts of care and affecting the providers by limiting their decision-making prerogatives and by limiting the traditional reimbursement models for health and mental health care (see Table 1-1). Social work is thus affected by a lessened demand for inpatient services; a perceived change in the value of central departments, which has characterized social work growth in health care for the past 35 years; and a shift in control of health care services from providers to insurers (Rosenberg & Weissman, 1995). Health care is now conducted in a competitive marketplace. Academic centers compete with community hospitals on the basis of cost and must find other ways to fund their educational missions and provide free and subsidized care for the poor (Blumenthal & Meyer, 1996).

Competition can provide for a delivery system of unprecedented quality and efficiency, but some populations are at risk for lesser-quality care. People who are chronically ill; frail elderly people; and poorly educated, low-income workers will not have the resources to choose providers and will receive care of inferior quality (Blumenthal, 1996). Managed care companies avoid such enrollees unless the companies can make a profit and only if the coverage plan calls for high reimbursements. For example, in the Oregon plan Medicaid rates are sufficiently high to attract quality physicians as plan providers (Bodenheimer, 1997).

Table 1-2 provides an overview of the stages of managed care market evolution. In stage 3 there are strong incentives to purchase managed care plans influenced by the demands of business to control costs. Market penetration ranges from 31 percent to 50 percent. Marginal providers either merge with others or go out of business,

TABLE **1-1**

The Changing Paradigm of Health Care

	1960	1980	2000
Marketplace	Independent providers	Early provider networking	Managed competition
Insurance	Indemnity insurance	Mixed insurance, HMOs, and PPOs	Managed care
Reimbursement	Charge based/per diem	Cost based/DRGs	Capitation and direct contracting
Core provider	Hospital	Medical center	Health care system
Service area	Neighborhood	City/town	Region
Care components	Inpatient services	Inpatient/outpatient	Full continuum of care
Physicians	Solo practices	Group practices/ overspecialization	Employed physicians/ rising demand for primary care

NOTES: DRGs = diagnosis-related groups; HMOs = health maintenance organizations; PPOs = preferred provider organizations.
SOURCE: Staff notes, Mount Sinai Health System.

and a smaller number of organizations emerge as dominant. Physician groups grow rapidly, forming independent practice associations, each with a utilization management system and frequently linked to hospitals. Regional systems develop, and providers begin to form alliances with payers. In the more mature stage of the managed care marketplace there is an increase in direct employer–provider contracting. The managed care penetration rate exceeds 50 percent with strong organizations

TABLE **1-2**

Stages of Market Evolution

STAGE 1: UNSTRUCTURED	STAGE 2: LOOSE FRAMEWORK	STAGE 3: CONSOLIDATION	STAGE 4: MANAGED COMPETITION
Independent hospitals Independent physicians Unsophisticated purchasers HMOs and PPOs offered as benefit options	HMO or PPO enrollment balloons Health plans retain large networks Excess inpatient capacity develops Hospitals remain profitable Loose provider networks form Payments are based on discounts, per diems Employers encourage enrollment	Employers reduce number of managed care options A few large HMOs and PPOs emerge, enabling network consolidation, price pressure, and shifting of risk Hospitals rapidly organize into systems Group practices capitalize Specialist revenue declines Integrated systems form	Employers form coalitions to purchase health services Integrated systems manage patient populations Fully integrated financing and delivery system emerges

NOTES: HMOs = health maintenance organizations; PPOs = preferred provider organizations.
SOURCE: Staff notes, Mount Sinai Health System.

surviving in each market. Insurance plans look more like health maintenance organizations (HMOs) than like traditional insurers. Physician–hospital organizations expand, and large groups dominate the market. Generalist physicians control the capitated dollars. Each region has a number of competing provider systems with a solidified provider payer alliance.

It is during the latter two phases that social work is usually downsized or restructured as part of a cost-saving effort. Central departments are often reorganized, and some work processes are re-engineered. There is a body of literature emerging in the field that describes and quantifies these occurrences (Dimond, 1993; Plavnick, 1995; Rosenberg & Weissman, 1995).

There are numerous opportunities for social workers as the markets consolidate and move into managed competition. Social agencies can aggregate and join with health systems as partners in new ventures and can engage in the creation of new programs in ambulatory care and in the community (Rosenberg, 1994; Rosenberg & Holden, 1997; Simmons, 1994).

Health care is now more businesslike, whether for profit or under not-for-profit or public ownership. How much control is exercised by the central entity is predictive of the stage of market and managed care development and also is related to how responsive the delivery system is to local community needs and desires (Figure 1-3). Hospitals and health systems are more or less autonomous and responsive to community needs based on the network models used to operate and control the system. Social work is a frequently targeted cost reduction function in health but sometimes expands in managed behavioral health because of quality and cost factors.

Health systems exist along the continuum from low to high control of their hospitals, long-term care facilities, and physicians. Operating companies are highly integrated health systems; network models are usually aggregations of voluntary organizations.

FIGURE **1-3**

System and Network Models

Low Control → High Control

NETWORK	HOLDING COMPANY	OPERATING COMPANY
Lead coordination by tertiary-care medical center	Parent entity	Single operating entity with one board and one management team
Program of specific joint ventures	Centralization of planning finance and other management services	All assets owned by the company
Steering committee coordinates activities	New holding company controls hospital boards	Physicians are employed
Hospitals are automated	Financial entities are separate	Hospitals lose autonomy and independent governance
Business relationships with alternative delivery systems and physicians		Control of cash and financial obligations is consolidated
No cross-functional obligations		

SOURCE: Staff notes, Mount Sinai Health System.

TABLE **1-3**

Fee-for-Service System Versus Capitated System

	FEE-FOR-SERVICE SYSTEM	CAPITATED SYSTEM
Primary care physicians	35–50 MDs	50 MDs
Specialty physicians	175 MD specialists	50 MD specialists
Hospital beds	275	150
Use of alternative delivery sites	Minimal	Extensive
Annual budget, per member	$3,500	$1,500
Annual budget, per 100,000 covered lives	$350,000,000 + $200,000,000	$150,000,000

NOTES: Comparison of the two systems is made on the basis of 100,000 covered lives. MD = medical doctor.
SOURCE: Staff notes, Mount Sinai Health System.

Fee-for-service systems, compared with capitated systems, are usually far more expensive (Table 1-3). The move to capitated care means more primary care physicians, fewer specialists, fewer available beds but greater use of those beds through reduced lengths of stay, increased use of nonhospital delivery sites, and use of community-based organizations to provide care at home and in the community. Incentives are provided for physicians to conserve health resources, particularly hospital care, and to hospitalize people in the least-expensive site. Social work, deeply embedded in the inpatient services of hospitals, has been slow in developing ambulatory care models that respond to the capitated and highly managed system.

The utilization statistics of both hospital and ambulatory care explain why the growth trend in health care spending has been reduced (Figure 1-4). As care shifts from indemnity insurance to managed and capitated care, length of stay is reduced for those in the hospital, and treatment focus shifts to ambulatory care. Integrated systems reduce the use of hospital care. In many of these systems, social work care is supplemented by non–social work personnel, insurance company utilization reviewers, and length-of-stay or case managers. As length of stay drops, the discharge-planning function must be carried out in part in the hospital and, more frequently, in the community. Preadmission counseling is also reduced because patients enter hospitals on the same day as a necessary procedure rather than a day or two before. Social work practitioners are in the process of developing a functional and structural response to these changes in health care.

Medicare, Medicaid, and Social Work

The history of public spending for Medicare and Medicaid and its relationship to the growth of managed care cannot be explored here. Other writers have explained that linkage (Angell, 1997; Greene & Knee, 1996; Morgan, Virnig, DeVito, & Persily, 1997). Even with a reduction in the rate of spending for public programs, the Congressional Budget Office estimated that spending on both programs will double within a decade (Gramm, Rettenmaier, & Saving, 1997) (Table 1-4). The reduction in rates will have adverse consequences on the most vulnerable populations—elderly men and women, children, immigrants, young people, and poor people who are employed.

FIGURE **1-4**

Market Evolution: National Utilization Comparisons

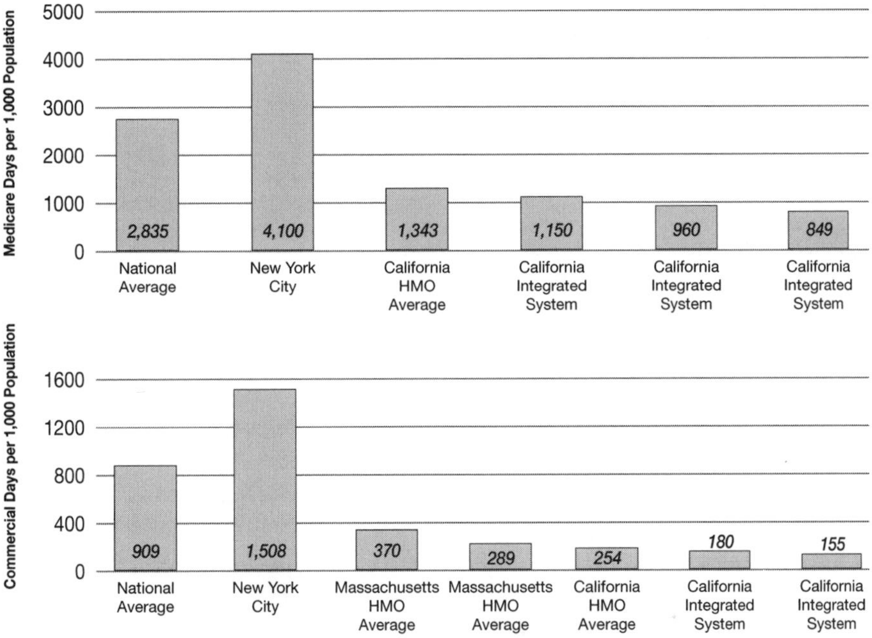

NOTES: In both charts above, moving from left to right, read the multiple measures for the same system as a comparison of less integrated and less managed systems with more integrated and more managed systems. HMO = health maintenance organization.
SOURCE: Staff notes, Mount Sinai Health System.

Let me describe managed care and its consequences for users of the health system. The term "managed care" is used to characterize a wide range of health plans that incorporate mechanisms to monitor and authorize the use of health services. Those plans usually incorporate negotiated payment methods and utilization controls. There is a change in benefits philosophy from an open-ended service benefit—where health and illness are viewed as an act of God—to a defined contribution approach—where behavior mediates health, risk, and illness.

Managed care is evolving (Table 1-5). Its functions, targets, and structure are changing as the markets mature, and it will continue to evolve as it solidifies its position as the organizing template of the American health care payment system. There are identifiable advantages to a managed capitated system. Hospitals, traditionally large employers of social workers, are affected by managed care: They begin by cutting costs, particularly those viewed as nonessential—those not mandated by law or regulation and those not deemed necessary for meeting mission, providing service, and enhancing revenue. Social work is frequently part of that third group and, even when not, social work is vulnerable in the next phase of cuts that usually involve restructuring or re-engineering work processes. Centralized social work departments are easy targets for consultants who perceive a multilayered group, with three to

TABLE 1-4

Medicare and Medicaid Spending Estimates

	1997	1998	1999	2000	2001	2002
Medicare	$209	$221	$223	$246	$270	$279
Medicaid	96	103	110	118	127	137

NOTE: Numbers are in billions of dollars.
SOURCE: Congressional Budget Office, 1997.

eight or more levels of staff who are more department and professionally related than team or functionally related and who are usually unclear about their contribution to the bottom line of the enterprise and to the quality of health care products. Social workers, in this phase of development in the managed care marketplace, are usually retained in discharge-planning roles, in psychosocial care coordination of chronically ill people, and in emergency departments, assuming multiple roles with patients having behavioral health problems and multiple management roles in health care settings and systems. As health systems mature, services will aggregate and integrate, fight for market share, and shift the risk from government to employers to health plans to providers and consumers. Social work services will shift to community settings, home care, and long-term care and to serving special-needs populations. The future integrated delivery system comprises hospitals, physician organizations, and ambulatory care centers and the management functions of finance, demand management risk, management plan administration, and information management.

The financial incentives for primary care and the reduction in hospital utilization and length of stay change as the market moves from a moderately managed utilization system to a more aggressively managed one (Figure 1-5). Physicians and hospitals risk financial gain or loss by how aggressively they manage care and apply the least costly resources to treat people under their care. Hospital and specialist physician risk pools are reduced in resources, primary care risk pools are increased, and profit is increased.

One outcome of managed care that shows promise of increasing the quality of health care is the increase in primary care. Schools of medicine are producing

TABLE 1-5

Managed Care Stages of Evolution

	STAGE 1: EVENT-DRIVEN COST AVOIDANCE	STAGE 2: VALUE IMPROVEMENT	STAGE 3: HEALTH IMPROVEMENT
Objective function	Price	Value and customer satisfaction	Health status improvement
Cost targets	Inpatient	Resources intensity	Health risks
Locus of control	External	Peer driven	"Contract" with family
Focal point	Inpatient hospital	Physician network	Home or neighborhood

SOURCE: Staff notes, Mount Sinai Health System.

primary care practitioners in increasing numbers and preparing them with a revised and creative curriculum for the challenges of primary care in the managed care marketplace.

Physicians and hospitals are competing for the capitated dollar, and so are home care and long-term care programs. For all professions working within a tightly managed care framework, professional behaviors may be compromised by business incentives. In mental health there are opportunities for social agencies to aggregate and provide the bulk of services to the chronically ill behavioral health population. Such conflicts will place pressure on the health and social work educational systems to provide teaching in ethical behaviors to effectively recognize and cope with these concerns.

To summarize the effects of managed care on the health care delivery system, we can note that managed care companies have used their market power to negotiate reduced rates from providers and to build networks that accept discounts to maintain access to patients (Smith, 1997), thus slowing the rate of inflation in health care costs. However, there are important and simultaneous trends that must be addressed and that have special relevance to future social work practice. According to Smith, these include

- the declining ability of health care providers to deliver uncompensated care
- the declining proportion of people with private insurance

FIGURE **1-5**

Distribution of the Health Care Premium under Managed Care

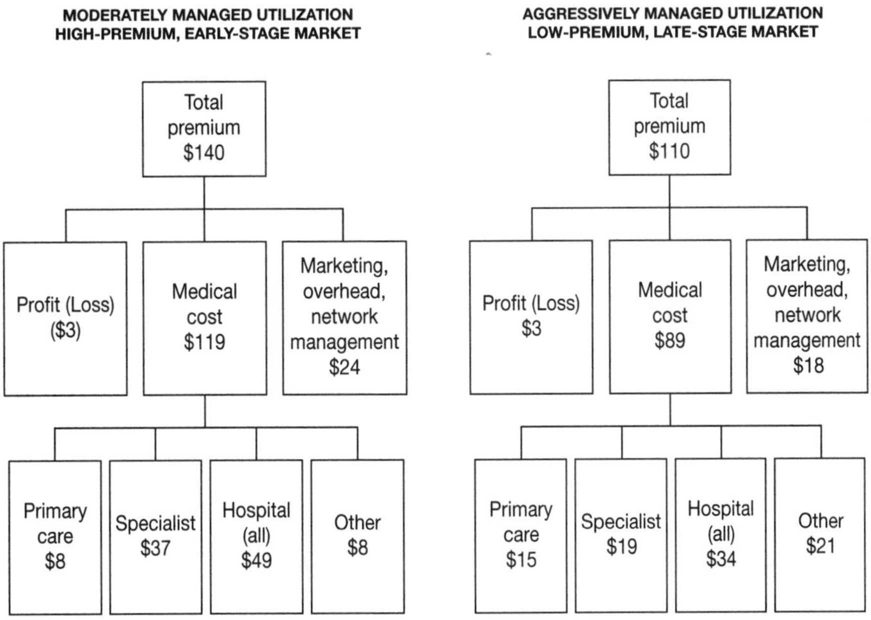

NOTE: Premiums are per member per month.
SOURCE: HCIA database; Milliman & Robertson's University Hospital Consortium actuarial cost model.

FIGURE **1-6**

Estimates of the Uninsured Population

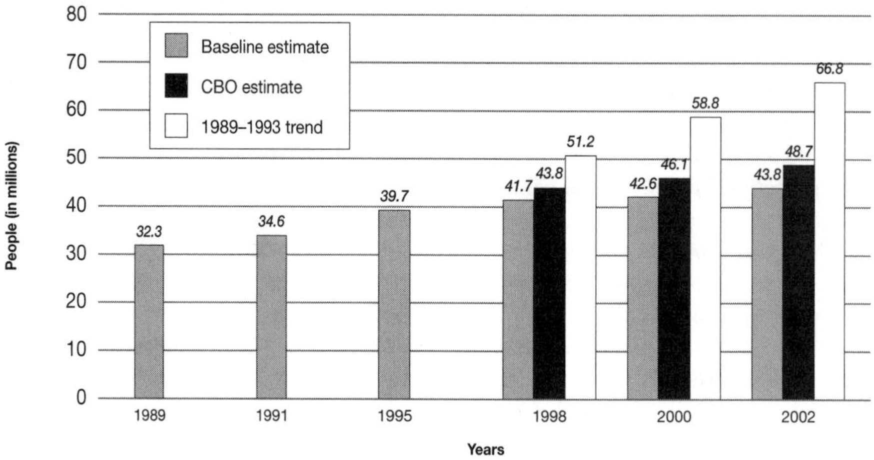

The light gray bars represent baseline estimates. The black bars represent estimates calculated on the assumptions that Medicaid enrollment will be frozen at current levels and that employer-sponsored insurance will decline according to projected estimates of the Congressional Budget Office (CBO). The white bars represent estimates calculated on the assumptions that Medicaid enrollment will be frozen at current levels and that employer-sponsored insurance will continue to decline at the same rate as during the years 1989 to 1993.

SOURCE: Congressional Budget Office, 1996.

- the continued growth in the uninsured population, especially children (Figure 1-6)
- the expected increase in the rate of inflation in health care costs
- budget reductions in Medicare and Medicaid.

Social Work's Place in Managed Care

Why has social work been unable to find a permanent and more fundamental place in health care? It has been difficult to find voices to support its services. Social work's objectives are frequently at odds with the prevailing culture of society. Rehr and Rosenberg (in press) pointed out that the lack of public recognition and status for the profession is based on several factors: Social work

- associates with poor and needy people who have little or no voice in society, and this is seen as functioning primarily in the welfare arena
- relates to physicians who hold the reins and are wary of competition in health care
- has not demonstrated its cost-effectiveness
- is criticized for not solving social problems that, in fact, require policy and program change and multidisciplinary investment
- has developed neither outcomes data to support best practices nor accepted quality management processes

- has not found an effective collaborative role with other health care professionals in addressing social health issues
- has been largely a charity- and government-supported service
- has its own internecine battles (for example, academics versus practitioners)
- has not been active in affecting public social health policy.

All of these factors have led to a general unease about the profession and uncertainty about its purpose and direction.

FUTURE DOMAINS IN SOCIAL WORK

Social work practice in health care will take place in the community as well as in hospitals. It will focus on the person, his or her social support systems, and on populations at risk. A mix of social services provision and short episodic and long-term counseling will prevail. Practice will take place in teams of multidisciplinary professionals and paraprofessionals. Social work services may not be centralized in the traditional sense, but social work consortia and coalitions will influence social work practice and institutional social health programs for vulnerable populations. Supervision as it is known today will not exist. Maintaining high standards of practice will require new modes of education and continuous learning. Social workers will need to be increasingly autonomous and self-directed. Practice will become standardized through quality studies that will guide the practitioner.

Community health programs are based on the concept of developmental provision, that is, as need is uncovered. Social work will help provide "those social utilities designed to meet the normal needs of people arising from their situations and roles in modern life" (Kahn, 1969, p. 36). Social work and other professions help provide the social architecture for enhanced community living.

The interactions among the increasing rates of societal changes—shifts in technology, greater population density, information overload, and stress—will play a role in creating new disease patterns. Social work practice will be based on the following concepts:

- An integral relationship exists between people's health and environment; just as confronting the actual infective and causative agents of disease is critical, so is confronting the changing social and physical environmental conditions that permit disease onset.
- Vulnerability to new waves of health risk is greater for economically disadvantaged people in every community, and improving living conditions becomes, by definition, a social health promotion strategy.
- Physical and social functioning of individuals in relation to their informal and formal networks is more significant than are disease patterns themselves.

Using social epidemiology and survey methods, health care social workers will be helpful in identifying and reducing health risks. As they contribute to health promotion, social workers will add to community strengths. In part, the move to this domain represents a return to social work's settlement house roots that emphasized amelioration and reform from an empowerment perspective, social science as an integral part of practice, a comprehensive response to complex problems and cross-functional program management (Harkavy & Puckett, 1994). Chavis (1993) stated that in this domain, social workers will

- respond fully to the organization mission, dealing with the constraints, while translating policy into programs that focus on individual need
- help institutional leaders develop the capacity to reach out to their communities and learn about their strengths, needs, and wants
- help institutions respond to the needs of communities by identifying models, distilling research knowledge, linking the institutions with others that have similar dreams, brokering resources with other institutions, developing the social technologies to be tested and refined, and engaging in an efficient collaborative planning process
- build the capacity of local institutions to initiate comprehensive programs
- increase the accountability of institutions
- increase citizen participation in and control over institutions.

COMMUNITY HEALTH PROGRAMS

The Mount Sinai Medical Center has created a community intergenerational program designed to link elderly people with latchkey children in the East Harlem community. This program, supported by a U.S. Department of Housing grant for Section 202 housing, is a partnership among the Mount Sinai Medical Center, the Greater Emmanuel Baptist Church, the Union Settlement Association, and the East Harlem Triangle. The program, staffed by retired business and professional people and the residents of Linkage House, provides important services for the children and meaningful intergenerational contact (*Aging Today,* 1997; Butler, 1997). Social work links the agencies through its community relations function, staffs Linkage House, and provides and coordinates the services. Social workers serve as president and members of the board of Linkage House.

Another social work program that has proven value and is community based is the East Harlem Cardiovascular Risk Reduction Program, funded in part by the State of New York. Social workers provide the organization and personnel to lead walking groups, offer health education, and work with *bodega* owners to change the kind of food offered in the community to include skim milk, low-cholesterol and low-fat foods, fish, poultry, and lean rather than fatty meats. Schools, churches, and other neighborhood organizations have combined efforts for a continuing campaign against smoking and for exercise. These programs have led to increasing collaboration with local community agencies, and there has been an increase in the numbers of medical school and hospital grants concerning health issues for people of color.

A third program was created by social workers in collaboration with a local high school, the Manhattan School of Science and Math. Gifted students are selected in junior high school and become Mount Sinai Scholars. They are offered an enrichment program, summer employment, and mentoring by medical students or faculty and staff of the Mount Sinai Medical Center. The lasting relationships formed with the mentors, combined with enrichment for the students and the faculty of the high school, have led to a successful program in which more than 230 children have completed or are attending school. Only two children have not completed the program. The first scholar entered the Mount Sinai School of Medicine in 1997's first-year class. This effort has been supported by the Commonwealth Foundation and the Edith K. Ehrman East Harlem Health Education Center.

NEW MODELS OF SOCIAL WORK SERVICES

Leadership matters, and good leaders will be critical to the future of social work in the new health care system. Social work roles and functions must be rethought. A new pattern for social work must be set. Leaders will have to share their visions and work effectively with other professionals as institutions expand their roles and functions in the ambulatory arena and in community-based services. Institutions are extending ambulatory linkages to primary care, home care programs, respite and hospice care, life care residencies, and nursing homes and affiliating with a range of community-based social agencies and hospitals. Because integrated ambulatory care is seen as cost-effective, financial support for services will be provided.

Social work's move away from its primary traditional role of working with hospitalized patients and families and of planning their discharge and aftercare is already in evidence. As financing of health services shifts to outpatient and community arenas, support for social work services is developing: insurers, government, and individuals recognize social work's value and cost-effectiveness. The new financial arrangements, however, demand that social work develop new organizational and service delivery and evaluation patterns (Plavnick, 1995). Reimbursement revenues are finite, and capitation and managed care benefits will fix the dollars available for care. Social work will have to document its claim to dollars with cost–benefit data.

Social work will be expected to develop new organizational arrangements that address the needs of diverse populations in diverse locations. Preadmission and fast-track triaging will be used to identify people with potential aftercare risks. Contractual arrangements with managed care organizations will set prescribed service allocations.

Social work leaders already are introducing models of mixed social work service that include combined salaried and private social services for private-pay and insured patients, coverage for clientele of group practice physicians, and community-organizing services and social work services for affiliated health care providers. In the institutions, social workers will be assigned to selected medical arenas (for example, patient-centered care units) to be available to clusters of patients with special needs, such as severely ill children in pediatric care and their parents.

Integrated Services

Social workers will serve as care managers, facilitating the use of services and resource allocation. As care managers, they will review service determinants to learn whether client–provider contracts with Medicaid and other insurers are being implemented or require change. Such individual and collective case reviews should lead to new knowledge and to development of new treatment models.

Social workers will become community-based clinicians with one foot inside and one foot outside the institution as they provide direct services and serve as consultants about the social health needs of clients within the community network.

Collaboration will lead to networking among social and health agencies, and services will be drawn from many sources. The health care system may support bundling of community and health services coordinated by hospitals. Consortiums with "packaged care" already are in the marketplace. Because of the breadth and scope of its practice—from services for the geriatric population to women's health to rehabilitation—social work will continue to contribute to the design, organization, and implementation of integrated services.

Cost-effectiveness of Services

Social workers will need to look at how their services can provide value and help reduce the provision of unnecessary and costly medical services. Worried well people, stabilized sick people, and those with social ailments will be redirected from medical care to less-expensive social services. Social workers can demonstrate that their services enhance physician productivity and efficiency, and they will have a responsibility to define vulnerable populations. High-social-risk screening will be expected. Preventive services and those that eliminate unnecessary hospitalizations will be offered. In offering health promotion and health education services in addition to counseling, social workers will have to demonstrate cost-effectiveness in developing a more motivated, educated group of patients. Social workers will assist caregivers in coping with the increasing responsibility for people who are elderly or chronically ill. Joint-degree programs will proliferate to prepare future health care social workers.

Shift in Focus

Social work will shift from a diagnosis and disease–illness focus to one that emphasizes individual physical and social functional capacities through the life cycle. Concentration on social risk factors as they affect health status will require specialized knowledge of the etiology, treatment, and consequences of disease and disability. Major emphasis will be on those risk indicators related to chronic illness in elderly men and women, people who have a physical or developmental disability, children who are acutely and chronically ill, and people who are terminally ill. The family or the informal network will be critical components affecting how a person copes with illness. Because resources for social work are diminishing in the formal service community, much care will be provided by family and will draw strongly on clients' informal support systems. Social workers can promote this involvement because they are trained as family-focused therapists. Involvement with patients will be limited to social diagnosis and motivation, discharge planning, support of home care, rehabilitation, and linkage with essential community-based facilities (Goldberg, 1995).

PRIMARY CARE

In the primary care setting, social workers collaborating with physicians and nurses will play an important role in developing and implementing screening mechanisms to identify people at risk for health and mental health problems. Primary care social work services will include

- case and care management services to ensure that people with illness follow through with their treatment recommendations or modify them in ways the patient and family need to adapt the treatment recommendations to their lifestyle
- coordination of health care and community support services
- continuity among continuing care and episodes of acute treatment in hospitals and long-term care facilities, home care, and community services
- direct behavioral health services as part of primary care.

The newer integrated primary care models use a screening questionnaire to identify physical and emotional difficulties. If the responses to the questionnaire indicate need for a behavioral health services, a provider is assigned with the primary care physician to do the initial consultation. Studies show that the diagnosis of depression is missed in 50 percent of the patients who see only a primary care physician and that only 50 percent of the patients who receive the correct diagnosis are appropriately treated (Mulrow et al., 1995). By combining a social worker and a primary care physician, one can increase the level of satisfaction among primary care physicians, increase patient satisfaction, decrease medical costs, and increase overall patient well-being. For those patients with such chronic illnesses as coronary disease and diabetes, who place significant demands on primary care physicians, using social workers to empower patients to be more effective at self-treatment may reduce physician cost and demand.

CARE OF CHRONICALLY ILL AND ELDERLY PEOPLE

Maintaining health and preventing further disability in chronically ill and aging populations will be the major business of clinical social work. Rowe (1997) and Rowe and Kahn (1998) presented a picture of those populations: In 1900, 4 percent of the U.S. population was over age 65; today it is 13 percent. Life expectancy at birth in the United States has increased from 47 years to more than 76 years and will likely reach 83 years by 2050. There is mounting evidence of a compression of morbidity in old age. The prevalences of several chronic disorders, including arthritis, dementia, hypertension, stroke, and emphysema, are falling. Eighty-nine percent of those ages 65 to 74 report no disability, and even after age 85, 40 percent of the population is fully functional. The proportion of elderly people living in nursing homes has declined from 6.3 percent in 1982 to 5.2 percent. Men who are 65 are likely to spend 12 of their remaining years fully independent.

Research programs supported by the John D. and Kathryn T. MacArthur Foundation and the National Institute of Aging have demonstrated substantial reversibility of loss of function with age as well as the limited impact of heredity on health and functional status in old age (Rowe & Kahn, 1998). These findings have led to optimism regarding our capacity to attain successful aging. Preventive gerontology now aims not only to retard disease but also to prevent functional decline. Health and functional status in later life are increasingly seen as being under our individual control (Rowe & Kahn, 1998). The stage is set for major community-based intervention studies designed to enhance older people's capability to avoid disease and disability and to age successfully. What a remarkable opportunity presents for the profession of social work.

Social workers will serve as care managers, assisting in the appropriate use of services. Care managers will review service determinants to learn whether client–provider contracts with Medicaid and other insurers are being implemented or require change. Such individual and collective case reviews should lead to new knowledge and to the development of new treatment models.

Social workers will become community-based clinicians as they provide direct services and will serve as consultants about the social health needs of clients within the community network.

QUALITY OF CARE

To be perceived by payers and clients as effective, social workers must conduct quality studies that answer the question of how much social work is necessary to provide a positive result as part of an interdisciplinary effort. Quality, defined as the degree to which health care services for individual clients and populations increase the likelihood of desired health and psychosocial outcomes and are consistent with current professional knowledge, can be defined and measured (Chassin & Sui, 1996).

Current research documents serious problems with quality. A study of discharge planning found that in 40 percent of patients discharged with a plan, one or more components of the plan were not implemented. Discrepancies were more likely among low-income patients, with less-than-adequate care provided and negative consequences resulting.

Quality *can* be improved. For many of our services, managed care is not the problem; quality is the problem. Quality problems come in three kinds: (1) overuse, (2) underuse, and (3) misuse (Chassin, 1991). Overuse of the health system is widespread and exposes people to needless risks. Twenty percent of health services provided are believed to be unnecessary. Underuse of care is also a quality problem. For example, patients entering the health system do not receive effective care for depression, on average, 58 percent of the time; women do not receive proper care between 45 percent and 65 percent of the time when mammography is indicated (Coyne, Fechner-Bates, & Schwenk, 1994). The 6.5 percent (Moore, 1998) of hospital patients who have preventable adverse drug reactions is an example of misuse of the system.

The goal is to determine the correct amount of social work services required to provide an optimum outcome. Social work must develop practice standards and guidelines based on outcome and process research studies. Best practices in social work must be codified and taught in schools of social work (Callahan, 1996; Ewalt, 1995).

Social Work Curriculum Changes

The conceptualization discussed earlier can help guide our educational efforts in preparing social workers to effectively enter future health care practice. The curriculum in schools of social work requires modification to prepare practitioners for the changing health and social services landscape, whether managed care is the continuing mode of delivery care, or a new delivery structure and philosophy emerge (Table 1-6). Curriculum changes may include

- an emphasis on community intervention and advocacy and a return to the settlement house roots of social work
- primary prevention, public health, and social epidemiology methods and knowledge as a base for understanding social support and population-focused practice
- quality studies that lead to practice standards and guidelines
- refined case and care management technologies
- a review of the importance of social justice and alignment with vulnerable populations as the sine qua non of practice
- continuing education learning centers for relicensing of social workers.

TABLE **1-6**

Current and Future Assumptions about Social Work

CURRENT ASSUMPTIONS	FUTURE ASSUMPTIONS
Institutional-based treatment	Community-based treatment
Directive care	Supportive care
Medical/disease-based focus	Health/prevention-based focus
Individual and family focus	Individual, family, and population focus
System focus	Community support focus
Employed by the hospital	Visitor to the hospital
Passive patient	Participating patient
Reactive patient	Advance-planning patient
Supportive episodic care	Supportive continuity of care
Treatment focused	Patient and family focused
Patient or client	Consumer
Discharge planning	Patient health care planning
Provider initiated	Patient and provider initiated
Efficiency/organizational	Effectiveness/individual
Fear and resistance	Trust and teamwork
Expedience	Creativity
Isolated care	Connected, integrated care
Individual patient focus	Family and community focus
Case management	Care management

SOURCE: Adapted from Volland, P. (1996). Social work practice in health care: Looking to the future with a different lens. *Social Work in Health Care, 24,* 35–51. Copyright 1996, The Haworth Press. Used with permission.

Conclusion

A technician is a person who understands everything about the job except its ultimate purpose and social usefulness.

—Sir Richard Livingston, chancellor of Oxford University, 1976

Over the years, social work has been distinguished by outstanding achievements and is now looked on as leading the way in maintaining the human aspect in an environment of increasingly impersonal care. Future roles for social workers relate to the "ultimate purpose and social usefulness" of professional activity. In the years ahead, the role and shape of social work will be determined largely by how creative social workers are in developing and implementing innovative social welfare programs that are effective and more humane.

Social work education has always been challenged to produce practitioners who understand the purpose and social usefulness of their work. In the health care field of practice, we have been part of a system that does not provide for those most in need of opportunity and care. Social work educators are challenged today to produce professionals who can provide quality services, create responsive programs, and provide policy analysis and research while the profession strives for more equitable institutional provisions for the population.

References

Aging Today. (1997, July/August), pp. 11–12.

Angell, M. (1997). Fixing Medicare. *New England Journal of Medicine, 337,* 192–194.

Blumenthal, D. (1996, Summer). Effects of market reforms on doctors and their patients. *Health Affairs,* pp. 170–184.

Blumenthal, D., & Meyer, G. (1996, Summer). Academic health centers in a changing environment. *Health Affairs,* pp. 200–215.

Bodenheimer, T. (1997). The Oregon health plan—Lessons for the nation. *New England Journal of Medicine, 337,* 651–655, 720–723.

Butler, R. (1997). Living longer, contributing longer. *JAMA, 278,* 1372–1373.

Callahan, J. (1996). Social work with suicidal clients: Challenges of implementing practice guidelines and standards of care. *Health & Social Work, 21,* 277–282.

Chassin, M. (1991). Quality of care. *JAMA, 266,* 3472–3473.

Chassin, M., & Sui, A. L. (1996). Academic quality improvement: New medicine in old bottles. *Quality Management in Health Care, 4*(4), 40–46.

Chavis, D. M. (1993). A future for community psychology practice. *American Journal of Community Psychology, 21,* 171–183.

Coyne, J. C., Fechner-Bates, S., & Schwenk, T. L. (1994). Prevalence, nature and comorbidity of depressive disorders in primary care. *General Hospital Psychiatry, 16,* 267–276.

Dimond, M. (1993). Cross-functional management: Strategies for changing times. *Social Work Administration, 19,* 1–2.

Ewalt, P. L. (1995). Clinical practice guidelines: Their impact on social work in health [Editorial]. *Social Work, 40,* 293.

Goldberg, G. S. (1995). Theory and practice in program development: A study of the planning and implementation of fourteen social programs. *Social Service Review, 69,* 615–655.

Gramm, P., Rettenmaier, A., & Saving, T. (1997). Medicare policy for future generations: A search for a permanent solution. *New England Journal of Medicine, 338,* 1307–1310.

Greene, R. R., & Knee, R. I. (1996). Shaping the policy practice agenda of social work in the field of aging. *Social Work, 41,* 553–560.

Harkavy, I., & Puckett, J. L. (1994, September). Lessons from Hull House for the contemporary urban university. *Social Service Review,* pp. 299–321.

Kahn, A. J. (1969). *Theory and practice of social planning.* New York: Russell Sage Foundation.

Kotelchuck, R. (1994). The New York City health system: A paradigm under siege. *Social Work in Health Care, 20,* 21–33.

Levine, C. (1997). *Home sweet hospital: The nature and limits of private responsibility for home care.* Unpublished manuscript, United Hospital Fund, New York.

Moore, J. D. (1998, April 20). Deadly consequences. *Modern Healthcare,* p. 12.

Morgan, R., Virnig, B., DeVito, C., & Persily, N. (1997). The Medicare–HMO revolving door—The healthy go in and the sick go out. *New England Journal of Medicine, 337,* 169–175.

Mulrow, C., Williams, J. W., Gerey, M., Ramirez, G., Montiel, O., & Kerber, C. (1995). Case finding instruments for depression in primary care settings. *Annals of Internal Medicine, 122,* 913–921.

Plavnick, C. (1995). Centralized vs decentralized rationale for a blended model. *Social Work Administration, 21,* 4.

Rehr, H., & Rosenberg, G. (in press). Social work and health care: Yesterday, today and tomorrow. In H. Rehr, G. Rosenberg, & S. Blumenfield (Eds.), *Creative social work in health care.* New York: Springer.

Richmond, J. B., & Fein, R. (1995). The health care mess: A bit of history. *JAMA, 273,* 69–71.

Rosenberg, G. (1994). Social work, the family and the community. *Social Work in Health Care, 20,* 7–20.

Rosenberg, G., & Holden, G. (1997). The role of social work in improving quality of life in the community. *Social Work in Health Care, 25,* 9–22.

Rosenberg, G., & Weissman, A. (1995). Preliminary thoughts on sustaining central social work departments. *Social Work in Health Care, 23,* 111–116.

Rosenberg, G., Weissman, A., & Auslander, G. K. (1997). International perspectives on social work in health care: Past, present and future. *Social Work in Health Care, 25* [Special Issue].

Rowe, J. W. (1997). The new gerontology [Editorial]. *Science, 278,* 367.

Rowe, J. W., & Kahn, R. L. (1998). *Successful aging.* New York: Pantheon Books.

Simmons, J. (1994). Community based care: The new health social work paradigm. In G. Rosenberg & A. Weissman (Eds.), *Social work in ambulatory care: New implications for health and social services.* New York: Haworth Press.

Smith, B. M. (1997). Trends in health care coverage and financing and their implications for policy. *New England Journal of Medicine, 337,* 1000–1002.

Volland, P. (1996). Social work practice in health care: Looking to the future with a different lens. *Social Work in Health Care, 24,* 35–51.

Suggested Reading

Association of Oncology Social Work. (1996). *Managed care: A survival kit for the oncology social worker.* Baltimore: Author.

Berkman, L. (1995). The role of social relations in health promotion. *Psychosomatic Medicine,* 245–254.

Brown, L. D. (1992, Winter). Political evolution of federal health care regulation. *Health Affairs,* pp. 17–37.

Cowen, E. L. (1994). The enhancement of psychological wellness: Challenges and opportunities. *American Journal of Community Psychology, 22,* 149–179.

Dorfman, R. A., Lubben, J. E., Mayer-Oakes, A., Atchison, K., Schweitzer, S. O., DeJong, F. J., & Matthias, R. (1995). Screening for depression among a well elderly population. *Social Work, 40,* 295–304.

Ell, K. (1996). Social work and health care practice and policy: A psychosocial research agenda. *Social Work, 41,* 583–592.

Fuchs, V. R. (1996). Health economics—The difficult choices. *Economic Times,* pp. 4–5.

Gager, P. J., & Elias, M. J. (1997). Implementing prevention programs in high risk environments: Application of the resiliency paradigm. *American Journal of Orthopsychiatry, 67,* 363–373.

Gillum, R. F. (1996). The epidemiology of cardiovascular disease in black Americans. *New England Journal of Medicine, 335,* 1597–1598.

Ginzberg, E., & Ostow, M. (1997). Managed care: A look back and a look ahead. *New England Journal of Medicine, 336,* 1018–1020.

Iglehart, J. K. (1996). Health policy report—Managed care and mental health. *New England Journal of Medicine, 334,* 131–135.

Kassirer, J. P. (1995). Managed care and the morality of the marketplace. *New England Journal of Medicine, 333,* 50–52.

Lawlor, E., & Raube, K. (1995). Social interventions and outcomes in medical effectiveness research. *Social Service Review,* 383–404.

Manton, K. G., Corder, L., & Stallard, E. (1997). Chronic disability trends in elderly United States populations: 1982–1994. *Proceedings of the National Academy of Sciences of the United States of America, 94,* 2593–2598.

Moore, J. D., Jr. (1997, August). The state of the uninsured. *Modern Healthcare,* p. 15.

Reinhardt, U. E. (1995, Spring). Turning our gaze from bread and circus games. *Health Affairs,* pp. 1–4.

Rowe, J. W., & Kahn, R. L. (1997). Successful aging. *Gerontologist, 37,* 433–440.

Schroeder, S. A. (1996). The medically uninsured—Will they always be with us. *New England Journal of Medicine, 334,* 1130–1133.

Shore, M. F., & Beigel, A. (1996). The challenges posed by managed behavioral health care. *New England Journal of Medicine, 334,* 116–118.

Specht, H., & Courtney, M. E. (1994). *Unfaithful angels: How social work has abandoned its mission.* New York: Free Press.

Tebb, S. (1995). An aid to empowerment: A caregiver well-being scale. *Health & Social Work, 20,* 87–92.

CHAPTER 2

Corporate Values and Managed Mental Health Care: Who Profits and Who Benefits?

Gerald Schamess

Managed behavioral health care has produced changes of astonishing magnitude in less than a decade. Mental health delivery systems and practitioner roles have been substantially transformed, and graduate schools in all the mental health disciplines are discovering that their traditional curricula no longer adequately prepare graduates for practice. The media, corporate leaders, policy experts, and government officials all agree that drastic change is necessary because health and mental health costs are increasing at a rate that, if not contained, will bankrupt corporations and government entitlement programs shortly after the year 2000. Accordingly, cost containment has become a national priority, not to say a new gospel. In a concerted effort to reduce costs, private and public institutions have enthusiastically embraced managed care, in many instances forcing employees into health maintenance organizations (HMOs) by offering no other insurance options.

Some nonprofit managed health plans (notably Kaiser Permanente and Blue Cross/Blue Shield) have maintained a somewhat tenuous existence, having reinvented themselves to conform to industrywide standards. Nonetheless, for-profit plans currently dominate the "industry," having achieved a dominant market share. The basic for-profit strategy has been to reduce premiums (sometimes below actual costs) whenever there is competitive advantage in doing so and to enroll as few seriously ill, or "high-risk," subscribers as possible. Market control is achieved through mergers, acquisitions, and affiliations designed to absorb competitors or drive them out of business. For-profit HMOs purposely create an intensely competitive environment in which nonprofit insurers must either match the benefit packages and premiums the for-profits offer or accept a significant loss of market share, thereby endangering their survival. Those strategies allow for-profit plans to control both benefit packages and premiums throughout the health and mental health care industry. Of course, those are fundamental business strategies, used throughout corporate America. Because those changes so profoundly affect client and practitioner well-being, this chapter will focus on how corporate values are reshaping the fundamental nature of mental health care throughout the country.

What Has Changed

Among the few things proponents and critics of managed care can usually agree on are changes that already have been implemented. For better or worse, the network

NOTE: Originally published as Schamess, G. (1996). Who profits and who benefits from managed mental health care? *Smith College Studies in Social Work, 66,* 209–220.

of public and private social, human services, and mental health agencies painstakingly built up over the past 60 years has been largely dismantled. In the process, organizations either become profit centers for insurers or disappear as distinct entities. Mergers, acquisitions, and affiliations create larger and larger "care" systems as for-profit managed health companies expand their market share. At least a few of us still remember that less than two decades ago, policymakers recognized that large human services organizations were bureaucratically top-heavy, slow to implement change, and unresponsive to patient and client needs. As a result, decentralization became a national imperative, and regionalized control was implemented in mental health systems everywhere. At present, this revelation has been forgotten, and we are rapidly rebuilding highly centralized caregiving systems under corporate rather than governmental bureaucratic control.

To reduce use of the most costly services, inpatient psychiatric care has been reduced to a minimum, now typically ranging from three to 21 days. Most managed plans actively limit longer-term inpatient stays (Trugerman, 1996), preferring to authorize repeated brief rehospitalizations, a policy that implicitly accepts that significant numbers of patients with serious mental illness will relapse regularly. Solo mental health practitioners have become an endangered species, and most who remain in practice actively compete for a limited number of places on managed care panels. For example, Pomerantz, Liptzin, Carter, and Perlman (chapter 37) note that in their independent practice association the provider panel currently includes 100 psychotherapists, with 175 others on the waiting list. Even when a panel has openings, acceptance depends on how well the applicant's practice profile conforms to the treatment protocols the insurer favors. Once accepted, practitioners contractually agree to accept payer decisions about the type, length, and focus of treatment they will provide to each patient or client. These decisions are made by case managers or gatekeepers employed by and responsible to the insurer (Munson, 1996). Because most insurers insist that psychotherapy be directed toward reducing "functional impairments" as defined in the *Diagnostic and Statistical Manual of Mental Disorders, Fourth Edition* (DSM-IV) (American Psychiatric Association, 1994), treatment is almost always conceptualized in biological and cognitive–behavioral terms.

In essence then, managed care reflects not only the triumph of corporate values and ideology over more humanistic ones but also the triumph of technological (managerial, biomedical) and cognitive–behavioral perspectives over competing explanations of psychological dysfunction. Other theories about etiology and treatment (for example, psychodynamic, gestalt, existential, humanistic) have been swept aside in the corporate search for simple, concrete explanations of psychopathology that better lend themselves to cost containment and product marketing. Note that in the corporate vocabulary, "dysfunction" replaces other terms such as "mental illness," "psychopathology," and even "emotional disturbance." The term "behavioral health care" is preferred throughout the industry because insurers refuse to authorize treatment directed toward modifying relationships, enhancing self-esteem, or promoting personality change. Although the term is neither value neutral nor atheoretical (personal communication with J. Drisko, associate professor, Smith College School for Social Work, Northampton, MA, February 26, 1998), most practitioners currently use it, having concluded that economic survival takes precedence over theoretical conviction. Judging by the treatment programs they currently offer, the majority of distinguished, long-term, psychodynamically oriented mental health facilities, even the most prestigious among them, have reached the same conclusion, evidently, for the very same reason. The threat of extinction is remarkably effective in eliminating theoretical paradigms that do not immediately increase the likelihood of survival, thus creating a challenging intellectual environment in which to offer health and mental health care.

The changes outlined above have profound implications for recipients of care, practitioners, and treatment institutions. Proponents of managed care contend that change is unavoidable and will ultimately benefit society as a whole. The immediate consequences may be disruptive, but new systems and policies are necessary to control costs and expand services (Elias & Navon, 1996). A certain amount of disruption, and the hardship that results from it, is necessary to make an outmoded, inefficient system of service delivery more responsive to the healthy discipline of free market forces. Managed care benefits society because it creates delivery systems that provide larger numbers of "consumers" (formerly, "patients" or "clients") with less restrictive, less stigmatizing, more cost-effective behavioral health care. Programs of care are developed and implemented on the basis of "best practice" protocols, which reflect quantitative outcome studies and insurer-constructed consumer satisfaction surveys. Within newly developing systems of care, consumer boards advise administrators and providers about service needs and participate in evaluating program efficacy. Insurers and health network managers confidently assert that their research demonstrates the cost-effectiveness, accessibility, and quality of the care that managed, for-profit, behavioral systems provide (Elias & Navon, 1996).

Managed care critics paint a dramatically different picture. They contend that professional standards, treatment procedures, and guiding ethical principles have been replaced by new standards and procedures designed to rationalize the pursuit of profit above everything else. Consequently, the overall quality of patient or client care has deteriorated, and mental health practitioners have been progressively disempowered. Moreover, professional judgments about treatment needs are routinely overruled by poorly trained, therapeutically inexperienced case managers who are paid by insurers to limit and, where possible, deny care.[1]

Critics go on to say that the dissolution of venerable, well-regarded social services and mental health agencies seriously undermines treatment opportunities for poor people, nondominant racial and ethnic groups, and patients with serious mental illness (Dumont, 1996). Simultaneously, the loss of these agencies diminishes the quality and availability of care for working and middle-class patients or clients who assume they have adequate insurance coverage until they attempt to use it. In western Massachusetts, for example, most HMO insurance guarantees that subscribers can use 20 outpatient psychotherapy sessions a year. Nonetheless, internal HMO policy limits patients and clients to between six and 12 sessions unless they or their therapists can convince case managers either that their conditions are life threatening or that they will require hospitalization if not offered longer-term outpatient treatment.

Critics also contend that because insurers typically refuse to pay for any services except face-to-face treatment contacts, children, elderly men and women, poor people, and people with serious and persistent mental illness are routinely denied necessary collateral interventions (see chapter 25). "Nonbillable" and therefore unreimbursable interventions include telephone check-ins; school visits; court appearances;

[1]In chapter 31 of this book, Munson correctly emphasizes the degree to which "managed cost company" policies are designed to exercise control over every aspect of mental health care: access to treatment, type of treatment, choice of therapist, determination of fees, confidentiality, supervision, and professional vocabulary.

collateral contacts with family members who have no psychiatric diagnosis; brokerage activities, such as assistance in arranging for housing, medical care, legal representation, or public assistance; and advocacy services. These limitations are of particular concern to social workers who treat clients with complex emotional, social, and environmental problems that require intervention beyond what can be offered in 50-minute, office-based interviews.

In managed care practice, productivity standards severely reduce the availability of graduate school internships, postprofessional in-service clinical supervision, and teaching seminars (Donner, 1996; see also chapter 44). To meet productivity standards, managed care companies shift responsibility for required postprofessional education to continuing education programs that provide the continuing education units necessary for licensure. This policy significantly reduces agency costs (and also responsibility for quality of service) because, invariably, individual practitioners pay for conferences and seminars out of pocket. Ironically, insurers and HMOs widely advertise that their providers are all credentialed at the highest level of professional licensure. Generally speaking, critics say, mental health rationing has become the norm for all but the very affluent as practice judgments are increasingly controlled by corporate insurers for whom cost containment and profitability take priority over any genuine interest they have in providing care.

From my perspective, profitability expectations are particularly problematic in mental health care because corporate managers, as a class of people, are not particularly knowledgeable about emotional problems or their treatment. Because sound treatment practice is not as well defined for mental as for physical conditions and because even physician managers often share the discomfort many Americans feel about mental illness (see chapter 33), even well-intentioned gatekeepers generally decide that the best treatments are those that use medication, psychoeducation directed toward compliance, and the expectation that patients and clients will pull themselves together and get on with their lives. Unfortunately, good intentions do not prevent harm. Moreover, it is reasonable to expect managers to educate themselves about the problems and programs they manage.

PROFITABILITY

Are there large profits to be made from privatizing health and mental health care? Indeed there are! In 1995 *The New York Times* published the 1994 salaries and stock awards to the chief executive officers (CEOs) of the seven largest for-profit HMOs (Freudenheim, 1995). The highest remuneration was $15.5 million, paid to the president and CEO of Healthsource of Hooksett, New Hampshire. The second highest was $13.7 million paid to the CEO of Foundation Health Corporation. The average for the seven CEOs was $7 million, and the lowest listed was $2.8 million. When we compare HMO salaries with those of *Fortune 500* CEOs, there is a startling discrepancy (Sloan, 1996). The two highest 1996 CEO salaries cited in Sloan's report were $3.36 million (AT&T) and $3.075 million (Sears & Roebuck)—less than one-half the average package that private health care CEOs earned two years earlier.

What have managed care CEOs done to warrant such generous rewards? Not surprisingly, they have produced huge profits. According to the brokerage house Smith Barney Inc., Healthsource's 1995 net income rose no less than 44 percent, while its earnings per share rose by 29 percent in the fourth quarter alone. Foundation Health's profits were "disappointing" given Smith Barney's prior estimates, rising by only 22 percent per share in 1995. Overall, the Standard & Poor's Health

Care Composite Index rose 57.8 percent in 1995, exceeding the unusually large 45.9 percent rise in the *Standard & Poor's 500* stock average by a very healthy (for the corporations, if not for their patients) 25 percent.

Utilization Policies

It is instructive to study how HMOs have limited utilization. Their strategies are based on standard business policies and procedures, which in this case they apply to tasks that do not lend themselves to business solutions. Among the strategies currently used are

- purposefully and systematically magnifying public and legislative alarm about the rising cost of health and mental health care
- purposefully and systematically using the media to promote managed care as the only viable approach to cost containment, while suppressing or disqualifying dissenting viewpoints
- denying insurance coverage to people with pre-existing conditions or to those who seem likely to use services extensively
- limiting or denying treatment entirely to people whose difficulties do not respond to the time-limited interventions prescribed in the standardized treatment protocols they use
- using prepackaged treatment protocols and multiple levels of bureaucratic decision making to overrule professional judgments about treatment needs
- increasing requirements for recordkeeping and report writing such that graduate-level clinicians spend enormous amounts of time doing work appropriate to insurance clerks, and such that institutions find it necessary to expand their bookkeeping and billing facilities (and costs) exponentially
- removing case managers responsible for utilization review from direct contact with both patients or clients and practitioners by providing access only through overloaded telephone lines (busy signals and complicated touch-tone menus having become the leitmotifs of behavioral managed care)
- requiring that clinicians (renamed "contract workers," "vendors," or "stakeholders") comply with insurer policies and protocols or find employment elsewhere (if they can)
- financially rewarding clinicians who are most successful at reducing utilization, and punishing those who prescribe "too much" expensive, specialized care
- implementing appeal procedures that are difficult to access, impersonal, time-consuming, and inherently frustrating for all but the most sophisticated and aggressive patients or clients
- using economic power to drive down reimbursement levels for billable hours to a level that makes it impossible for agencies to cover the cost of providing services if they offer a benefit package to practitioners.

There is nothing unusual about any of these practices. Every one is congruent with policies and practices used routinely throughout corporate America. They are equally applicable to making cars, running airlines, managing banks, and flipping hamburgers in fast-food restaurants. Basically, they allow health managers to define and defend advantageous market positions, reduce competition, lower the unit cost of "production" by reducing labor costs, and provide a relatively uniform product (that is, "quality treatment") that is easy both to advertise and to deliver. As in every branch of the insurance industry, profitability depends on attracting large numbers of subscribers while minimizing benefit payouts.[2] These and other similar practices allow American corporations to market goods and services that frequently are of marginal quality while simultaneously increasing production pressure on employees, reducing or freezing salaries (when adjusted for inflation, worker salaries in the United States were essentially frozen between 1987 and 1997 (Kilborn, 1995; Uchitelle & Kleinfield, 1996), reducing fringe benefits (especially health insurance), and undermining job security.

Even though these business practices are ubiquitous, they do not serve the best interests of either consumers or employees. Certainly they should not be used as a blueprint for providing mental health care. With the exception of medication, health and mental health care are not products that can be packaged and distributed in handy, throwaway containers. When such business practices define care, too many patients and clients simply become refuse—disposable because there is no profitable way to treat them. Professional social workers are well acquainted with America's disposable populations because those are the people who most frequently and most desperately require our services.

Are Profits and Caregiving Compatible?

As we contemplate these practices, it is worth emphasizing that America will not fully understand the nature of the current health care "crisis" until historians determine the degree to which it has been generated by changing demographic and structural factors (for example, an aging population coupled with a relatively low birth rate), and the degree to which it has been manufactured to provide insurers with unprecedented opportunities for profit. One does not have to be a student of ancient history to remember the "Gulf oil crisis" of the 1970s, during which oil company profits (and retail prices) rose exponentially. Today, however, it is difficult to find a reputable expert who expresses concern about the likelihood of an imminent global oil shortage. The aspirations of the Third World oil producers who collaborated to create oil-pricing and -exporting policy served oil company interests very well even though they probably did not intend to do so. The international crisis was real enough, but its resolution incorporated a successful corporate strategy for increasing oil company profits—a strategy that in all likelihood was purposely conceived and skillfully executed by the companies. Will today's health care crisis look similar to that 25 years hence? We just don't know.

In today's world of managed care, size and market control have become goals in and of themselves. At present, nine of the largest behavioral health plans are engaged in merger negotiations that, if successful, will reduce their number to six. In response, NASW has joined other professional organizations in a class-action suit

[2]Interestingly, Glasser (1998) described managed care as a giant Ponzi scheme in which health care insurers must constantly enroll new, relatively healthy subscribers or fail financially. Furthermore, he contended that insurers use premiums and copayments from new enrollees to pay current claims. As a result, when the percentage of yearly revenues allotted to patient care (the "medical-loss ratio") increases, as it inevitably will when patients with more serious health problems are enrolled, companies will either have to reduce benefits further or go out of business. I have no way of evaluating his line of argument, but it does suggest an intriguing area for future research and policy analysis.

(*Stephens et al. v CMG Health et al.*) claiming conspiracy to fix prices and restrict trade ("Health Care Mergers Decried," 1998). One company, Magellan Health Services, Inc., currently manages the behavioral health benefits of 60 million Americans (approximately 22 percent of the total population) and has revenues of $1.5 billion a year (chapter 37). Some experts suggest that within the next decade, five or six enormous insurance companies will control the entire U.S. managed care market (Trugerman, 1996). So much for regional control.

In considering health care managed by huge insurance entities, it is important to understand two fundamental principles that inform most corporate policy decisions. The first asserts that patients or clients receive too much treatment, especially from high-priced specialists (a category that includes clinical social workers). The second asserts that most health and mental health care practitioners are overpaid for the services they render.[3] These principles provide clear guidelines for containing mental health care costs, by reducing utilization rates, shifting patients and clients from more expensive to less expensive facilities and practitioners, and lowering payments to providers, for example. In return for stable or lower costs, employers direct health care premiums to insurers who agree contractually to provide care at a capitated rate (chapter 3). Even in the public sector, insurers often receive financial incentives when the utilization rate drops below contractually agreed-on levels. Typically, payers are unperturbed by the fact that insurers will apply 20 percent to 30 percent of premiums to administrative costs and profits. Apparently this is a "win–win" situation for everyone except the subscribers who are denied treatment.

As professional social work celebrates its 100th birthday, it is disheartening (not to say depressing) to hear our national leaders affirm publicly that corporate values and policies (exemplified by managed health insurers) not only represent our best hope for the profession's future but also offer a viable model for addressing and meeting client needs. If the idea were not so passionately held and earnestly presented, it would be nothing less than mind boggling, especially for a profession that claims a core value commitment to social justice. Social work practitioners consistently bear witness to the inhumane, exploitive, and often disastrous effects that corporate policies have on poor and working-class Americans. The official story, which states that corporate insurers and managers are benefactors to poor and working-class people, asks social work to do nothing less than ignore its history, literature, and values—not to mention 100 years of practice experience.

Those who believe that corporate intentions are reliably benign should recall the ferocious 1993 campaign that the insurance industry and medical profession mounted against the Clinton administration's universal health care proposal, a campaign that left some 30 million (and growing daily) mostly poor Americans without health insurance of any kind. Believers might also consider the current gyrations of the (still very profitable) tobacco industry as it tries to protect its profitability by denying legal and moral culpability for the health problems that arise as a result of cigarette use. And, for those who prefer examples from the health care industry, there are these: the ongoing investigation of the huge hospital chain, Columbia/HCA, for Medicare billing fraud as well as a variety of other illegal activities; the

[3]Policy initiatives that target overpaid social workers and clients who receive too much treatment leave most agency-based practitioners gasping for breath, especially in settings that serve impoverished, high-risk clients. In the eyes of managed care payers, who view us as vendors and stakeholders, however, our incredulity is simply "self-serving."

$1 million fine the Texas Department of Insurance levied against the Kaiser Foundation Health Plan in April 1997 to enforce better standards of care (Riester, 1998); or the ongoing investigation of the Oxford Health Plan for exaggerating its profits in reports to stockholders and concurrently delaying payments to service providers.

In citing these examples I am well aware that as individuals, many managed care trustees, CEOs, and administrators are decent, well-meaning people genuinely (at least, in their own eyes) devoted to providing "quality" health and mental health care to their subscribers. Unfortunately, their individual decency obscures the effects that the policies they implement have on patients and clients. From the corporate policy perspective, there is nothing even remotely personal in for-profit managed care policies. Whatever terms we use to describe subscribers, the corporate perspective focuses on the "medical-loss ratio; that is, that percentage of yearly revenues allotted to patient care" (Glasser, 1998, p. 37). Apparently, the dichotomy between individual motivations or attributes and the structural implications of corporate policy is confusing to policymakers and the public at large.

Most Americans and many social work spokespeople are inclined to view the examples cited above as aberrations from an ideal free market norm. Unfortunately, "aberrations" of this kind occur with sufficient frequency throughout the economy to support the argument that profits occupy a much higher position in the corporate hierarchy of values than does human well-being. I'm not even sure this particular point of view is controversial, at least at the higher levels of corporate decision making. The privileged place that profit occupies in the American economy is reflected daily in how shareholders reward or punish corporations on the basis of their profit statements and in standard practices such as downsizing.

We cannot rely on corporations to demonstrate genuine concern for human well-being, or (especially when profit margins are threatened) even to explain their policies and practices with any degree of honesty. "Fiduciary responsibility" requires corporate trustees to do everything possible to preserve capital and increase revenues, and the CEOs they hire do nothing less. In chapter 6 of this book, Havas comments that as long as we persist in thinking about health care as a business, we have no reason to complain about the "bottom line being paramount." Accordingly, if social work accepts that real politics and contemporary financial realities require us to work collaboratively with managed care insurers and HMOs, we should also commit ourselves to advocacy on behalf of clients and practitioners as well as to proactive efforts toward reshaping national policy. Moreover, we should have no illusions about whom we are climbing into bed with or about how our new partners are likely to use us, should their profit margins decline. Of course, social work is far from immune to the financial pressures currently reshaping society. Ultimately, almost all of our funding comes from corporate and government sources.

What Is Happening to Relationships in Managed Mental Health Care?

Given what is said above, it should come as no surprise that I have grave misgivings about corporate America's ability (at least in the 1990s) to provide effective and appropriate treatment for people with emotional problems. Above and beyond the policies that corporations implement to ensure profitability, we should also consider their attitudes about human relationships. During the past five years, wave after wave of layoffs, coupled with record-breaking corporate profits, leaves little doubt when opportunities present themselves, contemporary corporations consistently choose profit over people—at least to the degree outside forces (for example, unions, government regulators) do not prevent them from doing so. Interestingly, a number of colleges and universities, following the lead of their corporate board members, have recently pursued similar policies. Extremely high expenditures for new technology (such as hardwiring campuses, computer networks) are routinely approved by university trustees. Simultaneously, expenditures for faculty and staff are viewed with concern. The rationale is that technological costs are predictable, fixed, and beneficial over time, but employee salaries tend to increase yearly in relation to seniority and inflation, thereby burdening university income and endowment. From a contemporary corporate perspective, even in higher education, automation and other forms of technological innovation are almost always preferable to expenditures on "human resources."

In March 1996 *The New York Times* (Uchitelle & Kleinfield, 1996) listed 15 major companies that had publicly announced their intention to eliminate a total of 662,900 jobs between 1992 and 1996. These layoffs involved between 13 percent and 35 percent of their work forces, mostly relatively well-paid, white-collar, middle-level managers. *Newsweek* magazine (Sloan, 1996) commented on those layoffs in an article titled "Corporate Killers: The Hit Men":

> You lose your job, your ex-employer's stock price rises, and the CEO gets a fat raise. Something is just plain wrong when stock prices keep rising on Wall Street while Main Street is littered with the bodies of workers discarded by big companies like AT&T and Chase Manhattan and Scott Paper. Once upon a time, it was a mark of shame to fire your workers *en masse*. It meant you had messed up your business. Today, the more people a company fires, the more Wall Street loves it, and the higher its stock price goes. (p. 44)

Apparently, both the *Newsweek* and *The New York Times* articles were precipitated by Pat Buchanan's early success in the 1996 Republican Party presidential primaries. Before the positive voter response to Buchanan's campaign, which challenged established business practices (especially the relationship between downsizing and free-trade legislation), the litany of layoffs was reported routinely and factually on the business pages with barely a yawn. With few exceptions, no one in the media seemed to think layoffs were worthy either of editorial comment or serious investigative reporting, and no one except union leaders and a few liberal legislators publicly expressed outrage. It took a significant threat to the established power structure within the Republican Party to awaken political and media concern.

Although downsizing is done in pursuit of profits, it has a second important implication for health care policy. By eliminating large segments of their work forces, many of the most respected corporations in America shatter the illusion that there is a meaningful human relationship between workers and corporate entities. Downsizing demonstrates that employee loyalty, service, and productivity are of little consequence in the competitive marketplace. From my perspective, the callous disregard for employee well-being implicit in downsizing disqualifies corporations from a primary role in providing health care, particularly to people in emotional distress. If one believes, as I do, that actions speak much louder than words, there is no way to reconcile downsizing with genuine concern about the health and mental health either of employees or of the "insured lives" covered under managed care contracts. The underlying corporate assumption is that both the recipients of care and the workers who provide it are "human resources," accordingly to be used as needed in pursuit of profit and then discarded once they have outlived their usefulness. It is a profoundly exploitive assumption, implying that people have no value simply as human beings and acquire value only when they become "resources"—that is, useful in advancing corporate objectives. In corporate America, value is an economic rather than a human attribute.

Human services practitioners cannot ignore the devastating economic and psychological effects downsizing has had for millions of workers and their families. Given the events we are currently witnessing, it is incomprehensible (if not immoral) to transform the essence of health and mental health care by reconfiguring it as an industry and entrusting its management to yet another group of corporate directors and CEOs whose value systems predispose them both to ignore the human meaning of relationships and to sacrifice patient and client well-being on the altar of profitability. There are a great many things, mostly technological, that corporate America does extremely well. Caregiving is not among them. If they do nothing else, downsizing policies should make that very clear to all of us.

Complexities Implicit in Caregiving

Of the many possible motivations for providing care to people who suffer from serious emotional problems, the pursuit of profit is among the most dismal. Practitioners have known for generations how difficult it is to maintain a reasonable balance between self-interest and patient or client need in working with people with mental illnesses or emotional disturbances. When practitioners minimize the importance of self-interest and self-care, they become vulnerable to despair, helplessness, and burnout. When they become too invested in personal self-interest, they exploit or abuse their patients and clients in a variety of ways, indifference and fee gouging being prominent among them.

Reform and More Reform

Over the past 30 years, practitioners have recognized many of the excesses built into the solo practitioner–specialist–teaching hospital model of mental health care (for example, inflated incomes for those in positions of power and authority, inpatient stays of inordinate length, and training at the expense of patient care). Did that model of care need to be reformed? Indeed it did! Can it be reformed by corporate executives for whom profit is the fundamental criterion of success? I don't think so. In and of themselves, high profits and high CEO salaries do not make it impossible for private corporations to provide humane, inclusive, thoughtfully conceived mental health care. What make it impossible are greed; dishonesty; opportunistic profiteering; the tendency to view subscribers as means toward an end; unwillingness to recognize the depth and complexity of psychological difficulties; and reliance on quick, simple, technological fixes advertised as "quality care."

Mental health care needed reform before the for-profit managed care companies took over the field. Now it needs reform again. At present, the constructive changes corporate policy and technological innovation can affect have, for the most part, been incorporated into human services systems. Time-limited psychodynamic and cognitive–behavioral models of psychotherapy are widely accepted and routinely used, brief hospitalization has become the norm, home and community-based care programs are expanding, increasingly sophisticated psychotropic medications provide symptomatic relief for many conditions, and the cost of "care units" in different settings has been significantly reduced. Moreover, most agencies and practitioners now recognize the importance of cost containment.

Given these changes, it is past time to regulate for-profit managed care companies to promote and protect public well-being. Better yet, it is time to introduce a rational, universal coverage, single-payer system. A recent research report (Beinecke & Perlman, 1996) found that in Massachusetts the managed care company that took over the Medicaid system in 1992 spent "about *six* times what Medicaid spent for administration before managed care" [italics added] (p. 16). That 600 percent increase represents an enormous amount of money *not* being used on behalf of people who seek and need mental health care. Moreover, the comparison speaks volumes about the relative cost-effectiveness of "bloated, inefficient" government bureaucracies compared with "lean and mean," fiscally responsible corporate management systems. Dare I suggest that bloated, inefficient, private, managed care bureaucracies are purposely designed to frustrate subscribers and deny benefits? It is noteworthy that the much-maligned Canadian national health care program manages benefits for less than 40 percent of what private, for-profit insurers currently charge to manage benefits in the United States.

Implications of the Managed Care Vocabulary

People with mental illness or serious emotional disturbances should not be subjected to exploitation or profiteering from either the private or the public sector. Because typically they feel frightened, vulnerable, and helpless, as if they have lost control of their lives, patients or clients need compassionate relationships thoughtfully attuned to interpersonal conflicts, traumatic memories, and painful feeling states. And as we know, relationships are not what managed behavioral health is currently selling. In speaking about health care, Glasser (1998) described the issue eloquently: "In less than five years, managed care has managed to eliminate from the public-policy debate any and all words that describe suffering and disease" (p. 38).

Even though patients or clients use services, they are not, in essence, consumers.[4] Moreover, patient and client problems cannot be addressed effectively by providing

[4]In the managed care vocabulary, the term "consumers" is illuminating because it is ubiquitous. As every reader of *Consumer Reports* knows, informed consumers are well advised to be self-protective in dealing with marketers. In addition, the relationship between consumers and marketers is frequently adversarial in nature, especially when inferior products are advertised and sold at inflated prices. Given the widely acknowledged ongoing war between informed consumers and exploitive marketers, do we really want to promote a consumer–seller relationship between patients or clients and caregivers as a function of national policy? Do we really believe that trust is an outmoded concept in mental health care that can be replaced by technological innovation? Moreover, according to the *Random House College Dictionary* (1988), *consume* means "to destroy or expend by use . . . to devour," and a *consumer* is "a person or thing that consumes" (p. 289). Destruction, whatever its form, has no place in humane mental health care except in the eyes of corporate managers who think in terms of consuming and therefore destroying economic resources. Here again, there is a core conflict between an economic analysis and humanistic values. Needless to say, however, the idea that patients or clients are mental health consumers delineates a profitable new product line in a society determined to define everyone and everything in terms of consumption. "Consumption," as we commonly use the term, has an alternate meaning with a common root: "progressive wasting of the body," as in tuberculosis of the lungs (*Random House College Dictionary*, 1988, p. 289).

behavioral health "products." As the managed care vocabulary takes hold, some agency-based social workers have even begun to refer to themselves as "income producers," a depressingly accurate description. Because role functions are, in large measure, shaped by the names assigned to them, it is important to talk about psychotherapists, psychopharmacologists, case managers, community aides, and peer counselors as healers or helpers, not as contract workers, vendors, or stakeholders.

The terminology that corporations and practitioners use reflects underlying theoretical assumptions about the etiology of problems and the remedies deemed likely to ameliorate them. According to the *Random House College Dictionary* (1988), *healers* are those who "make whole or sound; restore to health, free from ailment" (p. 609); *vendors* are "people or agencies that sell" (p. 1459); and *stakeholders* are ones who "hold the stakes of a wager" (p. 1279). The different terms suggest that as a society, we are currently being sold a particular mental health care system without being given the opportunity for meaningful public discussion that would allow us to make informed choices along a range of possibilities. The corporate formulation views emotional problems in the context of functional impairments that require repair. In this formulation, repair is accomplished through the use of technologically up-to-date, aggressively marketed products designed to modify or eliminate particular symptoms. The humanistic formulation emphasizes the importance of trying to make people with emotional problems "whole" through meaningful relationships, self-understanding, an informed use of medication, and constructed and supportive communities of peers. The choice has become increasingly difficult because we can now, at least some of the time, suppress symptoms without in any way ameliorating the human suffering that elicited them (see chapters 14 and 33 of this book). Nonetheless, difficult or not, there is a choice, and informed public discussion is both a right and a necessity in a democratic society.

Conclusion

It is fortunate for all of us that change is in the wind. Managed care profits have dropped significantly in the past year, patients and clients are protesting more forcefully against callous and inadequate care, collaborations among professional groups are gaining momentum, the number of malpractice suits against HMOs and managed care companies is increasing rapidly, and media commentaries on health and mental health care have become more incisive and critical (see, for example, Glasser, 1998; Kilborn, 1998). For at least a year, federal and state legislators have been debating regulatory relief related to a range of widely perceived abuses, and President Bill Clinton signed a Health Care Bill of Rights for federal employees, Medicaid beneficiaries, and members of Congress in the spring of 1998 ("Three Ways to Manage Managed Care," 1998). If patients and clients, practitioners, and public interest groups work together, they can create a humane, efficacious, relationship-enhancing health and mental health care system that also is cost effective. The time is ripe; we need only the will.

References

American Psychiatric Association. (1994). *Diagnostic and statistical manual of mental disorders* (4th ed.). Washington, DC: Author.

Beinecke, R. H., & Perlman, S. B. (1996). Managed Medicaid: The Massachusetts experience. *Behavioral Health Management, 16*(2), 14–16.

Donner, S. (1996). Field work crisis: Dilemmas, dangers and opportunities. *Smith College Studies in Social Work, 66,* 317–334.

Dumont, M. P. (1996). Privatization and mental health in Massachusetts. *Smith College Studies in Social Work, 66,* 293–306.

Elias, E., & Navon, M. (1996). Implementing managed care in a state mental health authority: Implications for organizational change. *Smith College Studies in Social Work, 66,* 269–292.

Freudenheim, M. (1995, April 11). Penny pinching HMOs showed their generosity in executive paychecks. *New York Times,* pp. D1, D5.

Glasser, R. J. (1998, March). The doctor is not in: On the managed failure of managed health care. *Harpers Magazine,* pp. 35–41.

Health care mergers decried. (1998, February). *NASW News,* p. 1.

Kilborn, P. T. (1995, July 3). In the new work world, employers call all the shots. *New York Times,* pp. 1, 7.

Kilborn, P. T. (1998, May 17). Voter's anger at HMOs plays as hot political issue. *New York Times,* pp. NE1, NE22.

Munson, C. (1996). Autonomy and managed care in clinical social work practice. *Smith College Studies in Social Work, 66,* 241–265.

The Random House College Dictionary (Rev. ed.). (1988). New York: Random House.

Riester, A. (1998, February). Texas HMOs fined for violations. *Group Circle,* p. 3.

Sloan, A. (1996, February 26). Corporate killers: The hit men. *Newsweek,* pp. 44–48.

Three ways to manage managed care. (1998, June). *Consumer Reports,* p. 7.

Trugerman, A. (1996). All managed care is not equal. *Smith College Studies in Social Work, 66,* 261–268.

Uchitelle, L., & Kleinfield, N. R. (1996, March 3). On the battlefields of business, millions of casualties. *New York Times,* pp. 1, 26.

C H A P T E R 3

Mental Health Services for the Future: Managed Care, Unmanaged Care, Mismanaged Care

Jeffrey L. Geller

Mental illness services have progressed considerably since the mid-20th century, when book titles such as *The Shame of the States* (Deutsch, 1948) and *Every Other Bed* (Gorman, 1956) literally described both the locus and quality of treatment. The mental health care delivery system has moved from the asylum to the community, as described by Grob (1991) but, beyond simply translocating services, where are we now?

Clearly, we have moved to new models of mental illness services, new enough to require a contemporary umbrella label of "behavioral health care." These models include ever-increasing privatization and management and progressively decreasing autonomy and choices for patients. This movement, however, has yet to demonstrate short-term stability or long-term clear directions. Contemporary health care reform has been called "an uncharted odyssey" by Altman and Reinhardt (1996), privatization has been labeled a "fragile balance" by Dorwart and Epstein (1993), and managed care needs to be managed according to the Institute of Medicine (Edmunds et al., 1997).

As you read this history of and prognostication about managed mental health care, consider the following: Will these reforms truly be able to take on a preventive focus (Mrazek & Haggerty, 1994)? What efforts will managed care take to reduce (even better, to eliminate) the stigma of mental illness (Fink & Tasman, 1992; Rich, 1997)? Will managed behavioral health care even try to grapple with such clinical issues as violence in people with mental illness (Monahan & Steadman, 1994); the need for coercion in outpatient settings (Dennis & Monahan, 1996; Geller, 1986); or low-frequency, highly dangerous behaviors like firesetting (Geller, 1992)? Finally, is there a chance that managed psychiatric treatment can ever take a public health perspective (Levin & Petrila, 1996)?

Background

As of January 1995, of the estimated 185.7 million Americans with health insurance, about 58.2 percent (108 million) were enrolled in some form of specialty

NOTE: Originally published as Geller, J. (1996). Mental health services of the future: Managed care, unmanaged care, mismanaged care. *Smith College Studies in Social Work, 66,* 223–240.

managed mental health or behavioral health programs. The number is significantly greater when we include those in managed health care programs inclusive of psychiatric treatment—the health maintenance organizations (HMOs). This phenomenon is of recent origin, representing a rapid and progressive shift from indemnity insurance plans and fee-for-service medicine to managed systems of care.

Why has this occurred? Health care costs have been rising in the United States at alarming rates, and mental health care costs are no exception. In 1988, the direct cost of mental illnesses and substance abuse was $273.3 billion. The indirect costs of mental illness and substance abuse are even higher than the direct costs and disproportionately higher than other medical disorders. On the other hand, although mental disorders are treatable, a high percentage continue to go untreated.

Rising costs. Treatable disorders. No treatment for many. Excessive indirect expenses. Something had to happen. As Franklin D. Roosevelt said in 1932, "The country needs, and unless I mistake its temper, the country demands bold, persistent experimentation. It is common sense to take a method and try it. If it fails, admit it frankly and try another. But above all, try something" (Frank, Sullivan, & DeLeon, 1994, p. 855).

And try we do. In the mental health field, what we are currently trying is managed behavioral health care. We are participants in the end of the cottage industry of medicine and the onset of the industrial age of medicine. The industrialization of mental health care will mean that

- The providers of goods and services (psychiatrists, social workers, and other mental health practitioners who provide psychotherapy or psychopharmacology) lose control of the production of the goods and services.
- Because industrialization grows and blossoms on cheap labor, there will be the progressive deprofessionalization of the professions. Less-trained practitioners will replace better-trained ones. For example, MSWs, who replaced MDs, will themselves be replaced by BAs.
- Greater efficiencies will be repeatedly achieved, so that there will be a perpetual and progressive decrease in the numbers of providers, that is, practitioners. The ranks of those with more training will decrease at faster rates than the number of those with less training.
- Quality will suffer at first. Then, as the industry matures, quality will improve and should surpass its earlier levels.
- Greater efficiencies will mean that more people can receive the goods and services (mental health treatment) without an increase in overall costs (total health care costs).
- There will be progressively fewer organizations providing the goods and services (mental health treatment). Successful companies will take over less-successful ones. The small provider, that is, solo practitioner, will disappear.

This industrialization, as described by Nicholas A. Cummings (1995), the founding chief executive officer of American Biodyne and now president of the Foundation for Behavioral Health, portends major changes for the organization of mental health care and for the individual practitioner.

Before I discuss each of these anticipated changes in detail, two basic points need to be made to serve as the foundation. First, I need to define "managed care." For detractors, *managed care* means "care managed by someone else." For those seriously interested in managed care, *managed care* is "any measure, that from the purchaser's perspective, favorably affects the price of services, the site at which the services are delivered or received, or their utilization," or "an arrangement or system in which there are financial, administrative, organizational and monitoring constructs whose end is to minimize resource allocation and maximize efficiency and quality" (Croze, 1995).

Second, as Jay Cutler, director of government relations of the American Psychiatric Association, aptly points out, managed behavioral health care is a financial or Wall Street issue, not a health care issue (Sabshin, 1995). This revolution is not being lead by patients or practitioners, many of whom find the changes in psychiatric practice closer to revolting than to revolutionary. Managed behavioral health care is a revolution lead by the payers of health care, namely industry.

Organization of Managed Behavioral Health Care

An understanding of the development of the managed behavioral health care industry can be gleaned from an analysis done for the Substance Abuse and Mental Health Service Administration's Center for Mental Health Services (Freeman & Trabin, 1994).

EVOLUTION OF METHODS OF MANAGING BEHAVIORAL HEALTH CARE

Managing Benefits

Starting in the 1970s and continuing through the early 1980s, the principal methods for cost-containment were actuarial manipulations designed to manage benefits. Many different benefit packages blossomed, all with built-in elements to control both utilization and expenditures. They did so with little regard for the impact the benefit changes had on the indirect costs born by beneficiaries, employers, and the community. Furthermore, the changes were made without consideration of their effects on the displacement of care onto the general medical sector.

Modifications in benefit plan design included restrictions, exclusions, limitations, penalties, incentives, prior authorization, and retrospective denial. Access, in a radical shift, became directed by the least-trained professional (or even nonprofessional) in the group (Lazarus, 1995). The results were some short-term cost savings and cost shifting that benefited payers, that is, the employers who used these methods.

Managing Care

Leaders of the managed behavioral health care industry have advocated a shift from the manipulation of benefits to cost control through the proper management of care. By limiting authorization of expenditures to only those services deemed medically necessary and appropriate, delivered in the least-restrictive and -intrusive treatment setting, and only by previously designated qualified practitioners, the advocates of managed mental health care believe that the right care can be delivered to the right patients at the right time, in the right setting, by the right type of provider, in the right amount, and at considerable cost savings as compared with care that is unmanaged.

The techniques used to achieve this noble goal include management through contracting, profiling, credentialing, educating, and organizing a specialized, accessible, and interactive network of behavioral health care providers. Further methods for managing care include the mandated use of standardized pretreatment assessment and treatment planning methods. These are supported by standardized forms, restricted formularies, and outcomes management. One major casualty of these procedures has been confidentiality. Although some people are pleased with the results, others have indicated that providers "are being coerced into applying Band-Aids to cover emotional malignancies rather than reaching the root causes of psychiatric problems" (Levy, 1995, p. 35).

Managing Health

Those with even more progressive ideas about managed behavioral health care believe that disease management, demand reduction, health promotion, and wellness can emerge as the foci of the new managed behavioral health care industry. But public funding for these programs has never been impressive and is waning, and the private sector has yet to adopt them in any way beyond token efforts. HMOs and other capitation-based arrangements have fiscal incentives for using these strategies, but both efforts and results have hardly been impressive.

Methods to manage health include health advisors, individual health risk assessments, health education programs, self-help groups, financial incentives for meeting personal health goals, crisis and outreach services, and medical offset programs.

MODELS OF MANAGED BEHAVIORAL HEALTH CARE

There are many organizational arrangements for providing managed behavioral health care, and new ones appear often. Without a glossary of acronyms, it is difficult even to remember what the designations mean. Some of the more common arrangements are discussed below.

Carve-Out Programs

Managed behavioral health care carve-out programs are characterized by

- management teams devoted exclusively to mental health and substance abuse services
- case managers who are credentialed and work under the purview of licensed mental health providers
- the use of specifically developed case management criteria for level-of-care assignments (these address medical necessity and medical appropriateness)
- practice arrangements, for example, specialty behavioral groups staff models and preferred provider organization (PPO) networks that are supposed to provide a continuum of care, the availability of a full range of disciplines, and discounted fees.

The most common type of managed behavioral carve-out in 1994 was a contracted network of independent providers.

Because many behavioral health care networks of PPOs now include too many providers for each to receive regular referrals, only some of them can receive sufficient numbers of patients to build a real relationship with the managed care organization (MCO). Managed behavioral provider networks are therefore downsizing and will, in all likelihood, continue to do so. More volume will be channeled to more-effective providers, effectiveness being determined by practice pattern analyses done by the MCO.

Managed behavioral carve-outs may be offered on an administrative-services-only basis, a risk-sharing basis, or a fully at-risk basis. Administrative-services-only contracts involve all aspects of care management except final payment of provider bills, which is the responsibility of the insurer. At-risk offerings also include payment to providers, either with the risk shared among the managed care company and the providers or, in a fully capitated model, with all risks in the hands of the providers.

Staff or Clinic Model HMO

In this arrangement, therapists are employed on a salaried basis to provide treatment. HMOs are characterized by certain features that predate carve-outs and that have been borrowed by managed behavioral health plans. Features of HMOs include

- prepayment financing on a per-member per-month basis (capitation)
- payment for all levels of authorized care, often with a small copayment, and with every attempt made to substitute alternatives to hospitalization for inpatient care
- physician or behavioral health specialist gatekeepers
- population-based health care measures that assess the overall behavioral health of all covered lives.

The primary care gatekeeper model is the most common method used by HMOs to control utilization.

HMOs have suffered significant market share losses as managed behavioral carve-out offerings have grown. HMOs integrate mental health care with general health care (a real plus), but mental health needs are more easily underserved in HMOs than in the carve-out because the mental health dollars are more hidden in the overall HMO fee. Furthermore, the ratio of psychiatrists to members is typically considerably lower in HMOs than in other systems of care (McFarland, 1994).

In HMOs the question has arisen over whether this model allows sufficient checks and balances on the economic self-interest of providers. Consequently, the best patient care may be seriously jeopardized. Specifically, if the HMO has strong economic incentives to undertreat and if the providers' entire income is dependent on the HMO, then the provider is less likely to protest overly restrictive limitations on treatment.

Hybrid

A third type of managed behavioral health care delivery system that may serve the patient better than either of the above is a mixed, or hybrid, model in which groups and clinics are supplemented with a backup affiliate network of independent providers. But even here the system can "punish" the provider who refers out "too" often.

EAP-Based Programs

Corporate employee assistance plans (EAPs) are branching out into broader managed care functions. An employer can carve out its behavioral health care benefit to the EAP, and the EAP will perform all the functions of a carve-out vendor, such as oversight, network development, case management creation of a continuum of care, and utilization review. Essentially, a company is using its EAP as its own mental health carve-out provider.

Facility-Based, Integrated Delivery System Programs

Treatment facilities are becoming fully integrated delivery systems with a complete continuum of care. Many hospitals have to do this to survive. An example of such an arrangement is the physician–hospital organization (PHO). In this arrangement, behavioral health care is essentially carved-in with the psychiatrist and other mental health care professional groups (through any of several corporate arrangements) providing behavioral health care services and their management oversight (Pomerantz, Liptzin, Carter, & Perlman, 1994).

Why Did Managed Behavioral Health Care Grow?

The Tax Equity and Fiscal Responsibility Act of 1982 led to several new methods to control Medicare costs, the most well-known being diagnosis-related groups (DRGs) for reimbursement. With the end of cost-plus reimbursement, and its replacement with reimbursement based on diagnosis, hospital profits for medical and surgical treatment began to decline, and private investors became disenchanted.

The behavioral health care industry was basically untouched by DRGs, largely because psychiatric diagnoses were thought to lack sufficient power to predict the course of treatment. Entrepreneurs saw tremendous opportunities available in the relatively unregulated behavioral health care market. Consequently, large, for-profit chains of specialty psychiatric and chemical dependency hospitals began to build facilities throughout the United States.

By the early 1980s, employers, who were basically offering indemnity insurance plans, were becoming more concerned about fast-rising behavioral health care costs. Self-insured employers began to contract with utilization review companies in an effort at least to control unnecessary inpatient hospitalization.

Traditional benefits in indemnity plans generously reimbursed inpatient services. Reimbursement for outpatient treatments of all kinds was much more limited. For example, there was very poor reimbursement, if any, for such alternatives to inpatient treatment as partial hospitalization or day treatment. Behavioral health care companies recognized the limitations of the existing indemnity plans. They began aggressively to market their services by offering a range of lower-cost replacements for inpatient treatment and by promoting the continuum-of-care philosophy.

Other employers began to increase the attractiveness of HMOs by offering their workers lower employee contributions if they enrolled in HMOs. But HMO mental health and substance abuse benefits were traditionally less generous than those offered by indemnity insurance plans. HMOs tried to contain costs through access barriers and, some would say, undertreatment.

PPOs also began to develop in the early 1980s. These organizations were based on groups of clinicians who contracted to serve a defined population on a discounted fee-for-service basis. The PPOs provided little or no case management. With no control on utilization and fees generally rising faster than the rate of inflation, PPOs by themselves did not prove able to control costs effectively.

Other employers and insurance companies began to contract with utilization review companies to do telephone reviews with treatment facilities after a patient had arrived for admission. They performed a policing role but had only limited effectiveness in cost containment, and virtually no impact on enhancing quality of care. Reviews done only after admission simply proved to be too little, too late.

Of all these care arrangements and fiscal oversight schemes, managed behavioral carve-outs emerged as the clear victor, ready to prosper in the 1990s.

How Did Managed Behavioral Carve-Outs Grow?

Many companies in the managed behavioral health care industry had their beginnings in the early 1980s. They began as private clinics or informal networks of local providers in a small geographic area, with a few contracts to provide services to businesses and insurers. Some started as utilization review companies, gradually becoming more comprehensive by building a contracted network and beginning to manage a full continuum of care. During the 1980s, there was a proliferation of small managed care companies throughout the United States.

Between 1986 and 1992 managed behavioral health care companies grew rapidly. To gain competitive advantage during this period, companies had to implement aggressive sales and marketing programs. At the same time they had to build a functional operational infrastructure to handle rapid growth. This form of development was quite costly, and the pace meant that growth could not be adequately funded by company profits. Rather, behavioral health care companies needed venture capital. Officers of venture capital firms were pleased to sign on because they viewed behavioral health care as a major growth industry.

Between 1988 and 1997 there has been movement toward industry consolidation ("Trajectory of Managed Care," 1997). The number of managed care companies has been decreasing while each remaining company's market share has been increasing. Because of their size and ways of doing business, insurance companies have generally not been able to mount managed behavioral health care enterprises. So instead, large insurance companies have simply bought them!

One example is MCC/Cigna. Metropolitan Counseling Clinics, founded in 1981, was a national managed behavioral health care company with a network of providers and clinics throughout the United States. It was purchased by the insurance company Cigna in 1989. In 1995, MCC Behavioral Care covered approximately 5.2 million lives (Oss, 1995); by January 1998, MCC Behavioral Care covered 7.9 million lives (personal communication with Margaret Dickinson, assistant vice president, professional relations and network strategy, MCC Behavioral Care, Eden Prairie, MN, January 13, 1998).

Some of the larger, successfully managed behavioral health care companies remained independent of traditional insurance companies for longer periods of time. One example is Value Behavioral Health, formed by Preferred Healthcare and American PsychManagement. Before the merger, each of the companies largely focused on the managed indemnity market and contracted predominantly with large, self-insured employers. In 1995, they covered 13.1 million people (Oss, 1995). By January 1998, Value Behavioral Health, which had merged with Columbia/HCA on August 7, 1997, covered 23.5 million lives. Highlighting the rapidity of change in the arena, by late winter or early spring of 1998, Columbia/HCA will have sold Value Behavioral Health, ending this brief merger (personal communication with Judy Barber, vice president, marketing, Value Behavioral Health, Inc., Falls Church, VA, January 20, 1998).

A recent development in the consolidation of the managed behavioral health care industry has been the formalizing of relationships among managed behavioral health care companies, pharmaceutical manufacturers, and mail-order prescription management companies. One example is Medco Containment Services–Biodyne–Merck Pharmaceutical. Medco Containment Services was a highly successful mail-order prescription management company. In 1992, it purchased American Biodyne, Inc., to form Medco Behavioral Care (MBC). MBC was purchased by Merck Pharmaceutical in 1993. In early 1995, MBC covered 14.1 million individuals. But once again these trends prove not to be linear. In July 1995, MBC Management, together with Kohlberg, Krantz, Roberts and Company, purchased controlling interest in MBC from Merck, making MBC—which changed its name to Merit Behavioral Care—an independent company. As of January 1998, Merit Behavioral Care covered 22 million lives (Coughlin, 1997).

The Individual Provider

Within the new culture of managed behavioral health care, how will individual practitioners survive? For how many will the shift from practitioner to businessperson be too much (Stone, 1997)?

Nicholas A. Cummings (1995), whom I mentioned earlier, has outlined seven paradigm shifts that will be required of future mental health care providers to survive in the changing marketplace of mental health care delivery. His paradigms are worth consideration.

- **Paradigm Shift 1.** *Recent:* Few patients are seen but for lengthy courses of treatment, usually individually. *Future:* Many clients are seen for brief episodes of treatment, very often in nontraditional modes.
- **Paradigm Shift 2.** *Recent:* Treatment of patients is continuous, often weekly or even more frequently. *Future:* Treatment of clients is brief and intermittent throughout the life cycle.
- **Paradigm Shift 3.** *Recent:* The therapist is the vehicle for change, and emphasis is on treating the patient's psychopathology. *Future:* The therapist is merely a catalyst for the client to change, and the emphasis is on growth rather than cure.
- **Paradigm Shift 4.** *Recent:* The therapy is the most important event in the patient's life, and it is within the treatment span that the patient changes. *Future:* The therapy is an artificial situation like an operating room, and significant changes occur and keep occurring for the client long after scheduled therapy has been interrupted.
- **Paradigm Shift 5.** *Recent:* Therapy continues until healing occurs, and the patient is terminated as more or less "cured." *Future:* Therapy is the foundation for growth outside therapy; formal treatment is only part of the therapy process. The client can return to formal therapy as needed.
- **Paradigm Shift 6.** *Recent:* Individual and group psychotherapy in the office are the main modalities by which patients heal. *Future:* The client uses community resources, a better approach than limiting the healing process to the psychotherapist's office.
- **Paradigm Shift 7.** *Recent:* Fee-for-service is the economic base for practice, and the patient and therapist must constantly fight against limitations on benefits.

Future: Prospective reimbursement or capitation supposedly will free the therapist to provide whatever psychological services are needed by the client.

Note that in all of these paradigms there a shift from "patients" to "clients." This change in terminology was lobbied for by the social work profession. But it is coming back to haunt social workers. Why does someone need a master's degree to see a "client"? How far will the substitution of less-well-trained providers for better-trained (and presumably more-skilled) providers go (Karon, 1995)?

The Loci of Managed Behavioral Health Care

The modern era of managed behavioral health care began in the private sector, but these principles and practices have spread to the public sector. Public sector managed psychiatric care in the United States started through Medicaid Managed Care (U.S. House Committee on Ways and Means, 1995) but is spreading rapidly to Medicare Managed Care (Fox, 1997).

Medicaid Managed Care is being driven by the spiraling costs of the Medicaid program. Between 1985 and 1993, Medicaid costs tripled and the number of beneficiaries increased by over 50 percent (U.S. General Accounting Office, 1995). Medicaid Managed Care has taken place through states obtaining Medicaid waivers from the Health Care Financing Administration (HCFA). There are two basic types of waivers:

1. *Program Waivers.* Section 1915(b) program waivers allow states significant waiver authority, although these are not as expansive as Section 1115 waivers. Section 1915(b) waivers are limited in that they apply to Medicaid services furnished to Medicaid recipients. Program waivers do not allow states to cover traditionally non-Medicaid populations, modify the Medicaid benefit package, waive Section 1903(m) HMO provisions, such as enrollment composition and disenrollment on demand, and restrict access to family planning providers.
2. *Research and Demonstration Waivers.* Section 1115 waivers, sometimes called "research" or "demonstration" projects, are unlike Section 1915(b) waivers (which clearly provide for waiver programs to continue indefinitely if successful) in that projects under Section 1115 should, at some point, reach a conclusion. Generally, proposals for statewide reform under Section 1115 waivers have several common factors: The state wants to expand its use of managed care, it is expected that savings will be achieved as one outcome of increased use of managed care, these savings (plus savings from other state actions) are to be used to finance coverage for people previously ineligible for Medicaid, and the demonstration is expected to be budget neutral over the life of the project (generally five years).

Many requirements can be altered under Section 1115 waivers. These include

- statewide uniformity—permitting variations in the program in different areas of the state
- comparability requirements—allowing different benefits to be provided to one group and not another
- eligibility—permitting states to revise Medicaid eligibility standards and criteria

- provider choice or freedom of choice—allowing restriction of recipients' provider choice and requiring enrollment in managed care systems
- managed care organizations—permitting recipients to receive services through alternative delivery systems not recognizable under existing state and federal requirements (under Section 1115, states may, for example, contract with HMOs that have Medicare and Medicaid enrollments in excess of 75 percent and may limit Medicaid recipient disenrollments from HMOs to an annual "open season")
- reimbursement—allowing reasonable alterations in Medicaid payment requirements
- freedom of choice of family planning services providers—allowing states to limit people to receiving family planning services from providers within their managed care plans or systems.

Although Section 1115 authority is very broad, certain statutory and policy restrictions exist for state demonstrations. Statutory restrictions include

- services for pregnant women and children—states must provide medical assistance to pregnant women and children younger than age 19
- drug rebate provisions—states must provide medical assistance for covered outpatient drugs and cannot affect drug manufacturers' rebate provisions
- copayments and other cost sharing—states are prohibited from imposing copayments on categorically eligible people enrolled in HMOs
- nonemergency use of emergency room services—copayment restrictions prohibit imposing copayments on Medicaid-eligible HMO enrollees for the unauthorized, nonemergency use of emergency room services
- federal medical assistance percentage rates—the rate at which the federal government matches states' expenditures cannot be waived.

Some policy restrictions include

- reduced quality of care—programs or policies that inappropriately reduce access, benefits, or otherwise reduce quality of care cannot be approved (HCFA, in fact, requires the managed care systems to enhance access to quality services)
- budget neutrality—programs cannot cost the federal government more than the states' Medicaid plans would cost without waivers
- unnecessary utilization and access safeguards—safeguards against unnecessary use of services as well as assurances that payments are sufficient to enlist enough providers to make services as available as they are to the general population
- quality improvement—states are expected to enhance quality improvement plans.

The current state of waivers is unclear. Massachusetts has a waiver that, effective July 1, 1997, allows it to bill Medicaid for 30 days per episode, 60 days per year of psychiatric treatment in its state hospitals. This is a major break with the longtime Institution for Mental Disorders (IMD) exclusion that traditionally prohibited states from billing Medicaid for state hospital patients. On the other hand, the Balanced Budget Act of 1997 may eliminate the need for waivers in certain situations, allowing states to move some Medicaid populations into a managed system of care without federal approval ("Balanced Budget Bill," 1997; Bazelon Center for Mental Health Law, 1997).

Will these waivers work? Research into their effects has just begun. Some would say that, historically, the states' departments of mental health tried to do everything with nothing. Others would say that, contemporarily, the managed care companies appear to be trying to do nothing with everything. There must be a better way!

People with Serious Mental Illness

What about people with serious mental illness? Can managed behavioral health care meet their needs? We don't know.

Can states successfully integrate their historic, state-provided services into MCOs? We don't know.

Can we adequately differentiate between acute treatment and long-term care in those with chronic mental illnesses to prevent dumping? We don't know.

Can MCOs save money and appropriately provide care and treatment to those with chronic mental illness? We don't know.

Until now, have MCOs met the needs of people who are seriously mentally ill? No.

Until now, have MCOs refrained from riding on the backs of the states' departments of mental health? No.

Until now, has the shift to managed care and privatization improved the already compromised continuity of care in the public sector? No.

Until now, has managed care improved the quality of life of people with serious mental illnesses? No.

Until now, do we have any clear indications that managed care is better than what we had before for people with serious and persistent mental illnesses? No.

There are nascent research efforts (Callahan, Shepard, Beinecke, Larson, & Cavanaugh, 1995; Psychiatric Services Resource Center, 1997), but the data are simply too meager to support conclusions.

What's in the future? If all goes well, then people who have historically received very little (poor people and those with chronic mental illnesses) will get more, people who received a lot ("worried well" people) will get less, and both groups will be better off.

This could occur through the reform effort now known as "parity." A discussion of the almost 150-year struggle to increase the federal responsibility for people with chronic mental illnesses (Geller, 1994) and the most recent advances toward equitable health care coverage for this population (Geller, 1996) is beyond the scope of this chapter, but one point is important in the context of managed care for people with serious mental illnesses: There is an almost complete disconnection between health reform through Medicaid Managed Care and parity. Massachusetts, the first state to have a statewide, managed, Medicaid mental health carve-out (Elias & Navon, 1995) and to attempt to evaluate it (Callahan et al., 1995) will be the last of the New England states to achieve parity, if it achieves it at all (Flynn, 1997).

There should be no rushing to judgment, but advocates, patients, and family members in Massachusetts are all concerned (*Cutting Costs by Cutting Care,* 1997; Fendall, 1997; Flory, 1997). Jane Richardson's recent remarks are worth attention. Richardson, the mother of Diane Richardson who died February 4, 1995, on the psychiatric unit of Beverly Hospital (Massachusetts), lamented, "Danver's [State Hospital] smelled, it was old, and it looked dirty, but in retrospect, I saw a lot of staff members being compassionate. The [private] hospitals Diane has been in since then smell nice, but the care stinks" (cited in Bass, 1995, p. 40).

Matching the Systems of Care and the Practitioner

In reviewing the changes in the systems of care and the major life changes in mental health practitioners of all disciplines, are there goals on which those who manage the system and those who practice in it can agree? Let me suggest 10 actions:

1. appropriately deliver treatment (direct costs) to avoid subsequent adverse health effects (indirect and secondary costs)
2. provide preventive care and education to decrease treatment costs, morbidity, and mortality
3. innovate in service delivery patterns and systems that will improve patient outcome, lessen length of treatment, minimize removal of patients from natural environments to the maximal extent possible, and decrease iatrogenic morbidity
4. ensure access to treatment to all those who need care and eliminate stigma to facilitate this, while achieving a balance so that there is neither overutilization nor underutilization of care
5. develop consensual definitions of medical necessity and appropriateness
6. promulgate clinical practice guidelines that define standards of treatment and ensure that these guidelines recognize a relationship between a provider and his or her patient.
7. develop agreed-on outcome measures and mutually endorsed technologies to determine them
8. develop patient satisfaction measures and use them
9. find or create accrediting organizations and define accreditation standards (either free-standing or government regulatory agencies)
10. arrive at an ethos that company, provider, and patient agree on in defining the relationships among the three.

Until we can accomplish these or comparable objectives, advocacy groups may continue to suggest how to do it right (Bazelon Center for Mental Health Law, 1995) and bestow failing grades on efforts to date (Hall, Edgar, & Flynn, 1997), the federal government may continue to increase regulations through legislation (Moran, 1997), and providers may continue to feel squeezed to produce more with less ("Mass-[achusetts] Providers Question," 1996).

Editorial: When Less Is More, When Less Is Less

Let me conclude with an editorial, published in the American Psychiatric Association journal *Psychiatric Services* (Geller, 1995), that is both a call for recognition of where we have been as professionals and a plea for full participation in our future:

> Is managed behavioral health care new?
> Are fixed budgets, prospective payments, and carve-outs new?
> Are alternatives to inpatient utilization such as step-down units new?
> Are case managers new?

Are crisis intervention, admission diversion, mobile emergency services, or home-based specialing new?

Far too many persons would answer yes to some or all of these questions. The correct response to all of them, however, is no.

For between 100 and 200 years in most states, the state government has been running a carved-out, managed behavioral health care entity, generally known as states' departments of mental health. The departments received a fixed budget to provide all psychiatric care and treatment to a defined population. More services rendered did not accrue greater payments; less money spent in one area such as inpatient care meant more money available for other services; replacing costly providers (physicians and nurses) with lower cost providers (aides and technicians) meant greater economies; and annual performance evaluations compared dollars spent with services provided.

In all states, managed behavioral health care provided by the state went astray, and allocated resources became so inadequate for the population in need that services deteriorated to a nadir best labeled by Albert Deutsch as *The Shame of the State* in his 1948 exposé. There is a lesson here. Managed behavioral health care can mean efficiencies with more services available for more people. But it can also deteriorate to less, less, and more less.

Virtually all the alternatives to inpatient care now used by managed behavioral health care were developed in the public sector for the same reason managed behavioral health care has embraced them: to move the locus of care from costly inpatient to less costly outpatient services. There is a lesson here, too. We can get better services for more individuals with significant mental illnesses, or we can get less, less, and more less, leading to underserved and unserved people who populate our street corners, jails, and cemeteries.

Many say the public sector is disappearing. That's only true if you define the service system by the payer source. If you define the system by its procedures, personnel, and technologies, then the private sector is disappearing. The public sector service system has emerged as state of the art. We should give it the respect it deserves, and we should learn from its past errant ways.

It will surely be disastrous if managed behavioral health care becomes the next Shame of the States. The slope is a slippery one; we've been down it before. Let's manage not to do it again. (p. 1105)

References

Altman, S. H., & Reinhardt, U. E. (1996). *Strategic choices for a changing health care system.* Chicago: Health Administration Press.

Balanced Budget Act of 1997, P.L. 105-33, 111 Stat. 251, 787.

Balanced budget bill eliminates waivers, offers few Medicaid protections, standards. (1997, August 11). *Mental Health Weekly,* p. 102.

Bass, A. (1995, July 3). Deaths in the mental health system. *Boston Globe,* pp. 39, 40–41.

Bazelon Center for Mental Health Law. (1995). *Managing managed care for publicly financed mental health services.* Washington, DC: Author.

Bazelon Center for Mental Health Law. (1997, December 12). *Advocacy Alert,* pp. 1–2.

Callahan, J. J., Shepard, D. S., Beinecke, R. H., Larson, M. J., & Cavanaugh, D. (1995). Mental health/substance abuse treatment in managed care: The Massachusetts experiences. *Health Affairs 14,* 173–184.

Coughlin, K. M. (Ed.). (1997). *1998 Medicaid management behavioral care sourcebook.* New York: Faulkner & Gray.

Croze, C. (1995). Medicaid waivers: The shape of things to come. *Proceedings of the Fifth Annual National Conference on State Mental Health Agency Services Research and Program Evaluation* (pp. 324–338). Alexandria, VA: National Association of State Mental Health Program Directors.

Cummings, N. A. (1995). Impact of managed care on employment and training: A primer for survival. *Professional Psychology: Research and Practice, 26,* 5–9.

Cutting costs by cutting care. (1997, June). Quincy, MA: Advocates for Quality Care.

Dennis, D. L., & Monahan, J. (1996). *Coercion and aggressive community treatment.* New York: Plenum Press.

Deutsch, A. (1948). *The shame of the states.* New York: Harcourt, Brace.

Dorwart, R. A., & Epstein, S. S. (1993). *Privatization and mental health care.* Westport, CT: Auburn House.

Edmunds, M., Frank, R., Hogan, M., McCarty, D., Robinson-Beale, R., & Weisner, C. (Eds.). (1997). *Managing managed care.* Washington, DC: National Academy Press.

Elias, E., & Navon, M. (1995). The Massachusetts experience with managed mental health care and Medicaid. *Health Affairs, 14*(3), 46–49.

Fendall, S. (1997, Spring). MHMA wrapping up; Partnership starting up. *Advisor,* pp. 1–4, 13–16.

Fink, P. J., & Tasman, A. (Eds.). (1992). *Stigma and mental illness.* Washington, DC: American Psychiatric Press.

Flory, B. (1997). Will Massachusetts survive managed care? *AMI Messenger, 15*(4), 4–5.

Flynn, L. (1997, December 22). Equal coverage for mental illness. *Boston Globe,* p. A23.

Fox, P. D. (1997). Applying managed care techniques in traditional Medicare. *Health Affairs, 16*(5), 44–57.

Frank, R. G., Sullivan, M. J, & DeLeon, P. H. (1994). Health care reform in the states. *American Psychologist, 49,* 855–867.

Freeman, M. A., & Trabin, T. (1994). *Managed behavioral healthcare: History, models, key issues, and future course.* Rockville, MD: Center for Mental Health Services.

Geller, J. L. (1986). Rights, wrongs, and the dilemma of coerced community treatment. *American Journal of Psychiatry, 143,* 1259–1264.

Geller, J. L. (1992). Pathological firesetting in adults. *International Journal of Law and Psychiatry, 15,* 283–302.

Geller, J. L. (1994). A history lesson. *Psychiatric News, 29*(6), 10.

Geller, J. L. (1995). When less is more; when less is less [Editorial]. *Psychiatric Services, 46,* 1105.

Geller, J. L. (1996). Is the camel's nose under the tent? *Psychiatric News, 31*(23), 18, 34.

Gorman, M. (1956). *Every other bed.* Cleveland: World.

Grob, G. N. (1991). *From asylum to community.* Princeton, NJ: Princeton University Press.

Hall, L. L., Edgar, E. R., & Flynn, L. M. (1997). *Stand and deliver: Action call to a failing industry.* Arlington, VA: National Alliance for the Mentally Ill.

Karon, B. P. (1995). Provision of psychotherapy under managed care: A growing crisis and national nightmare. *Professional Psychology: Research and Practice, 26,* 5–9.

Lazarus, J. L. (1995, July). Managed care problems and solutions: Psychiatrists urged to take initiative in solving access, funding concerns. *Psychiatric Times,* p. 36.

Levin, B. L., & Petrila, J. (1996). *Mental health services.* New York: Oxford University Press.

Levy, M. I. (1995, July). Why we should "opt out" of managed care. *Psychiatric Times,* pp. 27–28, 34–35.

Mass[achusetts] providers question carve-out's spending reductions. (1996, September 30). *Mental Health Weekly,* pp. 1–2.

McFarland, B. H. (1994). Health maintenance organizations and persons with severe mental illness. *Community Mental Health Journal, 30,* 221–242.

Monahan, J., & Steadman, J. H. (1994). *Violence and mental disorder.* Chicago: University of Chicago Press.

Moran, D. W. (1997). Federal regulation of managed care: An impulse in search of a theory? *Health Affairs, 16*(6), 7–21.

Mrazek, P. J., & Haggerty, R. J. (Eds.). (1994). *Reducing risks for mental disorders.* Washington, DC: National Academy Press.

Oss, M. E. (1995). More Americans enrolled in managed behavioral care. *Open Minds, 8*(12), 12.

Pomerantz, J. M., Liptzin, B., Carter, A. N., & Perlman, M. S. (1994). The professional affiliation group: A new model for managed mental health care. *Hospital and Community Psychiatry, 45,* 308–310.

Psychiatric Services Resource Center. (1997). *Managed care and mental health services.* Washington, DC: Author.

Rich, F. (1997, December 28). Admit to psychiatric help; see most careers disappear. *Sunday Telegram,* p. C3.

Sabshin, M. (1995). *Annual report of the medical director May 1994–May 1995.* Washington, DC: American Psychiatric Association.

Stone, D. A. (1997). The doctor as businessman: The changing politics of a cultural icon. *Journal of Health Politics, Policy and Law, 22,* 533–556.

Tax Equity and Fiscal Responsibility Act of 1982, P.L. 97-248, 96 Stat. 324.

The trajectory of managed care. (1997, May). *Issue Brief, 9,* 1–4.

U.S. General Accounting Office. (1995). *Medicaid spending pressures drive states toward program reinvention* (Report No. GAO-HEHS-95-122). Washington, DC: Author

U.S. House Committee on Ways and Means, Subcommittee on Health. (1995). *Health Insurance Portability and Accountability Act (HIPAA)* (104th Cong., 1st sess.). Washington, DC: U.S. Government Printing Office.

CHAPTER 4

Managed Care, Mental Illness, and African Americans: A Prospective Analysis of Managed Care Policy in the United States

King Davis

Health Care Reform

In a series of presentations, letters, and analyses in 1993 (Bureau of National Affairs, 1993; White House Domestic Policy Council, 1993), President Clinton indicated that his rationale for shifting American health care policy toward managed competition was the increasing degree of health insecurity in the American population and the extent to which the system of care "is badly broken" (White House Domestic Policy Council, 1993, p. 1). Furthermore, in his message to the American people, Clinton concluded that the current health care system is overly complex with increasing costs, declining quality, and choice. In its place, Clinton proposed a national health care system based on a set of interlocking principles for reversing the decline in security and choice and the increase in complexity and costs. Clinton proposed that without a major change in health policy, 63 million Americans would be unable to maintain their existing health care insurance coverage (Bureau of National Affairs, 1993; White House Domestic Policy Council, 1993). Up to 37 million Americans were reported to lack health insurance coverage entirely, although many of these are families in which at least one adult is employed but cannot obtain coverage. Clinton reported that close to 25 million people had coverage that was considered insufficient to meet their family needs in a medical emergency (Bureau of National Affairs, 1993; White House Domestic Policy Council, 1993).

When the costs of health care in America are considered in the reform equation, the Clinton administration concluded that health care as a proportion of the gross domestic product (GDP) is rising at an unacceptably high rate (White House Domestic Policy Council, 1993). For the past decade, health care has consumed close to 15 percent of the GDP. (In 1995, total health care expenditures in the United States were $840 billion.) Projections show an increase to 20–22 percent of the GDP by the end of the decade. The ability to level these costs at around 17 percent of the GDP is dependent on the development of a global health care budget that Congress will pass and enforce. Without such efforts, the health care portion of the GDP could find its own ceiling in an open marketplace, perhaps in excess of 25 percent by the year 2010 (White House Domestic Policy Council, 1993). In addition

NOTE: Originally published as Davis, K. (1997). Managed care, mental illness, and African Americans: A prospective analysis of managed care policy in the United States. *Smith College Studies in Social Work, 67,* 623–641.

to the general rise in health care costs in the United States, taxes rose an average of 18 percent per annum over the past decade to meet the increased cost of Medicaid. As continued increases in health care costs and taxes are added to products and services, the competitive international market and sales position of American companies potentially decreases.

When American health care costs are compared with those of other industrialized nations, the disproportionate growth is more overt. Of seven highly industrialized nations, the percentage of their GDP consumed by health care is only one-half of the percentage spent on similar care in the United States (Bureau of National Affairs, 1993; Hurst, 1991; White House Domestic Policy Council, 1993).

The health reform package proposed by President Clinton (White House Domestic Policy Council, 1993) was designed to decrease the upward spiral in health care costs and the complex set of issues associated with a lack of coverage. However, that reform package and the strategies for moving it forward failed to win adequate support within Congress, the health professions, business, or the general public (Johnson & Broder, 1996). In the gap created by the failure of the Clinton health care reform effort, two events have occurred that are changing the face of health care delivery. First, private businesses have moved rapidly to develop and implement myriad health care cost-containment strategies under the broad rubric of managed care. These private companies require that their employees join approved managed health care plans, and they follow a series of processes designed to result in a significant reduction in health premium costs to the business. Second, by the close of 1996, the federal government had not yet passed a comprehensive policy to reform the ailing health care system in America. Despite the absence of overt government policy, the willingness of the federal government to grant states broad powers under Medicaid waiver programs, the shift in P.L. 93-222 (converting HMOs from nonprofit to profit status), and the subsequent rise of unregulated managed health care organizations seem to have brought about one of the most dramatic shifts in the financing, distribution, and delivery of health care in American history. For the first time in many years, the upward spiral of health care costs has declined. Physician incomes are down. Employed Americans and those receiving transfer payments are joining managed health plans at an accelerated rate.

The actions by federal and state governments and the private business sector are designed to achieve two very closely related goals in American health care underscored in the President's initial plan: (1) lowering the steep rise in costs and (2) restricting care to only that which is considered medically necessary. It would be difficult to argue against a public policy decision designed to lower the overall costs of health care in America, even if that policy were to reduce personal choice while maintaining high levels of equitable access and clinical quality. What is worthy of exploration and analysis is the prospective impact that managed health care reform policy is likely to have on the access to and quality of health care for particular groups of Americans who have historically been viewed as medically underserved. Although not identified specifically in the Clinton health reform package (White House Domestic Policy Council, 1993), medically underserved populations include African American, Hispanic, and Native American people, white people living in rural areas, and people with disabilities, as well as populations in poverty, in low-wage jobs, or who are otherwise unable to gain access to quality health care. In this chapter, the focus will be the prospective impact of managed health care reform on low-income African Americans with severe and persistent mental or physical illness, on their families and communities, and on their traditional community health care networks and providers. The chapter will define managed care and a number of its key processes designed to reduce the cost of health care.

Defining Managed Care

One of the dilemmas in understanding managed health care and its impact by race and class is the absence of clear conceptual or operational definitions (Randall, 1994). Currently, no single, universally accepted definition of managed health care is in use. It is easy without clarity of basic concepts and terms (Piotrowski, 1971) to assume that the term "manage" in managed health care connotes that services will be handled more efficiently, effectively, or carefully than services delivered in a fee-for-service plan.

Hurley, Freund, and Paul (1993) defined *managed care* principally as indemnity insurance plans with intensive utilization review systems to monitor access, cost, quality, and outcomes. The managed care industry (United Healthcare Corporation, 1994) defined *managed care* as a system of health care delivery that influences utilization and cost of services and measures of performance. According to this second definition, the goal is a system that delivers value by giving people access to better-quality, cost-effective health care. A third definition suggested that *managed health care* is any process, plan, program, or procedure that controls access, cost, quality, and outcomes (Davis, 1996). Although there are slight differences in these definitions, one clear conclusion is that managed health care is primarily a financial management strategy, whereby the optimum profit margin depends on the use of specific processes that confine clinical care to populations covered under the plan and limit individual care to procedures considered medically necessary and included in the benefit package.

Key Processes in Managed Care

Managed health care plans institute a variety of processes to ensure a balance between services that are covered and those actually provided. That balance is determined and maintained, at least partially, by medical necessity criteria. Medical necessity is a process for determining whether services demanded are "appropriate and necessary to meet basic health needs" (United Healthcare Corporation, 1994, p. 48). Medical necessity is based in part on the presence and application of nationally accepted guidelines, competencies, and standards to guide diagnosis and treatment. In those instances in which services are not considered medically necessary, the health plan can deny the consumer reimbursement. It is not clear what the medical necessity outcomes are when there are no acceptable standards, guidelines, or competencies for either a specific illness or for specific populations of consumers.

Another key process, often found in life insurance plans, is evidence of insurability and eligibility (United Healthcare Corporation, 1994). This process requires that the prospective consumer of services demonstrate "evidence of good health" and meet other qualifications related to the number of hours employed to be eligible for services under the contract.

Capitation, one of the more critical concepts in managed health care, denotes that a fixed amount of money has been negotiated to be paid to a provider on a regularly scheduled basis for health care delivered to all people covered under a contract (United Healthcare Corporation, 1994). *Copayment* (deductible) is a process in which an insured person must pay a specified portion of the charges before the plan will pay for the services. *Disallowance* is a process in which the payer refuses to pay for services provided based on the payer's interpretation of the benefit. *Disenrollment* is the process in which a person loses access to the health care plan and services for a variety of reasons. The authority to make disenrollment decisions is held by the managed care plan.

What is clear from those and related processes in managed health care plans is the belief that such processes will decrease the demand for services that are not medically indicated while also decreasing costs. Inherent in this set of processes is an effort to delimit choices by consumers or have consumers pay out of pocket for exercising choices. These policies are based on the belief that unlimited choices result in increased demand whenever consumers do not have to pay for these costs.

Each of these key processes suggests that health care is a commodity, subject to the same or similar market and fiscal forces as all other products and services. People who lack insurance, cash, credit, or transfer payments will be less able to participate in the open-market health system to acquire services at a level commensurate with people who have the financial resources. If health services did not so closely determine ongoing health, daily functioning, presence of illness, and the probability of mortality, this market force analogy would be considerably less important.

It is clear that people who lack access to quality health care are more likely to have undiagnosed illness, untreated disease, and higher rates of mortality at a younger mean age. The balance among health status, access, and race becomes a critical consideration under a managed health care policy in which the emphasis is placed on acute care, employment, and cost savings. It is important to explore differences in health status by race as well as the probable impact of managed care both as a financial and service mechanism and as a series of processes that affect the physical health and mental health status of underserved populations.

Health Care and Race

Historical and current data about the health status of American populations confirm that there are significant differences in prevalence and incidence of physical and mental health problems among groups based on color, income, and residence. Also noted are major differences in help-seeking patterns (Neighbors, 1986). In two special reports (Center for Health Economics Research, 1993; Robert Wood Johnson Foundation, 1991), people of color, particularly residents of inner cities, showed major disparities in their health status when compared with other populations. The disparities cover the range of disorders from high neonatal mortality rates per live births, higher rates of heart and circulatory problems, disproportionate rates of AIDS and related deaths, greater prevalence of chronic conditions, higher rates of edentulism, and higher rates of admissions to psychiatric facilities. The high incidence of substance abuse, physical injuries, and deaths from violence greatly distinguish neighborhoods and communities of low-income African American residents in terms of potential and actual costs of health care. According to some reports, substance abuse is the most significant health problem in the nation (Institute for Health Policy, 1993). Populations of people of color also have less access to health insurance and have a significantly lower proportion of health professionals within easy access from their neighborhoods.

From the time that state governments decided to provide and finance residential care for people with long-term mental illness, major public policy paradoxes have been identified and debated in regard to race and mental illness (Jarvis, 1844). The first of these paradoxes centers on the incidence and prevalence of severe mental illness in the African American population, and the second centers on the extent to which African American populations require and consume public or proprietary mental health services (Snowden & Cheung, 1990).

Historically, answers to the two interrelated sets of public policy paradoxes concerning race and mental illness have been more a reflection of the prevailing racial climate in American society at large than of objective epidemiologic or ethnographic data. A cursory review of the data on admissions to inpatient psychiatric facilities (Manderscheid & Sonnenschein, 1987; Scheffler & Miller, 1989; Snowden & Cheung, 1990) shows disproportionately high rates of admissions by race to all types of facilities. Those data (Manderscheid & Sonnenschein, 1987; Snowden & Cheung, 1990; Snowden & Holschuh, 1992) show that between 1980 and 1992, the rate of admission for all people to state hospitals in the United States was approximately 163.6 per 100,000. The rate for white people was 136.0, for Hispanic people it was 146.0, and for Native American and Asian people it was 142.0 per 100,000 (Manderscheid & Sonnenschein, 1987). During the years studied, the admission rate to state hospitals for African American people was 364.2 per 100,000 population.

When admissions to private psychiatric hospitals are considered by race, the rate for all people was 62.6 per 100,000, and the rate for white people was slightly above the mean at 63.4. The rate of admissions to private psychiatric hospitals for Hispanic people was 34.4 and for Native American and Asian people it was 29.6. The rate for African American people was close to the national mean at 62.9.

Admissions to general hospitals with psychiatric units showed similar patterns by race and ethnicity. For the population as a whole the rate was 295.3 per 100,000, and for the white population it was 284.9. The rate of admissions for Hispanic people was 227.0, and for Native American and Asian people it was 221.7. During the same period, 386.6 per 100,000 African Americans were admitted to general hospital psychiatric units. The national mean admission rate to Department of Veterans Affairs hospitals was 70.4 per 100,000, but African Americans had a rate of 118.2 per 100,000. No other racial or ethnic population approximated the African American admission rate to those hospitals.

When age is examined, the relationship between admissions to psychiatric hospitals and race is even more pronounced. For example, the rate of admissions to state psychiatric hospitals for African American men and women ages 18 to 24 was 598.0 per 100,000; the national mean was 163.6 (Manderscheid & Sonnenschein, 1987). The most excessive rate found was for African Americans between ages 25 and 44; 753 per 100,000 were admitted to state psychiatric hospitals (Manderscheid & Sonnenschein, 1987). Although admissions are not indicative of actual prevalence rates in the population, what is shown clearly is an inveterate pattern of service utilization differentiated by race and class.

To a great extent, access to and consumption of psychiatric inpatient services by African Americans has historically paralleled the prevailing theoretical views of their vulnerability and morbidity. During the colonial era, when African Americans were believed to be less susceptible to mental disorder, public policies extended inpatient services to free African Americans but denied similar services to enslaved African Americans. Given the numerical imbalance between free and enslaved African Americans at that time, the low utilization of existing services by slaves supported the hypothesis of lower susceptibility. The more recent idea that African Americans were more vulnerable to major mental disorder parallels the socioeconomic and political conflicts surrounding the abolition of slavery. As slavery drew to a close in 1863, public policies created separate mental institutions for African Americans throughout the southern and border states (Jarvis, 1844). As freedom for African Americans drew closer, it was predicted that a major increase in mental hospital beds would be needed to accommodate those who would suffer from post-slavery stress disorder. Data from the 1840 census were used to show that the frequency of mental illness was 11 times higher for free northern African Americans than for those in bondage in the South (Thomas & Sillen, 1972). Similar data were used to show that the ratio of serious mental illness in southern African Americans was considerably less than the ratio in southern white people; the reverse was found in Northern states.

At the other extreme in the policy paradox was the view current between 1945 and 1985 that African American and other urban populations were far more susceptible to major mental illness because of a greater frequency of poverty, life stress, and migration to urban areas. Those data and their conclusions were used by President John F. Kennedy to build his successful legislative rationale for the establishment of community mental health centers in 1963. The prevailing belief that African Americans were more vulnerable to mental illness resulted in policies that facilitated excess admissions from 1863 well into the 1990s. During this time, the number of African Americans admitted to various psychiatric institutions grew at a disproportionate rate, with a sizable number admitted involuntarily (Manderscheid & Sonnenschein, 1987; Ramm, 1989; Snowden & Holschuh, 1992).

Data drawn from the National Institute of Mental Health (Manderscheid & Sonnenschein, 1987) showed that African Americans were more frequently diagnosed on admission with severe mental illness than were other ethnic or racial populations. Admissions of African Americans to state mental hospitals showed that 56 percent of those individuals received a primary diagnosis of schizophrenia; only 38 percent of all people admitted received a similar diagnosis. Hispanic people, too, received a disproportionately high (44 percent) rate of severe mental illness diagnoses on admission to state mental institutions. Flaskerud and Hu (1992), Garretson (1993), Jones and Gray (1986), and Lawson, Heplar, Holladay, and Cuffel (1994) concluded that the primary reason for the disproportionate rate of severe mental illness diagnoses is errors made by diagnosticians who are unfamiliar with mental illness as it is manifested in populations of color.

Decades of knowledge in the literature on how African American populations consume mental health services show the following trends:

- African American populations with major mental illness drop out of services at a significantly higher rate than do white populations.
- African American populations use fewer treatment sessions for their mental health problems than do white populations.
- African American populations enter mental health treatment services at a later stage in the course of their illness than do white populations.
- African American populations underconsume community mental health services of all kinds.
- African American populations overconsume inpatient psychiatric care in state hospitals, using it at twice the rate of corresponding white populations.
- African American populations are more often misdiagnosed by mental health practitioners than are white populations.
- African American people are more often diagnosed as having a severe mental illness than are white people.

Managed Behavioral Health Care and Race

The data reflect a number of conclusions that may be helpful as the nation sets its course toward managed behavioral health care in the public and private sectors. First, it is clear that under the present and previous systems of care, African Americans with serious mental illness were not served well: Diagnoses were found to have been in error; admission rates were disproportionately high; involuntary admissions were used with great frequency; and the most severe mental illness labels were ascribed at a rate considerably higher than their expected frequency in the population. Of importance as well are the findings of different patterns of help seeking and help use on the part of African Americans, who tend to delay seeking help for psychiatric problems (as well as for major physical health problems) from formal health systems until conditions have become chronic and most other community and familial resources have been exhausted. African Americans also do not tend to remain engaged in outpatient services or use as many service units as other populations, although their diagnoses are more severe. Each of these conclusions portends important clinical and marketing issues for managed behavioral health care. As new managed care policies and services are being developed, there is a greater need to focus more attention on service issues and dilemmas related to race and severe mental illness. Although a key aim of managed care policies and procedures is to reduce unnecessary services and excessive costs, the role of race and service use remains poorly understood.

With the onset of managed care policy, the paradoxes associated with race and mental illness are likely to disproportionately affect low-income communities of color. For managed care to serve African American populations with severe mental illness effectively, there will need to be a significant focus on issues of access as well as quality of diagnosis and treatment. Too often, clinical issues are not examined from an ethnic or racial perspective because they do not fit the dominant cultural perspective. Even professionals who have been educated in urban areas with large concentrations of populations of color may be conditioned to assess consumers using standards and guidelines that are not culturally specific. In a behavioral health care environment that seeks to penetrate the African American mental health market, new service questions become relevant. They include the following:

- What factors explain the perceived differences in mental health service utilization patterns by race?
- What service design and delivery issues are pertinent to the provision of behavioral health care to predominantly African American Medicaid populations?
- What will African American populations expect from behavioral health services under managed health care?
- Are existing models of behavioral health care applicable to African American populations with severe and persistent mental illness?
- Are there clinical practice guidelines or standards that have been developed to support and measure clinical service outcomes to African American populations?
- To what extent is service utilization related to income and social class in African American populations?
- What mix of staff will be required to provide behavioral health care services to African American populations?

- What is the relationship between the conceptualization of severe mental illness held by African American populations and their use of behavioral health care?
- What are the help-seeking patterns used by African American populations to obtain behavioral health care?
- What roles do African American families and other social institutions play in determining help-seeking and services use of their relatives?

It is clear that poor African Americans are disproportionately diagnosed with high rates of severe physical and psychiatric illness that distinguish them in the health care marketplace. Flaskerud and Hu (1992), Jones and Gray (1986), and Lawson et al. (1994) concluded that those disproportionate rates of illness are reflections of diagnostic errors, cultural differences in language and symbols, and the training orientation of clinicians. The absence of culturally competent standards or guidelines for mental health care of African Americans contributes to the frequency of diagnostic and treatment errors (Davis, 1997). It could also be argued that the higher-than-expected frequency of severe mental illness, diagnosed on admission, results from the tendency in African American populations to delay help seeking until problems are more severe. Because of these distinctions, the needs and demands for services under any system of health care may push up the annual costs of caring for African Americans and, accordingly, negatively affect their access to care.

In a capitated environment, the probability that the cost of care will far exceed the contracted rate may eliminate any incentive for a managed care organization to serve the low-income African American population (Smith, 1994). The assumed relationship between race and higher per unit cost of care may delimit the access that poor African Americans have to managed behavioral and physical health care. Poor African Americans may also enter managed care systems with a plethora of preexisting chronic conditions, some of which are environmental, behavioral, or related to previous inadequate health and mental health care. Randall (1994) described what she termed "intergenerational illnesses" related to the continuation of life in high-risk environments in which successive generations of poor African Americans have been reared. In a managed health care system that puts the greater emphasis on acute conditions and infrequency of usage, poor African Americans with long-term illnesses may be denied access to care or disenrolled at a higher frequency than other populations as their demand for services increases. It also seems possible that, because of their higher frequency of illness and its chronicity, some African Americans would receive fewer services than their illnesses require as managed care systems give preference to groups with lesser illnesses (Randall, 1994). Snowden (1996) termed these processes "creaming and dumping."

One process that could be used to offset the potential for excess service usage by African Americans would be higher copayments. Copayments are designed to curb the demand for services by forcing the potential consumer to weigh the impact of the copayment against the impact on his or her life if the condition goes medically untreated. In instances in which government pays the copayment, there may be much less incentive to curb unnecessary medical and psychiatric visits by poor people. In instances in which copayments either are not paid by government or are increased because of frequency of demand, poor African American populations may be forced to forgo health and behavioral health benefits.

Another area of concern is the imbalance between prevention and treatment. In both physical and behavioral health care, it is evident that prevention of disease has not been stressed adequately for poor people. Blueford (1994), Smith (1994), and Weil (1994) indicated the value of identifying measures to prevent disorder and disease. In the most successful managed care programs for poor people, health promotion, health education, and early intervention have been shown to be cost effective (Bowles, 1994). Blueford (1994) indicated that changing long-term patterns of help-seeking, as characterized in African American populations, requires an intensive prevention and educationally oriented outreach service. He described the need to provide transportation that is available 24 hours per day, interpreters where needed, 24-hour help lines, community counselors, and intensive case management. When those preventive health care measures are applied in primary care, the numbers of emergency room visits and low-birthweight babies decline dramatically (Blueford, 1994). However, managed care organizations may not recognize or be willing to pay additional dollars for improving health care through promotion, prevention, and early intervention services to poor African Americans.

A basic dilemma for managed behavioral and physical health plans is determining the geographic location of services (Blueford, 1994; Weil, 1994). The majority of poor African Americans live in inner cities and rural areas. Such geographic areas lack adequate numbers of physicians, hospitals, outpatient services, integrated health systems, and public transportation. Each of these is in short supply, and health professionals are frequently unwilling to locate in rural or urban areas with a high concentration of African Americans. In rural areas the population base may be too minimal for managed care organizations to be profitable. Where medical personnel, population size, and transportation are all limited, poor African Americans may not be an attractive market for managed care to cover. Here, too, health status may suffer, and African American consumers may be forced either to travel long distances to receive care or to confine their requests for care to the most serious emergency situations. To serve poor African Americans adequately in reasonable proximity to their rural and urban neighborhoods, health and behavioral health organizations will need to offer transportation, home health services, satellite locations, and other approaches that reflect the needs of this market of consumers, even though such services may drive up unit costs.

Managed care processes are based on the development, maintenance, relevancy, and application of standards of care that fit a particular market of consumers. Randall (1994) believed that one of the serious dilemmas for managed care services to poor African Americans is found in utilization review. She warned that standards for service and utilization review may be biased toward European males. Standards of care may be insufficiently sensitive to the patterns of behavior and lifestyles of African Americans. Recent efforts by the Center for Mental Health Services (Davis, 1997) to identify the extent to which standards of care exist for African Americans have demonstrated an absence of standards, guidelines, or competencies specific to this population. As a result, poor African Americans are more likely to be denied services. Prospective reviews would deny services before they are rendered, leaving poor African Americans with the option of securing needed care at the point of service with their own funds or through added premium costs. Retrospective utilization reviews could deny reimbursement to the providers or consumers of service, thus potentially increasing their costs. In either of those utilization situations, poor African Americans would be disadvantaged financially and clinically. It seems unquestionable that there is a critical need for market-specific standards of care that take race, class, and ethnicity into consideration.

The ability of managed health care organizations to achieve their business goals and reduce the overall cost of health care supports their strategic emphasis on acute care and problem-focused services. The concept of medical necessity is designed to match the level of care needed with the level of care available and provided. No more, no less. With low-income African Americans, these expectations run counter to the data on current and previous health status and help-seeking behavior. A significant proportion of the adult African American population has a plethora of preexisting chronic physical conditions that may not prove responsive to short-term interventions. Differences in language, symbols, culture, conceptualization of illness and health, and help-seeking behavior may hamper obtaining accurate diagnosis, care, and aftercare services.

Essentially, managed health care is an indemnity insurance program designed to integrate various health care systems, providers, financing, and processes for full-time employees. In this insurance arrangement, various systems assume gradations of risk for an enrolled, insured population. Benefits and services are available only for individuals, families, and groups whose lives or health status are covered under a managed care product or plan. Usually, to be a "covered life" under managed care requires that at least one family member be employed full-time by an employer who agrees to offer health benefits. Alternatively, individuals and families can pay the out-of-pocket costs of managed health care in lieu of an employer's doing so. Chronically unemployed people, those who have lost jobs, and those in low-wage and low-benefit positions cannot afford to pay the out-of-pocket costs and therefore have no access to health care through managed health insurance plans. Historically, African American and Hispanic men have had higher rates of unemployment and, accordingly, are likely to have the greatest degree of health insecurity. African American and other women of color employed in service positions have a high degree of health insecurity as well. If the basis for distribution of health services within managed care maintains the link among health insurance, work, or transfer payments, unemployed African American and Hispanic men and underemployed African American and Hispanic women will continue to have inadequate, limited, or no access of any kind to health care (Leigh, 1994).

Clinical services under managed care need to be located within reasonable geographic distance to African American neighborhoods. Although the African American population has been noted for extensive migratory behavior over the decades, the majority of the population lives in or near urban areas. There is a discrepancy between where the African American population lives and where health care providers are located (Center for Health Economics Research, 1993). Providers are far more concentrated in suburban than in poor urban areas, making it vastly more difficult for inner-city and rural African Americans to obtain care. Access to care may require that African Americans expend additional dollars to reach managed care services. The presence of these additional costs may act as an indirect "managed" process that results in a lowering of demand for health care services under managed care. The dilemma for managed care organizations is identifying a means of getting physical health and mental health care practitioners in their provider networks and panels to locate services in or near low-income communities. A further dilemma under these circumstances stems from the realization that lower demand caused by differences in geographic location may result in short-term savings for managed care organizations or providers under capitated contracts. The ability to realize savings by not providing care may encourage managed care organizations to limit their efforts to serve low-income consumers within their own communities (Dawson, 1994).

The issue of choice seems to differentiate managed health care by social class. Initial resistance to managed health care by middle-class consumers was predicated on the loss of choice and selection of care providers or the inability to maintain services from existing providers. Lower-income African Americans may be willing to trade such choices for greater access while recognizing their lack of power to demand either. Upper-income classes with the resources to purchase services outside managed care plans do not have to trade either access or choice because they have the purchasing power to demand both. Middle-class populations may be willing to trade greater access for choice, while using their political power to maintain choice and variety. In the matter of choice, managed care companies may be more likely to respond to the needs of the middle-class consumer by expanding choices of providers while controlling access, a market strategy that may decrease services for the lower-income classes.

Human Resources Issues

Before the existence of managed health care, residents of African American communities received their health care through emergency rooms of general and teaching hospitals and from physicians willing to locate in their communities (Neighbors, 1986). Butcher (1993) believed that managed health care will destroy the traditional health care delivery system in African American communities and will severely displace African American physicians and other health care providers. Managed care networks invite health care providers to become part of their panels of providers. As a greater proportion of the population of employees join managed care organizations, their contracts may require that they use health care providers who are part of the managed care panels, or pay all differences in costs. A similar situation exists for recipients of Medicaid where those government-financed programs have been continued at the state level under managed care contracts with the private sector. African American health care providers who have not been accepted on managed care panels will not be able to continue providing services within these or other markets unless the consumer can pay out of pocket. Butcher (1993) reported numerous instances in which African American health care providers were denied participation on managed care panels and not given explanations for not being accepted. As more consumers become covered under managed care contracts, some African American health providers are finding that their fee-for-service practices are diminishing and in some instances closing entirely (Walton, 1994).

Managed care organizations place a premium on the credentials, background, and documented clinical experiences of potential panel members. Licensure, board certification, and an ability to show longitudinal data that verify successful practice interventions is required by many companies. Butcher (1993) noted that a smaller proportion of African American health providers are board certified or have automated information systems that allow them to provide detailed longitudinal data about their clients. It is also noted that a high proportion of African American health care providers operate as individual practitioners rather than in the group practices that are common and desired in managed care. As a result of a combination of these factors, African American health care providers may be excluded from joining managed care networks or may be asked to join in salaried positions. The potential impact of integrated managed health care on African American providers can be conceptualized as similar to previous efforts to vertically and horizontally integrate segregated school systems. It is reported that when public schools were required by law to integrate without regard to race, principals, teachers, counselors, and employees of formerly African American schools were displaced. Butcher's (1993) concerns that African American health care providers are being systematically driven from the market may result in a series of class-action lawsuits challenging managed care practices that appear exclusionary, discriminatory, and illegally in restraint of trade.

Before the introduction of managed health care, African American consumers obtained physical health and mental health care in a variety of ways. Their methods of accessing care often required them to travel long distances, wait for long periods of time, be treated in demeaning ways, and receive inferior services. Historically, African Americans were provided services under fee-for-service plans in which, as consumers, they had limited opportunities to voice meaningful complaints about the quality of services they received. Under a fee-for-service and publicly financed health and mental health care system, the health status and quality of life of poor African Americans were significantly lower than those of most other populations. Managed care processes have the potential for providing better-quality health care for poor African Americans through the emphasis on prevention, health maintenance, quality control, case management, and health education. Where managed care service efforts are based on knowledge of the cultural characteristics of the population and neighborhoods, quality of care may improve (Bowles, 1994). Of importance, too, in improving quality of care for African American populations is the presence of consumer rating scales in almost all managed care contracts, including Medicaid. Consumer rating scales (linked to continued contracts for managed care companies) offer African American populations the opportunity to insist on quality care and the ability to change providers if the expected level of quality care is not reached.

Conclusion

Managed health care as de facto public policy is being implemented at the same time that significant changes in welfare entitlement policies are being reformed. As welfare is reformed there are corresponding changes in the Medicaid programs, whose costs have escalated dramatically over the past decade. Each of those reform efforts is tied closely to the reinvention of states' rights as a political strategy for increasing the degree to which state governments control resources from the federal government, which heretofore had required adherence to federal policy and spending guidelines. States' rights may be the nexus between welfare reform and health care reform. Concomitant with the shifting of federal dollars to the states will come transfer of authority to redesign Medicaid and the policies under which it operates in meeting the health care needs of poor African Americans. Because managed care has demonstrated an ability to save scarce health care dollars, a number of states have shifted their Medicaid programs to private managed care companies. In previous years, African Americans, without regard to income or social class, did not receive equitable services and access when states made decisions about the distribution of societal resources, benefits, and rights. The unfairness of local and state governments in their treatment of African Americans fostered a significant amount of ill will as well as federal suits designed to curb racial discrimination. The partisan support of managed care strategies and processes by conservative state and local governments and the simultaneous combination of changes in welfare and Medicaid may harm the acceptance of managed health care in African American communities.

The inveterate dilemmas and paradoxes concerning race, mental illness, and health care have not been resolved adequately. As new managed health care policies and services are being implemented, there is a great need to focus attention on the multiple issues cited here to reach, penetrate, and adequately serve African Americans with severe mental and physical illness. Although a prime concern in managed care policy is cost reduction, the role of race and service utilization remains poorly understood. As in earlier eras of change in public policy, the paradoxes associated with race are likely to have a disproportionate impact on low-income populations of color. Although there are initiatives that can diminish the potential negative impact of managed health care, there are also key processes within managed health care that bode well for African American consumers. If managed care organizations can and are willing to find creative ways to harness their prevention, early intervention, health maintenance, and educational strategies with the idiosyncrasies of the market of African American consumers, there is a strong possibility that the litany of health and mental health problems evident in fee-for-service health care will be diminished. Managed care systems will need to find alternative ways to provide holistic health care to people of color within reasonable proximity of where and how they live and die.

References

Blueford, J. W. (1994). A public sector HMO in a competitive market: Ensuring equity for the poor. *Journal of Health Care for the Poor and Underserved, 5,* 192–199.

Bowles, R. L. (1994). Managed care: Theoretical or practical. *Journal of Health Care for the Poor and Underserved, 5,* 173–177.

Bureau of National Affairs. (1993). *Description of the President's health care reform plan.* Washington, DC: Author.

Butcher, R. O. (1993). Managed care now and forever. *Journal of the National Medical Association, 85,* 505–507.

Center for Health Economics Research, Brandeis University. (1993). *Access to health care: Key indicators for policy.* Princeton, NJ: Robert Wood Johnson Foundation.

Davis, K. (1996, March). *Managed care and populations of color: A conceptual framework.* Paper presented at the Statewide Public Psychiatry Conference, Case Western Reserve University, Department of Psychiatry, Cleveland.

Davis, K. (1997). *Managed care bibliography and African Americans: Core competencies and standards for human resources* (Draft Report). Rockville, MD: Center for Mental Health Services.

Dawson, G. (1994). For African Americans, real health care reform or business as usual? *Journal of the National Medical Association, 86,* 893–895.

Flaskerud, J. H., & Hu, L. (1992). Relationship of ethnicity to psychiatric diagnosis. *Journal of Nervous and Mental Disease, 180,* 296–303.

Garretson, D. J. (1993). Psychological misdiagnosis of African Americans. *Journal of Multicultural Counseling and Development, 21,* 119–126.

Hurley, R., Freund, D., & Paul, J. (1993). *Managed care in Medicaid: Lessons for policy and program design.* Ann Arbor, MI: Health Administration Press.

Hurst, J. W. (1991, Fall). Refroming health care in seven European nations. *Health Affairs, 10,* 7–21.

Institute for Health Policy, Brandeis University. (1993). *Substance abuse: The nation's number one health problem, key indicators for policy.* Princeton, NJ: Robert Wood Johnson Foundation.

Jarvis, E. (1844). Insanity among the colored population of the free states. *American Journal of the Medical Sciences, 7,* 71–83.

Johnson, H., & Broder, D. S. (1996). *The system: The American way of politics at the breaking point.* Boston: Little, Brown.

Jones, B., & Gray, B. (1986). Problems in diagnosing schizophrenia and affective disorder among blacks. *Hospital and Community Psychiatry, 37,* 61–65.

Lawson, W. B., Heplar, H., Holladay, J., & Cuffel, B. (1994). Race as a factor in inpatient and outpatient admissions and diagnosis. *Hospital and Community Psychiatry, 45,* 72–74.

Leigh, W. A. (1994). Implications of health care reform for black Americans. *Journal of Health Care for the Poor and Underserved, 5,* 17–32.

Manderscheid, R. W., & Sonnenschein, M. A. (1987). *Mental health, United States, 1985.* Rockville, MD: National Institute of Mental Health.

Neighbors, H. W. (1986). Ambulatory medical care among adult black Americans: The hospital emergency room. *Journal of the National Medical Association, 78,* 275–282.

Piotrowski, Z. (1971). A basic system of all sciences. In H. Vetter & B. Smith (Eds.), *Personality theory: A source book* (pp. 2–18). New York: Meridith.

Ramm, D. (1989, Fall). Overcommitted. *Southern Exposure,* pp. 14–17.

Randall, V. R. (1994). Impact of managed care organizations on ethnic Americans and underserved populations. *Journal of Health Care for the Poor and Underserved, 5,* 225–236.

Robert Wood Johnson Foundation. (1991). *Challenges in health care: A chartbook perspective.* Princeton, NJ: Author.

Scheffler, R. M., & Miller, A. B. (1989). Demand analysis of service use among ethnic subpopulations. *Inquiry, 26,* 202–215.

Smith, M. D. (1994). Managed care and the poor. *Journal of Health Care for the Poor and Underserved, 5,* 147–154.

Snowden, L. (1996, June). *Impact of managed care on ethnic minorities.* Paper presented at the Managed Care and Ethnic Minorities Working Group Conference, Washington, DC.

Snowden, L. R., & Cheung, F. K. (1990). Use of inpatient services by members of ethnic groups. *American Psychologist, 45,* 347–355.

Snowden, L. R., & Holschuh, J. (1992). Ethnic differences in emergency psychiatric care and hospitalization in a program for the severely mentally ill. *Community Mental Health Journal, 28,* 281–291.

Thomas, A., & Sillen, S. (1972). *Racism and psychiatry.* New York: Brunner/Mazel.

United Healthcare Corporation. (1994). *A glossary of terms: The language of managed care and organized health care systems.* Minnetonka, MN: Author.

Walton, T. M. (1995). Challenges for health professions in the face of health care market reform. *Journal of the National Medical Association, 87,* 256–257.

Weil, T. P. (1994). Managed competition for the poor: More promise than value. *Journal of Health Care for the Poor and Underserved, 5,* 158–169.

White House Domestic Policy Council. (1993). *Health security: The President's report to the American people.* Washington, DC: Author.

CHAPTER 5

Medicaid Managed Care and Urban Poor People: Implications for Social Work

Janet D. Perloff

Managed care is rapidly becoming the predominant method of financing and delivering health care to Medicaid recipients. The shift from Medicaid fee-for-service arrangements to managed care has important implications for the health care available to low-income and uninsured people living in U.S. cities. It also presents significant new challenges to the financial viability of urban "safety-net" providers—that is, the public hospitals, academic medical centers, community health centers, local health department clinics, school-based clinics, and other community-based health care providers that traditionally serve residents of low-income urban communities.

Social workers in direct practice and management positions in urban hospitals, clinics, and managed care plans, as well as in policy development and advocacy positions, have many opportunities to influence the transition to Medicaid managed care in cities. This chapter aims to help equip social workers for broad-scale implementation of Medicaid managed care by describing its theoretical basis and development; presenting reasons for its apparent popularity; and analyzing its likely effects on access to care, the long-term viability of urban safety-net providers, and social workers with Medicaid clients. Steps are identified by which social workers can support clients in the transition to Medicaid managed care and work for the preservation of access to care for disadvantaged urban populations.

Medicaid Managed Care

THEORETICAL BASIS

Enrollment of Medicaid recipients in managed care reflects the widely held belief that managed care can improve health care access while also promoting cost containment and federal and state budget control (Edinburg & Cottler, 1995; Keigher, 1995). Medicaid managed care seeks to bring increasing numbers of recipients into health care delivery systems that are subject to "the new economics of managed care" (Shortell, Gillies, & Anderson, 1994, p. 48), which is based on the fact that

NOTE: Originally published as Perloff, J. D. (1996). Medicaid managed care and urban poor people: Implications for social work. *Health & Social Work, 21,* 189–195.

care is provided to a defined number of enrollees at a fixed rate per member per month. Under capitation-based health care, all revenues are earned "up front" when contracts are negotiated. All system components—including hospitals, clinics, imaging centers, and primary care physicians' offices—are transformed from revenue centers to cost centers; these cost centers need to be managed within the capitation-based budget. In theory, these arrangements create incentives for keeping people well and, when they become sick, for treating them at the most cost-effective location on the continuum of care and in the most cost-effective manner. These arrangements also create incentives to underserve patients.

TYPES

Medicaid managed care plans vary in the strength of their incentives for cost containment. Three major types of Medicaid managed care plans are (1) fee-for-service case management, under which the state pays a health care provider a monthly case management fee to perform gatekeeping and service coordination for each person enrolled; (2) fully capitated systems, under which the state pays a managed care plan, usually some form of health maintenance organization (HMO), a preset, or capitated, rate for each person enrolled, and the plan is then at risk for paying the costs of providing a comprehensive package of services to its enrollees, usually including inpatient, specialty, and primary care; and (3) partially capitated systems, under which the state pays a managed care plan a capitated rate for each person enrolled, but the plan assumes risk for the costs of providing a more limited package of services, usually excluding some specialty and inpatient care but including at least primary care services (Perkins & Rivera, 1995). Fully capitated systems contain the strongest incentives for cost containment; therefore, states are placing the greatest emphasis on developing and enrolling Medicaid recipients in fully capitated plans. As a result, fully capitated systems are the fastest growing type of Medicaid managed care, covering an estimated 63 percent of all Medicaid managed care enrollees in June 1994 (Lewin-VHI, 1995).

GROWTH

Recent increases in the number of Medicaid recipients enrolled in managed care have been dramatic. In 1983, 750,000 Medicaid recipients—3 percent of the Medicaid population—were enrolled in managed care. In 1994, about 7.8 million recipients—23 percent of all Medicaid recipients—were enrolled in managed care. Between 1993 and 1994 Medicaid managed care enrollment grew 63 percent, from 4.8 million to 7.8 million recipients (Kaiser Commission on the Future of Medicaid, 1995).

Currently, the populations being enrolled in Medicaid managed care are primarily children and adults receiving Aid to Families with Dependent Children and other low-income pregnant women and children. Historically, elderly and disabled Medicaid recipients have been excluded from Medicaid managed care because of their complex service needs, technical challenges in setting appropriate capitation payments, and difficulties finding plans willing to serve these populations. However, the high cost of the care of these Medicaid recipients has increased state interest in serving elderly and disabled people through managed care arrangements (Lewin-VHI, 1995). Some states have also begun to enroll special subpopulations of Medicaid patients in managed care, including patients with AIDS, substance abuse problems, and serious and persistent mental illness (Kaiser Commission on the Future of Medicaid, 1995; State of New York, 1995).

The pervasiveness of Medicaid managed care is indicated by the fact that as of June 1994, all states except Alaska, Connecticut, Maine, Nebraska, Oklahoma, Vermont, and Wyoming had some form of Medicaid managed care program (Kaiser Commission on the Future of Medicaid, 1995). In many states, Medicaid recipients voluntarily enroll in a managed care plan. However, mandatory Medicaid managed care programs are more attractive because they are more likely to yield cost savings (U.S. General Accounting Office [GAO], 1993). Many states are presently requesting and receiving federal approval to implement mandatory Medicaid managed care plans, and indications are that mandatory enrollment of Medicaid recipients in managed care plans will grow exponentially over the next several years (Holahan, Coughlin, Ku, Lipson, & Rajan, 1995; Kaiser Commission on the Future of Medicaid, 1995; Lewin-VHI, 1995).

Empirical Evidence and Implementation Issues

States are enthusiastic about the promise of Medicaid managed care for improving access, costs, quality, and health outcomes. However, the empirical evidence about Medicaid managed care is equivocal. Several reviews of empirical studies concluded that some versions of Medicaid managed care bring improvements in utilization, costs, and access over traditional fee-for-service arrangements (Fox & McManus, 1992; Hurley, Freund, & Paul, 1993; Lewin-VHI, 1995), but others concluded that the available evidence does not support many of the claims about cost savings, improved access, or improved quality (Freund & Lewit, 1993; Rowland, Rosenbaum, Simon, & Chait, 1995).

In the absence of definitive empirical evidence about its impact, Medicaid managed care is perhaps best viewed with a mixture of optimism and caution. Four questions are central to whether state Medicaid managed care initiatives can achieve their full potential: (1) Are managed care plans adequately prepared to meet the unique, pressing, and often complex health care needs of urban poor people? (2) Is the supply and distribution of primary care in cities adequate to ensure that Medicaid recipients enrolled in managed care will be able to find care? (3) What is the future of the health care providers who have traditionally served low-income urban residents? and (4) Will Medicaid recipients be adequately prepared to choose among managed care plans and to protect themselves against managed care's potential for aggressive enrollment and underservice?

HEALTH CARE NEEDS OF URBAN POOR PEOPLE

Cities have high incidence rates for health problems such as low-birthweight babies and infant deaths, measles, tuberculosis, AIDS, and sexually transmitted diseases. Many of these problems, particularly those affecting low-income women and children, are concentrated in the most socioeconomically disadvantaged urban communities (Fossett & Perloff, 1995). These urban residents live in states that are the most eager to enroll in Medicaid managed care plans.

Little empirical evidence exists about the impact of Medicaid managed care on service utilization and health outcomes of high-risk populations. Research is needed to fully assess the effects of managed care on urban Medicaid recipients and to develop systems of care that produce the best health and mental health outcomes for these clients. However, the available empirical literature provides reasons to be cautious about the likely impact of Medicaid managed care on service utilization patterns and health outcomes for high-risk, multiproblem, chronically ill, and more expensive patients (Fossett & Perloff, 1995). Most managed care organizations are accustomed to serving employed, low-risk populations and have little experience with providing support services such as outreach, case management, transportation, and other psychosocial services that are beneficial to high-risk populations. In addition, because managed care organizations, especially those participating in full capitation programs, face strong financial incentives to limit utilization, patients enrolled in these plans may encounter difficulties obtaining the full range of health and related social services. As a result, patients needing these services have frequently not fared well in managed care arrangements (Schlesinger, 1986, 1989).

URBAN PRIMARY CARE SUPPLY AND DISTRIBUTION

There are reasons to be cautious about whether the supply and distribution of primary care in low-income urban neighborhoods will be adequate to meet the needs of Medicaid recipients (Rosenthal, 1993). Most of the nation's metropolitan areas are richly supplied with doctors and hospitals, but embedded in them are areas that lack health care resources adequate to serve the needs of their residents (Fossett & Perloff, 1995; Ginzburg, Berliner, & Ostow, 1993). This maldistribution originates, in part, because private physicians and other health care providers tend to select locations that enable them to attract a large and profitable clientele. As a result of the limited profit-making potential of poor neighborhoods, these areas have historically had very few private health care providers such as office-based physicians or private community hospitals.

The shortage of physicians is aggravated by the fact that many physicians in metropolitan areas do not accept Medicaid patients or limit the number of Medicaid patients they treat (Perloff, Kletke, & Fossett, 1995; Perloff, Kletke, Fossett, & Banks, 1995). The lack of private providers is made worse by some providers' personal inclinations to avoid crime, AIDS, and racial and ethnic diversity, as well as to avoid the challenges posed by patients beset with complex and often unyielding social problems (Physician Payment Review Commission, 1993).

Because many low-income urban neighborhoods already lack an adequate supply of health care providers, there is ample reason to be pessimistic that Medicaid managed care will improve the quantity and quality of health care available in these neighborhoods (Fossett & Perloff, 1995). In theory, Medicaid managed care tries to use the payment system to improve access to care in underserved communities. States set capitation rates at a level that will improve the attractiveness of the Medicaid population to managed care entities and then use mandatory enrollment to ensure HMOs a large and lucrative Medicaid market. It has been argued that the resulting competition among managed care organizations for contracts to serve Medicaid patients will improve the range of available health care alternatives.

However, managed care plans will face equally strong financial incentives to avoid making large investments in developing the health care provider supply. States may set capitation rates at levels that make it attractive for managed care plans to enroll Medicaid recipients, but the supply of care providers in many low-income urban neighborhoods will be inadequate to support mass mandatory enrollment.

Without sufficiently generous capitation payments or other financial incentives, managed care plans will be unlikely to foster significant improvements in the underlying supply of care providers.

URBAN SAFETY-NET PROVIDERS

With little access to private physicians and other health care providers, residents of low-income urban communities have come to depend on urban safety-net providers (Fossett & Perloff, 1995). The safety net includes public hospitals and clinics run by cities or counties and also academic medical centers that have historically tended to be in or near urban communities so that physicians, nurses, social workers, and other professionals in training could serve the needs of disadvantaged patients in exchange for rich learning opportunities. The clinics run by county and city health departments, the community health centers funded by federal grants, and the variety of family-planning and other community-based agencies that are supported by a mix of private and public resources have also become important elements in the urban health care safety net.

Safety-net providers offer many features that are valuable to urban poor and uninsured people (Fossett & Perloff, 1995). Providers are often close by, enhancing the probability of their use, and many offer a wider array of enabling services (including outreach, case management, and follow-up) and support services (including transportation, translation, and child care), which are important complements to medical services.

However, managed care organizations will be selective in forming networks, including only those providers who can be successful in keeping down the costs of care. Such network selectivity is likely to result in excluding or drastically reducing the role of the urban safety-net providers in the care of Medicaid patients. Some characteristics typical of safety-net providers may make them less than attractive as network providers for managed care organizations (Fossett & Perloff, 1995). Safety-net providers are often in poor financial condition, undercapitalized, outdated and in disrepair, inefficiently run, lacking in adequate information and management systems, and incompatible with both the mission and the management style of fully capitated health plans. Given the potentially high costs of working with these providers, managed care organizations may not be eager to include them in their managed care network.

Some safety-net providers have benefited from far-sighted and effective leadership and are prepared to be successful in a managed care environment by creating their own managed care plans or securing contracts as providers within the networks of private managed care plans. More typically, however, safety-net providers have had very little experience with managed care. These providers are accustomed to fee-for-service revenues and, in some instances, contributions to their budget from state or local appropriations. For safety-net hospitals, Medicaid's disproportionate share payments, which are made to hospitals that serve more than their share of poor and uninsured people, provide a vital subsidy. Accustomed to the world of fee-for-service with a subsidy, these providers lack experience in competing for patients; their inexperience places them at a competitive disadvantage.

Recent evidence suggests that Medicaid managed care is shifting patients away from urban safety-net providers, although the consequences of this redistribution of patients are not fully understood (Henneberger, 1994; Peck & Hubbert, 1994; Sack, 1995; Winslow, 1995). However, there is ample reason for concern. Exclusion of safety-net providers from managed care networks has the potential to disrupt existing arrangements that residents of underserved neighborhoods have made to obtain care and to shift these patients into the care of providers less responsive to their unique and often complex needs. In addition, the loss of Medicaid patients to managed care plans represents a significant loss of revenues for safety-net providers. Medicaid revenues are used by these agencies and institutions to subsidize the care they provide to the uninsured population. The loss of these revenues will limit the ability of these agencies to care for uninsured people in the future.

RECIPIENT PREPAREDNESS

Medicaid managed care is a significant departure from the way recipients have received care in the past and will require a reorientation to the health care system (Perloff, 1993). For the first time, Medicaid recipients will be asked to select a health plan and a primary care provider, limit their use to certain providers, and obtain authorization and referrals before using certain services such as emergency rooms or specialists. Medicaid recipients will need a lot of information if they are to make informed choices about both plan and provider and to be fully prepared to use the health care system in new ways.

In addition, state agencies will need to ensure that Medicaid recipients are protected from overly aggressive marketing by managed care plans (Perloff, 1987). Medicaid managed care plans face strong incentives to earn the up-front revenue from recipient enrollment. Very rapid build-up in Medicaid managed care enrollment and practices that may even be fraudulent can therefore be expected as plans maneuver to lock in enrollees (Gottlieb, 1995; Pear, 1995). In addition, without adequate monitoring by state Medicaid agencies, enrollment can rapidly outstrip the capacity of managed care organizations to provide needed services (Fisher, 1995). Finally, state agencies will need to ensure that both quality assurance mechanisms and legal protection are in place to protect Medicaid recipients from managed care's inherent incentives to underserve (Perloff, 1987).

Roles for Social Work

Developments associated with Medicaid managed care will have a significant impact on low-income and uninsured people living in cities and will also pose challenges for institutions traditionally serving this population. Social workers have many opportunities to shape the Medicaid managed care debate and to influence the outcome of these developments.

DIRECT PRACTICE AND MANAGEMENT

Social workers in direct practice can play an important role in helping clients develop the skills needed to obtain health care in the managed care environment. Social workers in settings in which the Medicaid eligibility of clients is being established will have the important task of informing and educating clients about various choices related to their coverage. This role will be particularly important in states implementing mandatory Medicaid managed care plans because, in most instances, clients failing to choose will automatically be assigned to a health plan and a primary care provider. Although the results of automatic assignment may be acceptable to clients, better choices would seem likely to result with client input.

Given that managed care plans have strong incentives to enroll patients and therefore may market themselves aggressively, social workers should place a high priority on helping clients fully evaluate managed care plans and choose the plan through which they will be best served. Clients may face choices between managed care and fee-for-service plans and from among an array of health plans and providers. Carefully assessing a client's situation and helping him or her fully understand and consider the options will improve the probability that good choices are made. For example, noting the existence of transportation barriers or an excellent relationship with a particular primary care provider will improve the likelihood that these situational factors will influence choice.

Social workers will need to be familiar with the rules of Medicaid managed care in their state to help educate clients about new care-seeking requirements and to ensure that these requirements do not become barriers to appropriate care seeking. Changes in care-seeking rules include the requirement to contact one's selected primary care provider before visiting specialists or emergency rooms and, in some states, the possibility that health care previously obtained from public health clinics or community-based agencies (such as immunizations or family-planning services) must now be obtained from one's managed care plan. Clients may also need support to ensure that they are not being underserved by a plan. Social workers can identify instances of potential underservice, compile data documenting such problems, and intervene with managed care plans and state and local Medicaid agencies on behalf of clients whose rights may have been violated.

The informing, educating, and advocating that may be required of social workers in a managed care environment will sometimes put health care social workers at odds with the goals and values of their employers (Cornelius, 1994; Ross, 1993). Social workers will find themselves advocating additional services for a client in an environment that places a premium on cost minimization. Social workers in supervisory positions in hospitals, clinics, and managed care organizations will need to be prepared to help staff social workers satisfactorily resolve such dilemmas arising from the new economics of managed care. To some extent, such dilemmas are inherent in Medicaid managed care. For this reason, social workers outside of Medicaid managed care will have a particularly important role to play in ensuring optimal health outcomes for clients. Because of their independence from the health care system, social workers in other settings—child welfare agencies, community-based social services agencies, mental health agencies, and schools—may be in the best position to help clients judge whether their health care needs are being met, to recognize aspects of Medicaid managed care that are working, and to identify and work toward remedies for aspects that need improvement.

POLICY DEVELOPMENT AND ADVOCACY

As was the case during the recent federal health reform debate, social workers should be actively trying to influence Medicaid managed care policy development. State Medicaid managed care initiatives entail a planning process, submission of applications for waivers to the federal government, and in many cases passage of state legislation. These and subsequent stages in the policy development process present numerous opportunities for public comment, testimony, and advocacy. Social workers and organizations representing the profession can also take part in emerging coalitions of providers, consumers, and other health and welfare advocates who are committed to sound planning and implementation of state Medicaid managed care initiatives, ongoing monitoring of the impact of managed care, and change.

In the attempt to influence the shape of Medicaid managed care, social work should make efforts to ensure that vulnerable populations will have access to health care. Social workers should be strong advocates for the development of state-level information systems that will monitor the ability of managed care plans to meet recipients' needs and that can produce timely indicators of access problems. Social workers should also advocate for policy proposals that will give managed care plans strong incentives to develop new capacity in underserved areas, including advocacy for payment of higher capitation levels to plans that propose to increase capacity in specific ways. In addition, ensuring access will require strong and continuing advocacy for federal and state policies aimed at developing the supply of primary care providers in underserved communities. Existing federal programs such as the Migrant and Community Health Centers Program and the National Health Service Corps should be preserved; creative new state and local capacity development initiatives should be developed and supported.

High priority should also be given to supporting policy proposals that strike a reasonable balance between protecting the financial viability of urban safety-net providers and fostering cost containment through competition in local health care markets. For example, California's proposed mandatory Medicaid managed care initiative, which was implemented in 1996, recognizes that safety-net providers have little experience with and lack adequate preparation for managed care, that they are extremely vulnerable to the loss of Medicaid and disproportionate share revenue that may result from increased competition, and that they will need insulation and time to adapt if they are to survive and continue to meet the needs of Medicaid recipients and the growing uninsured population (GAO, 1995). Features that would mitigate some of the harsher effects of managed care on safety-net providers (some of which are included in California's and other state Medicaid managed care plans) include requiring or creating strong incentives for the inclusion of providers in managed care networks; providing technical assistance to providers in key areas such as risk-based financing, negotiating contracts, and developing effective information systems; and ensuring that there is an ongoing subsidy for the services these settings provide to the uninsured population. In the absence of such features, Medicaid managed care will pose a serious threat to the future of urban safety-net providers, to social workers practicing in these settings, and to the people they serve.

References

Cornelius, D. (1994). Managed care and social work: Constructing a context and a response. *Social Work in Health Care, 20,* 47–63.

Edinburg, G. M., & Cottler, J. M. (1995). Managed care. In R. L. Edwards (Ed.-in-Chief), *Encyclopedia of social work* (19th ed., Vol. 2, pp. 1635–1642). Washington, DC: NASW Press.

Fisher, I. (1995, August 28). Forced marriage of Medicaid and managed care hits snags. *New York Times,* pp. B1, B5.

Fossett, J., & Perloff, J. (1995). *The "new" health reform and access to care: The problem of the inner city* (Background paper). Washington, DC: Kaiser Commission on the Future of Medicaid.

Fox, H., & McManus, M. (1992). *Medicaid managed care arrangements and their impact on children and adolescents: A briefing report.* Washington, DC: Child and Adolescent Health Policy Center.

Freund, D., & Lewit, E. (1993). Managed care for children and pregnant women: Promises and pitfalls. *Future of Children, 3,* 92–122.

Ginzburg, E., Berliner, H. S., & Ostow, M. (1993). *Changing U.S. health care.* Boulder, CO: Westview Press.

Gottlieb, M. (1995, October 2). A free-for-all in swapping Medicaid for managed care. *New York Times,* p. A1.

Henneberger, M. (1994, June 30). New York hospitals fight to retain Medicaid patients. *New York Times,* p. A1.

Holahan, J., Coughlin, T., Ku, L., Lipson, D. J., & Rajan, S. (1995, Spring). Insuring the poor through Section 1115 Medicaid waivers. *Health Affairs,* pp. 199–216.

Hurley, R., Freund, D., & Paul, J. (1993). *Managed care in Medicaid: Lessons for policy and program design.* Ann Arbor, MI: Health Administration Press.

Kaiser Commission on the Future of Medicaid. (1995, April). *Medicaid and managed care: Policy brief.* Washington, DC: Author.

Keigher, S. (1995). Managed care's silent seduction of America and the new politics of choice [National Health Line]. *Health & Social Work, 20,* 146–151.

Lewin-VHI. (1995, February). *States as payers: Managed care for Medicaid populations.* Washington, DC: National Institute for Health Care Management.

Pear, R. (1995, April 24). Florida struggles to lift Medicaid burden. *New York Times,* p. A2.

Peck, M., & Hubbert, E. D. (1994, July). *Changing the rules: Medicaid managed care and MCH in U.S. cities.* Omaha, NE: CityMatch.

Perkins, J., & Rivera, L. A. (1995, March). EPSDT and managed care: Do plans know what they are getting into? *Clearinghouse Review,* pp. 1248–1260.

Perloff, J. (1987). Safeguards are needed for Medicaid HMOs [Editorial]. *Chicago Sun-Times,* p. 38.

Perloff, J. (1993, April). *Medicaid managed care for women and children: What have we learned?* Paper presented at the National Conference on Managed Care Systems for Mothers and Young Children, Baltimore.

Perloff, J., Kletke, P., & Fossett, J. (1995). Which physicians limit their Medicaid participation and why. *Health Services Research, 30,* 9–26.

Perloff, J., Kletke, P., Fossett, P., & Banks, S. (1995, June). *Medicaid participation among urban primary care physicians.* Paper presented at a meeting of the Association for Health Services Research, Chicago.

Physician Payment Review Commission. (1993). *Annual report to Congress.* Washington, DC: Author.

Rosenthal, E. (1993, October 17). Shortage of doctors in poor areas is seen as barrier to health plans. *New York Times,* p. A1.

Ross, J. (1993). Redefining hospital social work: An embattled professional domain [Editorial]. *Health & Social Work, 18,* 243–247.

Rowland, D., Rosenbaum, S., Simon, L., & Chait, E. (1995, March). *Medicaid and managed care: Lessons from the literature.* Washington, DC: Kaiser Commission on the Future of Medicaid.

Sack, K. (1995, August 20). Public hospitals around the country cut basic service. *New York Times,* pp. 1, 24.

Schlesinger, M. (1986). On the limits of expanding health care reform: Chronic care in prepaid settings. *Milbank Quarterly, 62,* 189–216.

Schlesinger, M. (1989). Striking a balance: Capitation, the mentally ill, and public policy. In D. Mechanic & L. Aiken (Eds.), *Paying for services: Promises and pitfalls of capitation* (pp. 186–214). New York: Jossey-Bass.

Shortell, S. M., Gillies, R. R., & Anderson, D. A. (1994, Winter). The new world of managed care: Creating organized delivery systems. *Health Affairs,* pp. 46–64.

State of New York. (1995, March). *The partnership plan: A public–private initiative ensuring healthcare for needy New Yorkers* [Section 1115 waiver application]. Albany: Author.

U.S. General Accounting Office. (1993). *Medicaid: States turn to managed care to improve access and control costs* (Report No. GAO-HRD-93-86). Washington, DC: Author.

U.S. General Accounting Office. (1995). *Expansion of California's Medicaid managed care program* (Report No. GAO-HEHS-95-87). Washington, DC: Author.

Winslow, R. (1995, April 12). Welfare recipients a hot commodity in managed care now. *Wall Street Journal,* p. A1.

CHAPTER 6

Managed Care: Business as Usual

Eva Havas

Managed care can perhaps best be described as what happened on the way to not providing a national health care policy. It is the continuation of the posture that to establish a national health care system in the United States would be un-American, and so the United States continues to be one of two Western industrialized nations (along with South Africa) that do not provide health care coverage for all its citizens. Initially this was largely because the American Medical Association (AMA) succeeded in convincing the American public that national health care equaled socialized medicine. As public sentiment began to support broader coverage, in the 1960s the AMA threw its support behind Medicare and Medicaid, two federal mandates that would insure the most vulnerable populations in the United States. Sadly, this subverted the movement toward universal coverage so that millions of Americans to this day remain uninsured or underinsured.

In the 1980s and early 1990s, momentum again grew for changes in medical care as awareness increased that 40 million Americans were uninsured, and as more and more middle-class Americans undergoing downsizing lost medical coverage or knew someone who had. Moreover, corporations were increasingly disenchanted with the health care options for their workers as costs continued to rise. Although President Bill Clinton's health care initiatives, based on a managed care model, went down to defeat thanks to the insurance industry and the negative advertisement campaign featuring Harry and Louise, within a few years, without benefit of public discourse or debate, managed care seemed pervasive in the health care arena.

In the most fundamental sense there are two basic problems with managed care. The first problem results from the lack of a comprehensive U.S. health care policy, and the second results from the fact that managed care epitomizes health care as industry or business rather than health care as a basic right. Although rarely noted, these two problems are interrelated and determine the very nature of health care in this country. Even when noted, they are assumed to be givens rather than determinants that should be questioned. Thus, despite health care being viewed as part of the social welfare system in the human rights sense—something necessary to a person's well-being—the provision of health care is not considered a part of the pact between government and its citizens. Unlike universal systems such as education or social security, health care is distinguished as a "benefit" to be negotiated by individuals, except for programmed mandates like Medicare and Medicaid. Further, it is negotiated largely with private vendors, that is, employers and insurance companies.

This continues the long tradition in the United States of social welfare being first and foremost a history of private initiatives. The New Deal was born, providing its broad range of public benefits, only when the problems experienced by "average" Americans became so massive that the private sector was overwhelmed. The history of health care similarly has been largely a private venture, with government interceding only when it was deemed necessary to protect those who could not protect themselves. The New Deal, for all its comprehensiveness and despite discussion at the time, did not provide Americans with universal health care coverage. This was for the same reason that universal health coverage would fail time and again, that is, reform in the sense of governmental initiative and programs comes in response to widespread need but also to prevent more fundamental change (for example, welfare rather than income redistribution). Hence the leftist critique that the New Deal "saved" the country from socialism.

Until the advent of Medicaid and Medicare, it was not generally the government that intervened to protect people's health but rather private insurance. Health insurance is seen largely as a positive benefit because it affords people better protection than they could afford on their own, but it is generally forgotten that long before the advent of "managed care," insurance shaped the kind of care Americans received by setting the parameters of care. Insurance companies have tended to favor hospital and "cure" based care; in fact, Blue Cross was developed during the Depression years when hospitals were losing money because of people's inability to pay. Since the advent of insurance companies, their role has always meant that the kind of health care most Americans receive has never simply been the result of the interaction between doctor and patient, but rather has been influenced by what care was reimbursable. It is in this same time frame that the original health maintenance organization (HMO)—Kaiser Permanente—was founded, although it would be decades before HMOs became prevalent.

Although public support for universal health care has waxed and waned over the years, the above-noted long-standing opposition of the AMA, the power of the insurance industry as well as other industries that profit from the current system, and American distrust of "big government" involved in something as private as health care have also worked against the creation of a national health care system. Moreover, reforming health care is a complex task, and the political process that prefers simple solutions at the same time that it favors vested interests mitigates against meaningful reform. The most basic questions that must be asked, therefore, are whether health care is too important to leave to the current marketplace/political processes and whether the present system is worth saving.

Regardless of managed care, the present health care system with its reimbursement formulas favors high technology, high-intervention care while tending to ignore the fact that the greatest improvements in people's health have come about through public health measures such as improved basic hygiene, better sanitation, cleaner water, and better food (Dubois, 1959; McKeown & Lowe, 1974). Many diseases today are "diseases of civilization," caused both by lifestyle and by environmental problems. Public health measures clearly would be more effective than after-the-fact (of disease) palliative measures, but public health measures are not favored by health care as industry. As the population lives longer, we are more and more plagued with chronic diseases that similarly do not lend themselves to high-tech solutions, although high technology may prolong the lives of people who would previously have died from their conditions. With no real debate on such issues, however, we continue to downplay preventive or even maintenance medicine and to extol corrective medicine.

These issues have been meaningfully confronted neither by the health care system in general nor by managed care in particular. Thus the fundamental issue that must be faced in any discussion of managed care is that managed care truly does represent business as usual in the health care field. The form may differ, but the context remains the same. Indeed, perhaps the best that can be said for managed care is that it lays bare the basic premises of our health care system. It is a system without a vision beyond the bottom line or even, ironically, a clear mission or purpose. Although early HMOs, upon which managed care systems are largely based, at least in theory promoted prevention, for example, by encouraging annual physicals and well-baby visits, current managed care operations have introduced added layers of bureaucracy that intervene between patient and medical care provider and whose primary purpose is to discourage access and to control providers. In theory managed care could lead to more efficient care by bringing "discipline to a pattern of practices that at the margins provided little value for money" (Mechanic, 1997, p. 1810), and by promoting an opportunity and structure for evaluating intervention. In reality the emphasis has been on managing care to promote the bottom line. It has not been so much care that has been managed then, but rather the costs of care.

It is not at all clear that managing costs is as easy as it first appeared to be—when HMOs began aggressive marketing to younger, healthier members, such consumers allowed lower costs. As members have aged, and as managed care has taken over more of the marketplace, it cannot be as selective in terms of subscribers; further, in order to be competitive the level of choice in critical markets has had to approach those of traditional indemnity plans, with similar costs (Fisher, 1998; Freudenheim, 1997). The hard truth is almost inevitable—costs can only truly be managed if there is a rational health policy in place that focuses on prevention and quality because in the long term this is one of the surest places to look for savings. Additionally, profits must be examined—when CEOs continue to make six- and seven-figure salaries, when drug companies and all those affiliated with the medical business are concerned with profit margins, health care costs will inevitably rise despite any initial savings that come from controlling access and types of service. Moreover, as long as insurance companies remain an integral part of the health care industry, insurers, despite their nonmedical backgrounds, not only influence the kind of care people receive but also are additional components of the health care industry that need to make money.

It is not being argued that costs should not be a factor in determining the kind of health care system we want, but rather that cost, like other aspects of the health care system, should be subject to public discussion and debate. Countries that have national health care systems also take cost into account, but within a framework of establishing medical and health policy. Thus, there is a need in this country to have a vision of the kind of health care system we want, to establish priorities, and to discuss costs in that context. What is most ironic about health care in the United States is the widely ignored fact that this country fails to provide coverage for everyone or even some of the most basic health measures (like universal childhood immunization), despite spending more on health care than countries with systems that ensure everyone coverage.[1]

[1]The United States spends 50 percent more of its gross national product (for health care) than the average of all other industrialized countries. The average per capita expenditure in the United States in 1990 was $2,000, compared with a per capita average of $1,000 for industrial competitors (Hartman, 1993).

Most basic to understanding this irony is not simply our failure to establish a comprehensive health care policy, but also our failure to understand the nature of business. If health care is a business, then the emphasis will be on care that provides the most profit rather than on care that might make the most medical sense. High-tech interventions, common in managed care, are clearly expensive but profitable. A visit to a physician costs only the physician's time, the overhead involved, and the bureaucratic costs if the visit is covered by insurance. On the other hand, a visit involving surgery creates business not only for the surgeon but for all the personnel involved in the hospital operating room, for the hospital supply companies producing the needed equipment, for the drug companies providing anesthesia and medication, for the hospital stay, and so forth. It needs to be recognized that "the acquisition and management of capital has become as central to hospital policy-making as it is to corporations in other fields" (Stevens, 1989, p. 4). This orientation inevitably promotes those interventions that yield the most profit and whose costs can most easily be passed on. As with hospitals, so with managed care: "Much of what passes as managed care today... [is] managed profit or managed greed..." (Goonan, Gordon, Jankins-Scott, Kaplan, & Rabkin, 1997, p. C2). The problem is not only that high- rather than low-cost intervention is encouraged in such modalities, but also that those patients will be favored whose coverage allows such intervention. Moreover, high-tech interventions are necessary after disease has set in and so perpetuate the curative approach. Ironically, in the long run this approach is more costly because not only is there little emphasis on prevention, but there also is less emphasis on early diagnostic procedures and well-established relationships with physicians that would allow early detection of disease.

There are additional problems with the health-care-as-industry approach. Just as President Dwight Eisenhower warned in 1961 of the dangers of a military–industrial complex, there are dangers inherent in a medical–industrial complex that go largely unnoted and unrecognized (Relman, 1987). This medical–industrial complex abounds in opportunities for conflict of interest: proprietary hospitals and nursing homes, as well as private diagnostic laboratories all lend themselves to having as their goal the making of money rather than the patient's well-being. Clearly, in an age when tobacco companies and lawyers still collude to hide the impact of smoking on a person's health or when the effects of toxic waste and pollution still go largely unacknowledged, it would be naive to assume that corporate interests (read "medical–industrial complex") and patient interests are the same. The situation is all the more complicated when physicians, who are supposed to be advocating for their patients, have vested interests in the proprietary ventures for which they work and in which they invest.

It is not as if the past were all good. The health care system, like so much else in people's collective memories, was never quite as good as we now remember it. This may make reform more difficult as collectively we tend to forget that "Dr. Welby" was, after all, a television show rather than reality. Health care has always been rationed in this country, both in terms of geographic access (for example, with rural areas being underserved) and economic access (for example, with poor people dependent on charity). Middle-class people had the health care they could afford, which rationed care just as the lack of access rationed it for others. The difference between now and then, however, lies in the changing ideology of medicine, its core values, and to some extent its structure.

The Hippocratic Oath, with its caveat of doing no harm, made medicine seem a noble profession. Even if that were not always the case, physicians, in the prevalent ideology at least, were viewed as motivated by compassion and altruism. Dr.

Welby represented the ideal, someone concerned with the whole family, who took the time to listen and be involved. Medicine changed as specialization became more prevalent, and physicians dealt less and less with the whole person and more and more with the person's parts. This was true even before the pervasiveness of managed care, and was part of the emerging commoditization of medicine. Once people became parts the business ideology was easier to establish—decisions being made were no longer personal or about people, they were about body parts and could be made in the same manner, and with the same considerations, as decisions in the auto repair business might be made.

Karl Marx's concept of alienation is relevant here. As the solo practitioner has become somewhat of a relic, medicine is more and more often practiced in larger bureaucratic settings. The solo practitioner was likely to know his or her patients well, and the motivation for going into medicine was at least in part to establish relationships with others and to do good. Larger settings mean that more people come between doctor and patient; the more people involved, the less personal the relationship and the more other factors can intervene, like the bottom line. Marx argued that a core problem of capitalism was the alienation that resulted when workers became part of the production process, with no real control over their work. Materialism, commodities, things, take on a life of their own and become more important than people. Similarly, in medicine the technique and the production line have become more important to many than the art of healing.

Medical care at its best involves many different components: knowledge that allows practitioners to make an accurate diagnosis; skills involved in the actual practice of medicine; the ability and knowledge that translates into advice for the patient such as when high-tech interventions are called for or when more modest interventions are indicated, at least initially; and when lifestyle changes are necessary. It is the rare decision that is clear-cut; most involve the art of medicine, knowing the patient, and what would work best for that particular individual as well as what is medically possible. Most fundamental in this process is the diagnosis, a diagnosis that depends largely on what the patient relates. Ironically this basic feature is being short-changed in modern medicine, as physicians are increasingly pressured to see patients for shorter periods of time. One study shows that the average time given by internists for new patients is 11 minutes and the average time for hospital patients is four minutes (Inui & Frankel, 1991). This lack of time clearly mitigates against caring, compassionate relationships, affects the very quality of diagnosis (Scott, Aiken, Mechanic, & Moravcsik, 1995), and serves to enhance the alienation noted above.

Although the structural settings of most current medical practice mitigate against longer physician–patient contacts, organizational settings could be arranged to reward different behaviors that would ensure more consistent human care (Howard & Tyler, 1975; Levine, 1975; Mechanic, 1997). This would not only enhance patient satisfaction but also produce more accurate diagnosis, ensure greater compliance, and thus most likely result in cost savings in the long run. Even though less time with a patient might seem to increase profitability, Balint (1973) argued persuasively that patients who are not heard by physicians come back time and again, so that in the long run it would be better for the patient and less expensive for the system to take time initially. Yet as medicine becomes more and more infused with market ideology it is difficult to justify changes in practice: How does the interest of the institution get separated from the interest of the patient? How can it be ascertained whether surgery on an outpatient basis, with no regard to a person's support system or resources, ultimately shortens a person's life? How does the effect of spending more or less time with patients become quantified? It is easier to stress productivity measured in terms of how many people are being seen per hour. Physicians now have thousands in their "panel" if they work for an HMO and schedule patients on the average of every 10 or 15 minutes (included in which is the time for notes, conferring with others, and breaks). They are further pressured by a capitation system that discourages procedures such as extensive diagnostic tests.

The implications for managed health care as business are ominous for patients and for those providing care. The goals and values of business differ fundamentally from the goals and values of social welfare conceived of as a human right. Indeed, social welfare institutions at their best buffer the effects of a market economy and also provide those services deemed necessary for a civil society. Thus services such as those provided by the police, firefighters, and the multitude of personnel who maintain the society's infrastructure are viewed as essential to the well-being of the public. Similarly, the benefits derived from universal compulsory public education are viewed as vital for the continuation of a democratic society. Other countries have concluded that health care also provides such a necessary service, that not only is it a basic right but that the society as a whole derives benefit. A healthy populace yields a more productive work force—Kaiser Permanente, after all, was started to ensure a rapid return of workers who fell ill or were injured on the job.

The United States, however, has opted for a residual approach to health care, that is, those covered through government policy are those who "qualify" through low income, age, service in Congress (their comprehensive coverage is somehow not deemed a threat to the free market), veterans' benefits, and the like. Others must fend for themselves, which generally means obtaining benefits through place of employment. Clearly low-paid and part-time workers are at a disadvantage here, and they make up a large segment of the uninsured. Moreover, hospitals that used to provide free coverage do so less and less, "dumping" patients and meeting their obligation to the disadvantaged population by accepting Medicaid patients.

The problem is not solved when someone is covered by a health plan, which increasingly means a managed health care plan. Managed care, it must always be remembered, means managing *cost:* It is not a system of comprehensive care for the patient. It is a system that seeks to limit what care will cost; the most basic means for this is limiting access and limiting what services the physician can provide. This is accomplished through an intricate and increasingly complex referral system which in practice means that people other than the primary care physician are making decisions about a patient's care (people who are often euphemistically called "case managers"). This further bureaucratizes medicine and increases the alienation of both patient and provider. It also means that the relationship between providers and consumers becomes more adversarial, as consumers try to obtain more services and providers try to block them. If the managed care plan is for-profit, these issues are only exacerbated.

As access continues to be a problem, neglect will become more prevalent. Unfortunately, it will be the kind of neglect that is hard to prove in a court of law, so the situation will not be remedied through high-profile lawsuits that build momentum for change. It is the kind of neglect, for example, that comes from poorly servicing chronic conditions, from not providing care for nonemergency conditions, from discouraging people's access, from ignoring the effects of illness both on the patient and the family, from sending people home from the hospitals earlier and earlier, from having people rely on family and friends to provide care that formerly would have been provided in hospital. Even in the hospital, shortages of staff have meant that outsiders provide care that previously would have been provided by nursing staff. Whatever lawsuits do result, it may well be that insurance companies have built in the costs of fighting them, just as car companies have done (Dowie, 1991).

It is hard to overestimate the effects of managed care on the average consumer. There have been many anecdotal horror stories, but the true impact of managed care is perhaps best measured by the alienation that increasingly permeates medicine and affects the quality of any care that people receive. To the extent that the relationship between patient and provider becomes adversarial, the cooperation that is key for compliance with "doctor's orders" is lacking, as is the discourse necessary for accurate diagnosis. Moreover, an adversarial relationship—or no real relationship at all—adds stress to the patient despite our knowledge of the negative role of stress in both causing and exacerbating illness.

As the nature of medical care, which is increasingly a misnomer, becomes bureaucratized and "managed," one very real danger is that both providers and consumers may accept the impersonal nature of medicine and expect nothing more. There is undoubtedly a day-to-day wearing down of providers and patients that managed care can count on to limit the kind of care patients will seek or physicians will provide. Such a lowering of expectations is more damaging than any overt regulations or intricate referral systems. Certainly a consumer of health care who is "dis-eased" is not in a position to be a forceful advocate, and providers inevitably become worn down by unresponsive systems. Moreover, care is compromised as "short-cuts" are taken, as increasing amounts of "care" are given on an outpatient basis without regard to a patient's ability to cope, and without an assessment of whether adequate supports exist to deal with postintervention effects. Previously, this might have been considered negligence because it compromised patient care; now it is considered prudent because it is efficient and acknowledges the bottom line. In this manner, medical "care" becomes part of the problem rather than part of the solution.

We pride ourselves in this country on having the world's finest medical care, but if this boast has any validity, it is only on the outer fringes of medicine where a complicated technological intervention may save a person's life. For the average patient the very nature of health care in this country, it ahs been argued, mitigates against quality care. The art of medicine has become lost as medicine has become dehumanized and bureaucratized. Medical care becomes yet another arena in our society where people must fight to obtain what they need rather than being able to count on relief or solace.

The best hope for change may be in an alliance between consumers and the medical profession itself. Physicians have always been part of an elite profession that afforded great autonomy, with the ability to make clinical judgments independently. In the past, the profession has carefully controlled the number of doctors who would be educated, thereby limiting competition. Until rather recently, it has also been able to determine the structure under which care is given. Now physicians are being asked not to monitor themselves but to be monitored by others who lack their education and expertise. Even if the physician has a vested financial interest he or she may not wish to be accountable to the fiscal manager and the CEO rather than to the profession and to the patient. Also, physicians' satisfaction with their work decreases as that work is increasingly determined by "outsiders."

The present form of accountability makes fiscal concerns paramount and has the corporation determining what health care should be provided. Even at its best such care represents a "corporate paternalism" that is "removed from the doctor and the hospital administrator; it's now the insurer or the CEO of some large corporation . . . telling us that they're acting on our behalf" (Goonan et al., 1997, p. C2). It is a system that is "increasingly based on profit and a price competition and patients have . . . less and less of a voice" (p. C2). Physicians also have less of a voice; the question is not only whether physicians will revolt against this, but also whether that revolt will lead to more humanized care or simply a larger piece of the managed care pie for the physician. One way in which managed care has achieved savings is through what is paid to providers. Critics of managed care in the New York region have argued that managed care "is essentially discounted fee-for-service medicine" (Fisher, 1998, p. 27). Physicians clearly can limit their opposition to this fiscal reality or, as happened recently in Boston, can join with the wider medical care community to protest "the corporate takeover of medicine" (Lasalandra, 1997, p. 4) that is robbing medicine of its "soul" (Hilzenrath, 1997, p. B11).

It is not yet clear whether the medical community is ready to confront the reality that for meaningful change to occur the debate on health care must be reformulated, taken from those who believe medical care services are "mere commodities and regard suffering as an investment opportunity" (Lown & Fagin, 1997, p. A19). It cannot be assumed, as so many hospital administrators have done, that there is no inherent conflict of interest between serving the interest of the corporation and serving the interest of the patient. This entails beginning to look at health care in a social services or social welfare sense rather than as part of the economic marketplace and recognizing the differences in the two approaches. It also entails confronting the ideology and alienation in current medicine noted earlier. It means asking whether insurance companies, who provide no medical services per se, should play such a major role in our health care system. It also means questioning the effect of current mergers. As such mergers accelerate "the odds are that the most gains . . . will accrue to the stockholders and managers . . . not to the patients who seek treatment or to the health care professionals and personnel . . . who care for these patients" (Ginzberg, 1997, p. 1812).

Reformulating the debate in health care is all the more difficult given that managed care has emerged triumphant with so little debate. It is also made difficult by the fact that historically the nation has been concerned with how health care is financed rather than how it is delivered (Stevens, 1971). To slow the momentum of managed care legislative regulations will only be putting fingers in the proverbial dike; to really slow the momentum will require nothing less than confronting our basic values as a society and deciding whether we truly believe that medicine should be a business. If it is a business then the bottom line being paramount and "care" being determined by nonproviders is appropriate. If, on the other hand, we decide that medicine should be conceived of as necessary to a civil society then we must begin asking questions such as how health care can best be delivered, how our priorities are best determined, and whether the doctor–patient relationship is crucial enough to the medical process that its humaneness must be paramount. Most simply, perhaps, we must ask the question in terms of our own health and that of our families: Do we want the parameters of care set in corporate boardrooms? Do we want the decisions made by case managers who have no knowledge of us, or do we want to engage in dialogue with our primary care providers?

Although we have become obsessed over the cost of health care, and with managed care as a means of cost containment, we have not focused on the quality of health care, or on how to improve quality (Brook, 1997). We have failed to ask the even more basic question of whether high quality is possible in a business model of health care, or why, given how much we spend on health care, greater access and higher quality is not forthcoming. Ultimately our answer to the question of the kind of health care we want for ourselves and for our families and neighbors defines the kind of society we want to have. The question is too important to be answered passively, allowing managed care to happen without benefit of introspection or debate. Most basically it is our lives on the line, and it is all of us who will suffer if we fail to take control away from the corporate world.

References

Balint, M. (1973). *The doctor, his patient, and the illness.* New York: Pitman.

Brook, R. H. (1997). Managed care is not the problem, quality is. *JAMA, 278,* 1612–1614.

Dowie, M. (1991). Pinto madness. In J. H. Skolnick & E. Currie (Eds.), *Crises in American institutions* (pp. 20–35). Glenview, IL: Scott, Foresman.

Dubois, R. (1959). *Mirage of health.* New York: Harper & Row.

Fisher, I. (1998, January 11). HMO premiums rising sharply, stoking debate on managed care. *New York Times,* p. A1, A27.

Freudenheim, M. (1997, November 27). Baby boomers force new rules for HMOs. *New York Times,* p. A1, D2.

Ginzberg, E. (1997). Managed care and the competitive market in health care. *JAMA, 277,* 1812–1813.

Goonan, K., Gordon, S., Jankins-Scott, J., Kaplan, L. R., & Rabkin, M. (1997, June 1). Will care be there? *Boston Globe,* pp. C2–C3.

Hartman, A. (1993). Challenges for family policy. In F. Walsh (Ed.), *Normal family process* (pp. 474–503). New York: Guilford Press.

Hilzenrath, D. (1997, December 3). Doctors lash out against profit motive in health care. *Washington Post,* p. B11.

Howard, J., & Tyler, C. (1975). Comments on dehumanization: Caveats, dilemmas, and remedies. In J. Howard & A. Strauss (Eds.), *Humanizing health care.* New York: John Wiley & Sons.

Inui, T., & Frankel, R. (1991). *Do physicians' caring actions make a difference?* Stanford, CA: Center for Advanced Study in the Behavioral Sciences.

Lasalandra, M. (1997, December 3). Doctors protest against for-profit health biz. *Boston Herald,* p. 4.

Levine, S. (1975, November/December). Expanding the scope of health care. *Social Policy, 6,* 25–29.

Lown, B., & Fagin, C. M. (1997, December 27). Equity and quality are suffering in the corporatization of health care. *Boston Globe,* p. A19.

McKeown, T., & Lowe, C. R. (1974). *An introduction to social medicine.* Oxford, England: Blackwell Scientific.

Mechanic, D. (1997). Managed care as a target of distrust. *JAMA, 277,* 1810–1811.

Relman, A. S. (1987). The new medical industrial complex. In H. D. Schwartz (Ed.), *Dominant issues in medical sociology* (pp. 597–608). New York: Random House.

Scott, R. A., Aiken, L. H., Mechanic, D., & Moravcsik, J. (1995). Organizational aspects of caring. *Milbank Quarterly, 73,* 77–95.

Stevens, R. (1971). *American medicine and the public interest.* New Haven, CT: Yale University Press.

Stevens, R. (1989). *In sickness and in wealth.* New York: Basic Books.

CHAPTER 7

Is Managed Care the Way to Go?
Deciding Whether to Embark

Suzanne Gelber

More and more often, government officials and legislators are debating whether to use a managed care approach in health and human services systems directed either toward special populations or the general public. Managed care systems were originally developed for medical and behavioral health care, but they are expanding rapidly to child and family services, services for people with disabilities such as retardation, for multiproblem clients, and even for juvenile justice clients. A survey by the Child Welfare League of America (1996) found that 82 percent of states are considering or planning to apply managed care principles to child welfare services such as foster care and adoption. The goals of such approaches usually are to manage or reduce costs, to coordinate care using individually oriented service plans, to create an accountable group of organized delivery systems, to inject a mechanism for distinguishing excellence and inadequacy among providers, and to manage explicitly the quality of care and services provided for the dollars exchanged.

These are demanding objectives. Managed care is not necessarily a magic bullet that can instantly achieve those aims, which have eluded public systems for years. Managed care is only one approach—one technology that is popular today. It was developed to better manage medical care. Although it may be extended to human services such as child welfare, it may not produce the same results attributed to it in health care. Regardless, one knowledgeable commentator has described the momentum building to incorporate many human services under the umbrella of managed care as "an unstoppable steamroller." A surge toward managed care and more competition among services may yield better outcomes, but it may well leave some damage in its wake, particularly among our most vulnerable populations.

A variety of models characterize managed care implementation. For example, some states or counties have created their own managed human services networks using community mental health centers or federally qualified health centers as the fulcrum. Others have chosen to limit the public authorities' role to that of policymaker and quality reviewer. Some consciously adopt private-sector purchasing models, "outsourcing" management and purchasing functions to regional, public–private purchasing consortia selected by states, counties, and employers and often building

NOTE: Originally published as Gelber, S. (1997). Is managed care the way to go? Deciding whether to embark. In S. Scallet, C. Brach, & E. Steel (Eds.), *Managed care: Challenges for children and family services*. Baltimore: Annie E. Casey Foundation.

on earlier moves to privatize service delivery. The possibilities for enhancing coordination and improving accountability for performance have been addressed in many ways in the past. A new development, however, is the re-examination and reintegration of categorical agencies and the blending of their funds and provider networks. To some extent, states with Offices for Children (such as Massachusetts) tried this model years ago on a case management basis; now it is being linked to utilization review and network contracting.

This chapter delineates the information and steps policymakers must pursue to assess rationally whether their state, county, or community should implement a managed care approach in systems that serve children and families—and if so, how quickly to proceed. It provides guidance as to how to assess readiness for managed care, including gathering information and mapping the system, appraising internal capacity and using supplementary expertise, and evaluating available financial and system resources. Finally, it poses a variety of alternatives to monolithic managed care implementation that can affect a system's decision to embark on managed care.

Goals and Expectations

Unfortunately, an intent to embark upon a managed care initiative is too often declared before goals are discussed; stakeholders' divergent interests are resolved; and a set of policies regarding key, contentious issues have been promulgated. The magnitude of the changes involved, both policy and personal, often is not appreciated. The need to involve key stakeholders and participants is frequently ignored, only to surface after a crisis of confidence in governance has occurred. When this happens, often in a rush to implement before funds or political enthusiasm evaporate, the programs that result may be poorly conceived and contentious.

This phenomenon of rushing to change is not new to the public sector. A special challenge, however, lies in the possibility that poor decisions and poor systems may result in litigation. Badly designed systems can cause great harm to the vulnerable children and families they are supposed to serve or can create problems for providers, possibly leading to litigation. System users, advocates, or providers who feel that managed care approaches, systems, contractors, or technologies have been imposed inappropriately or have caused them harm might be expected to retaliate by suing the public authorities whom they allege acted without sufficient due diligence.

Delays caused by litigation, whether brought appropriately or inappropriately, may result in delaying the delivery of enhanced services for children and families. Even if the suits themselves prove unsuccessful, they can bring (and have brought) promising managed care initiatives to a grinding halt. Successful suits impose a costly price on people and organizations found to be at fault; the required redesign and rebidding of contracts for the initiative is quite expensive as well. Even more important, great and even tragic harm for which no damages can compensate may have been done to vulnerable people. Managed care approaches can succeed only when they are carefully planned and appropriate attention is paid to comprehending and incorporating stakeholders' perspectives and expectations.

The goals of managed care initiatives are complex and not always explicit. The values, the economic stakes, and the political objectives of various stakeholders can be diverse and conflicting. Such ambiguity and complexity of objectives can make it difficult or impossible to tell whether managed care initiatives are succeeding. Policymakers must clearly articulate specific, measurable objectives so that all stakeholders, including the public and the entities selected to manage and monitor the new managed care system, understand how and to what purpose scarce resources will be used and what must be accomplished or avoided in order for performance to be considered satisfactory.

However, policymakers—such as legislators, governors, or county commissioners—first must comprehend *why* things are done in a particular way and *how else* they might be done in order to determine effectively how they should be done in the future. Therefore, I will begin by identifying some factors that should be considered by policymakers as they set overall priorities and seek to address their many constituents' concerns.

Policymakers trying to consider the "big picture" face many competing priorities. They would want to be sure, for example, that the "overriding goals of protection and permanency" remain the hallmark of the child welfare services system (Institute for Human Services Management, 1996) and that the first responsibility of any such system, managed or not, is to ensure the safety of children. Placing a child in foster care or keeping a child at home while a family receives services are choices that must be available in any child welfare system. On the other hand, the choices may be different in the juvenile justice context. Because public safety is a primary goal in this system, intervention may be more oriented toward using a continuum of services, including out-of-home placement in secure programs when that is felt to be necessary for public protection. In a third example, mental health systems tend to feel that treating the child in the home or the community is the most critical goal for children with emotional disorders. These distinctions must be considered flexibly.

The goals and responsibilities of all the individual systems currently in place will not vanish under managed care. Building a successful managed care initiative requires policymakers to decide how to construct an all-inclusive services system that can encompass them. Each system responds to federal, state, and local decisions and may even reflect court mandates to organize and deliver services in one particular way. Deciding to change such systems simultaneously or sequentially involves reinstalling their objectives in a new way that neither violates legal or ethical responsibilities nor changes their text or interpretation.

Beyond such global concerns, decision makers must examine managed care approaches for state and local systems of care for children and families in light of many different objectives:

- holding down cost increases or absolute spending levels through the use of negotiation, competition, and capitation or performance-based risk sharing
- creating a system of continuous care and preventive services that cuts across categorical boundaries and creates multisource pooled funding for a designated population
- improving monitoring of and intervention in the quality of care and services
- expanding access to linked services, expanding the ability to link vendor and provider performance with compensation, and increasing the appropriateness and utility of services.

Not everyone subscribes to all of these goals, and many would include others on the list, such as protecting consumers' rights more proactively or saving service workers' jobs. Somehow, all these priorities must be built into any managed care system that seeks to combine and manage each or all of these systems for children and families.

Therefore, before beginning any effort to assess systems' readiness to convert to a managed care platform, policymakers must lay out certain essential factors:

- their vision of an ideal system
- the current care systems' objectives, capabilities, and weaknesses and state and federal entitlements and requirements, if any
- the key characteristics of the political and financial infrastructure supporting the categorical services
- the costs of the services and any existing cross-system financing capabilities or obstacles
- the strengths and weaknesses of managed care techniques and systems.

Policymakers must think through what changing to managed care will mean, theoretically and concretely. Decision makers must come to understand how managed care systems work and how they can fail. They must appreciate what they can and cannot accomplish using managed care approaches and how quickly results reasonably can be expected. If there is a preliminary match between system redesign needs and managed care capabilities, planning a new system can begin. The planning process takes time, but it can facilitate convergence of dramatically different goals and objectives, allowing all parties the space to negotiate and truly buy into the new system.

For example, an evaluation might determine that the primary problem of a system is that consumers are dissatisfied because the street-level staff with whom they come in contact are perceived as rude or ineffective in meeting their needs. This may result from poor training, lack of motivation, or disinterest in or disdain for consumer concerns. Addressing this primary problem may have little to do with applying managed care techniques; on the other hand, if consumer feedback mechanisms were built into managed care from the outset, these might contribute to resolving the problem. However, if the same assessment concludes that the primary problem is a lack of accountability and uneven provider performance, managed care mechanisms such as performance-based reporting and compensation might be effective in ushering in positive change.

All public agency contracts with private or internal managed care networks should include measurable outcomes (with variables and scoring defined in advance), such as those put forward by the Substance Abuse and Mental Health Services Administration (including its White Paper on Performance Measures and the Center for Mental Health Services Report Card). Both interim (process) measures and longer-term client and systems outcomes measures should be included. Grievance and appeal procedures should conform to state guidelines and be comprehensible in reading level and language. All contracts should have a "best practices" focus and reference, updated annually.

Assessing Readiness

The political will to initiate managed care usually precedes system readiness. No readiness assessment can succeed without an understanding of the steps involved and the intelligent use of valid data. The steps proceed as follows:

1. identifying, cleaning, and consolidating data on system resources, weaknesses, and utilization
2. clarifying the limitations of data in measuring actual readiness; for example, the age or comprehensiveness of the data may preclude accurate information

on which providers are currently in place and which have closed or even died

3. mapping the infrastructure and organizational components of the current system, including the current system's geographic catchment area
4. assessing the knowledge base, ability, and capacity of current staff to develop the plan for a new managed care system
5. identifying personnel, new contractors or entities, technologies, and financial resources that will be needed to implement the new system
6. evaluating the financial resources available to implement a new system that fills gaps in services and the sophistication of providers who would participate in the new managed care system
7. examining the willingness or obstruction to be expected regarding managed care from key stakeholders and determining whether objections can be neutralized or overcome within the time specified
8. evaluating legal frameworks (for example, procurement, federal guidelines, confidentiality, and provider agreements).

The information-gathering and analysis phase of an appropriateness assessment is both inescapable and expensive. This process of accumulating and digesting data enables the state or county to be informed by an accurate and current understanding of the existing needs and systems and how they interact and are organized. Because human services and health care data are notoriously difficult to collect and interpret, expert assistance is often required to decide what kinds of data are available and valid enough to use and then to determine what the data mean.

GATHERING INFORMATION AND MAPPING THE SYSTEM

The data gathered should give policymakers access to information (minimally) about

- the population being served (or excluded)
- the providers who serve the populations under study (for example, through claims data) as well as those who could serve them (for example, those who are licensed)
- the administrative managers who finance and monitor service provision
- the funding streams and costs associated with the current systems
- patterns of service utilization.

The long-term starvation budgets affecting most human and health services in the public sector have taken their greatest toll on the most capital-intensive investments: management information systems (MIS) and other sophisticated technology. Utilization data may exist only at the facility or program level rather than for the system as a whole. Information about staff capacity and capabilities requires assessing current data on workloads and examining credentials that may be out of date. Discovering potential contractors, improving MIS capacity, and exploring alternative plan designs and their implications involve gathering information from often unpublished or informal sources at the national, regional, and local levels. It is critical to understand where the pockets of information are and to weave them together to tell the system's complete story. It is also critical to be open to and engage in interagency cooperation rather than competition—for example, to share data, expertise, staff, or financing.

For example, looking only at easily obtainable hospital data such as average lengths of stay, admission rates, or cost per admission tells a partial story. Policymakers need to understand existing referral and use patterns in the area, to what extent hospital admissions occur because of a lack of residential or outpatient programs, and how often admissions occur after or during outpatient care. But answering the latter question, although it sheds light on how and why providers are used, involves determining a common but confidential client identifier that can track episodes of care by client or finding another way to link data across systems, manually if necessary. This capability is not built into many information systems.

Similarly, there can be extensive problems with the routine data that are collected: Confusion in coding the diagnosis for a discharge is common, making it difficult to separate psychiatric and substance abuse admissions. The extent to which medical admissions need to be analyzed is often not obvious either, and the problems involved in integrating multiple data sets by user or user cohort are not easy to solve.

Many states and counties have data on the same person in multiple health care and human services systems, but they lack the ability or willingness to match episodes of use by client name. The data systems themselves are not user friendly; many are cumbersome, categorical, antiquated, and subject to strict confidentiality provisions. Expecting them to yield useful and usable information sufficient for a complete and unbiased description of current system functioning may be unreasonable or may require significant allocation of priority and time.

In light of these endemic problems, decision makers must provide adequate funding and time for this step. At least they must proceed far enough to decide whether the necessary data exist and simply need to be organized or whether it is really hopeless to rely on existing data systems. In the latter case, the decision process will be far more speculative, begging for a pilot-site approach that includes gathering information on which to base future decisions. In some places the problem is not insufficient MIS capacity; the capacity may be there, but people may not be using it or may not understand it. Building the capacity to use information is as important as building information systems.

State and county decision makers must determine whether the available staff can address their data and information needs or whether they must hire additional staff or look to an outside contractor to find, interpret, and report the information needed to describe the system. Such a contract, too, must be well thought through.

In one recent state government managed care project, the state determined after much debate and a change in political parties that managed care could introduce positive change in the Medicaid system. A bidding process ensued to identify a consultant to assist with this profound change. However, the winner proposed such a small consulting budget that it was entirely consumed by the tremendous effort required simply to put together an accurate system description from more than 20 separate sources of data. Once that effort neared completion, the state had to go out to bid again for additional consulting services and a new consultant. The entire process cost more than twice the original estimate and also led to an unplanned 15-month delay that forced postponement of savings and considerable opportunity costs.

Had the state spent more time initially in assessing and preparing its data set, the whole process could have proceeded more efficiently and swiftly. Consulting fees could have been reserved for the more challenging project of helping the state to plan a well-engineered service system.

APPRAISING INTERNAL CAPACITY AND USING SUPPLEMENTARY EXPERTISE

The next questions involve the degree to which internal administrative and technical resources suffice for the tasks to be accomplished. It will be critical to assess skill levels honestly and realistically; failure to do so will lead to excess costs and disruption. Do available staff have the skills needed to implement and manage the type of managed care system under consideration for children and families? Are there sufficient staff internally or through interagency staff sharing who are skilled in designing and negotiating vendor services contracts, managing information systems, or monitoring and evaluating outcomes? Then, to what extent could current staff be trained for new roles in a short period of time, and for which functions does it make more sense to hire new staff or contract for expert assistance or technology? Do the public or private providers have the capacity to do multiyear budgeting that would take into account the cost of converting the system, including the cost of retraining workers, converting management information systems, contracting for some services, and putting new services in place?

Many states and counties answer these questions without conducting any assessment, relying on unsupported assumptions about whether or not they can function as managed care entities or should seek an outside vendor for particular services. However, even a hint that the public sector assumes it cannot perform certain managed care functions internally serves to signal vendors that the time is ripe for seeking business from the state. Vendor staff may besiege startled bureaucrats and decision makers with unanticipated proposals, barely veiled inducements, reams of marketing materials, and offers to provide "free" consulting services. It is possible that these offers will serve as helpful guideposts in a wilderness of choices. However, there is also the chance that they will lead the state to make choices that benefit mainly or only the vendors.

The decision to bring in consulting assistance should be made only after assessing the capacity of internal staff. The amount of influence a consultant will have, the tasks to be assumed, and the time and money to be spent on consulting services all must be carefully considered and articulated. Failure to do so will result in confused responsibilities, neglected time frames, inadequate deliverables, and other undesirable consequences.

Prudence in purchasing is always the safest and surest position. In hiring any type of contractor (for example, as consultants, analysts, or vendors), decision makers must ensure that the processes put in place to identify potential external resources lead to the selection of people who are truly expert, competent, available, and ethical. Designating consultants is particularly sensitive. The supply of consultants with expert knowledge of managed care decisions and methods and children and families is extremely limited, and the group of such experts who also understand governmental operations, resources, and funding streams (and will work for government) is even smaller. State policymakers risk lawsuits if they yield to political pressure to hire "favorite consultants," unless such individuals or firms turn out to be acceptable after an objective assessment of available alternatives.

EVALUATING AVAILABLE FINANCIAL AND SYSTEM RESOURCES

Financial resources must also be carefully considered but in such a way that sufficient thought is given to innovative combinations of funding. Historically, service systems have used "silos" of categorical funds that are further divided by purpose into demonstration, research, and block grants; state or county general revenues; and foundation support. Attention must be given to consolidating and restructuring funding streams and service systems. However, sufficient money to meet the needs of clients and systems has rarely been available in the past, and the present and future are equally, if not more, questionable. Koyanagi (1995) and others have raised grave concerns regarding whether governmental appropriations (federal, state, and local) will be sufficient even to come close to supporting systems of care for people in need, regardless of whether they involve managed care.

The amounts of money states and counties can count on is one concern. Another is the permissible uses of funds. Different funding sources currently place different requirements on the use of funds. For example, grant funds distributed through the mental health system may require that systems use them only for in-home services for children with serious emotional disorders. Juvenile justice funds may be earmarked only for residential treatment, whether that is what children need clinically or not. Children eligible for Aid to Families with Dependent Children (AFDC) can be supported through Medicaid funds, but in some places non-AFDC children may qualify for such funding only if they are placed outside their homes. Needless to say, such restrictions are not common in managed health care systems that function on rational criteria.

State procurement laws may require contracts to go to the lowest qualified bidder or the least expensive of several "equally" qualified bidders. However, there may be subtle but important differences that may be particularly salient for certain stakeholders. For example, one contractor may be more "client friendly," but another may have a more proficient data system and superior implementation plans.

It is not clear that managed care can be as effective as many assume if these requirements are left in place rather than waived because they contradict the notions of "clinically necessary care" that are the basis of managed care protocols. If, as seems likely, federal mandates are restrained and resources migrate eventually to block grants, some (but by no means all) of these restrictions may ease. However, planners will still need to decide how to organize, authorize, and distribute funds. Policymakers will need to assess how much funding they expect and whether managed care techniques can be implemented adequately, given expected funding levels. This is a major issue that has derailed many hasty managed care initiatives.

The capacity of the service system to meet the needs of clients must be considered in relation to the funds that will be available to pay for those services. There is no point in planning an elegantly designed system if the providers who must offer newly linked services lack sufficient resources or sufficient understanding of managed care techniques to ensure their willingness and ability to participate. Any thorough assessment of readiness and appropriateness of managed care, therefore, must include an objective analysis of the strengths and weaknesses of care providers, many of whom may be unrealistically positive or negative about their ability to change their historical operating patterns.

This dispassionate assessment should address whether providers have the following systems in place and know how to use them:

- adequate network capacity to ensure clinically appropriate levels of care and timely referrals
- protocols for clinical and service-level decision making (few of the latter have been developed or standardized)

- financial and administrative systems and personnel to handle capitation, risk sharing, claims preauthorization or payment, and performance standard reporting
- credible audit and quality management systems and staff
- culturally sensitive education and outreach systems to ensure that consumers understand the services and how to access them
- systems to train and evaluate managed care providers and practitioners
- outcomes analysis, research, and management information systems.

If only some of the above prerequisites are present and adequate, policymakers must decide whether it makes sense to invest in bringing the inadequate components up to speed and in what period of time that can be accomplished. The providers themselves cannot be relied upon to make such a decision, as it represents a conflict of interest. This kind of assessment may also require outside consulting analysis and should be integrated into any consulting proposal.

INVOLVING STAKEHOLDERS

Even if all other conditions for managed care readiness are met, resistance among stakeholders such as clients, advocacy groups, and providers can stymie a decision to move toward a managed system of care. Policymakers are, therefore, well advised to involve stakeholders in the process of assessing a system's readiness for managed care. Numerous ways of obtaining stakeholder participation in managed care readiness assessments can be employed, such as

- representation of stakeholders on bodies charged with assessing the system's readiness
- holding public hearings throughout the state, inviting testimony on the system's or clients' readiness
- surveying key stakeholders on their assessment of the system's readiness
- having stakeholders review and contribute to requests for proposal or contract language.

Soliciting stakeholders' opinions about the system's readiness will not only provide valuable insight into what obstacles must be overcome if a successful managed care system is to be implemented, but it also will identify areas of potential conflict. Unhappy stakeholders have been known to pursue legal means of fundamentally changing or delaying managed care initiatives. Policymakers aware of areas of contention at an early stage can plan to work with stakeholders to satisfy their concerns, whether or not managed care is ultimately pursued.

Checklist for Overall Readiness

Policymakers may want to make use of the checklist below to assure themselves that they have done a thorough job of considering the appropriateness, capacity, design, and implementation issues. It is easy to neglect or be unaware of design alternatives, and it is important to be as certain as possible that choices have been made with full knowledge of possible consequences and of alternatives. Policymakers need to be able to make most, if not all, the assertions on the checklist in order to have a reasonable chance of success in restructuring their system. Insufficient information to make an assertion suggests the need to postpone a decision about managed care until that shortage can be remedied.

Many of the checklist's statements relate to issues of managed care implementation, but policymakers will need to think through these issues as part of the process of deciding whether to embark on a managed care system. Only by pondering what implementation requires can policymakers truly assess if their system is ready for managed care. This checklist is designed to expose policymakers to the complexity of managed care initiatives *before* a decision is made. (Each statement on the checklist is a simplification of the depth of examination required. Following the checklist, an example is provided.)

- ☑ We have determined through careful data collection and analysis that the weaknesses and configuration of the current service system for children and families can be improved through using managed care approaches.
- ☑ We have considered a range of managed care approaches and designs with the best available knowledge of their financial, political, clinical, and administrative implications and have decided that a given managed care approach or set of approaches will work best in our particular circumstances.
- ☑ We have made all our decisions using the best possible expert advice and oversight from people with the knowledge and experience to steer us appropriately and ethically.
- ☑ We have specified how and to what extent consumers, family, and community groups will be involved in deciding on, managing, and implementing the managed care restructuring we are undertaking.
- ☑ We have determined with whom sponsorship of and authority or liability for the new system will rest and how that entity will be accountable to the public, both on an individual and a systemwide basis.
- ☑ We have agreement on the populations to which managed care techniques will be applied.
- ☑ We have decided which techniques will be applied to which populations.
- ☑ We have agreement among all agencies (including purchasing offices) and funding streams involved that the system changes we are planning are appropriate and feasible in the time frame elected and that all possible negative consequences have been anticipated and planned for to the extent possible.
- ☑ We have determined that existing or expected financial resources are at least adequate to carry out the scope of changes that is planned or that we have contingency plans to limit scope through the use of demonstration and pilot sites if resources are inadequate.
- ☑ We know who will pay for the system, how much is due, and with what mechanisms and frequency payments will be made. Our MIS is capable of monitoring the flow of funds.
- ☑ We have decided how clinical and financial risk will be handled (that is, reinsurance, capitation, performance standards, grievance mechanisms, and so forth).

- ☑ We have a reasonable assessment of what we will spend and what we will save.
- ☑ We have determined that we either have, can build quickly, or can contract for the vendor capacity to manage and monitor a managed care system combined with likely restructuring of services and funding.
- ☑ We have decided who will administer and who will evaluate the system.
- ☑ We have criteria in place to evaluate and guide implementation.
- ☑ We have communicated beforehand clear evaluation criteria that we are capable of measuring at predetermined points during implementation and operations.
- ☑ We have determined how, by whom, and using what competitive processes managed care will be purchased (that is, through a purchasing sponsor, a state agency, or a consortium of funders).
- ☑ We have considered how to identify potential bidders and how to conduct a fair and open bidding process that will withstand court challenge. We have determined on what basis entities will be eligible to bid, whether or not they are existing state agencies. We know how we will select the winning bid and how we will conduct financial and operational negotiations, and we have staff or consultants in place to help us.
- ☑ We have demarcated the time frame for this change and determined whether or not it will be phased in, at first applying to just a few regions.
- ☑ We have assurances from all parties involved that the time frame proposed is at least feasible, even if challenging.
- ☑ We have adequate contingency plans to deal with obstacles.

AN EXAMPLE: EVALUATION

Consideration of each question may entail exploring multiple levels and decisions. An example follows to illustrate the complicated nature of deciding on and designing a managed care system, even when the team of policymakers is well prepared. The more specific the questions asked in addressing each issue, the more likely that the state or county as purchaser will be able to determine appropriate and feasible responses. Decisions to embark that are based on data and clearly specified objectives are both defensible and most likely to yield positive results in the short and longer terms.

The complexities of determining who will evaluate the managed care program and under what circumstances can serve as a good example of the levels of decisions often involved. General issues come first. Policymakers will need to decide who will be responsible for undertaking and managing the evaluation and what assistance will be available to help the evaluators understand the project and properly couch their findings. This first decision takes policymakers back to goals and objectives. If the evaluation is to serve as the basis for deciding on performance-based risk sharing, for example, it is especially critical to decide whether in-house staff, external consultants, or a task force combining the two will attempt the analysis.

Findings that are negative may well be disputed, requiring arbitration mechanisms. The evaluators must be extremely skilled and accurate in their observations and conclusions because of the likelihood of challenges. The evaluators will need access to timely and reliable information, program staff, and the perceptions of participants. Access will depend heavily on the respect accorded to them as unbiased experts.

Evaluators may be chosen through competitive bidding. In this case, criteria for their selection must be available beforehand in addition to the criteria they will be expected to use in their study. Time frames must be clearly specified so that results are timely enough to be of use in program enhancement and refinement. Funders may expect that they will have the ability to influence the way in which the evaluation is conducted, who conducts it, who interprets it, and what consequences it has. The scope and limits of such influence must be clearly understood.

Process questions must also be addressed or delegated. For example, what will the methodological approach be? What instruments or data sources will be used? How will data be analyzed and by whom? How will confidentiality be ensured? How will valid and reliable surveys or audits be conducted or integrated into the evaluation? Answers must be found also for the extent to which consumers and families will be involved in designing, implementing, participating in, interpreting, and disseminating the results of the evaluation.

Probably the most difficult questions will involve decisions to be made ahead of results, such as what rules will apply if results are ambiguous, contested, or exceedingly negative or positive, particularly if financial rewards or penalties are at stake. Exactly what type and level of negative findings will trigger program change, reconsideration, or even discontinuation? Clearly, if the evaluation has such serious consequences there may be pressures to come up with positive findings. (A decision may be made to treat evaluations as advisory only.)

In the case of one large managed care initiative undertaken by a nonprofit insurance carrier, evaluation was the cornerstone of substantial financial incentives. Results were often ambiguous, and the consequence was audits that had to repeated three times until challenges were satisfied. Decisions about who the final arbiter would be shifted constantly and caused repetitive rounds of reanalysis that cost the carrier a great deal of money, delayed payment of bonuses to the contractor, and ultimately resulted in changing the contractor, who is suing the carrier for abrogating the contract and drawing all those involved into a tedious lawsuit.

Making the Decision

Ultimately, deciding whether managed care is the right or wrong choice is the most critical decision to be made. For managed care to be the "right" choice, some minimum standards must be met. Baseline assessments must have shown that managed care can redress system weaknesses and that resources are either relatively sufficient or can be enhanced adequately within the time frame proposed. Policymakers must have determined that the managed care techniques to be applied can be carried out appropriately and will not produce untoward and unforeseen consequences, such as suicide attempts or embarrassing litigation. Realistic, staged performance expectations must have been established and systems must be in place to measure their achievement.

The system's state of readiness is not likely to be uniform. Therefore, the managed care decision need not be a yes-or-no proposition. There are options that can match managed care implementation to the system's level of readiness, allowing parts of the system or state that are more ready to proceed more quickly. Decision makers will want to consider questions about phasing in managed care, such as

- Should the managed care initiative be implemented as a pilot, a series of comparable demonstrations, or systemwide? If systemwide, can it be phased in by region?
- Is one part of the state or county more prepared than others, having a full complement of providers who can function along managed care lines?
- Should certain regions or populations be covered with special pilots or demonstrations, phased in consecutively, or entered into the equation all at once?
- Should implementation wait until all desired locations or populations are ready to participate, or should it begin in the most well-prepared sites or populations first?
- Should certain providers be mandated or given special participation consideration, even if they are unready, because they comprehend and have experience with a particularly difficult subpopulation or because they are the most culturally appropriate? If not, what will happen to these providers? Will they be given a timetable to meet in developing managed care capabilities, and will the entire system await their entry?
- Should subsidized or free technical assistance be given to designated community-based providers in order to bring them to the point where they can participate fully? How much help should be made available and for how long? At what point does the probation or preparation period end, and how should this be factored into the financial risk sharing embedded in the system?
- Should risk sharing precede full-risk capitation so that providers and managed care organizations have a chance to learn how to work together?

Conclusion

The adoption of a managed care approach to services for children and families may in the end be the right decision. However, without rational and valid consideration of the purposes it is to serve and, whether managed care is the right course to follow, the results are more likely to be equivocal or problematic than to be positive. The processes and issues described in this chapter require a significant investment of time and energy. However, failure to confront them may cause delay, dissatisfaction, and even tragedy as the project is implemented. Success depends on an initial decision set that delineates specific and measurable objectives through data-based planning and feasibility analyses.

It is troubling that the rush to managed care often has literally been a rush, with some programs covering large and complex-need populations (such as Medicaid) being converted to managed care by fiat or outsourced to an eager private vendor in six months or less. Little consideration may have been given to the impact of such a comprehensive change, to whether managed care is the appropriate vehicle to carry out certain kinds of changes and reforms, or whether there really is a good match between the problems identified and the solution proposed. Especially because the populations involved are so vulnerable and because certain kinds of decisions entail potential conflicts of interest, both ethically and financially, this hastiness carries grave risks.

If the difficult decisions discussed here are understood, made, and made well and the result is a decision to proceed with a new managed care approach, the challenging tasks of planning, designing, and implementing the new system can begin. Understanding that managed care is not a monolithic system but can be tailored to meet the idiosyncratic needs of each system is a step toward designing a system that can meet the needs of vulnerable children and families.

References

Child Welfare League of America, Managed Care Institute. (1996). *Survey on managed care and child welfare: Preliminary draft.* Washington, DC: Author.

Institute for Human Services Management. (1996). *Managed care and child welfare: Are they compatible? Conceptual issues in managed care for child welfare.* Bethesda, MD: Author.

Koyanagi, C. (1995). *Remarks.* Partnership for Change Conference, Washington, DC.

CHAPTER 8

Managed Care Challenges for Children and Family Services

Cindy Brach and Leslie Scallet

Managed care has captured the imagination of the health and human services world. It has taken hold in the health and mental health fields, and its impact on other systems that serve children and families is growing. The attraction of managed care for children and family services lies in its potential to further goals long promoted by these systems: reducing service fragmentation, increasing access to individualized care, establishing accountability, reducing costs, and stimulating the development of more appropriate and less restrictive community services.

However, just as managed care has the potential to serve children and families more flexibly and holistically, experience in the health care sector underscores significant risks:

- hurried implementation that may preclude adequate planning for the development or continuation of elements necessary for an effective service delivery system
- failure to blend funding streams and to integrate acute and extended care, which may create financial incentive for service providers to shift the costliest children and families from one system to another
- inadequate cost allocation models and capitation formulas that may result in over- or underfunding
- rigid adherence to a medical model of care that works against the "psychosocial–behavioral" model of care embraced by children's reform initiatives
- fiscal incentive to underserve combined with insufficient quality assurance mechanisms
- exclusion of providers (particularly indigenous community-based ones) that have expertise in children and families, and conversely, inclusion of providers whose technology and values are at odds with those of children's reform initiatives
- loss of opportunities for community residents to participate in the design and management of services that affect their neighborhoods and families.

There are lessons to be learned from health and mental health experiences that can make managed care work better for children and family services. This chapter

NOTE: Originally published as Brach, C., & Scallet, L. (1997). Cross-cutting issues. In L. Scallet, C. Brach, & E. Steel (Eds.), *Managed care: Challenges for children and family services.* Baltimore: Annie E. Casey Foundation.

highlights five challenges facing those dedicated to the welfare of children and their families who also want to make the most of the opportunity managed care presents: (1) the speed with which managed care is moving through the various systems that serve children and families, (2) the emphasis that has been placed on outcomes, (3) the participation of clients in the design and implementation of managed care policies and programs and the importance of ensuring client protection, (4) the need for the development of culturally competent systems of care, and (5) the potpourri of legal considerations that accompany managed care initiatives. By analyzing the experiences of the health and mental health fields, we hope to promote intersystem learning that will aid those contemplating managed care initiatives in children and family systems.

Speed of Change

The breakneck speed at which managed care is proliferating puts at risk the fragile progress to date in creating child and family systems and instituting quality improvements. Financial considerations and ideological beliefs about the superiority of the private, for-profit sector have been the driving force in the creation of public managed care programs, and there is a fear that cost reduction goals are eclipsing quality improvement goals. For example, Medicaid capitation programs, with savings as their primary goal, have outpaced primary care case management programs, which are more likely to include improving accessibility as a primary goal.

With cost control as the impetus, fiscal administrators are making decisions about the structure of managed care programs, but administrators committed to systems of care often have not participated in planning managed care initiatives. The budget offices and Medicaid agencies that have been the driving forces are generally housed in departments separate from the agencies chiefly responsible for children and families. Managed care program designers have not adopted a client orientation, and they are relatively inaccessible to advocacy groups. Only a few places have established a process for substantial stakeholder input, but that number is growing as it becomes clear that any group that does not buy into a program may contribute to closing it.

One important lesson from the implementation of managed care in the health care sector is that although they want to "do right" by children and families, public officials often do not possess the skills needed to become "smart purchasers." The pace of change outstrips knowledge and resources. For example, the ability to accredit new organizations and providers lags behind a constantly shifting industry. Public managed care initiatives often rely on a few devoted public officials who, however tireless, cannot keep up with the range of capabilities they need to master.

The provider community also needs time to adjust. Managed care organizations (MCOs) may have little experience in dealing with the needs of multiproblem patients. They need adequate time for planning, obtaining client input, and developing quality assurance systems (Rowland, Rosenbaum, Simon, & Chait, 1995). In the case of traditional providers, long-established approaches to delivering services must change. For example, current treatment planning and clinical skills in the child welfare industry may not meet the new demands imposed by managed care. Unless given time to learn, the provider community is likely to become unstable, creating vacuums in the services delivery system.

Outcomes

As government increasingly contracts with for-profit organizations, the ability to specify in advance the results expected becomes essential. For-profit organizations cannot be expected to exceed the literal specifications of a contract (Donahue 1989). Increasingly, as they find themselves competing with for-profit organizations, nonprofits cannot continue to do so either. No longer can contractors be relied on to do right by their clients when the provisions of a contract are vague.

Contracts have been vague in the past, in part because there is disagreement about what the outcomes should be. Lack of specificity has allowed programs to appear to be meeting all constituents' demands. If the outcomes for which contractors are being held accountable are spelled out, then difficult questions must be answered: Is the juvenile justice system trying to rehabilitate offenders, or is it chiefly punishing and incapacitating them? At what point should the child welfare system give up on family reunification and seek a permanent alternative? Managed care, with its emphasis on outcomes, may force policymakers to come to terms with competing agendas within their own systems.

In addition to surmounting the difficulty in defining desired outcomes, the technical hurdle of measuring outcomes must be met. Government needs to be able to hold contractors and subcontractors accountable for outcomes as the public sector stops dictating how programs are administered. Yet many outcome measures in use today pertain to the individual child or family and do not measure how an organization or system is functioning. There are other concerns about outcomes measurement. For example,

- Can client improvement and treatment effectiveness be quantified? What happens when the results of successful interventions appear in the long term rather than the short term?
- Which outcome measures are appropriate for managed care? For example, if a contractor is in control of the decision to readmit a client to the hospital or to remove a child from his or her family after a reunification attempt, do recidivism rates measure contractor performance?
- Do outcome measures look at the typical experience at the expense of special-needs children?
- Are existing measures appropriate for various cultural groups? The unique culture, situation, and life experiences of the client are integral to outcome and should be taken into account.

The state of the art in outcome measurement varies among the different family- and child-serving systems. The health care sector has the most well-developed instruments, but even these tend to be geared toward measuring personal health status rather than the overall health care system. Attempts to address public-sector concerns, such as the revision of the National Committee for Quality Assurance's Health Plan Employer Data and Information Set (HEDIS) to include Medicaid recipients, demonstrate the unevenness and gaps in measurement knowledge.

In the behavioral health field, there has been a flurry of outcome measurement activity. Several groups, including the American Managed Behavioral Healthcare Association and the Mental Health Statistics Improvement Program, have developed report cards—a set of indicators that reflect the performance of an organization or system. The proliferation of performance measures, however, has introduced some confusion into the field about the differences among the measures and has provoked questions about which should be used. The U.S. Substance Abuse and Mental Health Services Administration funded an effort led by the Institute of Medicine to bring together measurement-defining organizations to clarify the distinctions among the measurements, but securing consensus around a single set of outcome measures was considered unrealistic.

Outcome measurement is less developed in the child welfare field than in the health and behavioral health fields. The measures used, such as length of stay in out-of-home placements, have been criticized by some as being too coarse and creating incentives to return children to their families prematurely. Measurement of client satisfaction, widely used to guard against underservice in health and behavioral health programs, is a less-dependable barometer of programmatic success in a system characterized by involuntary services and resistant clients. Those who would like to give managed care a chance argue that perfect outcome measures are not necessary at this stage—once the child welfare system has mastered the primitive measurements currently available, the demand for better measures will emerge.

The impact of outcome measures depends on how incentives are structured to promote particular outcomes. Incentives can be structured to promote reductions in service, but they also can be structured to hold contractors accountable for the safety of children in their care by linking penalties to subsequent incidents of abuse and neglect. Resistance to outcome measurement is understandable because it pushes the child welfare system to face its limitations—admitting that there are failures (just as some sick children will die in the health care sector, some children in the child welfare system will die) and that scarce resources can be stretched only so far.

Concern for quality under managed care has given rise to a demand for accountability, but the emphasis on outcome measurement is not without its price. Pressure to produce credible outcomes has been placed on ill-prepared providers. All too quickly, organizations are being asked to demonstrate that they can achieve results. Outcome measurement is sophisticated and expensive to implement, yet organizations have been made to feel that outcome measurement is the admission price to participating in managed care. Many of today's child and family services providers will need help building the infrastructure necessary to produce reliable information on outcomes.

Client Participation and Protection

Clients have fought long and hard to gain a measure of control over decisions made about their lives. Managed care threatens client gains by imposing a new decision-making process. Many decisions are made by someone who does not know the client or by a provider whose incentives have changed because of the assumption of risk. As the roles of provider and insurer become increasingly integrated, clients cannot count on providers to be their advocates. Even when providers are not at financial risk, they may worry about jeopardizing their relationships with MCOs if they repeatedly appeal denials. A provider, of course, has the option to continue to provide treatment even after an MCO has denied payment. Although there may be both a moral and a legal duty to provide clients with appropriate treatment, requiring providers to deliver unlimited amounts of uncompensated care is not a sustainable public policy (Appelbaum, 1993).

Managed care in the health and behavioral health sectors has also been associated with a loss of client choice. Restrictions are often placed on who can deliver care. The fact that such choice is relatively unknown in some of the other child- and family-serving sectors, where providers are routinely assigned, does not mean that choice is not an important value to be built into a managed care system. There are a variety of mechanisms that can preserve or create choice in managed care, such as making participation in a program voluntary or contracting with more than one MCO. Both voluntary programs and creating competition among MCOs encourage quality because dissatisfied enrollees can leave the program or go to another contractor.

Current managed care programs often lack client protections. For example, complaints about Medicaid managed care include

- continued use of generic drugs when name brands are prescribed
- failure to use appropriate specialists instead of generalists
- lack of grievance procedures
- dearth of client education.

Evidence of managed care's deficiencies is not strictly anecdotal. For example, analysis of the Medicaid Competition Demonstrations indicates that the proportion of children with a visit to a specialist declined an average of 53 percent after enrollment in managed care (Newcheck, Hughes, Stoddard, & Halfon, 1994). Another study of 59 health maintenance organizations (HMOs) revealed that although most plans offered a liberal range of the types of ancillary services needed by children at developmental risk (for example, home health care, mental health care, occupational therapy), access to the services was limited by discretionary decisions of plan administrators (Wehr & Jameson, 1994).

The Federation of Families for Children's Mental Health (1995) has laid out principles for family involvement in the development and operation of managed health and mental health care systems for children and youths. This can serve as a checklist for ensuring a strong client voice.

☑ Family members must be part of the decision-making team responsible for managed care system development in both the public and private sectors.

☑ Families must receive the information and training to empower them to advocate for themselves.

☑ Families must have a definitive role in the development of their child's care plan and service needs.

☑ Providers in the managed care system must be prepared to allow families to participate at whatever level they feel comfortable.

☑ Managed care systems must support the principles of wraparound and cover the nontraditional services designed and delivered through this approach.

☑ Managed care systems (both public and private) must have a comprehensive and easy-to-use appeals process for families.

☑ Money needs to be set aside by the managed care system to support and train family organizations as client-based entities that have a key role in monitoring the managed care system, as well as to be involved in complaint review and policy development.

Public involvement in managed care planning can begin at the earliest stages, with allowing client and family participation in planning groups and advisory boards and providing opportunity for public comment on managed care plans. Public input needs to be ongoing. The Bazelon Center for Mental Health Law has recommended a number of mechanisms to achieve ongoing public involvement (Koyanagi, 1995):

- Set up a state-level client-oversight board to review implementation of state managed care.
- Require MCOs to establish client advisory boards.
- Require both MCOs and appropriate state agencies (for example, Medicaid, mental health, child welfare) to conduct client satisfaction surveys on a regular basis.

Government officials also need to ensure that client rights, such as freedom from discrimination and the right to receive appropriate treatment even if other services have been refused, are protected under managed care. Grievance procedures with time frames for dispute resolution must be installed, and clients must be given information on how to file grievances. Protection against abuses, from marketing ploys designed to induce disenrollment as a result of costly service utilization or difficult behavior, needs to be established.

Cultural Competence

The public sector has long struggled to develop appropriate programs for its culturally diverse populations. Efforts to develop culturally competent programs for children and families in public programs need to be maintained. *Cultural competence* refers to the ability to honor and respect the beliefs, interpersonal styles, attitudes, and behaviors both of clients and of the multicultural staff who are providing services (Roberts et al., 1990). Culturally competent systems of care acknowledge the importance of culture, assess cross-cultural relations, are alert to cultural differences and their repercussions, and adapt services to meet cultural needs (Cross, Bazron, Dennis, & Isaacs, 1989).

Concern has emerged that managed care will lead to a "one size fits all" approach to service provision that ignores the complexity presented by America's wide range of ethnicities. Of special concern is the high out-of-home placement rate of children in nondominant racial and ethnic groups. Although managed care has the flexibility to institute service adaptations to reunify families or provide home-based services, managed care programs must become sensitive to the meaning of behaviors in particular cultures and take the time to develop trust and productive communication with families.

To move toward cultural competence, experts agree that there must be an organizationwide commitment. A clearly established policy to provide culturally competent services must be accompanied by specific changes in practices in such areas as assessment, outreach, family involvement, staffing, use of translators, caseload, and training and support (Roberts et al., 1990). Pursuit of cultural competence cannot be put on a separate track but must pervade all responsibilities and activities undertaken by an organization responsible for managing care. There must be a philosophical and policy commitment to cultural competency at all levels of the organization, from the top management to the front lines. Tools for assessing organizations' cultural competency can be a useful departure point for cultural competency activities. However, they are not designed to be used in isolation but should be used as part of a broader effort to achieve cultural competency, and with the guidance of experienced cultural competence experts.

The first step to becoming culturally competent is the ability of individual providers to identify the culture and language of clients. This information should also feed into data systems that can support analysis of utilization patterns, outcomes, and client satisfaction to determine if there are differences among groups. Developing sensitivity to the varying needs and strengths of particular cultures is the next step. However, sensitivity must be followed by the acquisition of knowledge about the cultures of clients served and the creation of skills to provide care based on that knowledge. For example, being aware of linguistic needs must lead to working effectively with interpreters, hiring bilingual and bicultural staff, and taking the time to develop trusting and productive communication with clients. Similarly, having diverse staff members does not necessarily mean an organization is culturally competent. Cultural competence requires staff to be able, for example, to interpret the meaning of behaviors of people from different cultures and to obtain cooperation with treatment plans or alter treatment plans to reflect the client's culture.

As MCOs continue expanding their business into the public sector, they will encounter more culturally diverse populations. As part of their process of becoming culturally competent, MCOs will have to share the scarce culturally competent resources among themselves. Traditional providers have been known to borrow staff from each other to meet a specialized need, such as sharing the services of a Spanish-speaking therapist with experience in childhood trauma. MCOs may have to broker such resources or risk not being able to provide culturally competent services. Care should be taken to preserve the culturally competent capacity already developed. As the trend in the provider community toward larger organizations continues, the viability of small, community-based organizations that have developed specialization in cultural competence is threatened. These organizations are also threatened by managed care's reliance on educational standards and accreditation to ensure quality because staff with cultural expertise may lack professional qualifications.

MCOs can learn to become culturally competent. They may not have the public sector's experience in serving culturally diverse populations, but competitive forces can create the incentive to learn. In areas where managed care programs are voluntary or where multiple MCOs are competing for Medicaid enrollees, some MCOs have aggressively recruited culturally competent staff and increased their training activities. An example of an MCO's increasing its cultural competence is provided by California Kaiser Permanente. Kaiser pursues MediCal enrollment by advertising in multiple languages, developing services that meet the population's needs, relocating clinics to reduce access barriers, and contracting out for such services as visiting nurses when the in-house array is insufficient.

Competitive forces, however, cannot be relied on to achieve culturally competent systems of care. Public agencies issuing requests for proposals can specify standards for culturally competent care, such as documentation of linguistic appropriateness, staff training on cultural competence, and use of organizational policies and procedures that support competency practices. To date, cultural competence requirements have rarely been incorporated into contractual language, but California is one state developing standards and addressing these issues. For example,

California's managed Medicaid program requires that MCOs use enrollees' preferred language when there are at least 3,000 people eligible to enroll in the service area who prefer that language. Just as with outcome measurement, groups are forming to propose cultural competence standards for use in managed care, such as the National Latino Behavioral Health Workgroup.

Outcome measurement can be used to monitor an organization's cultural competence. Population profile data, such as language needs, utilization patterns, length of stay, and client satisfaction, can be used by policymakers to flag areas needing attention. For example, short lengths of stay for a particular cultural group might indicate an organization's inability to serve that group adequately. Furthermore, service outcomes for nondominant culture groups can be compared among organizations. Culturally competent organizations would be expected to achieve better results because they have been able to communicate more effectively and develop more appropriate interventions.

To ensure that adequate input from diverse clientele reaches MCOs, often located far from the site of service delivery, public-sector payers can consider requiring community participation in an MCO's development of a managed care program. MCOs may be required to develop a staffing and program plan based on an analysis of the population profile.

The proportion of people of color in this country is growing (by the year 2000, 33 percent of the population under age 19 is projected to be members of nondominant racial and ethnic groups). Cultural competence will be an increasingly central part of any plan or system claiming to provide comprehensive care.

Legal Issues

Managed care brings with it a set of new legal considerations. Contract negotiation has become a highly prized skill, as public payers enter into contracts with MCOs and MCOs in turn contract with providers. There is a danger that parties entering into contracts may not realize the full ramifications of the services they are obligating themselves to perform. When devising contracts, both parties must learn how to take into account consent decrees, existing laws and regulations, as well as their own responsibility toward public populations.

Disparate power between negotiating parties can give rise to antitrust suits. For example, a group of physicians has charged a company with violating antitrust laws by pressuring it to accept unconditionally the HMO's contract terms. In another antitrust case, doctors and hospitals have been accused of operating a monopoly that tried to keep out lower-priced managed care plans. Lawsuits alleging conflict of interest or improper procurement practices are also proliferating among states and would-be contractors as MCOs contest the awards of contracts to competitors.

Managed care has also brought a new twist to malpractice lawsuits. Are providers liable for discontinuing treatment or failing to treat people when the MCO denies treatment? Court decisions predating managed care indicate that once a patient is accepted for treatment, health care providers have an obligation to furnish all necessary care; however, providers cannot be expected to provide unlimited amounts of uncompensated care (Appelbaum, 1993). A new form of defensive medicine may develop wherein providers appeal all denials of treatment by MCOs in an attempt to protect themselves from liability. When the provider and the MCO are one and the same, matters are further complicated. What is the liability of a provider, at risk for the cost of services, who reduces the amount of services provided in order to save money? States can retrieve money from MCOs for contract noncompliance, but are clients also entitled to enforce the contract under which services are being provided? Who is responsible for providing and paying for services ordered by a court, such as civil or community (outpatient) commitment?

Major legal changes must be made at all levels of government if managed care's full impact is to be felt. Federal waivers of the Medicaid, Child Welfare Services, and Foster Care and Adoption Assistance programs are necessary to free funding from its regulatory strictures. State and local agencies may find it necessary to streamline their procurement processes, which often are rigid and impede public organizations' ability to adapt to quickly changing circumstances. For example, some states are prohibited from entering into contracts for longer than one year, but contracts that short can lead to major disruptions in the services system and fail to provide incentives for contractors to make long-term investments.

Public agencies also may face a complete overhaul of their contract-monitoring functions because the complexities of managed care contracting and application of legal and contract provisions to subcontractors require increasing sophistication. Personnel systems also may face fundamental restructuring because managed care may involve increased privatization. To avoid costly delays and lawsuits, public officials proposing managed care initiatives that will replace publicly provided services with contracted services should engage labor leaders in discussions early in the planning process. A variety of strategies address the issue of displaced employees, such as mandating employment of displaced employees by contractors, offering displaced employees first consideration for employment by contractors, reassignment to other public agencies, working within attrition rates, retraining employees, or assisting them with career planning (O'Leary & Eggers, 1993).

The child welfare system, operating under a high level of legal mandates, introduces additional complexity. Courts have authority over child placement that is outside the managed care entity's control. The few operational child welfare managed care programs have been small enough to work closely with judges who have cooperated with preplacement assessments and recommendations. These interventions, however, are being operated by traditional providers rather than by national managed care entities. Furthermore, some judges, even without managed care, make their own treatment and placement decisions without following recommendations of child welfare workers. Managed care providers could find themselves responsible for care planned and ordered without their input.

MCOs are learning to interact with court systems. For example, MCOs have been known to approach the court on behalf of an enrollee facing charges for driving while intoxicated, letting the judge know what alternative services could be provided through the MCO. Experience gained from the health care sector can be applied to other child- and family-serving sectors. For example, MCOs covering youths who become involved in the juvenile justice system could use presentencing assessments as a means of developing options for the courts. Incentives, however, must be in place to motivate MCOs to divert children from detention.

References

Appelbaum, P. (1993). Legal liability and managed care. *American Psychologist, 48*, 251–257.

Cross, T., Bazron, B. J., Dennis, K. W., & Isaacs, M. R. (1989). *Towards a culturally competent system of care.* Washington, DC: CASSP Technical Assistance Center.

Donahue, J. (1989). *The privatization decision: Public ends, private needs.* New York: Basic Books.

Federation of Families for Children's Mental Health. (1995, Summer). Principles of family involvement in the development and operation of managed health and mental health care systems for children and youth. *Claiming Children,* pp. 10–11.

Koyanagi, C. (1995). *Managing managed care for publicly financed mental health services.* Washington, DC: Bazelon Center for Mental Health Law.

Newcheck, P., Hughes, D. C., Stoddard, J. J., & Halfon, N. (1994). Children with chronic illness and Medicaid managed care. *Pediatrics, 93,* 497–500.

O'Leary, J., & Eggers, W. (1993). *Privatization and public employees: Guidelines for fair treatment.* Los Angeles: Reason Foundation.

Roberts, R., Barclay-McLaughlin, G., Cleveland, J., Colston, W., Malach, W., Mulvey, L., Rodriguez, G., Thomas, T., & Yonemitsu, D. (1990). *Developing culturally competent programs for families of children with special needs.* Washington, DC: Georgetown University Child Development Center.

Rowland, D., Rosenbaum, S., Simon, L., & Chait, E. (1995). *Medicaid and managed care: Lessons from the literature.* Menlo Park, CA: Kaiser Commission on the Future of Medicaid.

Wehr, E., & Jameson, E. (1994). Beyond benefits: The importance of a pediatric standard in private insurance contracts to ensuring health access for children. *Future of Children, 4,* 115–133.

PART **TWO**

State Privatization Case Study

Managing Organizational Change: The Massachusetts Department of Mental Health Experience in Preparing for Managed Care

Eileen Elias and Marc Navon

Organizational change is one of the most significant challenges facing providers of health services in a rapidly changing health care environment. Market forces have driven massive restructuring of the health care system. Purchasers of mental health care are more sophisticated, demanding accountability for quality and cost containment to a degree never before imagined (Hammer & Champy, 1993).

Managed care has been the catalyst for these changes. Although the private sector is not immune to these pressures, managers in the public arena face daunting service, political, and fiscal challenges as they grapple to manage organizational change in transforming a traditional service system into one that can function within today's health care environment. The public outcry for more accountability and the streamlining of government has accelerated this restructuring.

State mental health authorities are more like buses than sports cars—they function best when not required to turn quickly. Inflexibility, unresponsiveness, the absence of consumer focus, obsession with activity rather than result, and inefficiency depict many government health care agencies (Essock & Goldman, 1995). These organizations work within a fixed budget and must navigate the state bureaucracy, accurately reading and capitalizing on changing political winds and setting a course for change without becoming grounded on bureaucratic shoals.

By describing the principles and action steps that drove the restructuring of the public mental health system in Massachusetts from 1991 to 1996, this chapter tries to answer the following questions:

- What challenges do health care managers face in restructuring a public system of care?
- What are helpful strategies, and where are pitfalls?
- How can change be accomplished effectively?

The Massachusetts process entailed managing the transition from an outdated, fragmented, and inefficient state hospital–based system to an integrated, comprehensive community services system better able to meet consumer need within the context of profound service, political, and fiscal challenges. The advent of managed care as it was mandated by the legislature made Medicaid, rather than the Massachusetts Department of Mental Health (DMH), the steward of mental health care services in the commonwealth.

NOTE: Originally published as Elias, E., & Navon, M. (1996). Implementing managed care in a state mental health authority: Implications for organizational change. *Smith College Studies in Social Work, 66,* 269–292.

The change process began in 1991 with a vision articulated by the newly appointed DMH commissioner that based on principles of consumer empowerment, community-based organized systems of care, the flexible use of resources, and accountability. This chapter describes the common challenges managers face in the change process, how the DMH approached those key issues strategically, and the critical role of leadership in producing positive reform. Although the restructuring process occurred within a specific public system, the central themes are applicable to other public and private systems.

Historical Context

By statute, the DMH provides services for citizens with long-term or serious mental illness, early and ongoing treatment of mental illness, research into the causes and treatment of mental illness, and emergency and crisis mental health services, and ensures a comprehensive service system. Massachusetts has a population of about 6 million people, and an estimated 44,730 adults are diagnosed with serious mental illness (Regier et al., 1988). The DMH services system is based on the assessed needs of about 80,000 children and adults. Its budget for fiscal year 1996 was nearly $520 million.

A severe budget crisis in Massachusetts and a tide of demands for change led to the election of Republican Governor William F. Weld in 1991 with a mandate to streamline state government. Responding to this mandate, Weld formed a special commission on consolidation of facilities charged with providing a blueprint for consolidating existing public health facilities and ensuring consumer access to quality services. The commission recommended closure of nine public health hospitals, including four DMH hospitals.

In June 1991, Weld appointed Eileen Elias, a DMH area director, as DMH commissioner. In her previous 25 years of work in the private and public sectors serving mentally ill people, Elias used a vision of change—a systems approach to providing consumer-based care by integrating inpatient and community-based services.

Elias initially found the DMH to be a highly centralized service system controlled by a central office largely out of touch with local needs. Budget cuts amounting to $55 million had undermined fiscal support of community services. A disproportionate share of the DMH budget was tied to maintaining antiquated state hospitals (Leadholm & Kerzner, 1995). The system was characterized by a limited focus on the needs of consumers and their families at the local level; decimated accountability structures (licensing and quality management staff had been laid off, there was no consistent set of objectives and time frames by which to hold managers accountable, and providers had no performance standards); and inpatient, emergency, community support, rehabilitation, and housing services were fragmented. Six percent of DMH priority clients served in inpatient settings annually used 42 percent of the agency's resources. At least 750 DMH inpatients awaited community placement. Statutorily required area board roles and responsibilities were poorly defined, and consumer participation was inadequate. Collaboration among the DMH and other state child- and adult-serving agencies lacked standardization and clear expectations, with agency "turf" boundaries often hindering effective services delivery. And the legislature had mandated the state's Medicaid agency to implement managed care for mental health without the DMH's involvement.

In response to the agenda for change necessitated by the administration, by the legislature, and by consumer needs, Elias worked intensively with all mental health constituents, developing and articulating the vision of change and challenging them to help develop the restructuring blueprint. She communicated around the state by telephone, memo, and meetings explaining to constituents that the DMH had to become more proactively involved in the restructuring process to ensure that consumer need would be preserved as a priority. The alternative would be draconian cuts in services.

The new structure was to evolve into a community-based, integrated, comprehensive system of care accountable for access, quality, and cost and was to assess and meet consumer needs continually. This restructuring encompassed an inclusionary planning process needed to create a comprehensive, integrated spectrum of community—rather than institutionally based services. The new system—the "Comprehensive Community Support System" (CCSS)—was to help constituents understand that this system would be the basis for managed care and would preserve access and quality, rather than sacrificing it in the name of saving dollars.

Vision drives action; it includes both deeply felt values and a picture of the organization's focus (Belasco, 1990). The efforts to define this vision culminated in a forum held at the State House in September 1991 to stress the importance of the restructuring. Eight hundred people attended representing all vested interests in mental health: consumers, family members, legislators, DMH staff, providers, trade organizations, personnel from other human services agencies, academics, and advocates. The statewide CCSS committee and five task forces were formed to work on implementing the agenda for change, based on the Governor's Special Commission on Consolidation of Facilities report mandating that the DMH carry out state hospital closure and the transfer of inpatient acute care to more appropriate and expanded community care as well as the legislative mandate to Medicaid to implement managed behavioral health.

The subgroups completed their work in January 1992, defining the standards necessary to plan the new system. This work, documented in a manual called the *Green Book*, advanced public managed care as a tool. The manual was designed as a resource guide for local planning participants and provided standards for the CCSS by defining the mission, values, and structure for re-engineering the services system.

Restructuring Steps

Six steps defined and carried out the restructuring. From 1991 to 1996, these steps helped the DMH expand its role as the advocate for consumers with mental illness in the changing health care world by

1. articulating and maintaining principles directing the process
2. ensuring support
3. maintaining an inclusive, participatory process
4. providing ongoing education and training on restructuring, including an aggressive public affairs strategy
5. ensuring a balanced staff representing the private and public sectors that would support the public–private partnership germane to the initiative
6. engaging in a partnership with Medicaid and other health and human services agencies.

STEP 1: GUIDING PRINCIPLES

A set of four guiding principles was developed to direct the local planning process undertaken by all stakeholders; those principles were key to following through with system reform steps:

1. supporting consumer empowerment and reducing stigma
2. developing an organized system of care
3. using resources flexibly
4. demanding accountability.

Principle 1: Consumer Empowerment and Stigma Reduction

Consumer empowerment is a national self-help movement that empowers consumers to help change the existing mental health system to become more responsive to their needs and to help address the stigma of mental illness (Leete, 1988). It was essential that consumer empowerment drive the restructuring process. The historic emphasis on provider need rather than consumer need would have negated this restructuring.

The concept of consumer empowerment permeated the restructuring; each new DMH policy was so directed. Clear vision, strong leadership, and the development of trust with an initially wary consumer population were necessary. Consumers were assured they were not being patronized for ulterior, self-serving motives. The creation of an Office of Consumer and Ex-Patient Relations throughout the system built trust. Consumers were also actively engaged in policy development at all levels of the organization. Credibility was achieved by frank, open, two-way communication. The focus on consumer empowerment was grounded in the conviction that people with serious mental illness have the same rights and responsibilities as others. With the new vision, the fragmented system of care tied to fitting consumers into programs evolved through the locally based planning processes.

Four years into the restructuring process, the DMH's focus on consumer empowerment became evident when an internal report of patient deaths and suicides was released in an information request. The data indicated that deaths in the state mental health system had risen by 79 percent between 1991 and 1993. When this information reached the public, it was used as evidence that the DMH restructuring was detrimental to seriously mentally ill people. The commissioner was called to testify and explain the statistics to the legislature's House Post-Audit and Oversight Committee. Hundreds of consumers gathered at the State House to support the DMH restructuring and gave the message that they would not be forced back into state hospitals. Elias explained that in 1992 the criteria for reporting client deaths were expanded to include a broader range of people having contact with the DMH. Although the increase in the reports of death resulted from this expanded method of collecting data, various mental health advocates and the main Boston newspaper continued to use the data as "proof" that managed care was the cause of increased deaths.

To deal proactively with this issue, Elias sought an independent group of researchers and others from the federal government which commissioned them to investigate further the reported increase in deaths and its relation to the restructuring. The team's report revealed an actual *decline* in the rate of consumer deaths from 1991 to 1993 (Critical Incident Reporting Task Force, 1996).

Principle 2: Organized System of Care

An organized system of care is an integrated financing and delivery system using multidisciplinary providers selected by quality and cost management criteria. It incorporates continuous quality improvement and incentives to provide appropriate and required acute and continuing care and is accountable to consumers and purchasers for quality, cost, and outcome criteria (England & Goff, 1993). The DMH implemented this organized, integrated system of care as the basis of restructuring. Medical, psychiatric, rehabilitative or vocational, and social support services and non–mental health services are integrated to attend to consumer need.

The organizational structures of the DMH and its citizen advisory boards were also defined to direct the process of change. Under the guidance of area directorss, CCSS planning and implementation occurred. The area directors were responsible for ensuring consistency across the area's CCSS sites and were held accountable to the central office, which monitored performance.

Developing the CCSS with consumer input sent a strong message to providers urging a change from program-oriented practice patterns. Creative diversionary, outreach, supportive education, employment, and housing services were established to help consumers live effectively in the community—a goal consistently articulated by consumers.

Principle 3: Flexible Use of Resources

One of the basic ingredients of managed care is the ability to use funding, staff and other resources flexibly and cost effectively. Historically, resources were allocated by the legislature through the DMH to fund categorical programs such as state hospitals and community mental health centers. This prevented flexible, innovative use of resources to meet consumer need. The DMH changed the categorical account structure into flexible allocations to support CCSS development by

- consolidating facilities and further downsizing through FY 1996, redirecting $70 million to enhance community services
- reducing administrative costs and reinvesting in such accountability systems as licensing, quality management, utilization management, and human rights—all of which were decimated during the budget cuts of 1990–91.

Dollars were used more flexibly both to change residential services provision so that it emphasized support services and to initiate a variety of home-based wraparound services to help the child remain at home. Similarly, resources were heavily invested to expand contracts with clubhouse programs and other community-based services to help consumers live more independently (Elias & Navon, 1995).

Principle 4: Accountability

A good managed care program must have systems in place to account for access, quality, and cost-effectiveness. Accountability was achieved through consistency in communication, planned follow-through, and policies and procedures that ensured access to and quality of services. When the DMH set out to accomplish an objective, it communicated its intent and, with stakeholder participation, laid the foundation to make it happen. In the fishbowl environment of this public bureaucracy, accurate, up-to-date information was made available. Criticisms based on anecdotal information were evaluated objectively, and responses were formulated.

The DMH invested heavily in sophisticated management information systems to ensure state-of-the-art communication and data availability. Data were important in managing the change process and in demonstrating that increased access to community services reduced inpatient use and readmissions (Pallak, Combings, Darken, & Hence, 1993).

To foster credibility with constituents and the legislature, the DMH published regular reports that outlined statistics such as readmissions, living status, and engagement in community-based services. Monthly management reports provided data on categories such as employee use of sick time, residential census, and revenue collected by the areas. Actual performance was reported in relation to established benchmarks.

A consumer-oriented total quality management approach to the delivery of mental health services was implemented to include the following actions:

- developing quality management and utilization management infrastructures that supported constituent involvement
- holding providers of public and contracted services accountable for self-monitoring and other quality management reporting
- instituting quality councils at the central office and field office levels
- creating medical director positions in each area DMH office to improve accountability for the quality of clinical care
- implementing performance-based contracting
- placing human rights officers in the field
- requiring DMH-contracted and -operated facilities to be certified by the Health Care Financing Administration (HCFA) and accredited by the Joint Commission on Accreditation of Healthcare Organizations (JCAHO). The southeastern area was the first public system of mental health to become JCAHO network accredited in the nation.

Strengthening the area and site boards empowered them to be watchdogs for the services system. Citizen monitoring processes in which citizens conducted onsite program visits enhanced the DMH's credibility. The Statewide Advisory Council developed a citizen's monitoring handbook that provided guidelines for citizens visiting residential programs to collect, record, and report on consumer service satisfaction.

Accountability was important with outside agencies. In dealing with Medicaid, the DMH was historically perceived as an agency that lacked accountability in its use of Medicaid resources. It was crucial to change this perception by developing a positive relationship with Medicaid because of the legislatively mandated managed care initiative.

STEP 2: ENSURING SUPPORT

The 80/20 rule suggests that 20 percent of people are open to change, and 80 percent will resist it by varying degrees (Oakley & Krug, 1991). An attractive new vision for needed change is not enough to make it happen—the manager of change must mobilize the support of the people both above and below and of external constituents (Hammer & Champy, 1993; Leete, 1988). Ensuring this support was the second step in the restructuring process; it helped overcome obstacles to change. The base of support included backing from the governor, the secretary of the Executive

Office of Health and Services, and the Massachusetts legislature. Other government agencies that were key in the restructuring process (for example, the departments of public health, education and training, social services, and mental retardation), consumers, legislators, advocates, providers, and all other stakeholders were also involved.

Support from the governor and the secretary for health and human services was necessary on several fronts. They shared the burden of managing change, serving as buffers when necessary and as advocates for the DMH. Tough problems, such as housing for people with mental illness in communities with a not-in-my-backyard mentality and restructuring of professional groups, pointed up the importance of working in a bipartisan manner to garner support from the legislature for DMH initiatives. Because restructuring included consolidating state hospitals and moving acute care to a network of public and private hospitals, the loss of union membership was perceived as a threat. Some used the media in attempts to thwart those changes. This dynamic was addressed by taking the following actions:

- Preparing employees for the changes—the human resources department worked extensively to prepare displaced workers for outplacement, and early retirement and severance packages were made available. In 1997, less than 6 percent of the 4,000 employees laid off were unemployed.
- Holding monthly advocacy breakfasts with 18 constituents from consumer, advocate, and public and private provider groups to ensure two-way communication regarding policy and planning developments. Differing views were expressed and addressed.
- Making necessary management changes in a time-sensitive manner. Some veteran staff approached the vision of change with skepticism: "I'll outlast this plan because it will die of its own weight." Key managers were asked about their attitudes toward restructuring, and their responses clearly indicated teamwork, willingness to support the new mission, contribution, and openness to sharing information. Personnel changes followed within 10 days after the commissioner took office.
- Engaging managers in the change process by ensuring a defined area–central office partnership. Managers were helped to share information and expertise by being brought together to identify the best practices, provide mutual support, and learn about what worked and what did not. The central office focused on standard development and technical assistance.
- Holding an annual Commissioner's Recognition Night, on which constituents were publicly recognized for outstanding performance. To emphasize their importance, these events were held in the State Capitol.

STEP 3: MAINTAINING THE PARTICIPATORY PROCESS

The third step involved instituting a participatory process grounded in the principles of consumer empowerment, shared accountability for outcomes, and the importance of all constituents in the process. To the extent that constituent input was sought, the DMH expected dissent from its staff, providers, consumers, advocates, and legislators. Dissent was sometimes subtle, sometimes very vocal; often it took the form of personal attack.

Critical to effective leadership is the ability to manage perception and withstand criticism. Strategies used to deal with this dynamic included open communication through the area directors to their citizen advisory boards and within all levels of the department. Consumers and other stakeholders were critical in garnering the support necessary to address significant resistance to change.

An example of the participatory process occurred with the restructuring of the services system through the closure of four state hospitals and the movement of the locus of care to community-based services. This precipitated an open rift between consumer and advocate camps. Specifically, consumers became vociferous in support of their right to have the community rather than the state hospital system as the focal point of the system of care. Family members, on the other hand, were alarmed by the perceived loss of a state hospital "safety net." It was critical to educate and assure advocates that the safety net could be transferred from the institutional setting to the CCSS. There would always be a need to maintain a critical number of state hospital beds for the most severely disabled people.

STEP 4: EDUCATION, TRAINING, RESEARCH, AND PUBLIC RELATIONS

The fourth step comprised educating and training all stakeholders about the restructuring initiative and the ongoing research and evaluation of its effects. People within and outside of the DMH were uninformed or misinformed about the role of managed care as a management tool in the transformation. Stakeholder dissent was based largely on anecdotal information. Through continuous formal training, educational workshops, and focus groups, stakeholders began to understand the principles that informed the restructuring steps. A series of training seminars was held statewide. Participants included all stakeholders. Sessions clarified the guiding principles and steps needed to implement the CCSS. Newsletters were published regularly by the DMH Office of Consumer and Ex-Patient Relations. Statewide information and training helped address anxiety. Other trainings covered topics such as quality improvement, case management, utilization management, clinical issues (for example, assessing and managing dangerousness and risk), human rights, and multicultural differences.

Two centers for excellence were funded by the DMH to provide research and evaluation and to further the field's advancements in treating mental illness. Restructuring research involved expanding it statewide. Clear expectations were set with researchers to ensure accountability and alignment with the DMH mission. The contributions of these centers advanced research in the field of treatment and rehabilitation at a time when other states were cutting back.

Maintaining an aggressive public affairs strategy was critical. The DMH executive staff worked with field managers to direct a strategy that would highlight positive changes in the system for consumers. Although the principal Boston newspaper was critical of the restructuring, local newspapers statewide were open to reporting on its strengths.

At the national level, the commissioner participated as a board member in the National Association of State Mental Health Program Directors as well as its Steering Committee on Health Care Reform. The DMH staff communicated to other states information about achievements and lessons learned from the public managed care initiative, and Massachusetts was perceived as a leader two years into the managed behavioral health initiative.

STEP 5: STAFFING BALANCE

Creating a balanced staff within the department was another factor in the restructuring initiative. Private-sector staff were recruited to balance those personnel who had been in the state system for significant periods of time. For example, the deputy commissioner for clinical and professional services and the DMH general counsel were professionals who had been in health care organizations in a variety of private-sector settings and were well versed in state-of-the-art managed care technologies. Unlike their veteran DMH counterparts, they had not worked in a government bureaucracy. There was a healthy push-and-pull dynamic between the private and public sectors. The aggressive "can-do" approach of the private-background personnel was balanced by veteran public-sector staff who brought forward valuable experience in navigating through the constraints peculiar to state agency work. Many of the restructuring initiatives could not have come to fruition without the mixed and complementary orientations of staff members and their skilled stewardship.

STEP 6: PARTNERSHIP WITH MEDICAID

It was crucial for the DMH to develop a working relationship with the state Medicaid agency. The relationship historically had been marked by mistrust and minimal collaboration. A joint planning and purchasing venture designed to use resources more flexibly and effectively was initiated. A strong alliance with Medicaid was needed for the following reasons:

- Medicaid was the largest purchasing source of mental health services in Massachusetts and was influential in deciding how those services were defined and delivered.
- The majority of DMH priority consumers were Medicaid recipients and directly affected by Medicaid policy.
- Medicaid was mandated by the legislature to embark on a managed care program for Medicaid-funded mental health services. This mandate did not obligate Medicaid to work with the DMH.

An agreement signed in October 1992 delineated roles and responsibilities for Medicaid's managed behavioral health care organization (MBHO) and the DMH in caring for shared mental health consumers. Medicaid was not a signatory to this agreement. The MBHO and the DMH jointly procured a statewide network of emergency services programs and established standards of care to upgrade this critical "front-door" service. Utilization management clinical criteria and protocols were implemented to guide decision making. Those protocols defined assessment, referral, and inpatient transfer procedures and criteria. Unprecedented, they defined the boundary between acute, medically necessary services provided by the MBHO and subacute or continuing care rehabilitative and social support services administered by the DMH.

As the Medicaid managed care program progressed, ambiguity as to which organization was the primary state mental health authority emerged. The DMH and MBHO had overlapping networks of acute care and duplication of case management services, undercutting the principle of flexible and efficient use of resources (Pallak et al., 1993). Continuity of care was an issue for the dually managed population: Inpatient readmission rates were more than double those of the population managed solely by the MBHO or the DMH. Data were not shared, and referrals were made increasingly on the basis of who paid their bills rather than on clinical need. The inability to share databases combined with complicated issues of interagency confidentiality impeded monitoring and evaluation.

In response, the DMH and Medicaid launched an initiative to improve the quality of acute mental health care and cost-effectiveness by more flexible use of combined resources. A framework document signed by the commissioners of Medicaid and the DMH in September 1995 committed the agencies jointly to plan, procure, and monitor a more fully integrated approach to the delivery of a publicly funded comprehensive services system, regardless of payment source. On behalf of the state, Medicaid contracted with a new MBHO to manage the entire acute care system. The DMH provided continuing care for consumers and held Medicaid legally accountable for provision of acute care, thus ensuring this one-tier system of care.

The interagency service agreement provided for the DMH to purchase acute care from Medicaid, according to specifications developed by the DMH. Those specifications included access, types of services, program standards, quality and utilization management expectations, reporting requirements, human rights procedures, critical-incident reporting procedures, and licensing along with other financial and service specifications. The system was based on DMH policies and regulations. The department was the single state mental health authority. This agreement preserved the DMH as the "executive director" of all public mental health care. This step required a major change in mind-set at the central and field levels: Managers were less responsible for day-to-day services system management and increasingly accountable to oversight of acute care delivered by Medicaid through its MBHO.

The mental health specifications incorporated into the MBHO contract were developed with the input of consumers, families, providers, and other interested parties, thus maintaining the principles of participatory process and consumer empowerment. For the first time, mental health consumers and family members participated in the Medicaid MBHO procurement process.

Benefits of this plan included an annually defined portion of savings generated from improved utilization management, maximized benefit eligibility, and reduced duplication of services. Those savings were used to expand the DMH continuing care system, which helped decrease use of the acute care system (Pallak et al., 1993).

As with any new initiative, there are risks that must be carefully assessed and managed. Relinquishing DMH's direct management of the acute care system to maximize resources and use them more flexibly was a source of concern. The participatory process established clear safeguards by incorporating DMH purchasing specifications into the MBHO contract, and the interagency service agreement with Medicaid, that delineated DMH oversight authority, helped ameliorate many of these anxieties.

Summary

From 1992 to 1996, the DMH restructuring initiative produced significant results. Resources were moved from antiquated, inefficient state hospitals to expand and to improve the amount and quality of community programs and to establish supporting infrastructures. The department reduced its use of inpatient care by 32 percent through closing four state hospitals and developing 1,600 residential units and 186 acute inpatient beds in 10 "replacement units" in general hospitals. These changes significantly increased the quality and cost-effectiveness of care provided to consumers.

The DMH evolved into a consumer-driven services organization with sound mechanisms for ensuring accountability and managing quality and with the flexibility to allocate resources according to local needs. It supported a managed system whose consumer focus promoted independence, community living, and services delivery. The DMH's standards of care—the bases of its quality and utilization management infrastructures—helped it evolve into an effective purchaser of behavioral health services.

The interagency service agreement between the DMH and Medicaid laid the foundation for this health care role. By moving to a one-tier system of publicly provided mental health care, the DMH linked the delivery of acute care and continuing community services, regardless of payment source. Specified savings are now redirected to the DMH to support services expansion and to reduce unnecessary hospitalizations.

The partnership between Medicaid and the DMH remains a priority. Continuing advocacy and clarity of principles are necessary to ensure that future decisions are not fiscally based. No matter the specific model of care (that is, carve-in or carve-out), it is imperative that the DMH remain the driver of the care system for mental health consumers.

Conclusion

Managers of change must establish a clear and energized vision based on principles that garner support and guide restructuring. The legacy left behind by this administration includes the focus on consumer empowerment, an organized system of care, the value of a participatory process, accountability systems, and standards of care. The evolution of a partnership with Medicaid has affirmed the DMH's role in overseeing a comprehensive, integrated system of care for mental health consumers.

Two years after the fact, this legacy continues. As an example, in 1998, the DMH and Medicaid used the previously developed behavioral health specifications in their request for responses (RFR) for HMOs. This was the first time such comprehensive and rigorous mental health programming requirements had been contained in a Medicaid RFR for its contracted full-service health plans. Purchasing specifications requiring services ranging from residential step-down care for adolescents to special care models for homeless people and for dually diagnosed populations were included. For many HMOs, those innovative, population-specific services presented programmatic and financial challenges.

The importance of leadership cannot be overemphasized—that is, the type of leadership that recognizes what needs to be done, accomplishes it, and ensures continuity to protect that work from being undone. In most situations, the leader must recognize that there is a limited period of time to effect lasting change.

References

Belasco, J. (1990). *Teaching the elephant to dance: The manager's guide to empowering change.* New York: Plume Books.

Critical Incident Reporting Task Force. (1996, January 26). *Report on Massachusetts Department of Mental Health Service recipient mortality (1991–1993).* Cambridge, MA: Evaluation Center at Human Services Resource Institute.

Elias, E., & Navon, M. (1995). The Massachusetts experience with managed mental health care and Medicaid. *Health Affairs, 14*(3), 46–49.

England, M. J., & Goff, V. (1993). Health reform and organized systems of care. In W. Goldman & S. Feldman (Eds.), *New directions for mental health services* (Monograph 59). San Francisco: Jossey-Bass.

Essock, S., & Goldman, H. (1995). States' embrace of managed mental health. *Health Affairs, 14*(3), 34–44.

Hammer, M., & Champy, J. (1993). *Reengineering the corporation.* New York: HarperCollins.

Leadholm, B., & Kerzner, J. (1995). Public managed care: Comprehensive community support in Massachusetts. *Administration and Policy in Mental Health, 22,* 543–552.

Leete, E. (1988). *The role of the consumer movement and persons with mental illness* (Switzer monograph). Washington, DC: National Rehabilitation Association.

Pallak, M., Combings, N., Darken, H., & Hence, C. (1993). Managed mental health, Medicaid and medical cost offset. In W. Goldman & S. Feldman (Eds.), *New directions for mental health services* (Monograph 59, pp. 27–40). San Francisco: Jossey-Bass.

Oakley, E., & Krug, D. (1991). *Enlightened leadership.* New York: Simon & Schuster.

Regier, D. A., et al. (1988). One-month prevalence of mental disorders in the United States. *Archives of General Psychiatry, 45,* 977–988.

CHAPTER 10

Privatization and Mental Health in Massachusetts

Matthew P. Dumont

I watched the process and effects of one small rivulet of the tidal wave of change in the privatization of mental health services in Massachusetts. As always, the social costs of this initiative were massive, immediate, and obvious, as was the protest against them. A coalition of public service unions, patient advocacy groups, patients themselves, and their clinicians devoted two years to organizing, educating themselves and the public, and lobbying legislators. Their efforts resulted in the enactment, over the governor's veto, of a bill that significantly slowed the process of privatization.

Although not the total moratorium desired by some of us, the law, drawn up as the Pacheco Bill, imposes on the state the obligation to demonstrate that actual cost savings would occur as the result of contracting with private corporations and it permits public servants, through their unions, the opportunity to compete with the private sector in cost containment and quality of services. There is also, for the first time, a legislative-monitoring function imposed on the private contracts that are signed.

Despite these minimal constraints on privatization, the Pacheco Bill was bitterly opposed by lobbyists for private interests and by Governor William Weld himself, whose philosophy of "entrepreneurial government" is based on the assumption that market forces bring efficiency, economy, and quality to public services. The leadership of his Department of Mental Health (DMH) operationalized his philosophy with a program based on downsizing (consolidating and closing) mental hospitals, laying off clinicians working in outpatient settings, and quickly contracting out as many direct or indirect services as possible. The central office of the DMH insisted that privatizing its programs would make them "equal to or better than" those provided by its own employees. The realities told a different story. The privatization of outpatient clinics in Massachusetts was associated with the laying off of 800 publicly salaried professionals. Contracts to private providers involved at least a 25 percent reduction in clinical personnel. In some cases, whole clinics were closed and others were consolidated. Patients accustomed to local, easily accessible centers or to home visits when they were housebound were often referred to larger and more distant facilities. It is not known how many patients subsequently dropped out of

NOTE: Originally published as Dumont, M. P. (1996). Privatization and mental health in Massachusetts. *Smith College Studies in Social Work, 66,* 293–303.

treatment, but observations from several facilities suggest that the number was high. Those lost to treatment were often those most in need—elderly men and women, disabled people, and socially incompetent people.

Community clinics used to be the first places contacted when patients became suicidal or psychotic. In the absence of such clinics, the emergency wards of general hospitals become the only recourse. There, after as much as a six-hour wait, a psychiatric resident who does not know the patient must evaluate his or her suicidal risk or other potential for violence. Errors are more frequent in such settings, with the attendant financial and human costs. This is on top of the inflated cost of any emergency ward visit which, through Medicaid or other insurers, is passed on to the general public.

The closing, consolidation, and privatization of state hospitals in Massachusetts has been even more devastating to patients. A century after the pioneering reforms of Dorothea Dix, impoverished people with mental illness are once again being found on the commonwealth's streets, in jails, and in shelters (the almshouses of the day).

In a nine-month period in 1992, at least 170 people were found to have been discharged to two major Boston shelters for homeless people. Following the closure of one state hospital, one of the shelters reported a 40 percent increase in the number of people with mental illness seeking admission (Massachusetts Human Services Coalition, 1992).

The private psychiatric hospitals or inpatient units of general hospitals that were expected to replace the state hospitals are themselves intolerant to these patients. They are disinclined to accept "disposition problems" who strain their utilization review guidelines. In some situations, they have already revealed their capacity to abuse public contracts through "creative accounting" and "case-mix management" techniques of questionable legality.

In any case, even when private facilities accept violent, disorganized, or homeless psychiatric patients, they do so only for brief periods, with the result that more patients are stuck in a useless, expensive, and demoralizing pattern of repeated admissions. The consequence is that greater numbers of psychotic people live on the streets and more deaths occur from exposure, suicide, or homicide. A major study of more than 9,000 patients with schizophrenia admitted to Danish psychiatric hospitals between 1970 and 1988 revealed that the effect of shortening first admissions from an average of 50 days to an average of 30 days doubled the suicide rate among such patients ("Gold Mine of Psychiatric Data," 1993).

It is hard to convey the depth of individual misery that resides in those realities. One year after I was laid off by the Massachusetts DMH from a clinic in which I had worked for 16 years, one of my former patients committed suicide. I had seen him through a series of crises for 15 years. He lived an isolated and paranoid existence. I may have been his only social contact, his only friend. He accepted my departure matter-of-factly but refused to go across the bridge from Chelsea to Boston to the mental hospital where he was told to "get his medicine." The home visits, the encounters in the street, the waves from the window—the whole pattern of informal and easy access that adds up to a community mental health program—was lost to privatization. I believe the loss killed him.

In August 1994, when hospital and clinic downsizing was already well established, the Boston news was dominated by two separate shootings of police officers. One of the officers was killed. In the media there were pictures of grieving families and fellow officers. Just behind the pathos and bitterness of those events was the information that in both cases the shootings were committed by "mentally deranged" people whose access to mental health care had been compromised by "lack of insurance" and unavailable public services. Privatization is a killer ("Gold Mine," 1993).

The phasing-down period in state hospitals scheduled to close is highly stressful for the patient population that is least easily discharged—the most violent and helpless patients. They may be transferred from one ward to another repeatedly before relocation to another institution. Hospital staffs face layoffs or a confused and demoralized "bumping" procedure. They tend to be dispirited, angry, and less motivated. In one institution, the consequence was a dramatic rise in the number of serious incidents, such as assaults, fires, suicides, and sometimes-fatal accidents. The overall frequency of incidents declined along with the numbers of patients in care (a fact reported with pride by the DMH), but percentages of dangerous incidents rose precipitously. With state hospitals closing, there are growing numbers of exhausted, guilt-ridden, and furious family members (generally mothers) trying to cope with the demands of former patients.

Increasing numbers of psychotic and homeless people on the streets and in shelters is accompanied by a greater risk of random violence and the spread of infection. But this is not the only burden to the community that results from privatization. Community-based mental health clinics are capable of detecting clusters of complaints that may be the first expression of a pathogenic point source involving heavy metal or organic solvent toxicity (Dumont, 1989). Larger and more centralized clinics cannot so easily determine that workers in a local factory are being exposed to neurotoxic substances whose earliest effects are irritability, insomnia, anxiety, depression, or acute psychosis. A community source of poisoning, such as the dust in a playground under a lead-painted bridge, may be detected through an unusual clustering of learning or behavior problems presenting at a local clinic and may be missed entirely by the staff of a more remote medical center.

In addition, when staff in privatized outpatient settings is paid solely on the basis of face-to-face encounters with patients, they are less likely to devote the time necessary to explore the source of clusters of complaints. It is more remunerative for private programs to place people on antianxiety drugs than to meet with community leaders, industrial hygienists, or union representatives about a focus of heavy metal or organic solvent toxicity—but it is far more expensive to the community. The lifetime costs of a single case of lead poisoning may be greater than the entire annual budget of a community mental health clinic. The smallest effort directed toward prevention and advocacy can save millions of dollars and avoid endless human misery and disability. Such efforts are not encouraged in private clinics (Dumont, 1990, 1992).

This is only one of the constraints under which mental health professionals are now operating. Practitioners face joblessness in greater numbers than ever before. Graduate programs in social work, psychology, and nursing continue to generate eager clinicians anticipating careers as psychotherapists. But jobs are less available, the private practice marketplace is already flooded, and private clinics are replacing long-term psychotherapy with brief, time-limited treatments dictated by third-party payment schemes. Managed care programs arbitrarily limit the numbers of sessions available to clients, and case management and drug therapy have replaced supportive psychotherapy for more seriously disturbed patients.

The increasingly scarce jobs for mental health professionals are themselves becoming more routinized, less thoughtful, less in practitioners' control—in short, less professional. At the very moment when a therapist has been able to establish a relationship with a brutalized child—at the moment when the child is beginning to open to another human being—suddenly an arbitrary, third-party constraint on the number of sessions paid for may force the termination of treatment.

Diagnosis-related groups or other formulas for controlling the extent and nature of privatized treatment do not permit individual professional judgments. Case discussions, when they take place at all, become meaningless exercises about arbitrary and fictive diagnostic categories (Dumont, 1987). There is no opportunity for a real and shared discussion about patients as human beings. Deliberations about ethics, mutual support, and peer supervision are out of the question.

Clinicians in privatized settings are often paid on a fee-for-service arrangement that compels them to think in terms of billable hours of direct service rather than the actual requirements of particular situations. Telephone contacts or discussions with family members, teachers, or other professionals are systematically discouraged. When incentive practice arrangements are built in, clinicians are actually paid on the basis of how much money they generate. This imposes a demeaning and demoralizing piecework mentality. Physiological measures of stress are higher when a task is rewarded on the basis of piecework rather than salaried (Johnson, 1989). In the absence of mutual support, this translates into higher rates of coronary heart disease, peptic ulcers, and hypertension as well as simple burnout.

A professional may try to keep his or her behavior independent of financial considerations, but a weekly or monthly "productivity" report relating to income or job security is hard to ignore, particularly when transmitted by an officious supervisor. Such regular feedback systems may even represent an operant-conditioning situation in which clinicians unconsciously make decisions based on productivity reports, while still believing that ethical or clinical considerations are guiding them.

In private mental hospitals, insurance and utilization review criteria result in patients being kept only as long as the coverage lasts, often being discharged on the day their insurance coverage runs out. Clinical staff must interrupt their treatment and swallow their anxiety about a possibly suicidal or homicidal patient being discharged prematurely. The burden of legal and ethical responsibility remains with the clinicians, but business managers make the decisions.

Privatization comes with a bit of contemporary cultural garbage, the mythology of management. Suffused with the arrogance and self-righteousness of a newly acquired vocabulary, holders of MBA degrees act like field marshals when confronting clinicians. They are armed with computers that generate and demand more information than is actually needed. They create their own reality and justify their own existence. Everything is reduced to millions of bits of yes-or-no decisions that mock the complexity and ambiguity of human suffering and of its relief.

Computerized information is a matter of counting and organizing isolated units. Mental health does not reside in such fragmented bits of data, and the treatment of mental illness cannot be understood within them. An hour with a person on the verge of suicide is not the same as an hour with a chronically psychotic patient or with an abused child. Managers and their computers end by redefining mental health considerations as financial ones. All patient sessions are seen to be the same. Each session generates the same amount of money, and the more money a clinician generates, the more competent he or she is thought to be.

This is all couched in a double-think mystification. During the hospital and clinic closings and layoffs in Massachusetts, central office managers were talking about "right-sizing" the system, "spreading hope," "accentuating the positive," and being "consumer driven." They instituted a "quality management" system relying on computerized printouts and slogans that belied the facts of the homelessness and violence that they had caused. Indeed, despite the Disneyland, happy-face vocabulary it used, the DMH successfully argued in court that it should have no responsibility for the care of patients who where thrown into the community after decades of residence in the state hospital system.

Along with the growing body of experience about the devastating consequences of privatization on mentally ill people and their families, there were widely reported instances of overt fraud in privatized settings. In addition, a Post-Audit and Oversight Committee report by the Massachusetts House of Representatives revealed that the reported "savings" of privatization did not, in fact, materialize (Massachusetts Senate, 1993). Such information, along with case histories and expert opinions, was part of an organized and eventually successful campaign to enact the Pacheco Bill.

As in all such campaigns, the campaign for the Pacheco Bill was made possible by building alliances among interest groups that were not naturally affiliated. Patients in a state hospital are usually a culture apart from and often in conflict with the clinical teams responsible for them. When privatization threatened to close a unit and cause layoffs in one state hospital, patients and staff mobilized to sign petitions, confront managers, and call legislators. The process was active, cooperative, and effective, and although not defined as a "mental health" activity, it had obvious benefits. Patients experienced a sense of participation in something outside themselves as well as a burst of self-esteem in its outcome. The discussions about mutual responsibility and the political economy governing their treatment (Who decides? Why?) was not a process of political education but a variety of psychotherapy.

The Alliance for the Mentally Ill (AMI), an organization of family members of psychiatric patients, was not previously in a confrontational position with the DMH and indeed was dependent on DMH funds for some of its staff expenses. In addition, it had so completely bought into the biological determinism of current psychiatric opinion that it tended to de-emphasize the psychosocial and rehabilitation activities of state hospital care. However, after many meetings AMI found itself in a solid alliance with clinicians and public service unions in challenging the privatization policies of DMH.

Indeed, after the publication of a leaked internal document from the DMH revealing a 79 percent increase in the death rate of its clients during the five years of privatization, AMI of Massachusetts called for the resignation of the commissioner. The official response to the revelations was that they represented "more accurate recordkeeping." However, reflecting the growing collaboration among advocates, legislators, and professionals, expert testimony was provided to an investigative committee of the Massachusetts House of Representatives that upheld the validity and gravity of the increased mortality rates resulting from DMH policies.

The activism surrounding the privatization struggle in Massachusetts was focused on local, narrowly defined issues, but it was not lost on some of the people involved that the broader political and socioeconomic context of privatization was relevant and profoundly significant. It was obvious that the shift from public responsibility for human services to a market-driven system of managed care was part of a wider and reactionary political agenda. A Republican governor with White House ambitions was lauding entrepreneurial government and advocating tax reductions for corporations and banks in the face of massive cuts in social programs. This reflected a systematic and coherent right-wing policy guided by the interests of finance capital.

Although it was not an issue that most mental health professionals and advocates were conversant with, some argued that an analysis based on historical and political–economic considerations was unavoidable. This state of affairs is the end result of a long process in the history of commerce. It reflects the ultimate destruction of any social function to capitalism as a consequence of the inflated value of finance capital, as credit itself has become the sole source of profit and the only substance of exchange. Fernand Braudel's (1984) exhaustive history of capitalism finds that profitability expands like an inverted pyramid as investments move inexorably from agriculture to manufacturing to commerce and, finally, to credit. It is more profitable and less risky to make olive oil than to grow olives. It is still more profitable to be involved in the trade of olive oil than in its production. But most profitable of all is to lend the money so that others can do the growing, manufacturing, and trading.

The trend over time for more investment to be made in banking (the provision of credit), rather than in other levels of business activity, creates an increasingly inflated and unstable situation. Like an inverted pyramid expanding ever more rapidly at the top, it is destined to collapse, and once it does it will be beyond repair. Our current economy is one in which automobile companies make higher profits by lending the money for buying their cars than in their actual sales. The distribution of credit cards, like a gigantic Ponzi scheme, is the most profitable activity for banks. The consequence of lowered interest rates is not greater investment in manufacturing and trade but leveraged buyouts of one company by another or, worse, the inflationary and meaningless investment in currency itself. Each day, the trillions of dollars exchanged in currency markets alone represent more goods and services than actually exist in the world.

These trends make this era of capitalism unique; so much capital at so high a return in profit is invested in so much insubstantial fluff, so far removed from human needs or appetites. It is no longer possible even for a war to give our economy a semblance of vigor. War used to be "good" for capital because profit resides in the gap between use value and exchange value, and nothing expands the latter or destroys the former more effectively. But when an economy such as ours is completely involved at the level of credit, even a war, as costly as it is, cannot breathe life into it. In short, after about 500 years, capitalism is now choking on an oversupply of overinflated credit.

That is why the privatization of public services is a desperate initiative. Banks must keep their capital moving if the economy is to appear alive. No longer able to invest in factories for a useless war machine and with the housing market exhausted, banks have turned to education, health, transportation, waste management, prisons, and mental health. But does not the government have an ongoing responsibility for basic human needs? Apparently not. It is not that the government lies, which it does. It is not even that the government lies all the time. Government *is* a lie. This is one of the implications of Braudel's (1984) history. What has masqueraded as an instrument for dealing with shared human needs or at least for balancing the appetites of various interest groups in some approximation of human need is actually, always and everywhere, the instrument of commerce. Government, in a capitalist society, *is business.*

When business became so desperately dependent on credit manipulations that traditional public responsibilities had to be privatized to justify the further expansion of credit, government accommodated by merely selling those responsibilities.

The private corporations taking over public institutions have to borrow money at prevailing interest rates to develop the mechanisms and personnel necessary to operate them. The media, itself an instrument of capital, cooperates by depicting public agencies as inept and their employees as corrupt, lazy, and self-indulgent. Lowering taxes is presented as the major justification for privatization, and in the process public service unions (the most vigorous sector of the dwindling labor movement) are systematically destroyed. The driving force and major purpose of the privatization of human services is to give banks new markets in which to invest their capital.

The fact that so-called "nonprofit" institutions are given contracts for what were once public administrations of schools, highways, clinics, and prisons should not confuse the issue. Institutions that are not apparently or nominally for-profit have always functioned as conduits for funds transferred from the public sector into banks and other lending institutions that are very much *for* profit. The trustees of universities, medical centers, and foundations control billions of dollars of investment capital, and they are generally the directors and executives of enterprises deeply involved with the direction of that money (Hancock, 1989).

This complex ecology of deception and greed surrounds and dictates the function of people and institutions that unwittingly serve finance capital. Traditionally defined responsibilities of local and state government are everywhere being put up for sale in tune with the banking interests that control economies and governments throughout the world (Brecher, 1993). When schools, highways, prisons, waste disposal, and water supply systems are taken over by private enterprise (whether profit or nonprofit), loans must be floated to the contractors for start up and sustaining expenses. Those loans are repaid to the lenders (always for profit) out of the pockets of the people at prevailing interest rates.

The experience in Massachusetts demonstrated a successful alliance of mental health professionals, trade union activists, and advocacy groups against the privatization of mental health services in the state. Such alliances are being forged elsewhere in regard to this and other issues. They will find common ground in a shared struggle on a broader front, evolving into a new and vigorous manifestation of progressive activism.

References

Braudel, F. (1984). *Civilization and capitalism: XV–XVIII centuries* (3 vols.). New York: Harper & Row.

Brecher, J. (1993, December 6). Global village or global pillage? [Editorial]. *Nation,* p. 685.

Dumont, M. (1987). A diagnostic parable: A review of DSM-III-R [Readings]. *American Orthopsychiatric Association, 2,* 9–12.

Dumont, M. (1989). Psychotoxicology: The return of the Mad Hatter. *Social Science and Medicine, 29,* 1077–1082.

Dumont, M. (1990). Managed care, managed people, and community mental health [Editorial]. *American Journal of Orthopsychiatry, 60,* 166–167.

Dumont, M. (1992). Privatization of mental health services: The invisible hand at our throats [Editorial]. *American Journal of Orthopsychiatry, 62,* 328–329.

Gold mine of psychiatric data discovered in Danish registry. (1993, March 26). *New York Times,* p. A4.

Hancock, G. (1989). *Lords of poverty: The power, prestige, and corruption of the international aid business.* New York: Atlantic Monthly Press.

Johnson, J. (1989). Collective control: Strategies for survival in the workplace. *International Journal of Health Services, 19,* 73–79.

Massachusetts Human Services Coalition. (1992, December 16). *State House Watch, 10*(19), 1.

Massachusetts Senate, Post-Audit and Oversight Committee. (1993). *A review of DMH policy planning and implementation during the closing of Northampton State Hospital.* Boston: Author.

CHAPTER 11

Massachusetts State House Oversight Report: Excerpts Regarding Medicaid Implementation

Gerald Schamess and Anita Lightburn

In September 1996 a committee of the Massachusetts House of Representatives Post-Audit and Oversight Bureau completed a preliminary review of Department of Mental Health (DMH) client deaths and investigations between 1990 and 1994. That review was published in a report from the bureau (Massachusetts House of Representatives, 1997). The reason cited for the review was that

> In June, 1995, the Bureau learned of information compiled by the DMH in response to a Freedom of Information Act request, indicating a 79% increase in DMH client deaths between 1990 and 1994. This information, coupled with a HPAO [House of Representatives Post-Audit and Oversight] Bureau review of DMH mortality and death investigations, prompted the House Audit and Oversight Committee ("the Committee") to hold hearings. The Committee held two public hearings at which the Commissioner and Director of Internal Affairs appeared on the issue of deaths and death investigation. The Bureau did an extensive review of mortality information for the 1990–1994 period with a follow-up for 1996 and 1997. (p. 1)

In accord with a legislative mandate, in 1992 the public mental health system in Massachusetts was restructured under a managed care model. In 1995 DMH Commissioner Eileen Elias appeared before the House Post-Audit and Oversight Bureau to testify about the reported increase in the mortality rate for clients under DMH care (see chapter 9). In defending department policy Elias explained that the expanded 1992 criteria for reporting client deaths included a broader range of people having contact with the DMH, and that the increase in the reports of deaths was likely a result of the wider data collection method, she noted that neither mental health advocates nor the media accepted that explanation. Instead, they continued to use the data as proof that the managed care restructuring initiative was linked to greater numbers of patient deaths. Elias sought an independent group of federal investigators to deal proactively with this issue and also commissioned them to investigate the reported increase in patient mortality and determine whether it was related to the restructuring initiative. The team's report (Critical Incident Reporting Task Force, 1996) revealed an actual *decline* in the rate of consumer deaths from 1991 to 1993.

Because the Oversight Committee's report (Massachusetts House of Representatives, 1997) is based both on its own investigation and on a review of the previous

Human Services Resource Institute (HSRI) report, the highlights cited in the bureau's report are reproduced below.

- Between 1990 and 1994, DMH data officially recorded 910 client deaths. Between 1991 and 1993, the DMH officially recorded 542 client deaths.
- The DMH's federally funded private consultant's report stated that between 1991 and 1993, the DMH recorded 674 client deaths, or 132 more deaths than the 542 deaths the DMH had previously claimed for the audit period. The consultant's inquiry of the DMH and Department of Public Health mortality statistics revealed an additional 884 DMH client deaths that were not recorded by the DMH between 1991 and 1993. Thus, according to the DMH's consultant, the DMH's total number of client deaths for 1991 to 1993 was actually 1,558 (Critical Incident Reporting Task Force, 1996).[1]
- Although the DMH's private consultant's report reveals an underrecording of client deaths from 1991 to 1993, the consultant's report also demonstrates unilateral discrepancies with the DMH's official mortality statistics for the same audit period. Were 542 deaths recorded between 1991 and 1993, as stated in the original DMH statistics from June 1995, or were 674 deaths recorded, as stated in the consultant's report? Either way, these discrepancies undermine the DMH's claim that mortality recordkeeping has improved.
- Of the deaths per year, the DMH fully investigated only 25 percent or fewer between 1993 and 1995.
- The average length of time for the DMH to complete a death investigation *tripled* from 1993 to 1995, according to 96 completed death investigations received by the bureau for that audit period. Specifically, the DMH required an average of 70 days in 1993, 135 days in 1994, and 184 days in 1995.
- Despite claims of better recordkeeping and an expanded definition of a DMH client, the DMH did not explain the sharp rise in DMH client deaths.
- The 96 DMH investigative reports received by the bureau were often incomplete and not uniform.
- DMH death investigations were often inconclusive and failed to provide the basis for meaningful corrective actions. One DMH death investigation contradicted the death certificate's official finding.
- During the audit period, the DMH completed fewer death investigations and took longer to complete those that were actually finished.
- The bureau's review of 96 investigative reports of deaths found 65 deaths for which the circumstances were potentially avoidable.

The Post-Audit and Oversight Bureau's report also addressed the issue of the DMH's expanded data-collecting activities (Massachusetts House of Representatives, 1997):

> The House Post-Audit and Oversight Bureau (the Bureau) analyzed the DMH's claim that the 79% increase in client deaths was due to better

[1]The House Post-Audit and Oversight Bureau has confirmed the theoretical assumptions of the report in a telephone interview with Stephen Leff, principal investigator and director of the Evaluation Center at HSRI. However, the bureau did not have access to HSRI's original data to verify the accuracy of the numbers published in the report.

> record-keeping and data collection capabilities, as well as other information relating to the deaths of DMH clients. The Bureau's preliminary fact finding found no documentary support for DMH's claim that better record-keeping was responsible for the increase in the number of reported deaths. During the period audited, the Bureau found that DMH had produced inconsistent information, a lack of uniformity of investigative reports, and unenforced and irregular investigative procedures. Also, the Bureau found no support for DMH's claim that changes in protocol made in 1992 increased the number of deaths reported, nor did the policy changes result in expanded Office of Internal Affair's (OIA) responsibilities. *The Bureau's preliminary fact finding raised questions about DMH's capacity to oversee its own death investigative process, and a performance audit was undertaken to fully examine DMH processes and decision making.* (p. 3, italics added)

In a letter dated May 23, 1997 (Massachusetts House of Representatives, 1997), the current commissioner, Marylou Sudders, detailed the DMH's ongoing efforts to address the findings reported in the investigative report. Commissioner Sudders reported to the committee's director and general counsel on "revised regulations," "organizational changes," "significant improvements in eliminating the backlog of investigation reports," and current efforts to monitor services purchased from more than "200 providers." She concluded with the following statement: "The Department remains committed to improving its direct care system and its accountability to the public. I look forward to working with the House Post-Audit and Oversight Committee and staff on the implementation of specific recommendations" (p. 5).

References

Critical Incident Reporting Task Force. (1996, January 26). *Report on Massachusetts Department of Mental Health Service recipient mortality (1991–1993).* Cambridge, MA: Evaluation Center at Human Services Resource Institute.

Massachusetts House of Representatives, Post-Audit and Oversight Committee. (1997, May). *Preliminary review: Department of Mental Health client deaths and investigations.* Boston: Author. (Available from the House Post-Audit and Oversight Bureau, Room 146, State House, Boston, MA 02133-1053)

C H A P T E R **12**

Mental Health and Substance Abuse Treatment in Managed Care:

The Massachusetts Medicaid Experience

James J. Callahan, Donald S. Shepard, Richard H. Beinecke, Mary Jo Larson, and Doreen Cavanaugh

Use of managed care is increasing, although it has not been definitively proved to be a means of controlling rising health care costs (Dickey & Azeni, 1992). First adopted by business, managed care is now being seized upon by state Medicaid programs (Freund & Hurley, 1995; Hurley & Freund, 1988). More than 5 million Medicaid beneficiaries—15 percent of the Medicaid population—were enrolled in managed care in 1993, 20 times the number enrolled in 1981 (Freund & Hurley, 1995). New waiver activity under Section 1115 will lead to an estimated Medicaid enrollment in managed care of close to 8 million people when implemented (Helf, 1994).

Medicaid managed care programs aim to control costs by producing more appropriate patterns of health care use (Giles, 1993). These plans vary along the dimensions of enrollment (voluntary or mandated), organizational structure (use of intermediary health maintenance organizations [HMOs], individual practice associations, preferred provider organizations, or benefit carve-outs), the range of services covered, and methods of payment (fee-for-service, capitation, or negotiated contract) (Hurley & Freund, 1988; Medicare and Medicaid Managed Care, 1993). State programs also vary by the specific subgroup of enrollees that participate. Most programs enroll Aid to Families with Dependent Children (AFDC) recipients, and a few serve disabled people (Center for Vulnerable Populations, 1993).

Despite this widespread adoption of managed care, however, specialty managed mental health programs within Medicaid are still somewhat uncommon (Helf, 1994; Lurie, Moscovice, Finch, Christianson, & Popkin, 1992). Uncertainty about costs and about the responsiveness of mental health services to financial incentives have been particular concerns (Arons, Frank, Goldman, McGuire, & Stevens, 1994). The most common approach to mental health treatment within Medicaid waiver programs is to include only limited acute treatment within the managed plan and to rely on state mental health or substance abuse (MH/SA) systems for more intensive treatment (Helf, 1994). Studies have found that prepaid or capitated payment systems reduce hospitalization among people with serious mental illness without consistent evidence

NOTES: Originally published as Callahan, J. J., Jr., Shepard, D. S., Beinecke, R. H., Larson, M. J., & Cavanaugh, D. (1995). Mental health/substance abuse treatment in managed care: The Massachusetts Medicaid experience. *Health Affairs, 14,* 173–184. ©1995 The People-to-People Health Foundation. All rights reserved. An earlier version of this chapter was presented at the 7th Biennial Research Conference on the Economics of Mental Health, NIMH, Bethesda, MD, September 1994.

of ill health effects (Cole, Reed, Barbigian, Brown, & Fray, 1994; Reed, Hennessy, Mitchell, & Barbigian, 1994; Wells, Manning, & Burciaga Valdez, 1989).

Massachusetts was the first state to introduce a statewide specialty mental health managed care plan in Medicaid. When begun, it was the largest managed care program with capitated mental health care (Lewin-VHI, 1995). Beginning July 1, 1992, the state enrolled approximately 375,000 disabled (mostly Supplemental Security Income [SSI]) and nondisabled Medicaid (mostly AFDC) recipients in a managed care program under federal 1915 waivers. For managed care enrollees, medical and surgical care is coordinated by primary care clinicians, but MH/SA care is managed as a benefit carve-out by a private company, First Mental Health, Inc. (doing business in Massachusetts as MHMA). This chapter reports on the first year's experience of enrollees in the MH/SA managed care program (MH/SAP).

The state's Division of Medical Assistance (DMA) contracted with MHMA to change existing utilization patterns by reducing average length-of-stay in bed-days per recipient; reducing admissions to overnight care (hospital inpatient and nonhospital residential) through the use of aggressive case management, outpatient care, and nonresidential settings; contracting for cost-effective services with a network of credentialed providers (expanded to include nonhospital residential providers); and using competitive rates. An incentive structure is designed to reduce costly admissions while allowing widespread use of less expensive MH/SA treatment. MHMA allows ambulatory mental health and alcohol abuse treatment providers to provide up to eight sessions of ambulatory care per year without prior approval. Beyond eight sessions, providers must develop an approved treatment plan and receive authorization for a specified number of additional sessions.

All 24-hour services require prior approval. When approval is granted, it generally is only for a few days, and additional days require an extension. Both ambulatory and 24-hour services are paid on a fee-for-service basis, but expenses (providers' time to develop and gather necessary information, develop treatment plans, and telephone MHMA) are not reimbursed separately.

Methods

Our report is based on an evaluation that was prepared to meet the Health Care Financing Administration's requirement that an "independent review" of the program be submitted for the waiver to be renewed. The review must examine costs and access and must ensure that Medicaid enrollees are not significantly worse off under the waiver than before. We refer to this requirement as "relative quality."

MEASURES

Access was evaluated primarily by examining penetration rates for MH/SA services overall and by type of service. The overall penetration rate was the proportion of enrollees who used any MH/SA service during the fiscal year. Additional measures concerned answers to questions on access from a random survey of providers. Relative quality was measured by the proportion of discharges followed by readmission to 24-hour care within 30 days of discharge and by answers to questions on quality in the provider survey.

To gauge the impact on costs, we compared total actual expenditures for MH/SA care with costs that were predicted absent the new Massachusetts program. Predicted service expenditures without managed care were estimated by calculating expenditures per enrollee from fiscal years 1990 (the year ending June 30, 1990) through 1992 by eligibility category and type of care, and expressing all values in constant FY 1993 dollars to adjust for inflation. This adjustment was based on the medical care component of the Consumer Price Index, the best available measure of overall medical care prices. Fitting trend lines to the results, regression analysis predicted values for FY 1993. Aggregate service expenditures, assuming there was no managed care, were estimated by multiplying actual enrollment in each category by predicted FY 1993 costs per enrollee. Predicted (based on past trends) and actual administrative costs were added to predicted and actual service expenditures, respectively.

DATA

The utilization and cost analyses were based on fiscal year reports for periods before (FY 1990 through FY 1992) and after (FY 1993) managed care was introduced. These included aggregate summary reports of expenditures and enrollments, aggregate summary reports of selected items with comparable data for the two periods, and Medicaid-paid claims for overnight care for FY 1992 and FY 1993. The process evaluation was based on reviews of documents, personal interviews with key informants in 43 organizations, and telephone interviews with a stratified random sample of 98 providers. The informant interviewed was the person identified as having the most working contact with MHMA. Usually this was a top clinician, but occasionally it was an administrator.

Results of the Analysis

Table 12-1 shows Medicaid costs for MH/SA treatment with and without the managed care waiver. Table 12-2 shows the results of the cost adjustments for FY 1990–93. As intended, the program sharply reduced expenditures for 24-hour care.

DISABLED AND NONDISABLED ENROLLEES

The MH/SAP uses two risk categories to determine the prepaid per capita monthly payments to its private contractor: (1) the disabled eligibility group (SSI and Medical Assistance only) and (2) nondisabled eligibility groups (primarily people on AFDC, but the category includes refugees and Medical Assistance clients under age 21).

Actual expenditures per enrollee were 37 percent lower for people with disabilities, 16 percent lower for people without disabilities, and 27 percent lower overall (Table 12-3). However, the decline in costs within each eligibility category was partly offset by an increase in the percentage of enrollees who had disabilities, from 14.4 percent in FY 1992 to 16.1 percent in FY 1993 (Table 12-2).

TWENTY-FOUR HOUR AND AMBULATORY CARE

We decomposed the savings between 24-hour care and ambulatory care, again comparing predicted and actual values (Table 12-4). Of the $57 million savings from reduced provider payments for direct services, $44.2 million (78 percent) was cut from 24-hour care (hospitalization, detoxification, and residential care) and $12.6 million (22 percent) from ambulatory care. We further decomposed the savings within each type of care. Compared with predicted values, the number of

TABLE **12-1**

Medicaid Costs for Mental Health and Substance Abuse Services with and without the Managed Care Waiver, FY 1993

TYPE OF COST	AMOUNT ($ MILLIONS)
Predicted Medicaid costs without waiver	
Administration in Division of Medical Assistance	2
Payments to providers	208
Subtotal	210
Medicaid costs with waiver (actual)	
Administration in MHMA and Medicaid	11
Payments to providers	151
Incentive payments to MHMA	1
Subtotal	163
Dollar savings	47
Percentage savings	22

NOTE: MHMA = First Mental Health, Inc., doing business in Massachusetts as Mental Health Management of America.
SOURCE: Massachusetts Division of Medical Assistance and authors' calculations.

TABLE **12-2**

Expenditures for Mental Health and Substance Abuse Care for Medicaid Managed Care Enrollees by Fiscal Year ($ Millions)

	1990	1991	1992	1993
Direct services payments, by eligibility group				
With disabilities	48.6	64.2	87.1	71.0
Without disabilities	73.8	89.2	97.4	79.8
Total administrative expenses	1.7	1.7	1.8	12.0
Inflation and enrollment				
Boston medical care services CPI	177.4	196.6	219.2	237.4
Total enrollment[a]	311.1	360.6	378.5	375.4
Percent with disabilities	14.3	13.6	14.4	16.1

NOTE: CPI = Consumer Price Index.
[a]Thousands of people, average number.
SOURCE: Massachusetts Division of Medical Assistance and authors' calculations.

TABLE **12-3**

Predicted and Actual Direct Services Expenditures Per Enrollee, FY 1993

ENROLLEE	$ PREDICTED[a]	$ ACTUAL	$ CHANGE	% CHANGE[b]
With disabilities	1,854	1,172	–682	–37
Without disabilities	303	253	–50	–16
Total	553	402	–151	–27

[a]Without managed care, adjusted for trends, inflation, and disabled enrollment mix.
[b]Calculated prior to rounding per enrollee expenditures.

TABLE **12-4**

Sources of Savings by Component, Predicted versus Actual, FY 1993

	SAVINGS		
INDICATOR	DECLINE (%)	SHARE (%)	AMOUNT ($ MILLIONS)
24-Hour care expenditures	38.2	78	44.2
Number of admissions	7.2	12	6.9
Length of stay	12.3	21	12.1
Mix of settings (impact on cost per day)	9.1	15	8.8
Price per day	16.4	29	16.4
Ambulatory care expenditures	12.9	22	12.6
Inferred number and mix of services[a]	5.7	9	5.3
Price per service	7.7	13	7.3
Subtotal, direct services expenditures	27.4	100	56.8
Administration	NA	NA	−10.0
Total	22.3	NA	46.8

NOTES: "Predicted" carries forward trends in utilization and applies them to actual shifts in enrollment and an overall 8.3 percent rate of inflation. "Share" is based on total savings in direct services expenditures. NA = not applicable.
[a]Inferred from difference between changes in expenditures and the overall rate of inflation.
SOURCE: Massachusetts Division of Medical Assistance and authors' calculations.

24-hour admissions fell by 7.2 percent, and length of stay declined by 12.3 percent. Savings from the mix of settings (reducing cost per day by 9.1 percent) were the result of transferring some days of care from hospitals ($475 average per day) to non-hospital facilities ($130 average per day).

The savings in price per day resulted from the fact that MHMA paid less per day than the evaluators' estimation of what Medicaid would have paid without the waiver. Had FY 1993 rates been held to the levels of FY 1992, FY 1993 prices would have been 7.7 percent below expected levels. In fact, the actual price savings (16.4 percent) were much greater. MHMA's use of its market power thus was one of the major sources of savings, reducing expenditures by $16.4 million below what was expected. Overall, all of these changes in 24-hour care are consistent with the goals of the MH/SAP.

Actual expenditures for ambulatory care, before any adjustments, fell by 1.2 percent, from $86 million to $85 million. When adjusted for enrollment, utilization trends, and inflation, however, FY 1993 expenditures were 12.9 percent below predicted levels. MHMA paid outpatient providers using the same fee schedule rates that Medicaid had used in FY 1992. The absence of any inflation adjustment was equivalent to a 7.7 percent price reduction below expected levels, or a savings of $7.3 million. There was a $5.3 million decline from use and mix of services. Within that total, $2.5 million was probably the result of a change in payment procedures.[1]

[1]MHMA included payments to psychiatrists and other professionals as part of the hospital fee in 1993, whereas they are included in what is counted here as outpatient care in 1992. Assuming that there was one health professional visit for every three days of inpatient mental health care and that these visits were paid at $70 (the approximate payment to psychiatrists), this shift would cause an apparent decline in "outpatient" visits of $2.5 million (108,555 inpatient mental health days divided by three days per visit times $70 per visit equals $2.5 million).

The remaining $2.8 million reduction was a 3.0 percent decline in outpatient use or mix of services below predicted values. It should be noted, however, that these predicted values were based on a 3.9 percent annual increase in use per enrollee (standardized for enrollment mix). After adjustment for everything except trends, outpatient visits were 0.9 percent above predicted levels. That is, although outpatient services continued to increase, the rate of increase was below recent trends.

MENTAL HEALTH AND SUBSTANCE ABUSE SERVICES

Compared with inflation-adjusted 1992 values, mental health costs per enrollee declined by about 19 percent (from $446 to $359) and substance abuse treatment costs declined by 48 percent (from $82 to $42). In both cases, reductions in 24-hour care accounted for the greatest change: 30 percent and 67 percent, respectively. Outpatient care expenditures decreased by 9 percent for mental health, largely because reimbursement rates did not rise with inflation. Ambulatory substance abuse treatment costs rose 8 percent above inflation.

ACCESS

Utilization generally changed from FY 1992 to FY 1993 in accordance with the incentive structure described earlier (Table 12-5). For example, the proportion of enrollees receiving outpatient mental health clinic treatment grew by 10.6 percent. The overall volume of MH/SA ambulatory services per enrollee, however, fell slightly (3 percent) below expected values, a change that was not anticipated. Similarly, use of 24-hour care declined after adjusting for enrollment changes; admissions fell by 7.2 percent, and length of stay by 12.3 percent. Overall, expenditures fell much more among enrollees with disabilities (37 percent) than among those without (16 percent). Enrollees with disabilities tended to use more 24-hour care and more intensive ambulatory care than those without.

The total number of MH/SAP users per 1,000 enrollees increased slightly, rising from 212.7 in FY 1992 to 222.6 in FY 1993. The number of users of inpatient hospital services (except for services in psychiatric facilities serving people under age 21) fell, whereas access increased for freestanding and Level III detoxification centers, acute residential substance abuse facilities, methadone treatment, clinic treatment and consultation, and psychiatric day treatment. Level III detoxification centers and new acute residential substance abuse programs substituted for inpatient care. Also, the mix of program services changed. Of the 13 types of mental health services, six showed increases and seven showed decreases. In substance abuse, six of nine services showed increases.

The survey of providers asked respondents to compare access under managed care with access under the previous system. Their average score of 3.02 on a scale of 1 (worse) to 5 (better) was virtually the midpoint. In providers' aggregate opinion, therefore, there has been no change in access since managed care was adopted. Providers reported greater availability of diversionary beds and services ($M = 3.64$) but too few diversionary beds when compared with their assessment of need (mean, 2.20). Providers also reported that they thought lengths of stay had decreased ($M = 2.08$).

Providers of all types—inpatient, outpatient, crisis teams, and diversionary—reported that their clients have more severe problems than before managed care

TABLE **12-5**

Mental Health and Substance Abuse Care Users Per 1,000 Enrollees, by Type of Service, FY 1992-93

	USERS PER 1,000 ENROLLEES		
MENTAL HEALTH	**1992**	**1993**	**% CHANGE**
Inpatient mental health[a]	16.5	16.1	−2.4
Clinic treatment (outpatient)	118.5	131.2[b]	10.6
Clinic evaluation	67.5	70.8	4.8
Outpatient (hospital)	59.7	48.7	−19.2
Psychiatrists	32.5	28.6[c]	−12.0
Clinic medication	24.7	31.9	29.1
Crisis intervention	18.3	15.9[b]	−13.5
Psychologists	16.3	11.5[c]	−29.6
Home care	6.0	5.4	−10.5
Psychiatric day treatment	3.7	4.7	27.0
Clinic consultation	0.0	38.3	—[d]
Acute residential (children)	0.0	1.3	—[d]
Community health center	6.0	5.4	−10.5
SUBSTANCE ABUSE			
Inpatient	9.1	3.5	−61.2
Free-standing detoxification	5.5	7.9	45.2
Level III detoxification	0.0	2.4	—[d]
Acute residential	0.0	3.2	—[d]
Outpatient	9.6	9.2	−4.4
Methadone counseling	5.4	6.2	15.5
Methadone dosing	5.2	6.3	20.2
Acute residential (child and adolescent)	0.0	0.1	—[d]
Acupuncture detoxification	0.5	0.4	−13.7
Total, all services[e]	212.7	222.6	4.6

[a]This entry is the sum of two service types: "inpatient mental health" and "inpatient under 21." They are combined because payment categories shifted between 1992 and 1993.
[b]In 1993, emergency (crisis intervention) services for patients already in clinic treatment were paid as additional clinic treatment sessions.
[c]In 1993, payment for care to inpatients was included under facility reimbursement.
[d]Not applicable because new service.
[e]Users cannot be summed across service types because many users received more than one service during the year. This total is the unduplicated user rate calculated from paid claims.
SOURCE: Massachusetts Division of Medical Assistance and authors' calculations.

was implemented ($M = 4.09$). This finding is consistent with the program's goal of moving clients from inpatient hospital care to the least costly, most appropriate setting and with providers' reports of a trend toward more severely ill people in the community.

RELATIVE QUALITY

The 30-day readmission rate dropped slightly, from 19.9 percent in FY 1992 to 18.9 percent in FY 1993. Thus, overall, patients are not being readmitted more often than before managed care. There was a difference, however, between the group with disabilities, which had declines in readmissions within 30 days (25.8 percent to 22.7 percent), and the group without, in which there was an increase (11.1 percent to 13.4 percent). Child and adolescent patients, in particular, showed an increased readmission rate of 10.1 percent (up from 7.5 percent before managed care), a finding which raises a concern about lower-quality care for this group.

Providers reported that clinical quality was generally favorable on several dimensions: treatment recommendations (M = 3.80), aftercare plans (M = 3.54), length-of-stay decisions (M = 3.53), appropriate settings (M = 3.66), and overall assessment (M = 3.23).

Although all of these means are in a favorable direction, about one-fourth of providers felt that clinical decisions were usually inappropriate, and another fourth had mixed views. Children's inpatient providers were more critical of clinical decisions than were other providers, and treatment of children was cited more often as a problem area by providers in response to both the scaled and the open-ended questions.

The MHMA contract with Medicaid required the establishment of a quality assurance program, including a means of assessing client satisfaction. Because this process was just beginning at the time of this study, data were insufficient to evaluate consumers' opinion of the services.

MANAGEMENT ISSUES

Many informants reported continuing administrative problems with MHMA, including long delays in reaching the utilization review staff by telephone, excessive and time-consuming paperwork, conflicting responses from different utilization staff, differences between oral agreements and final written approvals, and slow or nonexistent transmission of paperwork to providers. As a result, nearly all providers reported that much more provider staff time was being spent administratively managing Medicaid clients than before the MH/SAP initiative, which required either hiring additional staff or diverting existing staff from clinical tasks. Compared with other managed care providers, however, MHMA was generally considered to be about the same or slightly better on the characteristics of quality of utilization review decisions (M = 3.45, on a scale of 1 [worse] to 5 [much better]), access for clients (M = 3.62), flexibility (M = 3.30), and promptness in making decisions (M = 3.19). The primary criticisms of the first year of operation were bureaucratic administrative procedures and problems reaching utilization review staff by telephone.

Discussion

Preliminary data for FY 1994 show that the savings from managed care have been maintained. Service expenditures per enrollee (current prices) were $421 in FY 1994, a 5 percent increase above the comparable amount of $401 for FY 1993. This increase was less than the rise in medical care prices in the Boston area and virtually equal to the target set by the DMA.

The MH/SAP represents a new generation of Medicaid managed care programs in several ways: It is a statewide program administered by a for-profit managed care company; it assumes financial risk for reducing expenditures, tracks both inpatient and outpatient utilization; covers both mental health and substance abuse treatment (thus creating the possibility of treatment integration); and includes all levels of mental health need, not just high-cost cases. The program significantly restructured the payer–provider relationship by instituting treatment protocols and contracting with a subset of providers. Selective contracting gave more control to the contractor over rates, treatment protocols, and client flow, thus enhancing the chance for savings and service coordination. We believe that selective contracting for inpatient providers could not have occurred had Medicaid not "privatized" the program. Political pressure to contract with "my hospital" was blunted when the decision was put into private hands.

We do not believe that costs were shifted to the alternative payers: insurance, the Department of Mental Health, or the Bureau of Substance Abuse Services. Recipients lacked private insurance and the purchasing power to pay for services directly. Among other public programs, the Department of Mental Health faced its own budget and bed constraints and also reduced the number of admissions it financed. The state's Bureau of Substance Abuse Services, a last-resort payer for substance abuse treatment, capped the total payments to each facility below its demand. Thus, all these facilities sought to use Medicaid whenever possible. Finally, bad debt pools also were tightly limited in Massachusetts.

The experience in the program's first year of operation reflects the incentives and administrative features of a carve-out program, the types of populations enrolled, the historical use pattern, and the competitive and well-developed mental health market in Massachusetts (Commons, Hodgkin, McGuire, & Riordan, 1994). That state is not typical of all states. It has a generous Medicaid benefit package for medical and mental health services, with good provider participation. Its per capita Medicaid expenses for substance abuse are about equal to those of the median state, and it had a history of rapidly rising mental health expenditures when the MH/SAP was introduced (Larson & Horgan, 1994). Other states cannot necessarily expect the same types of Medicaid cost savings if they implement a similar mental health managed care program. Nevertheless, there are lessons that can be put to use by other states.

First, the DMA chose a proactive approach with a private contractor, using detailed contracting specifications with reporting requirements on access assurance, service expenditures, and consumer compliance, which are closely monitored by the agency. Although even this monitoring did not produce quality control as rapidly as planned, the DMA's intense engagement with the contractor is clearly an ingredient linked to the program's success. The contractor, in turn, is credited with introducing new arrangements for the interagency collaboration and negotiation with the state MH/SA authorities.

Second, the financial incentives under the MH/SAP are different from fee-for-service and HMO-type approaches. MHMA receives a predetermined monthly payment and has a risk corridor in which it shares savings or losses, but the service providers continue to be paid on a fee-for-service basis. Thus, although the contractor has a strong financial incentive to contain costs, the providers do not have a direct financial incentive to withhold care because they continue to be paid on a fee-for-service basis.

Third, MHMA was able to control provider prices through selective contracting, particularly with hospitals. Service providers, therefore, must be more competitive than under the previous systems, a change that can translate into improved quality. The contractor has adopted more detailed recommended treatment protocols than were previously used. These protocols specify a certain standard of care, which at times requires higher quality than that which has been evident in the performance of providers in the fee-for-service system (for example, the guarantee of a psychiatric evaluation within a specified period for all 24-hour stays).

Fourth, MHMA showed its capacity to negotiate rates of payment that were below former payment levels based on historical costs. For inefficient providers, this is an incentive in the right direction to improve their cost performance. Lower fees, however, may lead to skimping on necessary or desirable services. Furthermore, the increased administrative burden (reported consistently by providers) may have caused them to emphasize administrative tasks at the expense of clinical tasks. This problem should be examined in future research.

Fifth, patients may be benefiting from the protocols and increased service coordination. Nonetheless, some advocates are concerned that providers may become more sensitive or responsive to MHMA than to the needs of their patients. The impact of "fourth-party" involvement in these types of situations is not necessarily obvious within the first year of operation.

Sixth, the MH/SAP had different effects based on disability status and age. Access for adult disabled enrollees increased, and that for adult nondisabled enrollees decreased. It is not clear why this change occurred. It is clear, however, that children and adolescents faced more problems under the MH/SAP than did adults: The 30-day readmission rate for children and adolescents increased sharply. Providers reported that the average length of stay was inadequate to provide sufficient assessment and evaluation services for the exceptional needs of some children. For certain children with complex needs, coordination among family, school systems, and perhaps other state agencies is required, but under the MH/SAP there is much less time and funding available for this. That could account for some of the reported problems.

The relatively favorable evaluation offered here presents a picture of the startup phase of the program. How the program will perform in the long run will require further evaluation.

References

Arons, B. S., Frank, R. G., Goldman, H. H., McGuire, T. G., & Stevens, S. (1994). Mental health and substance abuse coverage under health reform. *Health Affairs, 13,* 192–205.

Center for Vulnerable Populations. (1993, April). *Spotlight* [Newsletter]. Portland, ME: National Academy for State Health Policy.

Cole, R. E., Reed, S. K. Barbigian, H. M., Brown, S. W., & Fray, J. (1994). A mental health capitation program: I. Patient outcomes. *Hospital and Community Psychiatry, 45,* 1090–1096.

Commons, M., Hodgkin, D., McGuire, T. G., & Riordan, M. H. (1994). Paying for public drug abuse services in the six New England states. In G. Denmead & B. A. Rouse (Eds.), *Financing drug treatment through state programs* (Services Research Monograph 1, pp. 95–142). Rockville, MD: National Institute on Drug Abuse.

Dickey, B., & Azeni, H. (1992). Impact of managed care on mental health services. *Health Affairs, 11,* 197–204.

Freund, D. A., & Hurley, R. E. (1995). Medicaid managed care: Contribution to issues of health reform. *Annual Reviews of Public Health, 16,* 473–495.

Giles, T. R. (1993). *Managed mental health care: A guide for practitioners, employers, and hospital administrators.* Needham Heights, MA: Allyn & Bacon.

Helf, C. (1994). *Medicaid managed care and mental health: An overview of Section 1115 programs.* Washington, DC: George Washington University, Intergovernmental Health Policy Project.

Hurley, R. E., & Freund, D. A. (1988). A topology of Medicaid managed care. *Medical Care, 26,* 764–773.

Larson, M. J., & Horgan, C. M. (1994). Variations in state Medicaid program expenditures for substance abuse units and facilities. In G. Denmead & B. A. Rouse (Eds.), *Financing drug treatment through state programs* (Services Research Monograph 1, pp. 21–50). Rockville, MD: National Institute on Drug Abuse.

Lewin-VHI. (1995, February). *States as payers: Managed care for Medicaid populations.* Washington, DC: National Institute for Health Care Management.

Lurie, N., Moscovice, I. S., Finch, M., Christianson, J. B., & Popkin, M. K. (1992). Does capitation affect the health of the chronically mentally ill: Results from a randomized trial. *JAMA, 267,* 3300–3304.

Medicare and Medicaid managed care: Issues and evidence [Special issue]. (1993, Fall). *Health Care Financing Review.*

Reed, S. K., Hennessy, K. D., Mitchell, O. S., & Barbigian, H. M. (1994). A mental health capitation program: II. Cost–benefit analysis. *Hospital and Community Psychiatry, 45,* 1097–1103.

Wells, K. B., Manning, W. G., Jr., & Burciaga Valdez, R. (1989, December). *The effects of a prepaid group practice on mental health outcomes of a general population: Results from a randomized trial.* Santa Monica, CA: RAND.

CHAPTER 13

The Impact of Managed Care on Massachusetts Mental Health and Substance Abuse Providers

Richard H. Beinecke, Maury Goodman, and Amy Lockhart

Managed care is predicted to have major clinical, administrative, organizational, and financial effects on public mental health and substance abuse providers. However, especially in the public sector, few studies have been conducted and few data are available on the actual impact of managed care on providers.

To determine changes that providers were making in response to the Massachusetts Mental Health/Substance Abuse Program (MH/SAP), a statewide Medicaid managed care initiative, two telephone surveys were conducted of nearly the same group of a stratified, random sample of providers in program years 3 and 4. The consistent changes reported by every type of provider reinforce the hypothesis that a widespread transformation in clinical care and management is taking place and that providers are preparing for the next evolution into capitated systems of care. The changes being adopted by Massachusetts providers offer survival strategies for providers in other states at earlier stages of the managed care revolution.

Rapidly evolving are integrated systems of care that provide comprehensive, coordinated spectra of horizontally and vertically integrated services to targeted populations, often on a capitated basis (Egnew, 1995; Jackson, Beinecke, Bond, Seldon, & Van Tassel, 1995; Shortell, Anderson, Gillies, Mitchell, & Morgan, 1993). Comprehensive services, continuity of care, new financing strategies, and accountability are core functions of the new systems (Hoge, Davidson, Griffith, & Sledge, 1994).

There are many guides to managed care and agency and practitioner survival (for example, Giles, 1993; Jackson et al., 1995; Lowman & Resnick, 1994; Schreter, Sharfstein, & Schreter, 1994; Todd, 1994; Winegar & Bistline, 1994). Reviewing these guides suggests some of the changes that one might expect under managed care.

Clinical practice is beginning to change in response to the new environment. Among the changes, brief therapy is becoming more prevalent, and studies are starting to demonstrate its effectiveness (Giles, 1993; Hoyt, 1994; Stern, 1993). More home care and preventive programs are expected to be developed (Budman, 1995; Lima, 1995). Group therapy is predicted to be well suited to managed service systems (Mackenzie, 1995).

NOTE: Originally published as Beinecke, R. H., Goodman, M., & Lockhart, A. (1997). The impact of managed care on Massachusetts mental health and substance abuse providers. *Administration in Social Work, 21*(2), 41–53. Copyright 1996 The Haworth Press.

As managed care treats more public clients, more chronic patients are becoming part of these systems, and the ability of managed care providers to treat people with serious mental illnesses is being debated (Budman, 1995; Flynn, Panzetta, & Shumway, 1994).

Providers are expected to make organizational changes. Quality assurance, total quality management, and outcomes management are core components of most managed behavioral health programs, and providers are expected to have to increase their abilities to perform these functions (Nadzam, 1994; Nelson, Hartman, Ojemann, & Wilcox, 1995). There is much debate and still much uncertainty over how best to measure outcomes (Hohmann, Sederer, & Campbell, 1995). To meet managed care data requirements, providers are also expected to have to implement management information systems and continually upgrade them because developments in computer technology change quickly (Cagney & Woods, 1994; Trabin, 1995). Early indications are that mental health and social services organizations will follow the lead of health care counterparts and enter into more mergers or acquisitions than in the past, thus increasing in size and forming their own subnetworks of care (Ray, 1995).

Massachusetts Managed Care Initiative

In 1992, the Massachusetts Division of Medical Assistance (DMA) contracted with Mental Health Management of America (MHMA), a national managed care management company, to develop and operate the MH/SAP for Medicaid enrollees. These enrollees had the options of choosing a health maintenance organization (HMO) or receiving their primary care from one of the physicians participating in the Primary Care Clinician (PCC) program and receiving their mental health and substance abuse care through the MH/SAP. Approximately 75,000 people joined one of the HMOs, and 375,000 people chose the PCC–MH/SAP (Callahan, Shepard, Beinecke, Larson, & Cavanaugh, 1995). MHMA organized and contracted with a network of providers and expanded the continuum of services by funding programs such as partial hospitalization programs; other hospital alternatives, such as holding beds and crisis stabilization; family support teams; intensive case (clinical) management; and treatment team specialists. Although MHMA was partially capitated, providers were reimbursed on the basis of negotiated rates. MHMA managed this contract for four years. After a rebidding process, the Massachusetts Health Partnership began managing the MH/SAP on July 1, 1996.

Study Design

As part of an evaluation of the first two years of the MH/SAP (Beinecke, Cavanaugh, Callahan, Shepard, & Larson, in press; Callahan et al., 1995), telephone interviews with 90 MHMA providers in 1994 began to describe the impact of the MH/SAP on providers and suggested that providers were changing both their clinical practices and their organizations in response to the initiative.

We hypothesized that in response to the MH/SAP and other factors, providers would change their clinical practices through greater use of timely assessments, groups, brief treatment, episodic care, and medication consultations. We further hypothesized that providers would also be changing organizationally, perhaps by improving their management information systems (MISs), conducting more utilization review and outcomes measurement, expanding in size and in the continuum of services they offered, and affiliating with other agencies. They would be changing their reimbursement from fee-for-service to capitation. Providers predicted that these changes would have a negative effect on their financial health.

Questions were added to the provider surveys in years 3 and 4 of the MH/SAP to test our hypotheses. Eighty-eight MHMA providers were interviewed by telephone during November–December 1994, of whom 85 were the same providers interviewed a year earlier. Eighty MHMA providers were interviewed in December 1995–February 1996, of whom 75 were the same as a year earlier. In the original survey and, thus, the follow-up studies, providers were stratified by services type and services region, and a random sample was drawn from each group. The samples contained adult and child inpatient psychiatric providers, substance abuse inpatient (level 4) and residential (level 3) providers, substance abuse and child diversionary providers (residential services designed to prevent hospitalization), and outpatient clinics. In each organization we interviewed the person who had the most contact with MHMA (Beinecke, Goodman, & Rivera, 1995; Beinecke & Lockhart, 1996).

The strength of these studies is that they are beginning to collect longitudinal data from nearly the same cohort of clients. The limitations are that the questions addressed in this study began to be asked in detail only in year 3 and that only providers working with MHMA were interviewed. Although they were very knowledgeable and were assured of confidentiality, they may have had a bias in favor of the MH/SAP that was not shared by people outside of the network.

Results

Summaries of utilization and cost data and providers' views about the effects of the MH/SAP on quality, access, and administration help to explain why providers made clinical, organizational, and financial changes (Beinecke, Shepard, Goodman, & Rivera, 1997; Beinecke & Perlman, 1997).

CHANGES IN CLINICAL PRACTICE

During years 3 and 4 of the MH/SAP, providers changed their clinical practices each year in response to managed care in the predicted directions (Table 13-1). There were no significant statistical differences among the different types of surveyed providers. A widespread change in clinical practice was clearly taking place. Respondents were engaging clients more actively in the treatment process and were better informing them of their benefits and restrictions on benefits; there was more awareness of low-cost alternatives. Some providers had developed new programs in response to the MH/SAP, such as short-term residential treatment, day treatment, and partial hospitalization programs; specialized services such as women's programs; and additional outpatient services. Providers had also increased their expertise in multiple languages and cultural diversity by adding multicultural clinicians, had speeded up their diagnostic (including testing) and treatment times, had added paraprofessional services, and increased the skill levels of counselors.

In year 3, 49 percent of those interviewed believed that they had improved care, but 22 percent felt that they had hurt care, and 29 percent said that the changes had made no difference. In year 4, 60 percent of providers believed that the changes had improved clinical care, 8 percent said that the changes had hurt care, and 32

TABLE **13-1**

Changes in Clinical Practice: Years 3 and 4

METHOD	YEAR 4 (%) INCREASED	STAYED CONSTANT	DECREASED	YEAR 3 MEAN[b]	YEAR 4 MEAN[b]
Comprehensive assessments	21	68	11	3.35	3.16
Timely assessments	40	56	4	3.54	3.44
Crisis management and stabilization	31	67	2	3.49	3.35
Brief treatment	51	45	4	3.48	3.56
Episodic care	38	68	2	3.43	3.42
Group work	42	54	4	3.28	3.42
Family treatment	28	70	2	3.21	3.30
Prescribing of medications	26	71	3	3.31	3.44
Substitution of less intensive/less costly services for inpatient care	62	38	0	3.69	3.74
Preventive services	40	59	1	3.21	3.43
In-home services	45	49	6	2.91	3.45
Consumer-run services[a]	28	71	1	NA	3.32

NOTE: NA = not asked.
[a]Such as support groups, clubhouses, or Alcoholics Anonymous/Narcotics Anonymous.
[b]1 = activity has decreased a lot, 3 = it is about the same, and 5 = it has increased a lot.

percent felt that they had made no difference. A large number of respondents felt that the changes in year 4 had not had a major impact on services in the earlier years of the program.

A third of respondents in both years felt that they had made these changes primarily as a result of the MH/SAP, and nearly half believed that the changes were a result of both the MH/SAP and other factors, including limitations on departments of mental health and social services, the increase in the severity of problems in the patient population, the reduction in permissible lengths of stay, changes in treatment philosophy, and new medications.

ORGANIZATIONAL CHANGES

Providers in both years were changing their organizations in response to managed care, including the MH/SAP (Table 13-2). Contrary to expectations, similar percentages of each type of facility were making these changes. The only significant difference was that a higher percentage of outpatient facilities was collecting information on consumers' experiences with care. In year 4,

- Fifty-one percent of providers reported that they had increased in size, 32 percent remained the same size, and 17 percent decreased in size.
- Seventy percent had expanded the variety of services that they provided, 28 percent had made no change in types of services, and 2 percent had fewer types of services.
- Thirty-four percent had greatly added or strengthened their total quality improvement (TQI) or total quality management (TQM) program, 60 percent

TABLE **13-2**

Changes in Organization: Years 3 and 4

	MEAN	
METHOD	**YEAR 3**	**YEAR 4**
Size[a]	3.60	3.40
Types of services[b]	3.61	3.83
Merged, acquired, affiliated (% yes)	44	65
Total quality management[c]	NA	4.09
Management information system[d]	3.64	3.38
Utilization review data[e]	3.40 (85% yes)	3.46 (87% yes)
Measurement	3.61	3.46
Client experiences[f]	NA	3.60
Staff hours for paperwork[g]	3.46	4.00
Training and supervision hours[h]	NA	3.42

NOTE: NA = not asked.

[a]1 = substantially decreased in size, 3 = stayed the same, and 5 = substantially increased in size.

[b]1 = many fewer types, 3 = no change, and 5 = many more types.

[c]1 = strengthened not at all, 3 = strengthened somewhat, and 5 = strengthened a great deal.

[d]1 = no improvements, 3 = some improvements, and 5 = great improvements.

[e]1 = increased collection of utilization/service and expenditure data not at all, 3 = somewhat increased collection, and 5 = increased collection a great deal.

[f]1 = increased collection of information on clients' experiences with care or client satisfaction not at all, 3 = somewhat increased collection, and 5 = increased collection a great deal.

[g]1 = devoted many fewer hours each week to paperwork, utilization review, and TQM, compared with direct clinical care, 3 = no change in hours, and 5 = devoted many more hours.

[h]1 = devoted many fewer hours each week to training and paperwork, compared with direct clinical care, 3 = no change in hours, and 5 = devoted many more hours.

had somewhat expanded their TQM, and 6 percent had expanded it very little or not at all.

- Fifty-nine percent had made many or great improvements to or expanded their MIS, 26 percent had made some or hardly any improvements in MIS, and 15 percent had made no improvements at all.
- Twenty percent had increased by a great deal their collection of utilization/service and expenditure data, 70 percent had somewhat increased the data collection, and 10 percent had not increased this data collection at all.
- Nineteen percent had increased their measurement of services and client outcomes a great deal, 58 percent had somewhat increased measurement, and 23 percent had not increased measurement at all.
- Twenty-one percent had increased their collection of information on clients' experiences with care or client satisfaction a great deal, 65 percent had somewhat increased this collection of data, and 14 percent had not increased collection of client experience data at all.

Eighty-three percent had developed improved referrals and linkages with at least one other organization (Table 13-3). Sixty-five percent had contracted or otherwise affiliated with another organization. Twenty-seven percent had merged or acquired another organization.

TABLE **13-3**

Changed Relationships during the Past Year

	WITH NUMBER OF ORGANIZATIONS (%)			
RELATIONSHIP	NOT AT ALL	1	2–4	MORE THAN 4
Referrals and linkages	17	3	43	37
Contracted	35	14	33	18
Merged or acquired	73	10	15	2

Paperwork

Eighty percent of providers in year 4 were devoting more staff hours each week to paperwork, utilization review, and TQI, compared with clinical care. Fourteen percent were devoting the same number of hours as a year earlier, and only 6 percent were devoting fewer hours. On average, the surveyed providers were devoting an additional 42 more hours per week to these administrative tasks. Thirty-nine percent of providers were devoting an additional 10 hours or less each week, 35 percent were devoting 11 to 20 hours more, and 26 percent were devoting more than 20 additional hours. Providers varied greatly in size, and the range of reported additional hours was 1 to 450. Therefore, the exact numbers of hours should be viewed cautiously, although clearly more hours were being spent in these activities.

Training and Supervision

Fifty percent of providers in year 4 were devoting more hours per week to training and supervision, 38 percent were devoting the same amount, and 12 percent were devoting fewer hours. The amount of additional time was relatively small, an average of 12 hours per week. Eighty-one percent of providers devoted less than an additional 10 hours per week, 14 percent devoted 11 to 20 hours, and 5 percent devoted more than 20 hours per week to training and supervision. The range was 1 to 150 additional hours.

Reimbursement

Despite much discussion about capitation, most providers were moving very slowly toward it. On average in year 4, 80 percent of current provider contracts were fee-for-service and 20 percent were capitated or partially capitated (Table 13-4). Contrary to expectations, inpatient facilities did not have a greater percentage of capitated contracts than did other types of providers. In year 4, 35 percent of providers said that they were moving toward capitation, an increase from 22 percent in year 3. In contrast to year 3, when it was primarily inpatient providers who were moving toward capitation, in year 4 all providers had similar responses, thus suggesting more widespread changes. Thirty-one percent of providers reported that they were fully prepared to move to subcapitation or other risk-sharing arrangements in year 4, 54 percent were somewhat ready, and 15 percent were only a little ready or not ready at all.

TABLE **13-4**

Fee-for-Service and Capitated or Partially Capitated Contracts

	FEE-FOR-SERVICE (%)	CAPITATION (%)
Percent of agency's total contracts		
100	45	2
76–99	21	2
51–75	11	13
1–50	21	36
0	2	47
Type of facility		
All	80	20
Adult inpatient mental health	82	18
Child inpatient mental health	80	20
Level 4 substance abuse	67	33
Level 3 substance abuse	64	36
Child diversionary	75	25
Substance abuse diversionary	92	8
Outpatient	90	10

Consumer Input

Sixteen percent of providers in year 4 said that they had large amounts of valued and effective consumer input from Medicaid clients in their planning and policies (for example, decisions on program structure, hiring, training, and quality improvement). Twenty-six percent had some consumer input, 20 percent had a little input, and 38 percent had no consumer input. Compared with results a year earlier, 31 percent had greater input, 54 percent had about the same input, and 15 percent had less consumer input.

One-third of providers in both years felt that these organizational changes were primarily a result of the MH/SAP. One-third believed that they were primarily a result of other factors, including the general reimbursement climate, relationships with other managed care companies, services expansion and diversification, greater competition, and reviews by the Joint Commission on Accreditation of Healthcare Organizations. One-third said that their changes were caused by both MHMA and other factors.

FINANCIAL CHANGES

Many providers in the years 1 and 2 survey were concerned about the future. They warned that further reductions in lengths of stay, tighter restrictions on inpatient admissions, additional reductions in funding, and continued administrative burdens could hurt their organizations' financial status.

In year 3, nearly half of the providers reported that they were doing better financially than either before the MH/SAP or a year earlier. But one-quarter of providers were doing worse. In year 4, more than one-third of providers were financially better off than either before the MH/SAP or than a year earlier, although more than

TABLE **13-5**

Changes in Financial Status: Years 3 and 4

	METHOD	
	BEFORE MH/SAP (%)	ONE YEAR AGO (%)
Year 3		
Much better	0	1
Better	40	44
About the same	31	30
Worse	27	25
Much worse	2	0
Year 3 mean[a]	3.12	3.21
Year 4		
Much better	8	8
Better	30	28
About the same	24	35
Worse	25	24
Much worse	13	5
Year 4 mean[a]	2.93	3.07

NOTE: MH/SAP = Massachusetts Mental Health/Substance Abuse Program.
[a]1 = much worse, 3 = about the same, and 5 = much better.

one-third were doing worse than before the MH/SAP, and slightly less than one-third were doing worse compared with the prior year (Tables 13-5 and 13-6). Compared with responses in the year 3 survey, somewhat more agencies were doing worse, and more were doing much worse. No patterns by facility type were visible in either year.

One-quarter of providers in both year 3 and year 4 felt that their financial changes were primarily a result of the MH/SAP, one-quarter said other factors were

TABLE **13-6**

Changes in Financial Status, by Facility Type: Year 4

	MEAN[a]	
FACILITY TYPE	BEFORE MH/SAP	ONE YEAR AGO
All	2.93	3.07
Adult inpatient mental health	3.05	3.42
Child inpatient mental health	2.20	2.83
Level 4 substance abuse	2.50	2.50
Level 3 substance abuse	2.88	3.25
Child diversionary	3.14	3.00
Substance abuse diversionary	3.29	2.86
Outpatient	2.95	2.91

NOTE: MH/SAP = Massachusetts Mental Health/Substance Abuse Program.
[a]1 = much worse, 3 = about the same, and 5 = much better.

the primary causes, and half attributed financial changes to both the MH/SAP and other factors.

Providers said they were doing better financially because they had increased their volume of clients, in part because of higher Medicaid utilization as a result of being in the MHMA network; had expanded to offer a full continuum of services; had grown in size; had broadened their revenue sources, especially by serving more private and fee-for-service clients and having enhanced working relationships with managed care organizations and networks with other providers; and had incrementally improved their reimbursement rates, especially for medication consultations. They were also managing more efficiently by improving billing and collection, hiring new management, downsizing and belt tightening, and having greater reliance on fee-for-service clinicians.

Providers were not doing as well because they had increased costs associated with seeing more severely ill patients and providing more intensive treatment; had shorter lengths of stay that led to increased case turnaround and higher costs associated with this pattern of care; had reimbursement rates too low for some services; and had high administrative costs, poor cash flow, and unreimbursed care as a result of MHMA's prior approval and billing processes. The amount of free care increased, primarily as a result of having to keep clients because of a lack of placements, although MHMA would not reimburse for them. A number of agencies had lost federal, state, or city grants.

Discussion

The surveys confirm that to participate successfully in managed care, services providers must make widespread clinical and organizational changes and prepare themselves to move toward risk-sharing arrangements. As managed care spreads, there will be a substantial change in the way that mental health and substance abuse care are practiced and organized. The fundamental restructuring of the mental health and substance abuse delivery system taking place is similar to changes being made by hospitals and other health care providers. The surveys suggest trends for a future with fewer providers more closely affiliated with each other and participating in a limited number of managed provider networks. To survive, providers must make changes to improve management information and quality assurance systems and services as well as outcomes measurement as they move toward capitation.

The surveys showed that more providers than expected were doing well financially under the MH/SAP. Over time, however, providers and funding sources need to appreciate the many risks of managed care caused by more severely ill and costly clients, the costs of shorter lengths of stay and of additional management, and pressures to keep unit payments low. Some closing of inefficient or change-resistant providers is to be expected under such a system, but the danger is that better providers also will be lost or will have to reduce the quality of their care to remain viable. This outcome is not in the best interests of clients, the managed care organization, or the state. Such circumstances need to be monitored and managed carefully.

The effects of managed care initiatives may take some time to appear, so continuing studies of providers are needed. It took three years for the changes described in these studies to become widely adopted in Massachusetts. Creative and thoughtful management will help ensure that clients receive the services they need in this new era.

References

Beinecke, R. H., Cavanaugh, D., Callahan, J., Jr., Shepard, D., & Larson. M. J. (1997). Provider assessment of the Massachusetts Medicaid mental health and substance abuse program. *Administration and Policy in Mental Health, 23,* 379–391.

Beinecke, R. H., Goodman, M., & Rivera, M. (1995, May). *Evaluation of the Massachusetts Mental Health/Substance Abuse Program: Year three.* Boston: Suffolk University, Department of Public Management.

Beinecke, R. H., & Lockhart, A. (1996). *A provider assessment of the Massachusetts managed Mental Health/Substance Abuse Program: Year four.* Boston: Suffolk University, Department of Public Management.

Beinecke, R. H., & Perlman, S. B. (1996). *The MHMA Mental Health/Substance Abuse Program outpatient protocols: A provider assessment.* Boston: Mental Health Corporation of Massachusetts & Suffolk University, Department of Public Management.

Beinecke, R. H., & Perlman, S. B. (1997). The impact of the Massachusetts managed Mental Health/Substance Abuse Program on outpatient mental health clinics. *Community Mental Health Journal, 33,* 377–385.

Beinecke, R. H., Shepard, D. S., Goodman, M., & Rivera, M. (1997). An assessment of the Massachusetts managed Mental Health/Substance Abuse Program: Year three (fiscal year 1994). *Administration and Policy in Mental Health, 24,* 205–220.

Budman, S. H. (1995). Clinician update—New clinical challenges: Managed behavioral healthcare and the chronic psychiatric patient. *Behavioral Healthcare Tomorrow, 4,* 49–51.

Cagney, T., & Woods, D. R. (1994). Clinical management information systems. *Behavioral Healthcare Tomorrow, 3,* 25–31.

Callahan, J. J., Jr., Shepard, D. S., Beinecke, R. H., Larson, M. J., & Cavanaugh, D. (1995). Mental health/substance abuse treatment in managed care: The Massachusetts Medicaid experience. *Health Affairs, 14,* 173–184.

Egnew, R. C. (1995). Administrative and management issues in public–private collaboration. *Behavioral Healthcare Tomorrow, 4,* 25–29.

Flynn, L. M., Panzetta, A. E., & Shumway, D. L. (1994). Dialogue: Can managed behavioral healthcare plans serve the severely mentally ill? *Behavioral Healthcare Tomorrow, 3,* 41–48.

Giles, T. R. (1993). *Managed mental health care: A guide for practitioners, employers, and hospital administrators.* Boston: Allyn & Bacon.

Hoge, M. A., Davidson, L., Griffith, E. H., & Sledge, W. H. (1994). Defining managed care in public sector psychiatry. *Hospital and Community Psychiatry, 45,* 1085–1089.

Hohmann, A. A., Sederer, L. I., & Campbell, J. (1995). Dialogue: The rush to measure outcomes: Help or hazard? *Behavioral Healthcare Tomorrow, 4,* 40–46.

Hoyt, M. F. (1994). Characteristics of psychotherapy under managed behavioral healthcare. *Behavioral Healthcare Tomorrow, 3,* 59–62.

Jackson, V. H., Beinecke, R. H., Bond, R. J., Seldon, D. R., & Van Tassel, R. (1995). *Managed care guide for social workers in agency settings.* Washington, DC: National Association of Social Workers.

Lima, B. (1995). In-home behavioral care: The missing link. *Behavioral Health Management, 15,* 17–19.

Lowman, R. L., & Resnick, R. J. (Eds.). (1994). *The mental health professional's guide to managed care.* Washington, DC: American Psychological Association.

Mackenzie, K. R. (1995). *Effective use of group therapy in managed care.* Washington, DC: American Psychiatric Press.

Nadzam, D. (1994, July). *Outcome measurement and quality assurance: What does the future hold?* Paper presented at the Third Annual Treishman Center Conference, Clinical Technologies: Information to Improve Outcomes in Mental Health and Social Services, Cambridge, MA.

Nelson, D. C., Hartman, E., Ojemann, P. G., & Wilcox, M. (1995). Outcomes measurement and management with a large Medicaid population. *Behavioral Healthcare Tomorrow, 4,* 31–37.

Ray, C. G. (1995). Why CMHCs belong in networks. *Behavioral Health Management, 15,* 15–16.

Schreter, R. K., Sharfstein, S. S., & Schreter, C. A. (Eds.). (1994). *Allies and adversaries: The impact of managed care on mental health services.* Washington, DC: American Psychiatric Press.

Shortell, S. M., Anderson, D. A., Gillies, R. R., Mitchell, J. B., & Morgan, K. L. (1993). The holographic organization. *Health Care Forum, 36,* 20–26.

Stern, S. (1993). Managed care, brief therapy, and therapeutic integrity. *Psychotherapy, 30,* 162–175.

Todd, T. (1994). *Surviving and prospering in the managed care marketplace.* Sarasota, FL: Professional Resource Press.

Trabin, T. (1995). File update: Challenges in computerization across the behavioral healthcare industry. *Behavioral Healthcare Tomorrow, 4,* 1–7.

Winegar, N., & Bistline, J. L. (1994). *Marketing mental health services to managed care.* New York: Haworth Press.

PART THREE

Notes from the Field

A. Agency Perspectives

C H A P T E R **14**

The Corporatization of Mental Health Services: The Impact on Service, Training, and Values

Sue Matorin

In the multidisciplinary arena, the social work profession is unique. We address both discrete clinical issues and the larger sociopolitical valences that affect the lives of our clients. To illustrate, a middle-aged Hispanic grandmother presents to a traditional psychiatry outpatient clinic with symptoms of anxiety. Social work assessment reveals that she is grief stricken over the loss of her daughter to crack cocaine, struggles to raise a seven-year-old granddaughter, and futilely battles her landlord about rats in her small apartment.

For us as social workers, what are our options? We might use a medical model plan and provide symptom relief—assign her to a psychopharmacology "slot" and "medicate" her anxiety. Alternatively, we could address the psychosocial issues underlying her presenting symptom. We could intervene more comprehensively and assign a clinical social worker to provide a focused treatment that includes establishing a therapeutic alliance to address this client's grief, mobilizing her to improve the quality of her life for herself and her grandchild, and strengthening her to do battle with the landlord and the department of health.

This vignette illustrates the pressures on today's clinicians to provide expedient interventions. More important, it underscores our training challenge. We educators should teach the development of clinical skill so that trainees learn to competently identify categories of the *Diagnostic and Statistical Manual of Mental Disorders, Fourth Edition* (DSM-IV) (American Psychiatric Association, 1994) and the basics of psychopharmacology. Such skill, with its narrow focus on symptom reduction, however important, shortchanges clients and betrays our professional heritage. Expedient interventions that seem cost effective in the short term fail to address the effects of the broader societal forces that truly shape client lives and undermine their functioning.

The training challenge is especially critical at this moment. The corporatization of human services delivery has had a pervasive effect on the organization of health and mental health services, on training for clinical practice, and on the professional lives of clinicians of all disciplines. This chapter will describe a number of emerging salient themes and suggest ways in which we can both preserve professional values and proactively confront the challenges. The material focuses on the impact on the social work profession, but the experience is painfully similar for our colleagues in other disciplines.

NOTE: An earlier version of this chapter was presented at the Smith College School for Social Work Summer Forum on Welfare and Managed Care, July 1995, Northampton, MA.

For example, people with debilitating schizophrenia often negotiate stressful appeals two or three times to obtain Supplemental Security Income benefits. A young single mother of two children, barely subsisting on public assistance, suffers from a hypersweating syndrome that prevents her from participating in job training to achieve economic self-sufficiency. In an odd catch-22, despite the prevailing policy to encourage such a woman to become self-sufficient to reduce welfare rolls, Medicaid refuses to cover prescribed medications. She cannot afford the additional out-of-pocket expense on her tight budget. Patients who must rely on Medicaid transportation vans routinely arrive 40 minutes late for psychiatric appointments in a tightly scheduled clinic. Frail elderly men and women dependent on Medicare-funded home care to retain the dignity of independent living must now do battle with the very bureaucracy initially designed to provide them with a safety net.

These compelling ethical dilemmas are most productively addressed in the classroom—an arena in which to grapple with complexity. In the current practice climate, harried clinicians must act without the luxury of analysis.

In writing about managed care's "silent seduction of America," Keigher (1995) accurately underscored the powerful commercial forces transforming health care. In exchange for the reasonable goal of cost containment, the consumer "voluntarily" gives up free choice. The Commonwealth Fund launched a thoughtful study to analyze critical unanswered questions to guide us: questions about quality of care, effectiveness of plans, commitment to poor people and those with complex medical needs, preservation of professional autonomy, and attention to training so that talent in the long term is not siphoned off in the process of saving money in the short term.

Impact on Mental Health Practice: Loss of Autonomy, Symptom Focus, Dehumanized Care, and Inadequate Resources

Despite efforts by the current administration to expand benefits, people with serious psychiatric disorders continue to confront stigma and lack of parity in health coverage. For example, the prevalence of underdiagnosed and untreated depression, alcoholism, substance abuse, and schizophrenia and their cost to society have been well established; yet corporations continue to maneuver exceptions in the health coverage they provide employees to limit an adequate mental health benefit.

Clinical social workers are active players in the effort to widen access to treatment. They approach this issue somewhat less paternalistically than do members of other mental health disciplines: They press for self-determination and the client's right to refuse treatment and they encourage clients to think through risk–benefit ratios in the use of medications that can produce adverse side effects. Social workers struggle to balance society's need for safety with the individual client's right to freedom—a balancing act now at risk. Symptom reduction is the prevailing goal.

Mental health clinicians of all disciplines have generally responded negatively to managed mental health care. Most of them support sound efforts to curtail escalating health care costs. Managed behavioral health care could offer an opportunity to base treatment decisions on outcome data regarding efficacy and ensure a wise use of limited resources. For example, to preserve an inpatient benefit for future emergencies, a clinician could work toward a shorter length of inpatient stay and then transfer a client to community-based treatment. So what are the objections and resistance? Clinical decisions are now routinely challenged (Bollas & Sundelson, 1995;

Johnson, 1995; Shore & Beibel, 1996; Slosar & Lettieri, 1996; Warres, Soderstrom, Marcus, Berman, & Liebman, 1996). A potentially constructive conversation about resource utilization can deteriorate and become adversarial. Seasoned clinicians with deep clinical knowledge now find themselves on the defensive, justifying a treatment plan to a managed care representative unfamiliar with clinical complexity. They are conflicted about the intrusion on confidentiality as they are pressed to reveal data to justify care.

Clinicians experience pressure to discharge patients from the hospital prematurely, knowing full well the limited availability of adequate aftercare resources. Decisions are dominated by fiscal concerns rather than thoughtful clinical planning based on our knowledge of relapse prevention. Clinicians are not only experiencing a loss of the autonomy to which they have become accustomed; they are being asked to carry out clinical care that defies what they know about the time needed to form a therapeutic alliance with a person with psychiatric problems whose capacity to trust is often distorted by the illness. A reasonable time frame critical to establishing treatment compliance and follow-through is now truncated by the compressed way in which they are being asked to practice. We know that this is a myopic view of complex mental health problems that require clinical attention to multiple diagnoses; medications and aftercare, for which clients often lack insurance coverage; and skilled family intervention to reduce family burden and relapse risk.

Brody (1995) of Shephard Pratt Hospital and Fleck (1995) of Yale each wrote eloquently of the dehumanizing trends in modern psychiatry. Many of their points apply to a variety of clients in social work settings. Specifically, they each cite the emphasis on disease rather than on the person, the pressures of managed care, and the reductionist approach to the education of our trainees.

To help my own organization to better prepare for managed care, I contacted colleagues in benchmark states (Minnesota and California). Colleagues in leadership positions honestly revealed that managed care often reimburses for the cheapest intervention. The expected outcome—a revolving door of readmission—has become the norm. In a drive to contain costs, the State of New Hampshire attempted to restrict outpatient access to psychiatric medicines. Notwithstanding measurement of suffering in both human and quality-of-life terms, Harvard public health researchers (Soumerai, McLaughlin, Ross-Degnan, Casteris, & Bollini, 1994) documented New Hampshire's significant rise in emergency room visits and partial hospitalization services. That New Hampshire "initiative" actually cost the state more in the long term.

Fleck (1995) underscored that the pressure to discharge narrows practice to a goal of symptom reduction. As a result, clinicians ignore the psychosocial life of the client, his or her disabling DSM-IV Axis II personality disorders, and key family interventions that could reduce relapse risk and improve outcomes. Moreover, fragile patients are often shifted to lesser levels of care over the course of a week. Such "treatment" plans subject them to multiple separations and changes in treatment team at the point when they most need continuity.

Managed care companies portend to ascribe to the important concept of continuity of care in the treatment of psychiatric disorders. Toward this goal, clinicians are advised to transition the patient to the next level of care based on clear clinical criteria. In theory, this approach is reasonable. In actual practice, the clinician, pressed to discharge an inpatient from a costly facility to a less costly alternative, too often finds himself or herself provided with a list of nonexistent resources or inadequately trained community clinicians. Clinicians engage in time-consuming and futile searches for a competent adolescent psychiatrist, a clinician with expertise with substance abuse, or a day program for people with borderline pathology who engage in dangerous self-destructive behaviors. As a result, the clinician experiences the managed care company as primarily preoccupied with cost containment rather than appropriate utilization of quality resources.

Despite the rhetoric to shift funding from institutions to community-based services, many states have failed to do so, thereby leaving a wide gap between need and availability (Geller, 1995). For example, in New York, city and state officials agreed to fund supervised housing for homeless people with chronic psychiatric illness. As a result, a quality program that proved to be cost effective and of public health value enabled some people with serious psychiatric disabilities to leave the streets and begin reassembling broken lives. The fiscal arrangement has now collapsed, and governmental negotiations have become contentious.

Most clinicians wholeheartedly endorse the value of vertical care for patients—care organized on a continuum that affords easy access and includes a full range of services, that is, not just expensive inpatient arrangements but crisis services, mobile teams, day and partial hospital programs, education for families, and so forth. In fact, those arrangements are not new concepts, but instead are based on valuable community psychiatry models of the 1960s. Those earlier innovative programs are being recycled, with new descriptors such as "networks" and "alliances." Alliances between large groups of providers with differing areas of expertise potentially offer exciting opportunities in the care of people with serious mental health problems. In such an arrangement, one program need not offer all services but rather can draw on the strengths of another to offer the client care on a continuum. However, the merger mania sweeping many of our institutions fuels new language: "market penetration," "seamless systems of care," and "population care" (Saunders, 1997). Such words appear *au courant.* They have not translated into meaningful studies of consumer satisfaction regarding ease of access and quality. The driving force behind the buzzwords seems to emanate more from an efficiency perspective than the truly coherent service delivery policies that shaped earlier programming.

Additional Issues: Dumbing Down, Morale, Training Conundrums, and Dishonest Dialogue

A number of other troubling issues are emerging that affect the social work profession. In the frenzy to cut costs, institutions have followed a two-pronged strategy: (1) increase volume to generate revenue and (2) downsize staff to contain expenditures. More insidious than downsizing, however, has been the move toward "downsubstitution." To ally with the institutional mission to cut costs, social work administrators have replaced seasoned clinicians with "junior beginners" or bachelor's degree–trained case aides. Most people would agree that a case aide can be helpful to carry out delegated tasks of discharge planning under supervision, and that hiring aides could be a cost-effective use of resources. That reasonable cost containment strategy, however, should not be confused with the loss to programs when seasoned clinicians with expertise are replaced by novice social workers. Many institutions are experiencing a serious brain drain as clinicians with expertise are replaced in such a manner. Strikingly, downsubstitution occurs at the time when institutions are eager to capture a competitive market share by advertising "centers of excellence." Despite the hype, clients actually may receive care by novice staff.

This trend is compounded by a collapse of the infrastructure on which we have relied to support critical professional development. There is a serious organizational push to focus exclusively on productivity and dramatically reduce time designated for professional development, supervision and consultation, and in-service opportunities. Sadly, this push is occurring at the academic institutions that have so many intellectual resources to offer us. Social work educators realistically understand that the complexity of the practice world cannot be taught adequately in a two-year graduate program. The eradication of institutional intellectual support for new graduates, who confront a fast-paced, demanding practice arena, is alarming. Agencies managed by social workers who value professional development may now offer new graduates a steadier induction into the profession than do interdisciplinary settings, whose sought-after intellectual riches are now so much less available.

In the long term this change could have a profound effect on the refinement of our knowledge base in mental health care. Social work professionals now enter the field with less mentoring and exposure to expertise and with little support for their growth. We are in danger of experiencing a "dumbing down" of the profession. As I reflect on my entry into the profession, it seems a luxurious antique: role models and mentors; supervision by different disciplines; and encouragement to attend conferences and Grand Rounds, to publish, to participate in interdisciplinary research projects, to experiment with new models of treatment, and to take on a variety of cases for professional growth. One reviews such history with profound sadness but also a coldly realistic appraisal of the new climate, one that demands productivity but shrinks an infrastructure to promote functioning and growth.

In the drive to contain costs, institutions have embraced outside consultants—people with considerable business savvy who impose the principles of business management on clinical care. In reality, the care of a troubled person is far more complex than the production of an automobile; one can quite easily shave costs by using a somewhat cheaper carpet for a car interior. Cutting cost by shaving minutes off a complex clinical interview is another matter.

Two trends have emerged from the use of such consultation firms. First, they have almost uniformly misrepresented social work as cost ineffective. They have presented "discipline" identification as adversarial to the notion of "program" and have convinced institutions that staff should be program related rather than discipline related. Interestingly, this trend persists despite solid national data from the Society for Social Work Leaders in Health Care (SSWLHC) (1997) that has demonstrated the deleterious impact on social work functioning in institutions that have followed this trend.

Second, consulting firms have pitted nursing against social work. They have underscored the value of the nursing profession to institutions at the expense of our profession. Rather than assessing the differential strengths of our professions and the value to patients and families of interdisciplinary care, consulting firms have promoted nursing to assume program management responsibility. Hospitals have swept out seasoned social workers and replaced them with nurses, have embraced nursing case management models, and have recruited nurse managers rather than social workers to administer clinical programs.

Seasoned social workers with a solid professional identity can easily identify with program over discipline. Such men and women may welcome the chance to develop expertise with a specific population, are secure in their practice and unthreatened by the skills of others, and take pride in contributing to the overall fiscal viability of a program. Those experienced clinicians have often embarked on additional training independent of the work site.

These arrangements present an educational dilemma, however, for trainees and new graduates. Supervision by a psychologist who is skilled in psychological testing does not foster clinical social work skill. A nurse may know the side effects of an antidepressant but has little expertise teaching comprehensive psychosocial assessment or family treatment interventions. The absence of a social work leader to monitor productivity, to buffer staff from unreasonable demands, and to orchestrate an environment for professional growth may have more long-range negative effects on the profession's future health than can be appreciated by the current zeal to embrace a programmatic identity. The data gathered at the national level underscore the damage to professional identity and the dip in morale—factors that ultimately rebound negatively for institutions.

It is especially troubling that these management decisions too often focus on the fiscal aspect and are based on principles of business that do not easily translate to the complex clinical world. The current climate does not encourage honest dialogue to explore complexity and the implication of these decisions for the long term. To illustrate, Kolata (1998) reported the dismay of a physician who questioned a marketing effort to promote over other proven methods a specific cardiac procedure for the treatment of arterial plaque. He spoke anonymously, feared ostracism from colleagues for speaking out, and cited the strain of advocating caution in a climate in which colleagues were eager to jump on a financially lucrative bandwagon. This could be a parallel experience for many experienced social work administrators who courageously raise reasonable questions about issues described above.

To illustrate, I organized a conference in which a blended case management program combining social work and nursing was presented (SSWLHC, 1997). Fearful of job loss in institutions jumping on the case management bandwagon, and often now reporting to nursing or utilization review management, few in the social work audience questioned the role blurring described and the implications for our profession. For example, what is the impact on quality when nurses perform child abuse assessments and family counseling? Is it an appropriate function for a professional social worker to track the use of antibiotics in medical records? Is this a reasonable training environment for clinical social work interns?

In sum, the profession is taking a beating in the current climate. Our beliefs and convictions are being discarded as irrelevant to the fiscal decisions that dominate treatment planning. Our programs are being maligned or misunderstood. We are being misrepresented as ineffective, financially lavish, or both. We who question issues of quality and outcome are painted as out-of-date and are unfairly portrayed as defending "old" models of care. Many of us are being brutally tossed out by institutions to whom we have given years of loyal, dedicated service. Some of us who are "surviving" do so at the cost of our professional souls: We identify with "the enemy" and "retool" ourselves to ally with business rather than clinical interests. Joining with "administration," we abandon our leadership role as a supportive buffer and advocate for overwhelmed staff, instead becoming impervious to issues of morale as productivity pressures dominate the work.

But most alarming is that our profession is being defined for us. Institutions no longer support the notion of supervision for our young people or training to refuel our skills. Hospital chief executive officers, handsomely paid themselves, tell us that complex psychosocial practice can be delivered by cheaper, untrained case aides as a substitution for professional social work. We are informed that nurses are more equipped to deliver case management services than are we. Social workers are urged to embrace nursing case management, learn utilization review tasks with enthusiasm, and work interchangeably without question about our unique contribution to client care. Productivity pressures, the absence of time to reflect, the shrinkage of opportunity for professional development—all have had a deleterious effect on morale because clinical staff experience their current professional life as akin to piecework on an assembly line.

An Illustration

Recently I saved a life. I should have congratulated myself on a job well done—for my clinical skill with a patient and family in a compressed time frame and for my ability to work effectively with a physician despite the absence of an ongoing interdisciplinary relationship. The following vignette will demonstrate the variety of skills needed, the pace, the obstacles to mobilizing a less-expensive treatment in the community, the diminished joy of working in the current climate, and the lost opportunities to teach.

I took care of Mrs. E., a 50-year-old Hasidic married mother of nine children, for three months following a brief hospitalization for psychotic depression and a serious drug overdose. Because patients from other communities come to this teaching hospital for inpatient care, the organization of quality aftercare in their own communities may not be viable for more complicated conditions. Aftercare availability must be weighed, however, against a commute that can be cumbersome to effect a continuity-of-care plan.

Mrs. E.'s spotty attendance for weekly appointments was troubling. It complicated our effort to adequately monitor her functioning and adjust her antidepressant medication to achieve a better therapeutic outcome. She continued to suffer early-morning lethargy and had difficulty mobilizing herself to care for her husband and the four school-age children remaining in the home.

She was obsessively preoccupied with being a burden to her family because of her poor functioning. Impulsively, she took on the stress of a part-time babysitting job for four small children. Her judgment that this activity would "get her out of the house" was clearly impaired in light of the extent of her illness.

Because of the stigma of psychiatric illness in the Hasidic community, it was difficult to assess whether this patient's social withdrawal resulted from shame or was a symptom of her depression. I decided to engage the family more actively, both to elicit more data about her actual functioning and to mobilize support for her recovery. Toward this end I arranged a major meeting with Mrs. E.'s husband. I used psychoeducation to establish a thicker alliance with him and to reduce the patient's sense of burden, and I initiated extensive telephone contact with a grown daughter. These interventions seemed reasonable to ensure Mrs. E.'s more consistent contact with us, to teach the family to hold and supervise her medications to diminish suicidal risk, and to remain in more regular telephone contact with us.

The plan failed. Mrs. E.'s husband did alert me that she was again experiencing a resurgence of suicidal ideation. However, most puzzlingly, no family member accompanied her to the clinic. She arrived with a giftbox of chocolates for me, indicating a budding alliance. She admitted to suicidal ideation and demonstrated little insight regarding the wisdom of taking on a stressful job in light of her depression.

In the absence of accompanying family, a consulting physician and I convinced Mrs. E. to re-enter the hospital. In less than an hour (an extremely compressed time frame), we assessed risk, guided the patient to enter voluntarily rather than against her will, initiated discussion of an alternative treatment (that is, electroshock therapy in light of her failure to respond to medications), alerted her husband so that he could arrange care of their children after school and bring clothing to Mrs. E. at the hospital, completed numerous forms for the emergency room, secured an ambulance, and coaxed the anxious patient to ride with the drivers.

Throughout that effort, I was acutely aware that the cost-effective alternatives were available but that we were too pressed to mobilize them. Because the patient had Medicaid coverage and a concerned family to secure her medications, we might have considered ambulatory electroshock therapy, daily crisis intervention, and then day hospital care to obviate an admission. The physician, however, was hurrying off to other responsibilities, leaving little time beyond crisis intervention to explore options; because he and I had little prior collaborative experience, there was no opportunity to explore his reasoning or advocate options. I had other scheduled patients backed up in the clinic. There is no transportation arrangement from other communities to facilitate an ambulatory alternative. We took the expedient course and admitted the patient to the costliest end of the continuum of care.

The physician and I had no time to acknowledge a job well done despite the constraints. Sadly, the pressures outweighed the sense of accomplishment one should experience. The breathless pace leaves little energy to teach those skills to trainees. Such crisis practice is akin to a MASH unit without the "M*A*S*H" camaraderie. The gratification of pausing to reflect with a colleague or to conceptualize one's skill to teach junior colleagues is missing. This would have been a rich teaching case because it underscored the complex social work role and a broad knowledge base that encompasses psychiatric disease, medications, family interventions, and important cultural components. The joy of the work and the teaching are endangered species now, drowned out by productivity pressures.

Professional Response to the Turbulence

How should our professional voice respond to the turbulence? First, we can and should practice in a more cost-effective manner, monitoring ourselves and our programs for waste and arguing from a base of outcome data rather than outrage. We need competence in speaking the language of the economics people who currently dominate the dialogue.

We must use our expertise to help our institutions survive. Because we cannot divorce clinical practice from the economic pressures shaping institutional life, we need to be active players in contributing to the financial health of our organizations. Volume and productivity are vital to agency survival and should be the concerns of all staff, not just the harried administrator.

At Columbia University, students present me with many agency cases in which service is fragmented and wasteful. This is not money wisely spent, nor is this professional practice that promotes self-sufficiency. It is paternalistic and costly, and it perpetuates cycles of dependency on the "kindness of strangers." Because we live in an especially unkind time, we must work with families, not on them, and enable them to equip themselves to be in better control of their own destinies. We must monitor ourselves to practice in a fiscally responsible manner and orchestrate tighter collaboration among the many agencies that serve families with multiple problems.

In an editorial, Poole (1995) urged us to avoid self-righteous rhetoric and reflect on our accountability to our own practice. How have we contributed to the public's disillusionment with our social programs? How bureaucratically do we organize the agencies in which we practice? Do we streamline documentation, or do we swamp staff with unnecessary, outdated recording requirements? Do we identify our clients' strengths as well as their pathologies? Does our practice promote dependency, or autonomy? Do we learn short-term, focused, behavioral treatment models, or do we rigidly cling to a long-term, exploratory approach for all problems?

Second, we need to ally more with colleagues of other disciplines who share our humanistic values rather than present ourselves narcissistically as practicing on a higher moral ground. For example, an article in the *New England Journal of Medicine* (Ziv & Lo, 1995) described physician efforts to oppose the California proposition to withhold treatment from illegal aliens. The authors urged physicians to offer some free care, if necessary to offset cost, as an obligation of their profession.

Third, historically our profession is the most comfortable with consumer groups. We are thus in the strategically best position to join with such groups and support their efforts to solicit feedback about the quality of managed care programs. We are the best trained to engage the consumer in actively scrutinizing proposed plans. In New York, psychiatric trainees organized a "picnic for parity" to protest budget cuts in mental health. It was poignant to participate with a large turnout of consumers, many of them clients of day and outpatient programs.

Fourth, we cannot afford the luxury of persistent unfortunate splits in our ranks between "clinicians" and social policy advocates. The arduous effort to hold together a fragile coalition to achieve a social work license in New York State illustrates how easily we can fragment into territorial special-interest groups despite the high stakes. Our profession knows about the interface of individual client problems with larger economic and political issues and the role that money and power play in determining who gets what in our capitalistic marketplace. Our capability to simultaneously assess and intervene on the individual and societal levels is what makes our profession unique. Our education trains us to see through the argument that there are no resources for those in need. We know they exist, but access to them is controlled. We know health maintenance organizations will curtail access to complex care through gatekeepers under the guise of cost containment; we also know the chief executives of such organizations are reaping huge profits in a ruthless pursuit of greed. It is critical that we weave clinical, advocacy, and social policy threads into one fabric. We must be the first voice when inexpensive constricted "treatments" violate a patient's right to quality and adequate care, and we should stand tall for the psychosocial treatments that we know do work.

Fifth, contributing to those unfortunate splits is our phobic avoidance of research skills. Students who groan when I suggest a review of data to substantiate a model's efficacy trouble me. We cannot prevail in such a climate, and we seriously weaken ourselves professionally by this failure to embrace research. Students confuse the decision to have a research career with the need to master essential skills in program evaluation and outcome measurement.

Sixth, we should insist that dialogue include important value issues currently absent. Annas (1995) recommended ecological metaphors compatible with our profession. This approach expands the focus beyond disease to larger prevention and public health issues. The rhetoric about preventive health measures that could curtail escalating costs has not been matched by action ("Hospitals and Health Networks," 1997). We have not yet introduced and supported national comprehensive plans to address smoking, teenage pregnancy, hypertension, and archaic attitudes about death and dying—behaviors that add soaring costs to the health budget. Similarly, the economic foothold that drug dealing has in our society undermines community-based substance abuse treatment initiatives.

What structures perpetuate ill health and drive up the budget? In New York, for example, Republican Mayor Rudy Guiliani enthusiastically congratulated himself on lowering the budget and reducing welfare rolls. But children in the Bronx fend off rats in epidemic proportions. Do those children choose to live like this? Who chooses for them? What do the rat bites cost in economic and human terms? Deterioration of the physical plants in the public education system aggravates respiratory conditions. Asthma and emergency room visits are a way of life for many small children who attend schools that have chipped plaster and who live with parents who smoke.

Our professional mission is to raise these disturbing questions consistently and persistently to shape the dialogue and preserve client rights. Cornelius (1994) argued that social workers fail clients if we cave in and adapt to the trend toward corporate care. We must teach our students the clinical skill that integrates holistic health and wellness concepts with psychosocial and cultural components.

Seventh, we need to maximize the power of the word. Some of my students have been thrilled to have their letters published on the editorial page of *The New York Times.* Those letters eloquently present vibrant vignettes from the field to document the devastating impact of service cuts on the lives of clients.

Eighth, we teach interdisciplinary collaboration too tamely. To prevail we need to move well beyond our traditional teaching of how to speak up cogently in team rounds. Our trainees need to read the journals of other disciplines and recognize that others share our outrage at inadequate service. We need to connect with other colleagues who care about and advocate quality care. Splendid material in the *New England Journal of Medicine, The Lancet,* the *Journal of Nervous and Mental Diseases,* and the *Harvard Mental Health Letter* dovetails with our own thinking. We cannot afford to be sanctimonious about our values and outrageed as if we owned this property exclusively. One reason talking therapies are harder to justify than psychopharmacology treatments is because multidisciplinary turf battles have obscured and distracted us from outcome research. All disciplines are now paying a price for this "guild philosophy" of the past, as decisions about utility and modality are scrutinized by nonclinicians.

We return to our consideration of the Hispanic grandmother. Do we provide her with a 15-minute visit and a prescription for Ativan for the discrete symptom of anxiety? Do we "treat" the symptom, or the person? Do we ignore our psychosocial knowledge base and teach and defend that as adequate practice? Do we put on our professional blinders and convince ourselves that this is a level of quality we professionals should be proud to provide? Alternatively, do we draw on our expertise and skill to establish a critical alliance to achieve loftier goals: help her grieve her addicted daughter, so that she can raise her grandchild competently and avoid a costly placement and empower her to rid her apartment of the rats with which no city mayor himself would live? That vignette underscores how every clinical encounter in the current climate harshly challenges our ethical center: Do we cave in; do an expedient, minimalist job; address a discrete symptom; and shrink our sights? Or do we stand tall by our professional heritage; address the complexity of the client's life; and aim for an outcome that includes prevention of costly academic, social, and health problems for the grandchild? The 15-minute visit may seem efficient in the short term, but we know the unaddressed prevention issues will return to haunt us.

Our profession has never refused to address disturbing societal inequities. Historically, identifying clear, focused health goals and champions to promote them has brought remarkable advances ("The Unequal, the Achievable, and the Champion," 1995). I am optimistic that social workers will produce a generation of professional champions to prevail and that we will not be derailed from our center.

References

American Hospital Association. (1997). Human resources. In *Hospitals and health networks* (p. 10). Chicago: Author.

American Psychiatric Association. (1994). *Diagnostic and statistical manual of mental disorders* (4th ed.). Washington, DC: Author.

Annas, G. (1995). Reframing the debate on health care by replacing our metaphors. *New England Journal of Medicine, 332,* 744–747.

Bollas, C., & Sundelson, D. (1995). *The new informants: The betrayal of confidentiality in psychoanalysis and psychotherapy.* New York: Jason Aronson.

Brody, E. (1995). The humanity of psychotic persons and their rights. *Journal of Nervous and Mental Diseases, 183,* 193–194.

Cornelius, D. (1994). Managed care and social work: Constructing a context and a response. *Social Work in Health Care, 20,* 47–63.

The unequal, the achievable, and the champion [Editorial]. (1995). *Lancet, 345,* 1061–1062.

Fleck, S. (1995). Dehumanizing developments in American psychiatry in recent decades. *Journal of Nervous and Mental Diseases, 183,* 195–203.

Geller, J. (1995). When less is more; When less is less. *Psychiatric Services, 46,* 1105.

Johnson, L. D. (1995). *Psychotherapy in the age of accountability.* New York: W. W. Norton.

Keigher, S. (1995). Silent seduction of America [National Health Line]. *Health & Social Work, 20,* 300–305.

Kolata, G. (1998, February 10). Where marketing and medicine meet. *New York Times,* p. A14.

Pear, R. (1998, February 10). Home care denial in Medicare cases is ruled improper [Editorial]. *New York Times,* p. A1.

Poole, D. (1995). Editorial. *Health & Social Work, 20,* 243.

Saunders, S. (1997, October). *Population management in an integrated service delivery network.* Paper presented at the NASW New York State Conference, New York.

Shore, M., & Beibel, A. (1996). The challenges posed by managed behavioral health care. *New England Journal of Medicine, 334,* 116–118.

Slosar, J. R., & Lettieri, R. (1996). Financing mechanisms in the delivery of mental health care services: Widgets or wisdom? In *1997 source book for managed mental health care* (pp. 115–164). New York: Faulkner & Gray.

Society for Social Work Leaders in Health Care. (1997, September). *Easing on down the road: Reflections on a "blended" case management model.* Program presented at a meeting of the Metropolitan Chapter, New York.

Soumerai, S., McLaughlin, T., Ross-Degnan, D., Casteris, C., & Bollini, P. (1994). Effects of limiting Medicaid drug-reimbursement benefits on the use of psychotropic agents and acute mental health services by patients with schizophrenia. *New England Journal of Medicine, 331,* 650–655.

Warres, N., Soderstrom, P., Marcus, L., Berman, P., & Liebman, M. (1996). The impact of managed care and utilization review: A cross-sectional study in Maryland. *Psychiatric Services, 47,* 1319–1322.

Ziv, T., & Lo, B. (1995). Denial of care to illegal immigrants—Proposition 187 in California. *New England Journal of Medicine, 332,* 1095–1098.

CHAPTER 15

Managed Care and the Oppression of Psychiatrically Disturbed Adolescents: A Disturbing Example

Phebe Sessions

In recent years, I have listened to many clinicians tell troubling accounts of their experiences in attempting to provide ethical and effective care under the aegis of privatized, for-profit mental health services. The telling of an individual tale of oppressive mental health practices can lead to responses of disbelief and disqualification, generating questions about the generalizability of such practices and the integrity of the storyteller. We are living through a turbulent period in the organization and delivery of mental health services, with increases in the technical knowledge about caring for vulnerable populations and reduction in the autonomy of clinicians to practice what they know. In the context of dramatic shifts in the management and financing of services, we become uncertain about what and whom to believe. We understand that clinicians might feel reluctant to share their accounts because of the risk to employability and credibility. However, it seems increasingly important to encourage each other to share these stories and bring them into the professional literature, even if anonymously, to propel us out of our isolation and direct us toward shared analysis and action on behalf of our clients, our society, and our profession.

In his thoughtful essay on the capacity of managed care to address the needs of people with chronic mental illness (chapter 3), Jeffrey L. Geller asked and answered a series of important questions:

- Have managed care organizations met the needs of people with serious mental illness?
- Have managed care organizations refrained from riding on the backs of states' departments of mental health?
- Has the shift to managed care and privatization improved the already compromised continuity of care in the public sector?
- Has managed care improved the quality of life of people with serious mental illnesses?
- Do we have any clear indication that managed care is better than what we had before for people with serious and persistent mental illness?

To all of these questions, Geller responded no.

This chapter provides a case study of clinicians' experiences within an intensive residential treatment program for adolescent girls that justifies Geller's pessimism about the quality of care for troubled clients under privatized services contracted by a state department of mental health. As I was listening to the alarming story recounted here, the word that continually came to mind to describe these mental health practices was "oppressive." Many of the practices appeared to be a reinstitution of conditions that existed in the public-sector mental health system before the development of community mental health.

The Program

The setting was a long-term, locked psychiatric unit considered to be a link in the continuum of care between inpatient hospitalization and community-based, outpatient care for people with chronic mental illness. All the patients in this setting were teenagers who had been psychiatrically hospitalized or had failed at several other residential placements. Four of the teenagers were psychotic at the time of admission; most had experienced abuse and trauma and had diagnoses that reflected those experiences. Clients were involuntarily committed for assessed danger to self or others or were voluntarily committed by parents. None were free to leave. The services were administered by a private vendor under contract with a state department of mental health. The vendor had pursued the contract for these services after a previous vendor, a not-for-profit corporation, had been criticized by the state for excessive use of physical restraints in response to a high level of violence. The state department of mental health believed that the high level of violence was in part caused by the use of an "uncovering" mode of therapy that exposed clients to their traumatic histories without sufficient structure and support. The private, for-profit vendor outbid several not-for-profit vendors, promising to deliver more effective services at reduced cost. To pay for these services, the vendor would receive contract monies from the state department of mental health, 80 percent of the client's Supplemental Security Income (SSI) disability check for residential services, and Medicaid reimbursement for medicalized and clinical services.

The private vendor subsequently hired as clinical director a clinician with extensive background in practice within secure treatment facilities and in trauma work. The vision of the clinical director was to base services on a "resiliency" model, aligning with the teenagers' strengths and trying to link them to meaningful roles in work and social life. The model was based on the clinical director's concern that many teenagers who have endured long periods of institutionalization have come to depend on institutional life and to believe that they have nothing to give to others or to society. Drawing on their capabilities and engaging them in community activities are significant parts of the rehabilitation effort.

The program was to provide two hours weekly of individual or family therapy, two hours of group therapy, milieu meetings three times weekly, and an educational program for 16 patients. A program director would administer the unit; the clinical director would supervise the clinical services; four child care workers and a shift supervisor would care for the milieu; a psychiatrist and nursing staff would monitor medication; and a separate educational program would address educational needs. In case of violence—which all hoped would be a rare occurrence—staff could apply chemical as well as mechanical restraints, such as straitjackets, "papoose boards" to strap down patients and move them from place to place, and "patient restraints" or leather straps to tie them to their beds.

Program Implementation

The model was never fully implemented as designed, and that failure led to severe consequences for staff and patients. The most important value that guided clinical and administrative decisions was keeping the costs low. To save money, the program failed to provide many promised services, thus leading to deficiencies in numerous areas, including those detailed below.

INSUFFICIENCY OF STAFF

In contrast to the program design, there often were no more than two child care workers on the unit. On official forms secretarial and clinical staff were reported as child care staff covering during the day. On weekends, the program frequently had to rely on "relief" staff supplied by a temporary agency. The relief workers had little training for work with clients with mental illness and had no relationship with the residents. The program director was seldom on site more than one half-day per week, spending much time in budgetary meetings. The clinical director was required to perform the role of program director. The clinical director and the clinicians on staff also frequently had to perform the tasks of child care workers to protect the patients.

Frequently there were vacancies in the professional and child care staff for months at a time. Management was extremely slow in filling vacant positions, sometimes leaving professional and managerial positions open for six to eight months. In about a year's time, there was a 90 percent turnover of child care staff and an 80 percent turnover of professional staff.

Management resisted replacing or filling in for staff as a cost-saving measure. A dramatic example of this occurred after an incident in which a patient assaulted a child care worker and knocked her unconscious. While the staff person was rushed to the hospital, the clinical director asked management for a replacement staff person to be assigned to help with an extremely troubled milieu; management responded that the hospitalized staff person was still being paid until 11 PM and could not be replaced until the conclusion of her shift.

INADEQUATE PROGRAMMING

Because of the lack of staff, there was little for the patients to do outside of the clinical services and their educational program. Much time was spent watching television on two overcrowded sofas. The environment was extremely understimulating and boring, leading to a high level of interpersonal conflict and inappropriate sexualized activity. Efforts to engage the teenagers in volunteer activity to link them meaningfully with the community were thwarted by management because of lack of funds. Lack of physical education increased frustration and deprived the patients of any arena for physical activity; in its absence, tragically, assaulting staff became a sport.

EXCESSIVE VIOLENCE

The level of violence on the unit escalated dramatically, soaring beyond the level experienced by the previous vendor—a level that had been considered unacceptable to the state department of mental health. An "expected" amount of violence at this level of care is one to two incidents per month. On this unit, there were up to 90 incidents per month that led to the use of physical restraints. The clinical director herself reported having to intervene in as many as 30 incidents per month because of staff shortages. The rate of injury to staff similarly escalated; at one time, there were six staff with injuries severe enough to require treatment and counseling.

The violence on the unit was not only frequent, but it also was severe and life-threatening. One patient inserted batteries deeply into her vagina, requiring surgical removal. Another patient, while on one-to-one suicide precautions, evaded the child care worker watching her, created a noose with her sneaker laces, and nearly hanged herself from a window sill. One patient thought she would receive better treatment in a prison and threatened to kill her clinician in order to achieve a transfer. The threat to patients and staff was extreme and unremitting.

UNRESPONSIVE MANAGEMENT

Many grievances were filed by the staff about safety issues; for the most part, they were dealt with by denial, evasion, and "reframing." When case managers from the department of mental health complained about the quality of care, they were told that the program simply needed time to compensate for the deficits caused by the previous vendor. Because the services were desperately needed and there was a long waiting list for this level of residential care, critical case managers assigned by the state department of mental health could often be deflected. Nevertheless, numerous sources filed complaints with management about the poor quality of care and the level of violence, and a review by the licensing authority led to a directive to reduce the use of restraints. Child care staff and clinicians were ordered to rely less on physical restraints in response to threats and noncompliance. As a result, the concerns about safety among the child care staff increased and lead to resignations.

Some complaints were greeted with bizarre and mind-numbing denials. For example, the clinical director complained to management that staff were demoralized and disturbed by the actions of one client who regularly vomited on them as they walked down the corridor. Management responded to this expression of concern by denying that any such incidents were taking place, alleging that the staff were confusing this client with another client who three years earlier had been on a different unit and had a regurgitation disorder. When staff persisted with their perception of events, management insisted vehemently, "THERE IS NO VOMIT!"

Management retaliated against staff who complained about working conditions or the quality of care. Disgruntled employees who resigned in protest against conditions on the unit were confronted with rumors circulated by management that they had been fired as a result of their poor job performance. Child care workers were cautioned against leaving the unit and advised that they would be unable to find other jobs. Dissension among unhappy staff members was encouraged by management. Following a visit by a utilization reviewer from the department of mental health, the staff was reprimanded for disclosing an attempted hanging that had taken place on the unit.

DETERIORATION IN CLIENT BEHAVIOR AND WELL-BEING

Not surprisingly, the clients got worse. Clients who had never before engaged in violent behavior soon became violent in this context. Similarly, clients without a history of self-mutilation began cutting themselves. During an eight-month period of time, no clients were planfully discharged from the facility, although several left against medical advice.

One client who clearly was harmed by her stay on the unit was a 14-year-old girl who was placed in the secure residential facility for running away, rebelling against her custodial grandparents, and abusing illegal substances. She was the daughter of a woman with the diagnosis of bipolar disorder. The mother's mental illness had led to the daughter's placement with grandparents and to a succession of foster homes. Early in her life, the client had witnessed battering of her mother by a boyfriend; her mother was severely beaten while the child, then age eight, hid in the bushes. The frequency of violence on the unit was frightening to this client and caused flashbacks of her early trauma. During incidents of violence, the client was sometimes moved to a different part of the unit; however, she could still hear the violence even though she could not see it. This experience of helplessness and enforced passivity during episodes of violence to someone else led to overwhelming experiences of trauma re-enactment. The client's family was involved in her treatment and commuted long hours for therapy appointments. Good clinical work could not compensate, however, for the traumatizing effects of the environment, and the client's behavior deteriorated. Through the intervention of a concerned case manager who was her guardian, this client was briefly transferred to another residential facility where there was less violence and more substance abuse treatment. After some lobbying from the vendor, however, the client was returned to the unit, even though this unit lacked any substance abuse treatment program.

DETERIORATION IN STAFF MORALE AND PERFORMANCE

The staff suffered directly from physical violence and indirectly from reduced morale and lack of opportunity to develop and express a range of skills. The insufficiency in the number of staff meant that the staff were continually dealing with crises rather than with program development and that clinical staff were often rerouted from the jobs that they were hired to do in order to compensate for lack of frontline staff. The clinical director had been hired with the understanding that she was willing to leave a more lucrative practice for a less-than-full-time job in which she could implement a creative model of services. In fact, the clinical director was confronted with so many emergencies that her job was much more than full-time. She and other clinicians frequently covered for missing frontline staff. In addition to her supervisory work, the clinical director performed clinical services. She was on call every weekend and received between eight and 20 emergency and consultative calls during those weekends. After eight months of that weekend duty, she was denied permission to relinquish this responsibility for one day in observance of a religious holiday. This was hardly the job she had bargained for.

Finally, the need to keep costs low and to have on staff only people who would be responsive to management directives led to decisions to hire less-qualified people. During several job searches, professionals with substantial experience in residential treatment programs applied but were not considered. Preference seemed to go to less-experienced and more-malleable clinicians who were new to the field.

Frequent staff turnover, chronic states of emergency, and use of relief staff to fill in for absent or ill child care staff led to few opportunities to give staff the training they needed to learn intervention skills to prevent escalation in crisis situations. Staff were overexposed and undersupported. One staff member who was on one-to-one suicide watch was required to observe the client for an entire shift without averting her gaze or leaving her post. This job was so monotonous that the staff member was found carving herself with a piece of glass. Low investment in the staff made them vulnerable to adopting client behaviors.

Commentary

The implementation of these services was not only ineffective in helping patients; it also created conditions that could only be described as oppressive for staff and patients. The case study of this secure facility provides a compelling example of problems that can result from contracting out services to for-profit companies. The effects of privatization can be seen in poor quality of care delivered to seriously troubled young people, withdrawal of responsibility from state departments of mental health through the sale of services, gaps in the continuity of skilled care, and reversion to conditions that we may have believed had been eliminated or at least greatly reduced with the advent of community mental health.

To deepen my understanding of the meaning of such derailment in the purpose and quality of mental health services, I have used a framework of analysis developed by feminist political philosopher Iris Young (1990), which describes the nature and various manifestations of oppression in contemporary society. Young wrote about the goal of social justice, the underlying purpose of our profession, and the impediments to its achievement. According to Young, a society committed to social justice supports the institutional conditions necessary for the realization of the values of the good life, including opportunities to develop and exercise one's capabilities and express one's experience and to participate in determining one's action and the conditions of one's action. She also described five forms, or "faces," of oppression that interfere with the achievement of a just society: exploitation, marginalization, powerlessness, cultural imperialism, and violence. Each of these faces of oppression can be recognized in the case example presented in this chapter.

EXPLOITATION

Young (1990) derived her understanding of exploitation from Marxist ideas of class-based social practices of domination; oppression as exploitation occurs "through the steady process of the transfer of the results of the labor of one social group to benefit another" (p. 49). That is the conceptualization of oppression that is most familiar in this society, and it focuses on problems in the redistribution of (generally material) goods. For-profit companies reintroduce into mental health care the problems of exploitation that had lessened when federal and state governments were its major sponsors. In our present case example, goals of quality care were continually compromised by the need to produce profit. Profit was not reinvested into the program but was transferred into private ownership. The need to produce profit led to decisions that powerfully affected the working conditions in the unit. Having contracted with the state and with employees to provide in-depth services with sufficient professional and paraprofessional coverage, company management proceeded in the enactment of its program to cut corners at every opportunity, particularly in staffing. Inadequate staffing meant that no one could perform a job according to its formal job description; everyone's job performance had to expand in an effort to fill the need without any change in compensation. Furthermore, it appears that there was adequate funding from federal and state sources (SSI, Medicaid, and the state contract) to support a more effective program, had the need for a profit margin not drained critical resources. By engaging for-profit companies to provide mental health services to troubled teenagers, state and federal levels of government may be failing in their responsibilities to protect the public by regulating and counteracting the harshness of corporate-driven priorities.

MARGINALIZATION

Young (1990) defined *marginalization* as the process of expelling a whole category of people from useful participation in social life, and she suggested that it may be the most dangerous form of oppression in contemporary society. She challenged widely held assumptions that "moral agency and full citizenship require that a person be autonomous and independent" and argued against condemning people who are for any reason marginal to the economic order to lives of "uselessness, boredom, and lack of self-respect" (p. 59).

In the case study presented here, processes of marginalization can be seen in the efforts to undermine the goal of the clinical director to counteract the effects of institutionalization by engaging the patients in community life at whatever participatory level was possible. This was a primary goal for the clinical director when she assumed her position, and ostensibly, management agreed to it; but the goal was easily discarded by management when it came to applying funds to implementation. From an empowerment perspective currently advocated by patients' rights movements, this goal of linking patients to meaningful social roles is central rather than marginal. Dignity, conferred by access to social roles, cannot be divorced from mental and emotional health.

POWERLESSNESS

Young's (1990) discussion of powerlessness is based on her observation that "most people do not regularly participate in making decisions that affect the conditions of their lives and actions . . . in this sense, most people lack significant power" (p. 59). Young recognized a significant hierarchy in the workplace: The top level consists of managerial people with access to and control of material assets, and the next level consists of professional people with some degree of autonomy in work conditions conferred by technical expertise and with a good deal of respectability. The lowest level, the powerless, have little work autonomy, exercise little creativity or judgment in work, have no technical expertise or authority, and do not command respect. Young noted that professionals are often in an ambiguous position because they receive directives from managers above them and give directives to more powerless workers below them.

Mental health professionals have recently been decrying what they experience as an erosion of their authority and respectability, as the managers who control budgets exercise increasing control over decisions, including the prioritization of managerial concerns over technical expertise. This case study clearly demonstrates a profound lack of autonomy in the mental health professionals providing care. Their priorities in program implementation and clinical service are repeatedly undermined, even in such clear clinical areas as safety concerns and protection. They also are repeatedly called to perform paraprofessional tasks. Respect for technical expertise is undermined by hiring decisions that favor less-experienced practitioners, who may be more likely to accept managerial directives.

However, in keeping with Young's analysis, the workers who fared the worst in our case study were the paraprofessionals. The extremely poor work conditions resulted in a 90 percent turnover rate in a year. Paraprofessionals were overworked by patterns of insufficient staffing and were subject to a high rate of assault and injury. They were given little training to perform a socially vital role; whatever skills they did acquire through experience were not acknowledged because it was assumed that their roles could be performed by temporary staff with even less experience. Interpersonal support from professional staff failed to compensate for such hazards.

CULTURAL IMPERIALISM

Young (1990) defined *cultural imperialism* as the process by which "dominant meanings of the society render the particular perspectives of . . . a group invisible; at the same time, they stereotype a group and mark it out as the Other" (p. 59). Cultural imperialism can be seen in the weight of authority assigned to perspectives developed by people who are racially white, culturally European, religiously Christian, male, heterosexual, able bodied, and lacking the stigma of mental disability when their perspectives are not sufficiently contextualized or the dynamics of power between self and other ignored.

In the present case example, we see a sharp division between the mental health professionals and managers, who are presumed to hold all the knowledge, and the patients, who are exclusively defined by their disability. The language of psychiatric diagnosis delineates the patients' incapacity, and patients may come to understand themselves less and less in their own terms and increasingly in the deficit perspective of the *Diagnostic and Statistical Manual of Mental Disorders* (DSM). In the clinical director's efforts to introduce a resiliency orientation, we can see some effort to identify a way of thinking both about and with patients, which might elicit patients' own terms for understanding their pain and generate empowering alternative behaviors. Challenging the dominant perspective on psychiatric disability can enable the voice of the client to emerge, with her framework of analysis and understanding of solutions. Both the clinical staff and the patients, however, were thwarted in their efforts to check the total domination of professionalized discourse, and that interference left both groups demoralized and diminished.

VIOLENCE

According to Young (1990), violence in this society is most frequently understood to be actions taken by individuals as a result of their own moral and emotional deficits. The systemic nature of violence, including its social sources and effects, is seldom addressed. Violence also can be understood as a form of social oppression in that it occurs regularly toward members of specific social groups, particularly toward low-status or stigmatized groups.

This case study describes a clinical unit in which violence escalated in a way that engaged everyone in frightening and destructive interactions. That escalation of violence might be understood as a function of the individual psychopathology of the residents of the unit, or it might be understood as a function of the dramatic and cruel withdrawal of basic supportive services for these vulnerable teenagers.

The violence was not random; it became deeply ingrained in the unit's social organization in the absence of sufficient and generous caretaking. Who, then, do we see as the perpetrators? It would seem as though the patients, who may have initiated the individual incidents of violence, had the least power to effect change on the unit and to determine the policies and the climate of care that affected their safety and well-being. They are the recipients of institutionalized violence, and they show the effects of the violence that has been directed toward them both in the past and in the present in their specific behaviors. Even within their treatment facility, they continue to live with unremitting trauma.

Conclusion

The sad tale of this secure unit highlights the vulnerabilities of patients and staff when responsibility for providing critical mental health services is sold to the lowest bidder. Despite the best intentions of highly educated and knowledgeable professional people, the requirement to prioritize the bottom line subverts all other competing value systems and opens the door to severe forms of oppression enacted against troubled teenagers. By the time regulatory agencies intervene to stop the practices of one corrupt agency, contracts have shifted to others, and agencies have merged or been transferred to new ownership. The problems lie not with one agency but with the current defeat of a powerful public health philosophy and value system that could challenge and effectively balance commercial and corporate values.

Reference

Young, I. M. (1990). *Justice and the politics of difference.* Princeton, NJ: Princeton University Press.

C H A P T E R 16

Agency Mission, Social Work Practice, and Professional Training in a Managed Care Environment

Alan B. Siskind

The social work field is currently moving through a period of adjustment and some uncertainty brought on by significant changes in the environment in which we operate. These changes result from a complex mix of factors—social, political, and economic in nature. In this chapter I want to focus on one particularly important change in our environment that, although most clearly economic in character, possesses political and social dimensions as well. The recent rapid growth of managed care is having a major impact on how social work services are delivered to those who need them and is affecting the very shape of social work practice and education. I will address certain salient issues raised by the growth of managed care, and in doing so I hope to give a balanced picture that speaks both to the opportunities contained in the challenge that it presents to the status quo and to the ways in which it must be held accountable to standards of good and appropriate practice that we know promote the well-being of the people we serve.

Let me be clear from the outset about the perspective from which I approach and analyze the developments associated with managed care. I am the director of a large mental health and human services agency in New York City—the Jewish Board of Family and Children's Services (JBFCS)—as well as a part-time practicing clinician. I plan to ground what I write here in my experience at the agency for which I work, so it may be helpful if I include a few words about that agency. JBFCS is a voluntary, not-for-profit mental health and social services agency with origins in the Jewish tradition of responsibility for people who are sick and troubled. In accord with this tradition, JBFCS continues to uphold as one of its primary obligations service to the Jewish community and recognizes and fulfills a commitment also to extend services to the general community. Throughout its century-long tradition of service, JBFCS has been a pioneer in developing new programs to meet the changing needs of the community. Using a wide range of methodologies and intervention techniques, each year the agency serves more than 54,000 New Yorkers in 130 separate programs.

The emergence of managed care has ushered in changes that significantly affect the way provider agencies like JBFCS operate. As we assess and respond to these changes, however, it is important to bear in mind that periods of profound change

NOTE: Originally published as Siskind, A. B. (1997). Agency mission, social work practice, and professional training in a managed care environment. *Smith College Studies in Social Work, 67*, 16–19.

are nothing new. Such periods have frequently altered the shape of the agency's services in the past. Yet throughout its history, the agency has maintained a set of basic core values in terms of which our mission is defined. Thus, we have gone to great lengths to ensure that we do not compromise our commitment to quality care, accountability, innovation in program development, professionalism in supervision and consultation and, in an area in which we have worked to take the lead, training and research. Of course, preserving core values in the face of changing conditions can be difficult when the pressures of new demands and imperatives force us to adjust the way we pursue our mission. We preserve core values in spite of such difficulties, however, because the alternative is to lose our identity and, with it, our integrity.

Change sometimes has made our job as providers easier. Decades ago, when government seriously began to contract with voluntary agencies to meet community needs, many of us in the provider community adjusted how we pursued our missions, and we found that we were able to serve more people and serve them better. New sources of funding allowed us to expand and enrich our services and serve more diverse populations in the community. We learned that continually adjusting to new demands and looking for new opportunities served the community well and kept our theoretical and practical assumptions from becoming too rigid.

Now, with government support dwindling in an antitax political environment and competition for scarce philanthropic dollars increasing among a growing number of parties, we are at another turning point. It is clear that we need to adapt ourselves to the demands of the commercial sector—specifically, managed care organizations (MCOs)—in order to sustain and enhance our services. It is our hope that here, too, as we engage new sources of revenue, we will be able to sharpen our skills and do a better job for our clients. Social work education also is at a turning point, and it must adapt itself to ensure that new social workers are prepared for a new environment. Provider agencies have always collaborated with social work schools to make sure that students get the hands-on training necessary to complete their education. That partnership will be all the more important in the years ahead. At the same time, however, we all need to recognize that agencies have fewer resources and are facing more and more restrictions from managed care companies. The question of how managed care affects the partnership between service providers and social work schools is a serious one. After discussing the ways in which managed care has forced us, sometimes with positive results, to re-evaluate certain premises of how we have been doing business and how we understand the role of the social worker, I will take up the issue of this all-important partnership.

It is worth noting, before we look at the specific implications of managed care for how we operate, that the new environment is as susceptible to transformation as the one it replaces. In fact, managed care in the form of health maintenance organizations (HMOs) might not even exist in five or 10 years. As the elements, values, and assumptions of newly designed care systems are integrated into our work, there will be less need for MCOs to contain costs and challenge inefficient services. That is all the more reason for us to participate in the development of time-effective and cost-effective interventions consistent with responsible, sound service delivery and client advocacy.

Managed Care and Long-Held Assumptions

It is no secret that managed care has not been whole-heartedly embraced by many people in the business of designing and delivering mental health services. Indeed, I have heard managed care described as "an insurmountable opportunity." I think that is an effective expression of the ambivalence that I and many of my colleagues in provider organizations feel about this relatively new system. It has, on the one hand, the potential to advance our work by allowing us to serve more people in need; on the other hand, it has the potential to interfere with appropriate service. Managed care also is making the role of the social worker a more complex one, and this change, too, engenders some ambivalence.

The ambivalence we feel toward managed care is healthy, as long as we do not slide into either implacable hostility or dispirited resignation, for we are not powerless to shape the environment around us. As a profession, social work can and should be a major player in the evolution of managed care. We have to seize opportunities to make improvements and to help shape viable new services delivery models. The more we work with the system and help to find solutions, the more likely it is that our input will be heard when we need to challenge the system to advocate in the best interests of our clients and for appropriate assessment, goal setting, and treatment planning.

Let us turn now to a few long-held assumptions—assumptions about our clients, what they want, and how best to serve them—that have been put in question by the need to adapt to an ever more competitive commercial marketplace. The challenges to long-held assumptions initiated by managed care reflect the magnitude of the changes under way. Significant as these changes are, I would not say that managed care necessarily conflicts with the missions of provider agencies—but it does force us to re-examine how we are pursuing our missions and designing our services.

The first assumption relates to waiting lists and might be captured in this way: *Waiting lists are an indication of demand for our services and therefore prove our success.* We used to feel it was our job to provide services until we "fixed" as much as possible. That often took a long time. For instance, outpatient mental health counseling used to function with different expectations, and JBFCS outpatient clinics were highly respected for the thoroughness of care they offered. But our desire to provide thorough care meant that many in the community had to wait before they could be seen. In the past, we did not think that having waiting lists was a failure—frankly, we thought that having people waiting for us proved how valuable we were. Now, in a managed care environment, making people wait *is* a failure in a business or economic sense because the system will not allow it. The new system puts a premium on accessibility of care, and it promotes the idea that services should be available on request. MCOs have a responsibility to their customers, and they are not likely to maintain contracts with providers who keep those customers waiting.

There is also a clinical reason, however, that we should regard waiting lists as a failure. As we all know, so much in treatment is based on timing. Some of people's felt needs are constantly changing, and it is when the need is experienced that we have the opportunity, in terms of treatment, to have maximum impact. When one waits, the immediate crises may pass and the problems that motivated a person to seek our help may change in such a way that they are, at that point, less open to engagement in a helping process. This is something we knew all along. It has always been a key element of good practice to engage the client "where they are." It took new forces to make us apply this principle to the issue of ready access. What is a commercial imperative, from a business perspective, helped us to recognize a problem that we all knew was there, and we have been able to address the problem effectively.

A second assumption that has been placed in question might be stated simply as the following: *More treatment is better than less treatment.* Of course, people with severe disabilities will need long-term or intensive services—for example, adults with chronic mental illnes or children with serious emotional disturbances. There are also many people who can benefit a great deal from longer-term, insight-oriented help. However, for many other people, symptom relief can be enough to get them functioning again and may be what they really want and need. This is a particularly significant issue because, obviously, shorter-term treatment is less expensive for payers.

It is important to be attentive to what people want as we make our assessment of what they need. Those two considerations stand in a complex relationship, which is one reason the profession would benefit from the development of protocols around situations in which people need or want more or less treatment. We are seeing, and I think we will continue to see, that many clients are satisfied with time-effective treatment, whether individually or in groups. If they need to be seen over a period of time, it will most likely be intermittently, as they really need it, instead of once a week on a regular schedule. Not all clients will do as well under this arrangement; another group of clients will do just as well; and a third group will probably do better. Treatment decisions should always be based on assessment, but that assessment needs to take into account more fully and honestly what clients desire, their ability to use different kinds of treatment, and the usefulness of sharp focus in goal setting and treatment planning.

The third and final assumption I want to examine is this: *The provider always knows best and is in control of treatment.* That is no longer the case (if it ever was). One of the primary features of managed care is attention to customer satisfaction. In a field such as ours in which outcome can be so difficult to measure objectively, customer satisfaction becomes all the more important. It is also difficult to define. For one thing, the client is not the only customer. The client's payer is also a customer, and sometimes the client's family is a customer, too. It is clear, however, that we are going to be judged much more than we are used to on the outcome of services and on the client's satisfaction with the services we provide. We will need to spell out clearly the goals and expectations—both the client's and our own—or we and the client risk experiencing a sense of failure and defeat.

Clearly, assumptions are shifting, sometimes to the complete opposite of what we used to believe, and this shift is having an increasing effect on our day-to-day work as service providers. In general, I think the commercial marketplace will continue to support treatment services as long as their value is practical and observable and as long as they produce some kind of measurable results. But I also think we can expect to see the system evolve to include more in the way of less expensive case management services and less in the way of clinic services. Case management services done appropriately are good services. Social workers have always provided both treatment and case management services. If the system moves too far toward elimination of needed services, I believe that advocacy and political forces will help restore the system despite the costs involved.

Current Role of the Social Worker

Given the current trend, how has the role of the social worker changed? What do social workers need to know now that we are seeing more seriously disturbed clients and being asked to serve them with fewer resources in shorter periods of time? In the past, we spent time engaging willing clients and felt accomplishment with each new insight we offered, as long as it seemed to make a difference to the client. Now we have to address quickly the immediate problems of clients who, in some cases, do not want to be in treatment. Sometimes we need to choose from among many problems the client presents for a particular episode of treatment, leaving other problems for another time. An active selection process involving the client creates a focus and can be a useful intervention in and of itself. In the past, we tended to thoroughly assess all of a client's problems along with his or her strengths. Now our task is to focus more on a client's strengths and any other resources that might be available to mobilize the client and the client's support network quickly. Those other supportive resources might be mutual-aid or self-help programs (such as 12-step groups), church, neighbors, or relatives. From the beginning of treatment, we have to think about its end and our client's posttreatment needs.

If we are providing good, time-effective treatment, we need to find out right away what clients want from us, and we need to let them know at the outset what we expect of them. It is important to come to an agreement with each client about realistic expectations within a particular episode of treatment and to learn to think about the use of services periodically as needed in the future. We also have to deal with the logistics of payment up front. This may strike some of us as a less-than-ideal way of engaging a client but, with managed care, some important parameters of treatment are defined by clients' managed care companies. If treatment is covered for only 10 sessions or six sessions, then we need to make sure that clients are aware of those parameters and of their options before they leave treatment. Limits, as we all know, can be used to engage, mobilize, and share responsibility. This does not mean that when the limit is countertherapeutic or counterproductive we should not be honest with clients about this and do our best to arrange for appropriate care.

In the current environment, we also need to become more comfortable with a wider range of group treatment models. Group services can be an excellent modality for clients dealing with conflict and rivalry, isolation, and other communication issues, and therapists can really see what goes on. Clients also can see their own strengths and learn how they can be helpful to other people. Diversity issues, too, need to be dealt with, and therapists should be ready to discuss diversity issues with clients to encourage honest communication quickly.

Reconciling with the New Treatment Circumstances

Adjustments affecting clinical practice obviously carry implications for social work education and training. Some of these implications relate to curriculum—for example, techniques and methods associated with group and time-effective therapy—and will improve quality of care and our ability to reach more people in need. But managed care is having another effect on education and training, and if left unchecked that effect will erode quality of care and undermine our field.

When I spoke earlier of core values to which JBFCS has remained committed through periods of change, I included training, supervision, and research. Those are areas where the pressure to cut back is becoming increasingly intense. We continue to regard them as core values integral to our mission because a strong commitment to training, research, and good supervision leads inevitably to quality care. They do come with a cost, however, and one of the central challenges we face today is that the cost of maintaining quality is not reimbursable. As we struggle with higher productivity at a lower cost, the cost of quality gets paid for out of philanthropic funding. We are, therefore, put in a situation in which we subsidize MCOs for costs that legitimately they should pay—and we have not yet found an answer to this problem.

An additional and especially troubling concern for social work schools is that managed care providers generally allow only licensed professionals to treat patients they refer. In some cases, the companies may allow treatment by supervised interns, but we will probably continue to see fewer opportunities for social work interns in outpatient settings in which managed care is the funder. At JBFCS, for instance, less than one-third of our clients covered under managed care contracts are with MCOs that allow interns to see their "customers." (That number may be even smaller at other agencies.) Credentialing requirements imposed on service providers by MCOs are growing more restrictive, not less so. The implications for social work training are enormous and must be addressed by social work schools and providers immediately.

Managed care nonsupport of social work training (that is, not reimbursing interns) is *not* a situation to which we should adjust, because the future of the profession and quality care over the long term is at stake. In other areas, however, providers and schools need to work through problems together and find ways of adjusting to new realities. I think there are steps social work schools should be taking to accommodate new demands and client needs. Required courses in time-effective therapies, more work with groups, and training on diversity issues and on working with addictions, for example, will help prepare new social workers for a changing work environment.

The changes that providers have made in response to managed care help us increase our productivity and represent a new way of doing business in the marketplace. But it is not enough to learn how to serve more clients time effectively. Provider agencies also have to adapt to a different funding methodology—capitation. We are accustomed to a fee-for-service system that reimburses us for each unit of service we provide a client or for each day a client is in our care. In a capitated system—and that appears to be where we are heading—we can expect to receive a fixed annual amount for each person in a particular population; some people will require more services, some will require fewer, and some none, and it will be our job to serve the needs of that entire population.

One advantage of a capitated system is that we become our own gatekeepers and therefore have more control of resources and treatment planning. Once the third party has paid us our capitated rate, we have more freedom to make our own decisions about treatment for people covered by that payer. The payer's main concern is that its members, as a group, are satisfied with the services we provide and, therefore, are satisfied with the coverage from that particular HMO.

In a capitated system, however, we also assume more risk. Capitation does not work if every member of a covered population uses the most intensive treatment possible. It works when some members' lessened use of intensive services helps pay for those who need more. Planning for the rise of capitation is difficult because assuming that kind of risk is new to us. It requires that we as providers have an integrated continuum of services so we can offer each client the least-expensive appropriate service. If there are gaps in our continuum, then we must link up with other providers to form an integrated spectrum of services. For example, JBFCS has joined in a consortium of 16 New York City–area providers in an effort to develop an integrated continuum of services for adults with mental illness.

It is important to recognize that our attention to commercial principles represents a shift in our relationship with government. We can no longer assume in this environment that the public sector will endlessly support legitimate services. We need to be more competitive to get publicly supported business as well as business from the commercial sector. Given the late-1990s political climate, we need to continue to define and advocate for services that address client needs so we can help rebalance the system as it evolves to one that is appropriate and client friendly. Government has embraced the principles of managed care and is working in many ways to shift the burden of caring for our society's most vulnerable citizens from the public sector to the private sector. For example, New York State has been enforcing a mandate that all Medicaid-eligible citizens be enrolled in managed care plans. The initial target date was delayed, but a substantial portion of the state's Medicaid-eligible citizens are already enrolled in managed care plans. To continue serving these clients, we must have contracts with their MCOs, and we must adapt to the standards of those organizations.

There will be some exceptions to the state's mandate. There will be carved-out populations for whom different rules apply. The state is working with provider representatives to develop "special-needs plans" for certain populations (people with AIDS, adults with mental illness, and children with severe emotional disturbances) that cannot be served appropriately by HMOs or in shorter-term services. A lot of work remains to be done in this area to determine how carved-out services will be provided and how government will view and pay for these services. Most of us would agree that government has some basic responsibility to meet the needs of our most disabled citizens and the needs of uninsured citizens whom the private sector cannot or will not serve. We must work to keep government from shifting responsibilities for vulnerable people who realistically have no other means of support.

Aside from being a means of cost containment, managed care is really a challenge to the establishment. It confronts many of our long-held notions of high-quality care—and some of those notions, although sincerely believed, may never have been completely valid. Likewise, as managed care rapidly takes hold, it becomes a new establishment that needs to be challenged and held accountable. To the extent that the pressures of managed care will help us develop better and more-efficient treatment models, we must take advantage of our opportunities. At the same time, as social workers we have to take the initiative to be politically active and to challenge proposals, whether from the public or the private sector, that we believe will endanger appropriate care or further marginalize those populations for whom we have historically taken responsibility.

* * *

I believe that the core values of our profession provide the standard against which we must define our services to clients, our dealings with government, and our dealings with the commercial sector, and I am confident that if we continue to embrace those core values, what is best for the client will ultimately emerge.

CHAPTER 17

The Community-Centered Board Model of Managed Care for People with Developmental Disabilities

Stephen R. Hall

In recent years considerable attention has been focused on redefining the role of government in Americans' everyday lives. At the same time, managed care has emerged as a way to help people obtain the services they need at reasonable costs. These new ideas emphasize local choice and control; people within their own communities are thought to be better decision makers in every aspect of service delivery because they know and are directly accountable to their own communities. Where this new thinking has gone into practice, compelling examples of success have emerged (Berger & Neuhaus, 1977; Fukuyama, 1995; Putman, 1993). One example is the community-centered board model of managed care.

More than three decades ago, Colorado changed its government-controlled service delivery system for people with developmental disabilities to private, not-for-profit, local citizen-led boards of community leaders, including members of the medical, legal, education, accounting, engineering, and other business and commerce industries. People with developmental disabilities and parents of children with developmental disabilities serve on the boards. The boards manage the employment, residential living arrangements, and community well-being of local citizens with developmental disabilities. While spending far less than the government-controlled system, community-centered boards have delivered far more.

This chapter discusses a model for combining community-centered boards with a managed care structure to effectively deliver services to people with developmental disabilities. Colorado's community-centered boards are offered as a successful starting point for the implementation of this model.

Colorado's Community Board

Managed care provides an opportunity to do business differently—to improve services and supports for people with developmental disabilities and to contain both current and future costs. In Colorado, managed care did not result in people with disabilities being sold off to the lowest bidder. The work of Colorado's community-centered boards has led to many accomplishments:

NOTE: Originally published as Hall, S. R. (1996). The community-centered board model of managed care for people with developmental disabilities. *Health & Social Work, 21,* 225–229.

- The state is first among all states in taxpayer cost–benefit savings on the basis of total costs and community employment, supported living, and community participation outcomes (Braddock, Hemp, Bachelder, & Fujiura, 1995).
- The state is third among states in improving employment-related services and supports through policy changes (Hall, 1994).
- The state is seventh among states in moving people with developmental disabilities into their communities with supports from high cost–low performance state institutions (Braddock et al., 1995).
- The state is fifth among states in using federal funds for real homes in communities for people with developmental disabilities (Braddock et al., 1995).
- The state is 41st among states in spending for people with developmental disabilities (Braddock et al., 1995).

DESIGN AND RESPONSIBILITIES

Colorado's community-centered boards have been a single point of entry, one-stop-shopping model of managed care service delivery to people with developmental disabilities for more than three decades. Through well-developed resource coordination, people with disabilities and their families are carefully matched with service and support providers. Intake, referral, resource coordination, other forms of case management, quality assurance, cost utilization review, and outcome monitoring are the boards' responsibility.

PROBLEMS

The current Colorado Developmental Disabilities Services' slot-funding mechanism is the antithesis of managed care. Not surprisingly, long waiting lists for people without designated funding, or a "slot," and overfunding of people with slots are the result. In some circumstances, people with slots are overfunded as the positive effects of the providers' work mitigate the effects of the person's disability. Community-centered boards and providers cannot shift resources to others with greater needs or to others on the waiting lists who do not have a funded slot. This is not managed care.

Another attribute of the current system is inflexible, predesignated government funding streams that often dictate how services should be delivered without consideration for real measurable outcomes or whether the services should be delivered at all. Advances in community employment methodologies and community-living arrangements are challenging archaic funding mechanisms that help keep some people outside of society's mainstream. Funding streams were developed when sheltered workshop employment, large group homes, and separate transportation systems were the only options for people with developmental disabilities. As providers seek community employment alternatives to sheltered settings, real homes, and side-by-side relationships between people with and people without disabilities, they are continually thwarted by these funding mechanisms.

Further, there is a tendency toward programs instead of supports. "Program thinking" relies on treating people as a never-changing group that needs continuous intensive services in a program setting. Too often only people with the less-significant disabilities—those most like people without developmental disabilities—get real jobs, real homes, and a real life in their community. This program orientation is not compatible with managed care.

Integrating Community-Centered Boards and Managed Care

The switch to managed care for people with developmental disabilities can be seen as a frightening time to retrench and fortify defenses or as a once-in-a-lifetime opportunity for community boards to make long overdue changes. With funding already scarce and hundreds of people on waiting lists for services, the notion of managed care funding capitation coupled with a service-to-all mandate seems nearly impossible. Meanwhile, a growing number of people with developmental disabilities and their families and advocates are demanding equal access to the types of jobs, homes, and relationships available to other Americans. As a result, "special places for them" thinking must be replaced with supports that ensure an opportunity for everyone's presence and participation in the work and social fabric of the community. The challenge is to meet these demands with fewer resources. Some believe that community-centered boards are already providing a model of managed care (Colorado Department of Human Services, 1995).

COMPONENTS OF MANAGED CARE

Funding capitation with future funding increases based on general demographics, projected population increases, or disability incidence data is a key component of managed care. A second component is cost control, usually in the form of categorical block funding. Categorical block funding protects people with developmental disabilities, because funds for their services and support are never given to a government social services bureaucracy, medical care corporation, or other entity that bundles service and support funds with medical care funds for people with different needs. Funds designated categorically for people with developmental disabilities go exclusively to serve their long-term service and support needs.

A third component is the outcome orientation that replaces the process model. Instead of dictating to providers how and when dollars should be spent and mandating details for every process along the way, managed care focuses on real outcomes. Instead of funding a process or a particular treatment, managed care's funding flexibility, creative freedom, and accountability are tied to a predetermined outcome.

A fourth component is full service to everyone in need. Everyone should receive the services and supports they need within block-funding constraints. Individual funding caps or other means of cost control that may harm those who require extraordinary services and supports are not part of managed care for people with developmental disabilities.

SUPPORTS PARADIGM

In recent years there has been a distinct shift from a services orientation to a supports orientation. Whereas a services orientation is about programs and places that deal with personal deficiencies through prescription planning, a supports orientation builds on a person's strengths in the context of community settings (Figure 17-1). The services orientation is about intake, evaluation, determination of deficiencies, prescription programming, endless objectives, adjustment, and further evaluation. Day centers, group homes, sheltered workshops, segregated employment settings,

FIGURE **17-1**

Moving from a Services to a Supports Orientation

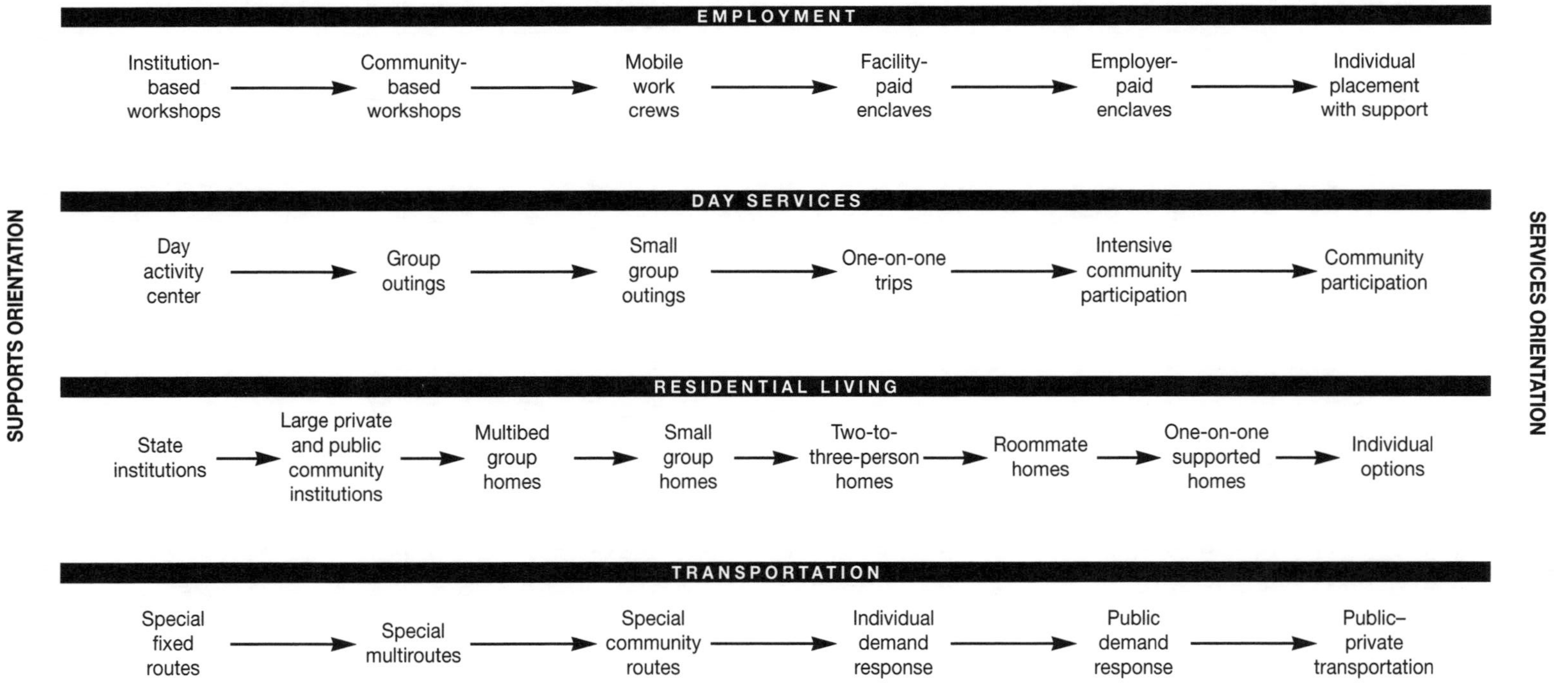
SUPPORTS ORIENTATION
SERVICES ORIENTATION
EMPLOYMENT
Institution-based workshops
Community-based workshops
Mobile work crews
Facility-paid enclaves
Employer-paid enclaves
Individual placement with support
DAY SERVICES
Day activity center
Group outings
Small group outings
One-on-one trips
Intensive community participation
Community participation
RESIDENTIAL LIVING
State institutions
Large private and public community institutions
Multibed group homes
Small group homes
Two-to-three-person homes
Roommate homes
One-on-one supported homes
Individual options
TRANSPORTATION
Special fixed routes
Special multiroutes
Special community routes
Individual demand response
Public demand response
Public–private transportation

field trips, and other activities in which people with developmental disabilities are in the same rooms at the same time are part of the traditional services delivery system.

The supports orientation, which began in the early 1980s, hinges on outreach, personal futures planning, and support management and includes supported and other forms of real employment, community-supported living arrangements, community participation, and other innovations that enhance the person's interdependence with people without developmental disabilities. The community-centered board model of managed care builds on the current movement from services to increasing options based on supports.

Although Colorado's community-centered boards have been leaders in cost-effective community employment and real community living for people with developmental disabilities (Braddock et al., 1995; Hall, 1994), most supports have been paid instead of natural. Natural supports are developed through reciprocal relationships between people with disabilities and people without disabilities (Figure 17-2). Instead of concentrating on deficiencies within the person with a disability as if the disability belongs solely to this person, the disability is viewed as a social construction that occurs when the person interacts with society in out-of-the-ordinary ways. The natural supports orientation moves from a "disabled person" reality to a "person with a disability" reality.

The role of social workers and other human services professionals in a natural supports orientation is to facilitate and interpret interactions in a manner that reduces or eliminates the definition of the person as "disabled." The orientation offers the opportunity to build community competence and participation of people without disabilities in the life of a person with disabilities to the extent that paid social workers and other human services personnel are needed much less often. Rather than hiring "friends" or "community connectors," social workers and other human services personnel build bridges to people in the community.

The natural supports paradigm may require extensive initial paid supports to move to nonpaid supports. Natural supports are the critical difference between a medical model of managed care and a community model of managed care. At first the promise of lower-cost supports to people with developmental disabilities seems easy enough. However, a "don't worry, we'll take care of them" attitude has led to increased costs within the community that, although far less than past institutional costs, are still growing. Another way to contain costs has been to put more people with disabilities into smaller rooms and pay those who oversee their well-being the lowest possible wages. A better way is to develop a community managed care system based on the pragmatic transition of funding from a services system to a

FIGURE **17-2**

Examples of Paid and Natural Supports

PAID SUPPORTS	NATURAL SUPPORTS
Employment training specialist	Coworker with consultation
Paid community provider	Nonpaid citizen relationship
Paid community supported-living specialist	Neighbor
Facilitated association membership	Unplanned associations

supports system that is fostered through professionals who can build interdependent relationships between people with disabilities and people without disabilities.

Community-Centered Board Model of Managed Care

The following are the key understandings of the community-centered board model of managed care:

- Supported employment, supported living, and community participation methodologies that engage people without disabilities in the habilitation process can deliver superior, cost-effective outcomes when compared to past congregate care and professionally staffed methodologies.
- An outcome orientation replaces the program orientation. Real jobs, relationships, homes, and community life replace the process orientation, which rewards "progress" within a given program.
- A shift from a service delivery or program orientation to a supports paradigm is essential. Rather than being seen as service providers, professionals are bridge builders who remedy the historic isolation of people with disabilities from those without.
- "Customer–provider" partnerships replace typical "professional–client" relationships. People with disabilities receive the services they want and are informed of all possible options. Customers and providers perform extensive redesign and systems review.
- Providers who deliver superior outcomes in a cost-effective manner are rewarded with stable and increased funding to serve more people with disabilities. Resources saved through provider efficiencies are used to solve the problem of waiting lists. No one profits at the expense of people with disabilities.
- No additional fees, sliding fee scales, user fees, or other customer payment mechanisms are used to provide or enhance supports. As taxpayers themselves, people with disabilities and their families are already paying on an income tax–graduated scale for needed supports.
- Slot funding, program funding, restricted funding, fee-for-service funding, and other mechanisms that limit provider activity to a prespecified process are replaced by block funding for specific outcomes across a range of living and community participation needs.

Conclusion

The community-centered board model of managed care works to replace antiquated funding mechanisms with flexible funds tied to real outcomes, allowing for a shift from programs rooted in mid-century ideologies to supports founded on the interdependence of communities. However, there is much work to be done by professionals who know how to build working and living relationships between people with developmental disabilities and people without disabilities.

Some believe that managed care can be used to infuse human services with a long overdue "natural marketplace" ideology. "Market forces," "survival-of-the-fittest competition," "natural market corrections," and similar statements promote a natural way to control costs. Often missed in this market panacea are the effects that multistate corporations with political buying power can have on local citizen-controlled human services delivery.

Colorado's community-centered boards have been a national model for superior, cost-effective services. These boards offer the benefits of both outcome-based management and close-to-the-customer reality. This model should be considered a historic opportunity to fuse the citizen-led independence of community-centered boards with the promises of controlled costs and real outcomes of managed care.

References

Berger, P., & Neuhaus, R. (1977). *To empower people: The role of mediating structures in public policy.* Washington, DC: American Enterprise Institute for Public Policy Research.

Braddock, D., Hemp, R., Bachelder, L., & Fujiura, G. (1995). *The state of the states in developmental disabilities.* Washington, DC: American Association on Mental Retardation.

Colorado Department of Human Services. (1995). *Proposed blueprint for change: Funding policy issues in developmental disability services.* Denver: Author. (Available from Developmental Disabilities Services, 3824W Princeton Circle, Denver, CO 80236)

Fukuyama, F. (1995). *Trust: The social virtues and the creation of prosperity.* New York: Free Press.

Hall, S. (1994). State improvement ranking: An analysis of states' services for citizens considered developmentally disabled who want to work. *Advance, 5*(1), 1–3. (Available from the Association for Persons in Supported Employment, 1627 Monument Avenue, Suite 301, Richmond, VA 23220)

Putman, R. (1993). *Making democracy work.* Princeton, NJ: Princeton University Press.

CHAPTER 18

All Managed Care Is Not Equal: The Relationship between Behavioral Cost and Care Management

Alisa Trugerman

The term "managed care" is being used to describe any and all attempts to control the costs and delivery of behavioral health services. The anxiety, fear, and anger experienced by many mental health practitioners come from the perceived threat that managed care will severely restrict access to care, that is, reduce patient referrals. Managed care is actually quite varied with regard to access, benefit design, network composition, quality assurance, and cost constraints. It is actually possible to manage "care" and reduce costs and also increase access to behavioral health services.

U.S. Behavioral Health, now United Behavioral Health (UBH), is a specialty vendor managing the mental health and substance abuse benefits for a wide variety of employer groups. Most of the employer groups have carved out behavioral health from indemnity, point-of-service, and preferred provider medical plans. Prior to UBH taking on their management, most groups spent 65 percent to 80 percent of the mental health and substance abuse dollars on 2 percent to 4 percent of their beneficiaries, and more than 70 percent of their expenditures were on acute inpatient services. To reduce the overall mental health costs, UBH asks employers to allow flexible benefit substitution that increases access to alternatives to hospitalization. Typically, after UBH begins managing the benefits, expenditures are reversed: 70 percent of the costs are on outpatient care, 30 percent on inpatient care, and there is an increase in beneficiaries (6 to 10 percent).

UBH offers a fully integrated behavioral health care program that includes precertification and concurrent review by care managers with a national network of providers. UBH operates a 24-hour, seven-days-a-week clinical intake service trained at the master's level to triage the needs of its membership and to make referrals. The network includes individual providers, groups, and facility-based programs. The individual practitioner network is interdisciplinary: 40 percent social work, 40 percent psychology, and 20 percent psychiatry. All providers are state-licensed mental health practitioners, have five years of postlicensure clinical experience, are members in good standing in the professional associations, and carry appropriate malpractice coverage. The credentialing process is rigorous, including a peer review of curriculum vitae and responses to the UBH application. The goal is to identify areas of clinical expertise to make the best possible patient–provider match at the onset of

NOTE: Originally published as Trugerman, A. (1996). All managed care is not equal. *Smith College Studies in Social Work, 66,* 261–267.

treatment. Facility-based programs include acute inpatient, partial and day treatment programs, crisis-respite beds, in-home services, residential care, and structured outpatient programs. All programs must be state licensed, accredited as appropriate by the Joint Commission on Accreditation of Healthcare Organizations or the Commission on Accreditation of Rehabilitation Facilities, maintain current liability coverage, and offer a continuum of care. Providers are recredentialed every two years in accordance with National Committee of Quality Assurance guidelines. There is also continuous review by care managers of the providers' assessment, treatment, and discharge planning. UBH staff conduct site visits and quality assurance reviews at high-volume providers.

Ongoing outpatient care and all intensive levels of care are managed by an interdisciplinary team of licensed mental health clinicians. Precertification and ongoing concurrent review with the provider network are the primary means of care management. The UBH guidelines of care have been developed in conjunction with the standards of practice by the American Psychiatric Association, the Academy of Child and Adolescent Psychiatry, and the American Society for Addiction Medicine. The basic philosophy of care is to use the least-restrictive level of care necessary to meet the patient's needs and to return the patient as quickly as possible to the community in which he or she lives, works, or attends school. All intensive cases are supervised daily by UBH staff psychiatrists with expertise in chemical dependency, child and adolescent psychiatry, gerontology, and psychopharmacology. Additionally, UBH has a dedicated child and adolescent care management team. Given the 24-hour availability of clinicians and the credentialing of a national network, access to specialty providers is quite easy.

An illustration that use of mental health care services can increase while providing a substantial cost savings through the consistent use of alternatives to hospitalization and increased outpatient care is UBH's management of the benefit for a large employer in the western United States. UBH assumed the management of the mental health and substance abuse expense benefit for all of the company's employees and dependents in January 1991. The total carve-out of behavioral health services ensures minimal bias resulting from the self-selection of benefit plan. To demonstrate cost savings through the use of alternatives in a preferred provider network, the data presented here compare the claims experience from 1991 to 1996 with the unmanaged experience for the three years prior to UBH management. The members within this sample are enrolled in non–health maintenance organization (HMO), managed medical plans (indemnity and point-of-service). It was not possible to obtain preimplementation data on HMO enrollees.

The average cost per member per month (adjusted) during the six years of UBH management was reduced from $15.45 to $10.95, 29 percent less than the three-year average before UBH assumed management of the benefit. This savings includes the additional administrative costs of UBH management (Table 18-1). There was an increase in utilization from an average of 7.49 to 9.31 percent, a 20 percent increase in the six years since 1991. Most interesting is that even with an increase in utilization, the per month (adjusted) cost during those six years decreased 11 percent, on average. The increase in 1993 primarily resulted from an increase in the UBH professional and administrative fees (Table 18-2).

In the six years from 1991 through 1996, the utilization of 24-hour care (days per 1,000), the average length of stay, and the per-member-per-month cost have decreased. Conversely, there has been an increase in the outpatient utilization (units

TABLE **18-1**

Mental Health Utilization, 1988–96

YEAR	MEMBERS	PATIENTS[a]	PAYMENTS ($ MILLIONS)	$/PATIENT	PMPM ($)	PMPM ($) (ADJUSTED)[b]	UTILIZATION (%)
1988	64,459	4,147	9,290	2,240	12.01	—	6.43
1989	66,754	5,577	13,130	2,354	16.39	—	8.35
1990	63,722	4,878	13,712	2,811	17.93	—	7.66
1988–90 average	64,978	4,867	12,044	2,475	15.45	—	7.49
1991	52,175	4,316	6,623	1,535	10.58	11.03	8.27
1992	53,910	4,621	6,316	1,367	9.76	10.30	8.57
1993	53,208	5,046	7,147	1,416	11.19	12.17	9.48
1994	52,016	5,187	6,081	1,172	9.74	11.01	9.97
1995	48,907	4,896	5,070	1,036	8.64	10.22	10.01
1996[c]	46,345	4,428	4,477	1,011	8.05	—	9.55
1991–96 average	51,094	4,749	5,952	1,256	9.66	10.95	9.31

NOTE: PMPM = per member per month.

[a]Patient count reflects outpatients, assuming the inpatient count is duplicative.

[b]1991–96 includes 100 percent of United Behavioral Health management fees.

[c]1996 data based on claims paid through September 30, 1997; no completion factors applied.

per 1,000) (Tables 18-3 and 18-4). The unit costs for inpatient and outpatient care are reduced by the UBH discounted fee schedule and in-network utilization. For those six years, under UBH management, approximately 25 percent of the costs for all services were for 24-hour care, compared with the experience of the previous three years, when 24-hour care accounted for approximately 50 percent of all costs. Thus, it has been possible to reduce the total cost of behavioral health care while

TABLE **18-2**

Mental Health Utilization, Year-to-Year Comparison, 1988–96

YEAR	MEMBERS	VARIANCE (%)	UTILIZATION (%)	VARIANCE (%)	PMPM ($)	VARIANCE (%)	PMPM ($) (ADJUSTED)[a]	VARIANCE (%)
1988	64,459	—	6.43	—	12.01	—	—	—
1989	66,754	4	8.35	30	16.39	36	—	—
1990	63,722	–5	7.66	–8	17.93	9	—	—
1991	52,175	–18	8.27	8	10.58	–41	11.03	—
1992	53,910	3	8.57	4	9.76	–8	10.30	–7
1993	53,208	–1	9.48	11	11.19	15	12.17	18
1994	52,016	–3	9.97	5	9.74	–13	11.01	–10
1995	48,907	–6	10.01	0	8.64	–11	10.22	–7
1996[b]	46,345	–5	9.55	–5	8.05	–7	—	—
1991–96 change	—	–5	—	4	—	–11	—	–2

NOTE: PMPM = per member per month.

[a]1991–96 includes 100 percent of U.S. Behavioral Health management fees.

[b]1996 data based on claims paid through September 30, 1997; no completion factors applied.

TABLE **18-3**

Mental Health Utilization, 24-Hour Care, 1988–96

	1988	1989	1990	1991	1992	1993	1994	1995	1996[a]
Actual									
Members	64,459	66,754	63,722	52,175	53,910	53,208	52,016	48,907	46,345
Patients[b]	271	315	292	171	170	187	161	137	134
Payments ($ millions)	4,763	5,607	6,078	1,815	1,561	1,905	1,183	1,133	917
Admissions[b]	327	404	433	261	231	270	232	199	193
Days[b]	8,376	8,134	7,439	3,652	3,267	3,892	2,528	2,125	1,602
Utilization analyses									
Days/1,000	130	122	117	70	61	73	49	43	35
Admissions/1,000	5.1	6.1	6.8	5.0	4.3	5.1	4.5	4.1	4.2
ALOS[b]	26	20	17	14	14	14	11	11	8
Utilization (%)	0.42	0.47	0.46	0.33	0.32	0.35	0.31	0.28	0.29
Cost analyses									
$/day	569	689	817	497	478	489	468	533	572
$/admission	14,566	13,879	14,037	6,954	6,758	7,056	5,099	5,693	4,751
PMPM ($)	6.16	7.00	7.95	2.90	2.41	2.98	1.90	1.93	1.65
PMPM ($) (adjusted)[c]	—	—	—	3.13	2.68	3.47	2.53	2.72	—

NOTES: ALOS = average length of stay; PMPM = per member per month.
[a]1996 data based on claims paid through September 30, 1997; no completion factor applied.
[b]Includes admissions to acute residential care.
[c]Includes 50 percent of United Behavioral Health management fees.

increasing access for beneficiaries by shifting the distribution of costs from 24-hour care to alternative levels of outpatient care.

In addition to utilization and cost analyses, UBH's extensive quality assurance program attempts to provide proofs of value to both payers and users of our services. The program includes a variety of activities to monitor the internal care management process and the provider network and to measure outcomes. Some examples of those activities are the following: UBH member satisfaction surveys; analysis of readmissions to understand the variables contributing to recidivism; monitoring of patients with chemical dependency for 12 months after intensive treatment to determine sobriety; and, in outpatient psychotherapy, the comparison of patients in the UBH Goal-Focused Treatment Planning and Outcomes (GFTPO) with a matched cohort on outcome ratings by patient and provider, symptom reduction, and length of treatment episode. Although beyond the scope of this chapter, preliminary results from GFTPO indicate that participation in goal-oriented psychotherapy reduces the incidence of premature termination (three sessions or less) and facilitates greater stabilization of the therapeutic alliance (as measured by the rate of return to the same therapist in subsequent episodes of treatment).

All "managed care" is not created equal. It is possible for managed behavioral health care companies to reduce costs without severely restricting access to care. This reduction is possible if 24-hour care is used only when medically necessary; lengths of stay are shortened; flexible benefit substitution allows for alternative outpatient levels of care; and providers agree to a discounted fee schedule. Rather than

TABLE **18-4**

Mental Health Utilization, Outpatient, 1988–96

	1988	1989	1990	1991	1992	1993	1994	1995	1996[a]
Actual									
Members	64,459	66,754	63,722	52,175	53,910	53,208	52,016	48,907	46,345
Patients[b]	4,147	5,577	4,878	4,316	4,621	5,046	5,187	4,896	4,428
Payments ($ millions)	4,527	7,523	7,634	4,808	4,755	5,242	4,850	3,937	3,560
Units	24,829	89,929	91,601	49,029	64,912	68,840	63,732	54,681	49,116
Utilization analyses									
Units/1,000	385	1,347	1,438	940	1,204	1,294	1,225	1,118	1,060
Average visits[b]	6	16	19	11	14	14	12	11	11
Utilization (%)	6.43	8.35	7.66	8.27	8.57	9.48	9.97	10.01	9.55
Cost analyses									
$/unit	182	84	83	98	73	76	76	72	72
$/patient	1,092	1,349	1,565	1,114	1,029	1,039	935	804	804
PMPM ($)	5.85	9.39	9.98	7.68	7.35	8.21	7.77	6.71	6.40
PMPM ($) (adjusted)[c]	—	—	—	7.91	7.62	8.70	8..40	7.50	—

NOTE: PMPM = per member per month.

[a]1996 data based on claims paid through September 30, 1997; no completion factor applied.

[b]Includes admissions to acute residential care.

[c]Includes 50 percent of United Behavioral Health management fees.

worrying about seeing fewer patients, practitioners concerned about referrals in the era of managed care would be wise to structure their practices to meet the needs of complicated patients in outpatient settings and to be prepared to handle more patients for shorter treatment durations.

The author expresses her appreciation for the synthesis of the data to William Goldman, senior vice president of medical affairs and quality assurance at UBH, and to Joyce McCullough, senior research analyst at UBH.

PART **THREE**

Notes from the Field

B. Practice Perspectives

Diabetes, Depression, and Despair: Clinical Case Management in a Managed Care Context

Joel Kanter and Madeline Silva

As managed mental health care has expanded over the past decade, the limitations of this approach have been outlined by many authors (Kanter, 1995b; Kramer, 1996; Shapiro, 1996). Two of the most common criticisms have involved the lack of adequate treatment for the most disturbed patients and the ineptness of the managed care reviewers. In this chapter, we will present the case report of a successful intervention with a severely disturbed and medically vulnerable man. The intervention was conducted with the support of the managed care department of a major insurer. In this situation, the needs of the patient and the insurer converged, and the social worker implemented a clinical case management[1] approach (Kanter, 1989, 1995a) that would not have been funded by traditional capitation plans. Although the situation is atypical, the report illustrates some of the potential benefits of case management intervention in a managed care environment.

Case Report

Paul, age 37, was referred to me (J.K.) three years ago by his psychiatrist on a general psychiatric ward in a local hospital when I was working as a case manager in private practice. Paul had been transferred to this ward from a medical unit where he had been admitted after a hypoglycemic diabetic episode. He had had insulin-dependent diabetes since age 30, and his diabetes had been out of control since the death of his father, who had become blind and lost a foot 20 months earlier as a result of diabetes. Living alone in his own apartment, he had been hospitalized at least six times in that period for both high and low blood sugar and had refused to allow home health nurses into his apartment. An adopted only child, Paul had apparently grown increasingly isolated as his mother, his main social support, became terminally ill with cancer. He had been employed as a mail clerk for a government agency but had obviously been unable to work for some time.

NOTE: Originally published as Kanter, J., & Silva, M. (1996) Depression, diabetes, and despair: Clinical case management in a managed care context. *Smith College Studies in Social Work, 66,* 358–369.

[1]Because there is considerable semantic confusion around the term "case management," we will use that term to describe a hands-on social work approach; we will use the term "care management" to describe the telephone and referral activities of managed care staff.

When his internist recognized that Paul's near-muteness and dramatic weight loss prevented effective medical intervention, he transferred Paul to the psychiatric unit where he was placed on antidepressant and antipsychotic medications. As he had no social support system and was uncommunicative, it was difficult to take an adequate history. His educational background suggested a severe learning disability or minimal brain dysfunction, but there was no evidence of prior psychiatric hospitalizations. His hospital psychiatrist quickly recognized that Paul's lack of social support would greatly impede effective discharge planning, and he asked me to evaluate Paul on the ward for case management services, especially finding him a supportive living situation.

When I met Paul on the ward, I was immediately struck by his emaciated body, disheveled appearance, sad and blank expression, and monosyllabic verbal responses. Diagnostically, it was impossible to discern whether he was suffering from simple schizophrenia, a more paranoid disturbance, or a severe depression. Organic brain syndromes were also a possibility. Yet, diagnosis aside, I had to consider how we could find a safe living situation for him in the next few weeks. This was complicated because Paul would tell me nothing about his financial situation: Did he still have a job? Any sick leave? Any funds in the bank? Without this information, case management planning was impossible. Aware that our dialogue would be very limited, I introduced myself, sat with him quietly for a time, and asked his permission to contact his mother (which had not been done by the hospital staff).

Two days later, Paul's aunt contacted the hospital. She told the staff that his mother had died the day before I saw him. She had been buried earlier that day, and the few relatives had chosen not to inform the hospital of her death until after the funeral. There were no relatives in the area. The aunt, who lived 200 miles away, had had little contact with Paul. No one in his family or in our community had had much, if any, contact with Paul in recent years. With the psychiatrist's permission, Paul's aunt visited the hospital to tell him of his mother's death. She was accompanied by an acquaintance of his mother, Mrs. T., who had been appointed both co-executor of the mother's estate (with the aunt) and the trustee for a trust established by the will to assist with Paul's care and medical expenses. Mrs. T. had not known Paul's mother well and had never met Paul but had agreed to serve as trustee when his mother prevailed on her after the death of Paul's father. Apparently, Paul's parents had also been quite isolated and had no good friends in the community, a fact that emerged when I learned more about the eight people who had attended the funeral.

Although Paul expressed little emotion about his mother's death or the fact that he was not invited to the funeral, I hypothesized that the death of his parents had considerable significance and proposed a graveside memorial service. This was held before his aunt—his closest living relative—returned home. Paul received a pass from the hospital to attend the service. We invited his aunt, Mrs. T., and three neighbors to attend—the only members of his network we could identify. At the cemetery, Paul also saw his father's grave for the first time, because he had not attended his funeral either. I read a few prayers and allowed Paul to meditate alone at the gravesite. Afterward, I went to lunch with Paul and his aunt. Paul was silent, but his aunt talked throughout the meal, expressing her belief that her sister's cancer could have been cured if the American Medical Association and the National Institutes of Health hadn't conspired to conceal the cure from the American public.

Paul returned to the hospital and improved marginally over the next few weeks. His weight stabilized, and he seemed more expressive nonverbally, although he still was largely mute. The insurer was demanding discharge. We still did not know if Paul had a job or any funds; he flatly refused to discuss financial matters during my frequent visits. By that time, we had learned about the trust that his mother's will had established and gained the support of the trustee in funding case management services when the estate cleared probate. With the trustee's support, I tried unsuccessfully to locate someone who would take Paul into his or her home informally because I knew that all formal residential programs would take months to evaluate and admit him. Finally, insurance mandated a discharge date, and although his psychiatrist and I did not know how he could cope in his own apartment, we decided that I would drive him to his home and see if we could somehow help him cope by having daily contact with him.

Paul was visibly anxious when I took him to his apartment and verbally expressed his hesitation about going home. When he opened the door, I was stunned by the disarray covering every inch of the apartment. Looking for a place to sit, I found nowhere to put the items that had been on the chair. Picking up the telephone, I could not get a dial tone—a very disturbing detail because I viewed telephone contact as essential. I was unclear whether the equipment was defective or the line was dead—and Paul would not tell me. When I called the telephone company from a nearby pay phone, they told me that service had been discontinued because the bill had not been paid for several months. It was a weekend and there was no way in which service could be restored for at least 48 hours. Mulling things over and looking at Paul's anxious, depressed, and uncommunicative state, I could not imagine how he could survive safely in the community. I called his psychiatrist to recommend readmission. Understanding my dilemma, Paul's psychiatrist called in a readmission order immediately, and I returned Paul to the hospital.

After another five days without much clinical improvement, Paul's psychiatrist spoke with a nurse care manager (M.S.) at the office of Paul's insurer. Her role is to develop special out-of-benefit treatment plans for patients with unusual medical conditions. Although Paul was obviously suffering from a severe mental illness, he was eligible for this assistance because he had a serious "medical" condition (diabetes) that had not responded to conventional medical interventions, and this condition had led to repeated hospitalizations that had been costly for the insurer. In a combination of self-interest and altruism, Paul's insurer, through the care manager, worked out a discharge plan whereby the insurer paid for him to enter a high-quality convalescent home, and it retained me as a case manager to find him a permanent living situation when his medical and psychiatric condition stabilized. Specifically, I was authorized to spend up to 20 hours monthly helping Paul; we understood that my activities would include developing a rapport with him in visits to the nursing facility, collaborating with the staff in the nursing facility, making telephone calls with possible residential providers and other collateral people, and preparing whatever written materials were necessary. I submitted a monthly diary of my services with my bill and called the care manager whenever I had a question about whether the insurer would support a given activity.

The nurse care manager had not made a similar plan for any other patient, but Paul's case was clearly an unusual one. In making this plan, she acknowledged that she discussed a budget for this intervention with her supervisor, using a formula that balanced the cost of the out-of-benefit services against his medical utilization in recent years.

Gradually, with the help of antidepressant medication and persistent social support, Paul's depression diminished, and he appeared to look forward to contact with me. I often took him out of the nursing facility, I bought him new clothes, and we sometimes ate at local restaurants. He continued to be evasive about his financial and vocational situation and seemed pleased at the care he was receiving in this facility. He initially was given a single room, and he enjoyed watching television all day, with meals brought to his bedside (a regression from the expectations on the psychiatric ward). I arranged with the nursing staff to transfer him to a double room so he would be less comfortable in the facility and more motivated to collaborate with me in finding an alternative.

Meanwhile, I did not have an easy time finding a suitable residential placement. The psychiatric programs were uneasy about working with a noncompliant person with insulin-dependent diabetes, and the geriatric placements were concerned about his psychiatric condition and his age. After two months I located a suitable foster home that would accept him, but then we discovered major problems in settling his mother's estate and funding the trust that would subsidize his placement. Without ensured funding, the foster home accepted another resident in Paul's stead.

Around this time, Paul had improved to the point where he was able to return to work. I called his supervisor, provided the company with adequate documentation of his medical and psychiatric conditions—documentation that helped them understand his lack of communication with them for more than four months—and negotiated a part-time return to work while Paul stayed in residence at the nursing facility. He clearly needed significant income beyond the small stipend offered by the trust to support a residential placement. Although he probably would have had little difficult retiring on disability, his resources would have been extremely limited and his quality of life would have been diminished.

Paul was ambivalent about returning to his job and expressed a wish to remain indefinitely in the nursing facility. After I conferred with the care manager, she agreed to take the unusual step of visiting Paul in the nursing facility and informing him that his stay in this facility was contingent on his participation in a plan that would return him to work and to independent living. If he did not wish to participate in this plan, his insurer would not continue its unusual, time-limited support for his care. Without a job, he would probably only be able to afford care in a less-desirable institutional setting.

That confrontation was a critical moment in Paul's recovery as he struggled with his regressive tendencies. Although angered that he would not be able to remain indefinitely in this institution, he agreed to return to work. However, he still would not collaborate with me about financial matters, and I had no assurance that he would pay his rent.

To obtain a residential placement, it seemed necessary that he have a financial guardian, but arranging for one posed further complications: Who would petition for guardianship? Who would pay an attorney to provide legal services? Who would serve as the guardian? Interestingly, the insurer agreed to pay attorney's fees, and I was charged by the insurer's legal counsel to retain an attorney competent in guardianship proceedings. I recruited the trustee to serve as petitioner, the attorney located a colleague to serve as guardian, and the guardian was finally appointed nearly eight months after Paul had entered the nursing facility.

Throughout his stay in that facility, I also had to address the problem of Paul's diabetes. I educated myself about the condition and consulted continually with the facility staff to encourage them to help Paul self-administer his insulin instead of doing it for him. If he could not self-administer his insulin, his range of residential options would be extremely limited, and he likely would require institutional care. As one might expect, skilled-nursing facilities are not equipped to help "thirty-something" young adults handle their own medications and go off to work each morning. This assistance was a particular problem, because shifts changed during the critical period when Paul had to be awakened to go to work, given his insulin, and encouraged to eat a healthy breakfast.

I was surprised to find myself constantly addressing diabetic emergencies. The first occurred when I visited Paul at lunch hour when he was beginning to eat from his lunch tray in his bed: After taking a few bites, he went into what I later learned was a hypoglycemic seizure and lost consciousness. I stayed with him though the seizure and then looked for a nurse. No one was working on his wing of the facility, and finally I called the front desk. Paul was taken to the local emergency room, but returned to the nursing facility several hours later. Acknowledging my own anxiety, I immediately knew that such incidents would cause major problems for most residential providers.

During his stay in the facility, Paul had at least four similar incidents. Two occurred while he was at work, and I learned that Paul had rushed out without breakfast on those mornings. On both occasions, I called and went to the emergency rooms. When the physicians could quickly diagnose the diabetic emergency and understand that Paul had adequate outpatient medical care and social support, he was discharged safely within hours once his blood sugar had stabilized. These incidents previously had resulted in hospitalizations of three to seven days, so the insurer's care manager was very appreciative of these cost-saving interventions. Over time, I learned more and more about diabetes and how uniquely it affected Paul.

Of course, there were significant psychological problems underlying all of these medical problems. Although Paul's depression remitted significantly over the six months after hospital discharge (and he gained back 30 pounds), his learning disability, isolative tendencies, and characterological difficulties came to the fore. He was manifestly dependent, avoidant, and passive–aggressive. Ambivalent about employment and residential placement, he repeatedly asked if he could stay in the nursing facility forever. I was amazed that a person of his age would want to share a room indefinitely with feeble and dying people. We struggled with his reluctance to go to work, administer his own insulin, or control his diet effectively—and the caretaking ethos of the nursing facility exacerbated the difficulties in addressing these issues.

After Paul had spent nine months in the nursing facility, I found a suitable "foster home" owned by a licensed practical nurse in a neighborhood Paul liked, and he was managing his diabetes more effectively. The guardianship was in place, but his mother's estate was far from being settled, and we needed a court order to release a small portion of the estate to enable Paul to move. This hurdle was cleared, too, and Paul moved into a new home.

More than four years have passed. Paul has remained in that home, with a dramatic reduction in the frequency and impact of diabetic emergencies (only one in the past year). Although a small stroke several months after his move from the nursing home disabled him for a short time, he returned to his job and continues to self-administer his insulin and oral medications. After the initial year, the insurer's care manager terminated my special contract. I continue to work with Paul through the support of his standard mental health benefits and with assistance from his trust. There are still many difficulties—especially his chronic tardiness on the job and his social isolation—but, overall, he enjoys better health and improved quality of life.

Discussion

Paul's medical and residential stabilization demonstrate the efficacy of a comprehensive case management approach that integrates psychological and environmental interventions in addressing both medical and psychiatric illnesses (Kanter, 1989, 1990, 1995a). In addition to addressing the objective realities of a life-threatening medical condition and the near-absence of social support, I had to contain my intense countertransference responses to Paul's guardedness, passive–aggressiveness, and seemingly self-destructive neglect of his own health (Kanter, 1988; Maltsberger & Buie, 1974).

Case management with Paul required many component activities, including engagement, assessment, planning, resource development, consulting with a variety of caregivers, psychotherapy, patient psychoeducation, and advocacy (Kanter, 1989). Yet, beyond these component elements, this intervention required a professional capacity to integrate knowledge from varying perspectives and operationalize this integration in pragmatic strategies (Kanter, 1996). For example, in working with Paul to prevent hypoglycemic emergencies, I had to both educate myself about diabetes and explore the complex psychodynamic factors involved with his difficulty in using seemingly simple, preventive dietary strategies. Then I had to understand the values and practices of the skilled-nursing facility to obtain its cooperation in helping Paul learn these strategies.

Also, I hypothesized that Paul's unique combination of self-neglect and intense dependency reflected unresolved conflicts about his recently deceased parents. Although Paul's capacity to use insight-oriented psychotherapy was limited, my ongoing support for his grieving processes, involving at least three visits to his parents' gravesite after the memorial service, helped him develop more collaborative relationships with his caregivers.

The experience with Paul has demonstrated that a managed care approach to case management can work to address effectively the needs of some people with chronic psychiatric and medical illnesses. Such an approach would never have been funded by a traditional indemnity approach to health insurance. The success of this intervention seemed dependent on the clinical knowledge, skill, and judgment of the insurer's care manager as well as on our capacity to develop an ongoing collaborative relationship (Mohl, 1996).

However, it is worth noting that these extracontractual services were made available to Paul only because he was a high-risk patient who had been a high utilizer of services. In contrast, I previously described a case management intervention with a treatment-resistant young adult with schizophrenia who had been isolated in her parents' home for several years (Kanter, 1995a). Although the intensity of my interventions in that situation was only a fraction of my activity in Paul's case, the client's background of low services utilization would have rendered her ineligible for the extracontractual benefits described above.

Furthermore, the insurer's cost–benefit assessment would support such an intervention only if the insurer had reasonable confidence that the insured would remain a beneficiary with the insurer for an extended period. In a competitive insurance climate in which employers, employees, and other insured people often change insurers, there will be less financial incentive for insurers to "invest" in their customers' health; keeping this in mind, policymakers should consider the value of supporting stable relationships between insurers and their customers.

This case report illustrates how managed care can function rationally to allocate limited resources in the shared interest of insurer and insured. Although such an intensive case management approach is not likely to become part of benefit packages, it can be a useful extracontractual option in selected high-risk cases. We hope that other insurers and case managers can collaborate in implementing similar creative approaches to maximize patient functioning while reducing long-term costs.

Commentary by the Care Manager

In the early 1990s, many large insurers with traditional indemnity products were beginning to feel the competition in the marketplace from managed care products. Until that time, care management had focused on controlling costs for patients with costly catastrophic illnesses. As competition intensified, care management programs began to target chronic illnesses that required costly interventions. This enabled care managers to develop innovative individual care plans that might more effectively address medical needs while containing costs. Paul's case was an early experiment in the care management of a patient with chronic medical and psychiatric illnesses.

Paul was initially referred to our medical care management unit from our company's psychiatric utilization nurse reviewer. She identified Paul's clinical instability and the interrelationship between his psychiatric diagnoses, social situation, and medical history, and she believed that he was at great risk for both medical and psychiatric recidivism.

When I spoke with Paul's community-based social worker and reviewed his hospital admission records, I learned that Paul's condition involved a major depression, an adjustment disorder to the loss of parents, borderline mental retardation, and mixed personality disorders. His medical history included many manifestations of Paul's inadequate management of his insulin-dependent diabetes mellitus, including hypoglycemia and insulin reaction, peripheral neuropathy, and seizures. A pattern of emergency or crisis management involving numerous emergency room visits and hospital admissions was evident.

His social worker and I discussed a range of treatment options of various intensity. After further discussions with the patient, treating physicians, and the employer group representative, I completed the cost–benefit analysis of a short-term care plan that would include transitional placement in a skilled-nursing facility to provide a safe living situation and an active diabetes teaching and monitoring program. I also developed a long-range plan that involved Paul's return to work and a move to a group living situation with home health care support. My company retained Paul's social worker to focus on the longer-range goals of providing Paul with counseling support on an as-needed basis and locating and moving Paul to a group-living situation with adequate support for his medical needs. Meanwhile, my role was to locate a suitable skilled-nursing facility, negotiate rates, and monitor the ongoing interventions. Through weekly contacts, the social worker and I pooled our professional expertise and resources to plan a strategy and address the various problems that arose over time.

Some of the major obstacles we addressed were

- finding a skilled-nursing facility located on a busline, with staff trained in diabetes management, that would take an adult patient with psychiatric difficulties

- obtaining permission from the insurer to provide extracontractual benefits that would enable us to implement the aforementioned plan
- educating Paul, his employer, his social worker, and the multiple caregivers and providers on handling medical emergencies and at the same time encouraging Paul to assume responsibility for his own health
- addressing a variety of legal and financial requirements for guardianship, estate settlement, and group home placement.

A review of the cost records for Paul's care indicates that his claims totaled $53,000 in the year before the case management program began (including hospitalizations, emergency room visits, professional fees, medications, and laboratory work); $84,000 in the year of the aforementioned intervention; $39,000 in the first year after; and $9,000 in the second year after. The costs in the initial year were perhaps twice what we expected because of the unforeseen legal problems we encountered around Paul's finances. In the next year, the majority of the costs resulted from Paul's stroke, another unforeseen occurrence. Yet, the dramatic trend toward cost reduction in this chronically ill man is clearly evident. Although our initial investment in these extracontractual benefits was higher than projected, Paul's clinical improvement and independent functioning and the long-term cost reduction have clearly justified our initial treatment plan. Without a doubt, the social worker's dedication, perseverance, and professionalism were the keys to the success of this individualized case management plan. I believe that this gamble in case management for chronic diseases became the model for the continuation and expansion of our company's chronic disease care management program.

References

Kanter, J. (1988). Clinical issues in the case management relationship. In M. Harris & L. Bachrach (Eds.), *Clinical case management* (New Directions in Mental Health Services, No. 40, pp. 15–27). San Francisco: Jossey-Bass.

Kanter, J. (1989). Clinical case management: Definition, principles, components. *Hospital and Community Psychiatry, 40,* 361–368.

Kanter, J. (1990). Community-based management of psychotic clients: The contributions of D. W. and Clare Winnicott. *Clinical Social Work Journal, 18,* 23–41.

Kanter, J. (Ed.). (1995a). *Clinical studies in case management* (New Directions in Mental Health Services, No. 65). San Francisco: Jossey-Bass.

Kanter, J. (1995b). Managed care and the seriously mentally ill consumer. *Arlington Voice, 4*(3), 3–4. (Available from the National Alliance for the Mentally Ill, Arlington County, VA, Chapter)

Kanter, J. (1996). Engaging significant others: The Tom Sawyer approach to case management. *Psychiatric Services, 47,* 799–801.

Kramer, P. D. (1996, January). What's news. *Psychiatric Times,* p. 4.

Maltsberger, J. T., & Buie, D. H. (1974). Countertransference hate in the treatment of suicidal patients. *Archives of General Psychiatry, 30,* 625–633.

Mohl, P. C. (1996). Confessions of a concurrent reviewer. *Psychiatric Services, 47,* 35–40.

Shapiro, J. (1996). The downside of managed mental health care. *Clinical Social Work Journal, 23,* 441–451.

CHAPTER 20

A Successful Short-Term Treatment Case in Managed Care

Sidney H. Grossberg

Clinical practice soundly based on ego psychology (Beres, 1956; Blanck & Blanck, 1974) emphasizes planful therapeutic management of the client–therapist relationship. In developing a treatment plan, the practitioner assesses the client's presenting problem, developmental level, personality structure, and previous relationship experiences as well as the conscious attitudes and responses the client evokes. Thorough assessment makes it possible to identify the kind of therapeutic relationship the client needs in order to change. That relationship can be focused and managed by

- increasing or decreasing the degree of dependency gratification
- increasing or decreasing expectations for self-responsibility (for example, acting appropriately in social and interpersonal relations, taking active responsibility for change in therapy, and so forth)
- altering the frequency and duration of interviews
- interspersing telephone and face-to-face interviews to provide more support or to encourage autonomy
- choosing a focus (that is, reality oriented, intrapsychic, or interpersonal)
- clarifying the nature and purpose of the relationship
- interpreting the client's needs, feelings, and demands as expressed toward the worker
- providing or withholding concrete services.

These recommendations provide useful guidelines for conducting short-term psychodynamic treatment under managed care.

In the case presented in this chapter, ego-supportive and interpersonal techniques are described. The treatment contract called for eight weekly sessions, and the focus was organized around Mr. X.'s statement that he uses marijuana as a tranquilizer for "being anxious." Exploration of the precipitating factors during the first interview indicated that Mr. X. had previously been able to give up marijuana at his wife's request and had started using it again because of anger about his unmarried daughter's pregnancy and the birth of his grandson. In that initial interview he also expressed concern about managing his anger and spoke of having put his fist

NOTE: Originally published as Grossberg, S. H. (1996). A successful short-term treatment case in managed care. *Smith College Studies in Social Work, 66,* 335–341.

through a wall. The consulting psychiatrist prescribed a mild, nonrefillable tranquilizer with the goal of weaning Mr. X. from marijuana until he could gain better control over the feelings and relationship problems that precipitated his renewed drug use. The clearly articulated, mutually agreed-upon treatment focus reduced his tendencies toward regression and dependency in relation to the therapist. In addition, inviting his wife and daughter into treatment when Mr. X. was ready to do so directed his adaptive efforts toward current interpersonal issues rather than toward re-experiencing and understanding the effects that his father's repeated beatings of him had had on his personality organization and functioning.

As treatment progressed, the following ego functions were strengthened (Beres, 1956):

- His relationship to reality improved as his daughter told him that the man who had fathered her child was more responsible and involved than he had previously thought.
- The combination of medication and help in verbalizing his angry feelings helped him regulate his drives, particularly anger, more effectively.
- His defensive use of projection decreased as he was helped to talk directly with his wife and daughter about their feelings and issues in relation to him and to each other.

The case also illustrates some transference and countertransference reactions during therapy that are common in managed care cases. Usually, an initial transference occurs wherein the therapist is seen as a warm, compassionate, giving authority figure who can fix things immediately—sort of an omnipotent mother, father, and teacher rolled into one. In short-term treatment under managed care, these transference reactions are contained by an explicit, goal-focused therapeutic contract that emphasizes the client's responsibility for working actively and quickly toward modifying the identified problematic symptoms. From this perspective, it follows that countertransference reactions can occur if the therapist is unconsciously "sucked into" fulfilling any of the roles described above. Other countertransference reactions occur if the patient or the patient's problems touch any of the therapist's past or current conflicts or if the therapist's need is to please the managed care company rather than to devote fully the therapeutic endeavor toward helping the patient.

Case Study

This case will be described session by session. As I look back over my treatment notes, it is quite striking how differently I handled this managed care case from similar cases not referred through managed care.

Mr. X. was referred to me by his Seattle-based, national managed care employee assistance program (EAP). He was entitled to eight sessions, and if additional help (other than diagnosis, assessment, and short-term crisis intervention) was needed, he would have to be referred to a different therapist. In that case my task was to find a therapist with whom he could use his insurance or health maintenance organization (HMO) benefits and who was expert enough to handle Mr. X.'s problem.

All I was told by the EAP case manager before my first interview was that this was a voluntary referral, not a job performance referral, and that Mr. X. had tested positive for marijuana in one of the company's mandatory drug screenings.

FIRST SESSION

Mr. X. was tall, age 40, with a physical resemblance to a football lineman; his demeanor was gentle, almost obsequious. He was dressed in work clothes. At our first session he read and signed the "Understanding of Confidentiality" agreement, which states that our sessions are confidential and that no one at his place of employment could receive information about our sessions without his knowledge and his written release of information. The Seattle EAP requires clients to sign this agreement at the beginning of the first session.

The EAP also requires answers to a few brief questions on a form that I choose to handle at the beginning of the first session. The questions are

1. Describe specific major problem(s), including those work-related and family-related, that have led you to seek help at this particular time.
2. If you have had previous treatment, give brief history and dates.
3. Has psychotropic medication been prescribed? If yes, indicate medication and dosage, date initiated, and name of prescribing physician.
4. Describe any indication of alcohol or chemical dependency in yourself or family members.

(It should be noted that some EAP and managed care companies originally were set up specifically to handle substance abuse problems. Over time, many of these companies have expanded to also cover mental health problems.)

Mr. X. had not received any treatment previously, nor was he on any psychotropic medication. He said he was here because he had been suspended from work for testing positive for marijuana. He had been smoking two to six joints per day. He had stopped drinking alcohol eight to 12 years ago, although his father is alcoholic.

He is on a point system at work for being late and sick, and when he was late recently he got mad at himself and started throwing things. Someone saw him and wondered if he was on drugs, so he was sent for a mandatory drug screening. He tested positive for marijuana.

Mr. X. is here voluntarily because he wishes to stop using marijuana. He wants to return to his job driving a taxicab rather than to the temporary office position into which he was put. He felt he had his usage under control, but he sees now that it does affect him.

When he indicated that he had stopped using marijuana for a while, I asked if he knew why he stopped and why he started again. I was trying to assess his capability for self-observation because he seemed to have difficulty expressing himself. I was uncertain about his perception of the sessions at this point. I wondered if he saw me as an agent of his employer, and whether, even though we had discussed confidentiality, unspoken concerns about privacy were affecting his ability to communicate verbally.

Mr. X. said he stopped using for the first time because his wife wanted him to stop. Then his 16-year-old, unmarried daughter became pregnant and delivered a son. He grew angry over that and anxious about how he would display his anger. He said he feels that now he uses marijuana as a tranquilizer for "being anxious." Marijuana is costing more now and not getting him as high. He stopped using last week, but when he gets anxious now, he gets angry. He even put his fist through a wall.

At this point our first session was coming to an end. Mr. X. had presented himself as a sincere but confused person wanting to save his job and stop medicating himself with marijuana but was frustrated over uncontrolled acting out of anxiety and anger. I suggested the possibility of a psychiatric evaluation, partly to make a differential diagnosis, partly to determine whether his anxiety and anger might cause further acting out, but mostly to consider a mild antianxiety medication during withdrawal from self-medication. My thinking was that medication might reduce Mr. X.'s need to use marijuana to deal with his anxiety while he worked toward expressing anxiety and anger verbally in psychotherapy. It might also help save his job. He accepted a psychiatric consultation.

Countertransference reactions during this first session included my reactions to the differences between my normal way of working with patients and the requirements I needed to fulfill to satisfy the managed care company.

SECOND SESSION

Mr. X. consulted with the psychiatrist. The psychiatrist's report came to the same conclusions I had, adding that Mr. X. had been using marijuana since age 15 and that his father had beaten everyone in the family, including Mr. X. The patient also had a mild sleep disturbance. A mental status examination proved normal, as did all other functions. A mild, nonrefillable tranquilizer was prescribed.

THIRD SESSION

Mr. X. began by saying he's sleeping better and not having nightmares about the fights he had with his brother as a child. He said he took another drug test on Monday so he could get back to his driving job and away from the company office where he is now working.

He began to discuss the problems he had with his daughter, who is living at home with her baby. He stressed that when she became pregnant he had started back on marijuana. He still won't talk much to her boyfriend, although the boyfriend and his daughter see each other and eventually plan to marry. He feels the boyfriend should be more financially supportive of his daughter's baby.

Mr. X. gets along with his daughter except when she feels she can do whatever she wants because she's now a mother. He wants her to be in the house on school nights. The daughter is a straight-A student and wants to go to college to be a speech pathologist. She has two more years of high school left.

Mr. X. said that his daughter will listen more to his wife than to him, yet his wife doesn't feel supported by anyone in their family. She works taking care of AIDS patients. He said his wife would like to come in also and that he would like that. He'd even like the family to be seen together, as there may still be a lot of hurt going on in regard to his daughter's pregnancy. He has "clammed up" at home and really can't talk to his daughter about this.

I said that rather than talking things out, he acts out his anxiety, hurt, disappointment, and anger by throwing things or punching the wall, or he clams up, or he uses marijuana. He agreed, and said that he and his father still don't talk to each other. His father still resents him for accidentally knifing his brother in the leg many years ago. We scheduled our next session as my ears perked up at learning about that obvious traumatic event from his past and the patterns through which affect was expressed in his family of origin.

FOURTH SESSION

Mrs. X. accompanied Mr. X. She said she thought his self-esteem was low because of his father and his childhood. She said he's always trying to prove himself to his father—a man who stands 5'8", weighs 300 pounds, and scares people. Mr. X. said his father would slug and backhand him, his brother, and his four sisters. His father beat up a sister for being a half-hour late coming home. He would hit the kids if he didn't think they were eating right. Mr. X. remembers getting knocked down again and again, until his father got tired.

When I asked about the knife accident, he said he stabbed his brother in the thigh. The brother had to spend 1½ years in the hospital or in bed at home. Everyone teased him about this, and kids in school seemed to pick on him or be gunning for him. He "had to" beat up a lot of kids and eventually dropped out of school in the 11th grade. He did have a close relationship with his mother and feels he still does.

Mr. X. said that although he doesn't hit, he yells, and once he starts he can't stop, so mostly he chooses not to start. He feels his daughter does not listen to him, so he shuts up.

Mrs. X. said she wondered if he is depressed when he gets quiet, but Mr. X. said he's not depressed. He feels people don't listen to him because of his lack of education. He never went back to school after the 11th grade. He said he's anxious because of a lack of education. He cannot write or spell. He said he was a fairly good reader, but this skill was self-taught. He has signed up for night classes, but he's been too exhausted to go to them. He's very embarrassed about his lack of education. This helped explain his discomfort in expressing himself verbally during our initial session.

FIFTH SESSION

Mr. and Mrs. X. came in together again. He said they have been talking about his feelings since our last session. He is thinking of going back to school to learn to write. Not being able to write has held him back from certain jobs and has made him feel totally inadequate.

Mrs. X. said her husband is talking more at home instead of isolating himself. He passed his second drug screening and is back driving his taxi. This has given him confidence. His employer has been supportive of him. Mr. X. said he has a good job and home and doesn't want to mess this up.

Mr. X. said he was afraid to get close to his daughter because he might let her down as his father had done to him. (I did not pursue his feelings about his daughter letting *him* down because I thought this would come out later.) When I asked him why he thought his father beat him, he said he thought there was something wrong with him (Mr. X.). Rather than pursue what he thought was wrong about himself, I proceeded (under the conscious influence of managed care) by asking, "I wonder what your daughter thinks or fantasizes she is doing wrong when you clam up because of your fear that you are letting her down as a father?" We also discussed his not talking to his daughter's boyfriend because he thinks that the boyfriend doesn't care enough about his daughter because he doesn't support the baby financially. He's never asked the boyfriend but instead assumes (through projection) that his own thoughts are actually the boyfriend's thoughts.

Mr. X. could see by his own identification with his daughter how his father made *him* feel and that he needs to share his thoughts and feelings verbally with her (and, let's assume, with others in his family and environment). Both Mr. and Mrs. X. wanted the daughter to come to our next session.

SIXTH SESSION

Mr. X. didn't come in or call. He called later to apologize and explain he had been asked to work late.

SEVENTH SESSION

Mr. and Mrs. X. came in with their daughter. The parents were able to talk with their daughter about how her pregnancy had made them feel, about her boyfriend, and about parent–child conflicts. Mr. X. talked about fears related to his lack of education and about not wanting to treat his daughter or let her down as his father had let him down. This was an excellent session in which each family member shared his or her projections and fantasies about what other family members think. There was much emotion, some tears, real openness, and a capacity to listen. I thought there was real empathy for each other.

EIGHTH SESSION

This was the final session, and all three family members attended. They said that our seventh session really opened up their talking to each other. The daughter especially began to discuss thoughts and fantasies she had about what her parents thought of her. Some of these were correct (disappointment in her pregnancy and fear she would drop out of school). She was able to point out to her parents the reality of her getting all As and her motivation for college. (Because of time constraints and not knowing what it would open up, I did not point out the connection among the father's dropping out of school in the 11th grade, the daughter's pregnancy, and the possibility that she would drop out also.)

Mr. X. has begun to talk to her boyfriend and has learned that he does want to marry her but needs to get through school so they can live better. He is working at a part-time job, but it is a low-paying one, and he doesn't have extra money for the child. He does buy small gifts for the child.

We focused again on identifying one's own feelings, being open and honest in expressing them, and questioning others about how they feel rather than assuming that other people's thoughts and feelings are the same as one's own.

Mr. X. is not using marijuana and is gradually cutting back on the mild tranquilizer originally prescribed (he has reduced the dosage from three to one tablet a day). He feels his thoughts are a "lot clearer" now. Mrs. X. was so happy with the increased communication, she is encouraging her husband to talk even more. None of the family members wished a referral for further counseling. She felt the downward spiral has stopped. They were headed upward and had learned a lot.

Conclusion

It is obvious that deep character change did not occur in the members of this multiproblem family. Nonetheless, they experienced the psychological benefits of talking about feelings rather than acting them out passively or violently; asking what others think or feel rather than accepting their projections as the only reality; recognizing and reconsidering the fantasy that others can read your mind and know what you want, feel, and think; and verbalizing their worst fears (for example, "I'm uneducated, stupid, and inadequate") and discovering that others are supportive rather than critical or demeaning. If Mr. X. and his family members continue to practice these principles, life may become more bearable for each of them individually and for the family as a whole.

References

Beres, D. (1956). Ego deviation and the concept of schizophrenia. In R. S. Eissler, A. Freud, E. Glover, P. Greenacre, W. Hoffer, H. Hartmann, E. B. Jackson, E. Kris, L. S. Kubie, B. D. Lewin, R. Loewenstein, M. C. Putnam, & R. A. Spitz (Eds.), *Psychoanalytic study of the child* (Vol. 11, pp. 164–235). New York: International Universities Press.

Blanck, G., & Blanck, R. (1974). *Ego psychology: Theory and practice.* New York: Columbia University Press.

CHAPTER 21

The Development of Self-Love and Managed Care—or, Reflections on Being a Tutor

Susan E. Weimer

Children referred for treatment at child guidance centers in recent years have come increasingly from chaotic and violent family situations. In these emotionally deprived children, disappointments and lack of trust are palpable and transparent, as is a raw, unsated, emotional hunger. Emotional starvation can manifest itself in a variety of ways: stealing, lying, and a presentation of what Winnicott (1945) referred to as a "false self."

One might ask what place love has in therapeutic relationships with such children when surely the goal is to stop them from lying and stealing? That is the response we would expect from a managed care company.

However, if one values developmental and dynamic theory, a clinical formulation of what is helpful with such children might differ radically from a managed care approach. Winnicott (1945, 1972) wrote extensively about the development of children, drawing on his work first as a pediatrician and then as a psychoanalyst. His most generative work focused on the mother–child matrix, that all-encompassing space in which the capacity for future relationships develops; not only the relationship the infant has with its mother, the primary object, but also the relationship the infant develops with itself and with others.

For development to proceed more or less intact, the mothering figure must first be "good enough," that is, must provide at least adequate care both in the external environment (that is, cleaning and feeding) and in the internal environment (that is, the emotional space in which concrete care proceeds).

Winnicott (1945) noted three developmental processes that start early. The first is integration of a sense of self distinct from other. Integration starts immediately, proceeds over time, and is fostered by "good enough" mothering, which involves feeding, bathing, and all the other aspects of caregiving. The second process is personalization, which involves the feeling that "one's person is in one's body" (p. 151). Personalization also occurs over time, as a child experiences soothing, nurturing, and satisfactory body care. The third process, which also starts early in life, is that of realization, which Winnicott defined as "the appreciation of time and space and other properties of reality" (p. 151). Those are the processes that must unfold progressively

NOTE: Originally published as Weimer, S. E. (1996). The development of self-love and managed care—or, Reflections on being a tutor. *Smith College Studies in Social Work, 66,* 342–348.

over time for "normal" development to proceed; they lay the groundwork for adequate internalized object relations.

Winnicott (1954–55) posited that those processes are necessary for a child to move through normal emotional developmental milestones, one of which he termed the "stage of concern." In that stage, the infant begins its journey from what he described as the "ruthless," or "pre-ruth," phase to the phase of "ruth," or concern for the other. Ruthlessness is marked by an absence of concern regarding the consequences of instinctual impulses. During that phase the infant expects release from instinctual tension (for example, to be changed or fed) as well as complete freedom of self-expression (crying), and places the object firmly outside of itself ("You! Care for me now!"). Winnicott noted that the change from ruthless to ruth happens over time and is not definitively established until a much later date in a person's development.

This model of adequate care, over time, provided by a mothering figure who is patient enough to tolerate ruthlessness is a model which, until recently, has been used to promote healing in children who suffer from early developmental deficits (for example, children who have been rejected, understimulated, abused, neglected, or seriously mistreated in other ways). Child therapists who ascribe to this treatment model view themselves as lending and reinforcing a caring attitude and a holding environment in which they can support the growth of integration, personalization, and realization. These are the ingredients of progressive development that eventually bring to fruition a secure real self as well as the capability for mature object love.

Using this model, a clinician working with emotionally deprived children might find himself or herself taking on the symbolic role of "parent" as protector; "parent" provides ego and superego supports. The treatment format may revolve for years around what could best be described as a "holding environment" (Winnicott, 1965). Although the physical holding of which Winnicott spoke may generally be absent, mirroring, supportive ego lending, and empathic caring are essential. These are love's building blocks. They are primary to the development of positive self-regard as well as object love.

In recent years, involvement with state and local child protection agencies has become more frequent as therapists grapple with the essentials: the safety and well-being of the child's total life and the provisions that make it possible for children to grow physically, emotionally, and cognitively in an average expectable environment. Therapists who formerly had (symbolically) taken on some part of the parenting process with at-risk children over extended periods of time are now asked to take a "bad seed" child and produce a healthy seedling in four to 12 sessions.

Case Example

José is an 11-year-old Latino boy whom I saw over a period of five years. When originally referred, at age eight, he lived at a local children's crisis shelter with a younger sister and brother. José and his siblings had been removed from their mother for the third time in their lives because of gross neglect. The staff at the shelter wanted an immediate evaluation, stating that they thought José was psychotic because of his provocative behavior and threats to kill himself.

There was no evidence in my first meeting with José that he was psychotic. Indeed, he presented as a likable, quiet boy who was reluctant to talk but who acknowledged that he had had a good time upsetting the shelter staff by saying he would kill himself. He knew it would upset them.

José related the precipitating factors that had landed him at the shelter. Their mother, an alcoholic, had "fallen down drunk" in the liquor store, and José had had to carry her home. During this same period, Maria had been raped at knifepoint by José's stepfather. All three children witnessed the rape. The stepfather had threatened to cut their throats if they cried or screamed. José stated that the stepfather forced the three children to watch the rape from under a bed. José, then seven years old, was helpless to defend his mother as she was raped on the floor.

To restrain his provocative behavior in the shelter, José had been wrestled to the floor and sat on, a method taught to the shelter workers by so-called experts in dealing with disturbed children. He became wild and, understandably, even more unmanageable when restrained in that fashion. The unmanageable behavior prompted the referral.

Despite José's history and reports from the shelter about his stealing, lying, and disruptiveness, I immediately took a liking to him. He spoke of feeling restricted at the shelter. He was used to being in charge of himself, his younger siblings, and his mother as well. His desire to play was initially constricted by his attempt to read me—to figure out what kind of play would please me. At the end of this initial session, he indicated that he would like to return to see me, and another appointment was made. We both ended this session feeling some degree of hope: for myself, that perhaps I could be of help to José; for José, that this was a good (safe and caring) place to be. However, because of a lack of local foster placements, José was placed elsewhere in the state before I could see him a second time as planned.

Three months later, when he was placed with a local foster family, he was re-referred. At that time, the state informed me that Maria had a "fatal illness" but that they were not allowed by law to tell me what that illness was. Maria had also filed a suit with the court to have her children returned. She was given 18 months to become sober and perform some tasks to indicate that she had become a good-enough mother.

During those 18 months, José's foster mother Lourdes brought him to appointments faithfully. José, who had initially presented as a quiet child, began to enjoy playing a variety of games. He created a form of basketball in which we shot baskets with checkers, using the space behind a wall map as the target area. I encouraged these occasional creative spurts as a vehicle for José to establish trust with me and a basic, positive sense of self.

During that time frame, José rarely acknowledged having a feeling and could not explore affects or conflicted areas of his life. This began to change shortly before his return to his mother, when he began to call me his "tutor." This puzzled me for a while. José has a reading problem for which he has received special help, and my initial reaction was that he must be using the term "tutor" to mean a general kind of helper, because at that point I had never actually helped him with his schoolwork.

As time passed, he also began to notice when I was late, when I was away, and when an interruption or intrusion by any other thought or person cast a shadow over our relationship and interrupted my focus on him. Clearly, as these transparent signs of attachment and neediness indicate, José had developed some level of relationship toward me. I had become an important object to him. On the eve of his return to Maria, a year and a half after our initial meeting, I tried exploring his feelings about leaving Lourdes. He responded that the good things about Lourdes were that she had provided him with food, clothes, a decent home, and rules—life's basic necessities. Maria had been unable to provide these, but she was his mother.

José denied feeling fearful about leaving Lourdes and returning to his mother, despite hugging a corner of the room with his back to me throughout most of that session. He was so ambivalent about his two mothers that he could neither express sadness about leaving Lourdes nor state that he loved her. If he said it, what would that imply about his feelings toward Maria?

For the first time in our relationship, he rejected me and my attempts to explore these feelings. He withdrew more and, following this initial sad silence, displayed contemptuous behavior by forcing air out between his teeth and maintaining a defiant silence. I suspected he was preparing for the emotional climate at home with Maria. That presentation followed my last stand at trying to help him connect affect with events. I had stated that it was alright if he loved both of his mothers. More to the point, he may have felt completely rejected by Lourdes and helplessly caught in the shuttle between his "real" and foster homes.

During the remainder of this session, silence reigned except for the defensive, contemptuous rejection of me, literally spitting me out between his teeth. I decided to use a paradoxical technique that had worked with other highly defended children, that is, benign ignoring. I sighed and said, "Oh, well, I guess I'll have to play by myself today because you aren't interested in turning around. If you decide you want to join me, just come on over. It's up to you." I took out a deck of cards and laid out a hand of solitaire. Out of the corner of my eye I saw José begin to turn around. As soon as I started, he was at my side.

"What game is this?" he asked.

"It's called 'solitaire,'" I said, "and you play it when you feel all alone. 'Solitaire' means 'by yourself,' and you look like you feel you're all by yourself today."

José's association must have been to prison, where his own father resides, for he replied, "Teach me how to play 'solitary.'"

I did. He asked me who had taught me how to play "solitary," and I told him that my own mother had.

"Is she still alive?" he asked.

"Yes," I replied.

"How old is she?" I told him. A new avenue then opened for us to begin to talk about Maria and Lourdes again and the "fatal illness" with which Maria had been struck. Unknown to me at the beginning of the session, José had recently been told that Maria had what he called "HB." He seemed unsure what that was and did not really want to discuss it in depth. However, we began to discuss what he did know about HIV and his mother's health in particular.

José's return to Maria was short lived, because as anticipated by everyone, she was unable to care adequately for her children. She also missed sessions for both José and herself. During his one-month stay with her, José continued to address me at times with a condescending attitude, and occasionally dismissed me with disparaging remarks, and his contemptuous air-through-teeth expletive. I thought of this as a borderline adaptation, as he was unable to juggle two, much less three, objects. Someone had to hang on the edge for a while, and his unconscious trusted I could manage that. He never completely abandoned the relationship despite several opportunities to do so. In fact, José eventually called the police on himself and his younger brother for beating up their mother. The two of them were removed from Maria and returned to Lourdes.

Children learn to survive, but not always adaptively. Although fighting with his mother may not have been adaptive, the fact that he himself called the police was impressive and speaks to a level of self-preservation and self-concern (Winnicott, 1972); of a desire to be safe, loved, and protected; and, perhaps, of a desire to punish as well.

After his return to Lourdes, José began to bring more of himself into the treatment. Why couldn't he live in my office? He fantasized what that would be like and more openly expressed his desires for security, safety, warmth, love, and stability. He began to use the game "Hangman" to express ambivalent feelings. Frequently the event that precipitated his interest in playing Hangman involved a situation in which he might have to share me with others. For example, his sister wanted him to invite her to a Christmas party José and I had planned. He was ambivalent about her joining us. That occasioned an attempt to explore with him what it would mean to share me (and the food) with his sister. He asked her because she asked him to ask—not because he truly wanted to include her. Although his foster mother saw such events as proof that José was selfish, I understood them as attempts to preserve an empathic attunement for himself.

In a drawn-out court case involving testimony from me and the Department of Children and Families (DCF), the children have remained in the care of Lourdes. Until recently, they saw Maria on a regular basis. Within the past month, however, Maria's HIV symptoms have increased. She developed pneumonia and a brain aneurysm. From what Lourdes has told me, Maria may also have developed Kaposi's sarcoma. The two younger children have cut off ties with her because of her chronic abuse of the daughter. José continues to want to see her, to get whatever he can from her. In this sense, he is ruthless in his quest for satiety and demands that she still provide him with good things. For him, for now, nothing, no one thing, perhaps no one person will ever be enough. Since his mother's rapid decline, José has again begun to pull away from me; he has occasionally shown contempt, but mostly appears sadly resigned.

I recently looked up the root of the word "tutor" in the dictionary and chuckled when I read the Latin translation—"to look after, guard." José continues to refer to me as his tutor and jealously guards his time with me. I dread to think of what may happen to José and his siblings (both of whom are also in treatment) now that managed care has taken over Medicaid in Connecticut. Does managed care have an interest in José's developmental needs? Will they care about his need for tutelage? Do they have any idea of what is meant by self- or object love, the time and involvement required in fostering basic healthy development? The answers to these questions seem self-evident. Our prisons are already filled with people like José. How many more Josés will the managed care system siphon off into the criminal justice system? Mind you, José's prognosis for the development of good-enough self-love is guarded at best. However, the first party we had late last fall was in honor of his report card: the first ever with no Fs. All of his As were in areas of "citizenship" and "respect for others."

In fact, the dichotomy between managed behavioral health and developmentally oriented mental health care is such that there is no common language, philosophy, or sense of mission that can bridge the chasm. As I wrote this chapter, I thought of the words of the Supremes' 1966 song, "You Can't Hurry Love." They are a far cry from those of Winnicott, but they bear a message just as wise and true. That song is an apt way to end my thoughts here on the development of self- and object love and the jeopardy we clinicians and our patients face when confronted by the limitations and dictates of managed care companies:

> I need love, love, to ease my mind.
> I need time to find someone to call mine.
> But mama said, "You can't hurry love.
> No, you just have to wait.
> Love don't come easy.
> It's a game of give and take.
> You can't hurry love.
> No, you just have to wait.
> You gotta trust, give it time,
> No matter how long it takes."

I resigned from the Child Guidance Center in the spring of 1997. José and I terminated shortly before my resignation. He was 13 and had talked on and off about wanting to stop during that winter. He was recovering from the shock of witnessing his foster father and foster brother shot (not fatally) during an attempted break-in at their home one night the previous autumn. DCF had also considered removing him for placement to a more structured setting prior to the shooting incident but eventually put this move on hold because we all agreed it would be too much of a disruption.

José's grades had plummeted following the break-in and assault. He had also been accused of stealing again, which he adamantly denied. Lourdes supported his protests of innocence and stood up for him in front of his accusers. During the course of the winter and spring, his school performance improved, and with much encouragement from me, Lourdes involved him in an after-school program. Thus, I eventually supported José's desire to terminate at this juncture. Aside from my impending departure, he had shown initiative in areas around school and peer relationships; he was speaking up for himself and verbalizing some sense of self in his need to explore other areas of the larger world, including an after-school basketball team. I have no further information about José and his development. As with all "tutors," I only hope the best for him.

References

The Supremes. (1966). *You can't hurry love.* Detroit: Motown Records.

Winnicott, D. W. (1945). Primitive emotional development. In M. R. Khan (Ed.), *Through pediatrics to psycho-analysis* (pp. 145–156). London: Hogarth Press & Institute of Psychoanalysis.

Winnicott, D. W. (1954–55). The depressive position in normal emotional development. In M. R. Khan (Ed.), *Through pediatrics to psycho-analysis* (pp. 262–277). London: Hogarth Press & Institute of Psychoanalysis.

Winnicott, D. W. (1965). The theory of the parent–infant relationship. In *The maturational process and the facilitating environment* (pp. 37–55). London: Hogarth Press & Institute of Psychoanalysis. (Original work published 1960)

Winnicott, D. W. (1972). Basis for self in body. *International Journal of Child Psychotherapy, 1,* 7–16.

C H A P T E R 22

Managed Care as a Transference Object: A Clinical Study

Roberta Myers

It is difficult to think about our clients' communications and issues when managed care demands intrude into the therapeutic setting and distract us from psychodynamic listening and intervention. I have been hearing a change in the way clinicians are thinking about their cases and the way in which they are listening to their clients. I have seen this change reflected in the content of professional conferences. Professional training seminars are steering therapists away from the necessity to listen for and understand the unconscious in managed care psychotherapies, and therapists are paying less attention to the unconscious determinants of their clients' issues. These changes have led me to think about the assumption that therapists have to abandon psychodynamic psychotherapeutic skills in managed care psychotherapy. With such an assumption, managed care demands are treated in a surface fashion, and their potential of holding unconscious derivative importance and meaning is ignored. It is my belief that this abandonment of psychodynamic psychotherapeutic skill is not necessary or helpful to clients or to the professional delivery of mental health services. These observations and reflections led me to write this chapter to illustrate the contribution psychodynamic understanding and method can make to managed care psychotherapies.

Some clinical literature has focused on the impact of managed care on the therapeutic alliance (Higuchi & Newman, 1994; Meehan, 1994); the therapeutic process (Busch, 1994); the confidentiality necessary for psychotherapeutic effectiveness (Bollas & Sundelson, 1995); the establishment of a therapeutic holding environment (Alperin, 1994); the timing of clinical interventions (Miller, 1994); the therapeutic impact of interpretation (Zuckerman, 1989); and on the transference, countertransference, and understanding enactments (Saakvitne & Abrahamson, 1994).

Some authors have suggested that the requirements of managed care and those of psychotherapy oppose one another. Shapiro (1995) examined the difficulties caused by the attempt to combine professional and corporate cultural values in managed mental health care. Raney (1993) concluded that reports about a client's psychotherapy are invalid as information loses its meaning outside of the therapeutic context in which it is obtained. He went on to suggest that the psychotherapy is destroyed when reporting requirements pressure the therapist to stop listening to the

NOTE: Originally published as Myers, R. (1998). Managed care as a transference object: A clinical study. *Journal of Analytic Social Work, 5,* 5–23. Permission to reprint granted by Haworth Press, Inc.

client's productions as "derivative expressions of arcane object relationships" (p. 35). Gray (1992) maintained that reporting requirements of utilization reviews damage the therapeutic alliance by creating what she called an "unanalyzable defect" (p. 154). Alperin (1994) concluded that managed care conflicts with the fundamental tenets of psychoanalytic psychotherapy: "Because of managed care's disregard for the treatment relationship, narrow focus only on the behavioral manifestations of symptoms and not on character pathology, preference for short-term approaches, and utilization review procedures, its basic principles are incompatible with those of psychoanalytic psychotherapy" (p. 137). Most authors point out the difficulty therapists have in staying within a psychoanalytic framework in managed care psychotherapies. A survey of the literature reveals that there has been little focus on clinical demonstrations of the maintenance of a psychodynamic psychotherapeutic process in managed care psychotherapies. Zuckerman (1989) approached this problem by describing a case in which the client's associations to her managed care company have transferential implications. Busch (1994) pointed out the importance of continuing to work with the client's and therapist's unconscious conflicts around managed care intrusion.

Apart from Zuckerman and Busch, it appears that what has been discussed is how managed care intrudes upon the psychotherapeutic process. What has not been discussed is how managed care intrusions call a therapist's attention away from therapeutic interest in the unconscious, including the transference. Both clients and therapists have transferences to managed care that, if clinically addressed, lead to a deeper psychotherapeutic experience that frees the therapist and client from the restrictions of managed care. This chapter will illustrate how a therapist, working through her own countertransference, struggles to maintain the ability to hear and work with clients' unconscious derivatives in managed care psychotherapy.

Shift in Clinical Attention

One of the most common clinical phenomena resulting from managed mental health care is that the managed care company requirements and the insurance benefit become a primary focus of attention. In a way, these become the new client in the treatment, and the therapy's focus shifts to the needs of this new client and away from the needs of the actual client. Those two clients' needs are often divergent, requiring quite different interventions. This is seen in the common managed care need for case reviews. Davidson and Davidson (1995) noted that a clinician faced with this managed care need is "now unable to satisfy, simultaneously, the two demands of protecting confidentiality and discussing the case in sufficient detail to satisfy the insurance carrier or their designees" (p. 454). Here, the needs of the managed care company and the client are in direct opposition with regard to confidentiality.

When the focus is taken away from the client–therapist interaction, the importance of the development and elucidation of the therapeutic transference is superseded by the managed care need for case reviews. The therapist is expected to conduct himself or herself as an authority figure, and active client participation is discouraged. Many times the clinician is expected to discuss clinical information with the managed care case manager directly by telephone. Again, there is conflict in several ways between serving the managed care needs and the actual client needs. Even if the therapist has first discussed with the client the information to be divulged, there is no guarantee that the therapist will not be expected to say more than has been agreed to. There is no opportunity to listen for the client's reactions in order to understand his or her clinical needs. Whether the reviews are verbal or in written form, the dates for completed reviews are decided unilaterally by the managed care company. Thus, no regard is given to the necessity of sufficiently working through any clinical issues that have arisen from the reporting requirement before any information is released. The external demands for action by managed care become more pronounced when a therapist confuses them with an anxiety-driven internal push for action, stirred up by managed care. This process can short-circuit the psychodynamic task of understanding.

In the shift away from the client's actual needs, interventions become focused on surface, conscious content and not on unconscious, derivative, transference-laden content. There is an open invitation from managed care for therapists to abandon the necessity to include the client's unconscious issues. The client's negative transference and resistance are not, therefore, interpreted but are externalized onto managed care and away from the treatment setting. This shift illustrates a collusion between the therapist and client in a struggle with managed care. Much has been written suggesting that negative transference and the accompanying resistance are among the most difficult issues for therapists to deal with. As long ago as 1905, Freud (1905/1953a) said that working with the transference was "by far the hardest part of the whole task" (p. 116). More recently, Gill (1979) also referred to the analysis of the transference as the most difficult aspect of analytic technique. Bird (1972) spoke of the "wear and tear of this abrasive experience" (pp. 278–279) as he referred to the effect on the therapist of the necessary involvement in the center of the client's transference. He suggested that therapists turn away from the handling of the transference in acts of "self-defense." We are vulnerable to the managed care invitation to avoid these difficult clinical issues. There is thus a danger that the therapist, in a desire to remain on the good side, splits the transference.

Therapeutic Listening

One of the tenets of psychodynamic psychotherapy is the importance of the unconscious in the genesis of psychological conflicts. Listening for derivatives of the unconscious in client material and understanding the concept of multiple determination (Waelder, 1936) are key components of psychoanalytic listening. Transference is thought to be an invaluable communication about the client's unconscious content, revealing the many determinants of the client's feelings and behaviors. Psychodynamic therapists are trained to listen with this clinical ear to everything the client brings into the session. We continually scan for unconscious meaning in the client's verbal and nonverbal productions. We also attend to the transference and countertransference clues in the relationship the client tries to establish with us. That therapeutic stance is necessary but also easily disturbed by myriad influences including transference and countertransference pulls.

At times, the therapist's attention is drawn away from the basic tenets of psychoanalytic listening, resulting in shifts from unconscious to conscious exploration and work. Some of those shifts are evident in the therapist's switch from an interpretive stance to a directive one. Others are evident in the therapist's or client's attempt to dilute the intensity of material with such mechanisms as splitting the transference. There are, oftentimes, attributions to externally based causality with the accompanying shift from unconscious to conscious exploration and work. Managed care offers clinicians and their clients a seductive way to collude consciously or unconsciously with the urge to keep difficult content out of the clinical moment.

It is commonly known that clients offer external and surface reasons for their actions and feelings. Freud (1915/1953b) helped us understand that what defines the unconscious is that it is out of a person's awareness. We cannot expect our clients to talk at a level of meaning beyond their conscious awareness. As a result, clients rely on our ability as therapists to understand the unconscious derivatives contained within their material. Psychodynamic therapists have felt reassured with the time-honored knowledge that unconscious meanings and transference meanings attach themselves to all sorts of things for expression, including external, factual events. Psychodynamic therapists have abandoned the either–or type of thinking in which something is either a fact or has psychological meaning. In fact, we spend much time in therapy helping our clients also achieve this level of development in their thinking.

Interpretation plays a significant and essential part in therapy because it is the therapist's tool for helping the client become aware of the archaic determinants of feelings and behaviors. When the unconscious content is brought to consciousness, the neurotic connections are interrupted. For example, external issues become more reality based without unconscious meanings attached.

Pull to Abandon Therapeutic Listening and Interpretation

As with many intrusions, the introduction of managed care into the therapeutic situation tends to draw therapists away from a therapeutic stance (Langs, 1973). When therapists abandon psychoanalytic listening, an understanding of the unconscious is lost. Under these circumstances, intrusions into psychotherapy can be considered only as external factors, disconnected from clients and their unconscious issues and conflicts. Inderbitzin and Levy (1994) have reminded us of the importance of making interpretive use of external reality when it intrudes into the treatment situation:

> The analyst helps the patient to explore how an external event is elaborated intrapsychically and becomes the subject of mental processes that reveal similarities to those conflicts and compromises that have been the focus of the day-to-day analytic scrutiny. Such grist for the mill becomes a means of demonstrating to the patient the unity and connectedness of mental life, at times providing the analysand with concrete and vivid examples that enhance his or her conviction about previous interpretive work. (p. 764)

When the external reality that is introduced into therapy involves the therapy itself, as in managed care intrusions, it is difficult for the therapist to maintain a clarity of clinical thought. As a result, the therapist may think of the intrusion in an external way, disconnected from the client and the client's unconscious conflicts and issues. There may be only a conscious, surface understanding between the client and therapist about the presence of managed care in the treatment. To forestall their own conflicted thinking, therapists may even make determinations about the managed care benefit ahead of time and without the guiding benefit of the client's associations. That happens regularly, for example, when a therapist views the amount of covered insurance funding available as synonymous with the amount of therapy needed. The therapist may also accept a surface understanding of the client's reactions to the various managed care events during the course of therapy. In summary, it is easy to view the events and reactions in managed care therapy simply as facts, forgetting to consider the associated conscious and unconscious emotional content.

Consider clients whose core issues center on feelings of disappointment and feelings of not having gotten enough of what they needed early in life. The typical presentation of such issues in therapy is both conscious and unconscious. The therapist begins to see, and helps clients to see, how clients experience those feelings transferentially every day in current life. To the extent that those feelings are unconscious and unresolved, clients must find an avenue of expression that will not be direct and conscious. The managed care process becomes an excellent vehicle for attachment of these feelings.

Clients with those problems bring to therapy unconscious transferential expectations of being disappointed and of not getting enough of what they need. My own personal experience is that when hints of this transference begin to show in the therapy hour, I know I have been given a direct interpretive way to help a client stop the unconscious repetition of painful feelings. I find it helpful to understand that the client's unconscious transference to me is no different from the unconscious transferences to others and no different from unconscious transferences to the managed care insurance and case managers. When I experience countertransference pulls to get more insurance coverage, it helps to consider the role responsiveness possibility in my reactions (Sandler, 1976). I explore the client's unconscious experience of me as a depriving figure and use the ample material in that situation to analyze and interpret the negative transference components that may have attached to the external reality of a limited insurance benefit. In that way, the use of the managed care experience shared by me and my client becomes an agent of change.

Case Studies

Some actual clinical material may be helpful in examining how the therapist begins to use the client's unconscious transference to managed care. We will look at two clinical vignettes drawn from psychotherapy cases involving managed care insurance.

MS. A.: NARCISSISTIC TRANSFERENCE

The first case is that of Ms. A., who began therapy with a traditional insurance plan that converted to a managed care form during the course of the therapy. This client came to therapy with a history of a relationship to a mother whom she felt had been self-involved, critical of the client, and unsupportive of the client's efforts to be different from the mother. In addition, the client had tremendous conflicting feelings about her early attachment to another family member as a substitute mother. When the client presented for therapy, she was depressed, felt poorly about herself, was isolated from others, and was experiencing conflict in her child-rearing responsibilities.

The following clinical material describes a point in the treatment when managed care had just entered the picture. The client spoke at that point about the managed care decisions regarding authorizing or not authorizing sessions as though the decisions were the same as her needing or not needing the therapy. We explored the determinants of this externalization. One involved the maternal transference she was experiencing to the case manager, in which the client felt she must "match" the view of the case manager, much as she had felt she had to do with her mother. Another involved her defense that her feelings and needs were not valid and acceptable unless they were validated by an outside source. In that way, she was able to avoid the possibility of experiencing as her own a feeling or need that was associated with painful disappointment by her mother and with terrible feelings about herself. The therapist's interventions at this point centered on interpretations both of the client's transference to the case manager and her defensive need to have the managed care company represent her needs, even when it was not an accurate representation. This client was clearly experiencing a negative maternal transference toward the case manager. It was possible to interpret the defensive function when we analyzed the way the client used the case manager's input. After such transference and defense interpretations were offered, the client disclosed that she anticipated the managed care company would authorize less than she needed; that idea would feel like proof that there really never is help and that nothing works, thereby evoking repetitions of her feelings and experiences in her relationship with her mother.

Later in the therapy, the client began the hour by bringing up the managed care company requirements for a clinical report. She said that the previous authorization expiration date was almost here and asked the therapist if she would call the managed care company and do the required clinical report to apply for further authorization of sessions. The therapist commented that the client did not seem to want to be involved. The client became tearful and said yes, she did not feel she should have to be involved. She repeated the managed care dictum that the therapist had to be the one who called the managed care case manager and wrote the report, and she added that she could not continue to come to therapy without this insurance benefit. The therapist noted aloud that, although the client felt she should not have to be involved with preparing the report, she also seemed to feel the therapist should be. The client responded with a teary and emotional tirade and said that the therapist was giving her an "attitude." She said that the therapist did not want to be involved and that the therapist was not interested in her or in what she needed. She asked why should the therapist involve herself with this because she obviously thought it was the client's problem and did not concern her? The therapist had never stated that she would not be involved in the authorization process, and there seemed to be a familiar transference theme in this material, so the therapist replied that the client seemed to want the therapist to conduct herself in a particular fashion (that is, telephone the case manager, write the report) so as to reassure the client against her feelings that the therapist's only interest in her was a self-interest. The client responded affirmatively and went on to talk at some length about the negative maternal transference. She reflected that she wanted to be able to find some way to avoid asking for things from the therapist where she had to be involved. The therapist offered the interpretation that she wanted to do so because when she tried to be involved and included she experienced the fear and anticipation that she would only be trying to involve herself with a person who was self-involved and disinterested in her.

Later, the therapist noted to Ms. A. that the therapist's observations were experienced by the client as if the therapist were saying "Get away and don't bother me" rather than heard as an invitation to understand something together or that they might work together as a team or as a "we." Ms. A.'s response to this transference interpretation was to say that, of course, when her managed care company said the therapist needed to telephone, it fit right in with her desire to stay uninvolved with the therapist. This led to a further unfolding of her fears of her desire to depend upon the therapist and to feel involved and attached. At that point, she was able for the first time to refer to an earlier session in which she felt she allowed herself to show a direct affection for the therapist but then felt shunned in the transference.

Therefore, the client's negative transference to the therapist was seen to be defended against by her use of the managed care requirements, although in the previous material the client's transference to the case manager and her defensive use of the case manager's input could be interpreted. When the therapist analyzed the client's "letter-of-the-law" way of looking at the managed care requirements, the negative transference that had been defended against could be elucidated and interpreted. This led to a deepening of the material and work.

In a subsequent hour, material continued concerning the client's long-held belief that to develop herself as an individual separate from her mother was selfish and harmful to her mother. As she recounted her defense of trying to remain passive and subservient, she again associated to the transference the passivity she had displayed around the managed care clinical report requests. She revealed the maternal transference both to the case manager and to the therapist as she talked about there being room for only one viewpoint about her case or else the other person (case manager or therapist) would get hurt. In her need to make herself passive and compliant, she felt she must view the therapist as the "expert" on her case. In that way, she unconsciously reached a compromise formation. On the one hand, she avoided the possibility of revealing herself as a separate individual with her own and perhaps different opinion (which felt dangerous as she equated being separate and different from the other with doing "harm" to the other) and of giving rise to painful, conflicted feelings of divided loyalty (something she had long felt between her mother and the family member who had felt like a substitute mother for her). On the other hand, she could serve the narcissistic transferential need that the therapist would only involve herself in such a requirement in a self-important and self-involved way, not wanting to be bothered by having to relate or be interested in the client and her thoughts. It became understandable that her desires for therapy were conflicted. She viewed her therapy as a way to achieve her goal of becoming a separate and happy adult individual, but at the same time she feared that achieving this goal would result in harm to and loss of the other. When this was understood in therapy, Ms. A.'s unconscious need to stay away from a certain depth in her treatment could be interpreted. Her associations included her desire to agree with the case manager's recommendations for less-frequent sessions versus more-frequent ones, as well as her anticipation of passively accepting the end of covered sessions as the end of treatment. As Ms. A.'s issues were interpreted, the neurotic connections were interrupted, and she was able to place more factual meaning and significance on the managed care decision; she began to feel that she would continue her therapy even if the managed care company stopped coverage of her sessions. As a result of this interpretive work, she eventually sought and obtained employment to cover such an eventuality.

When the next request for authorization occurred, the client for the first time involved herself in this process with the therapist. In a particular hour after completing the actual paperwork, Ms. A. spoke of feeling she never could have participated in such a way earlier in her treatment. Her associations to being a part of the report writing were that she had been afraid that she would find out something terrible and wrong about herself. She also talked about her fear that she would have found out that the therapist had her own ideas about the client that would have no bearing on how she felt about herself and would have no relation to what she had thought she had communicated to the therapist. She feared that she would find evidence that the therapist was just like her mother, in that the therapist would be adamant in her unattuned, self-involved, and unchangeable conclusions about the client.

Although primary attention has been paid here to the client's transference to the case manager, it is also important to speak to the parallel manifestation of the therapist's transference to the case manager. This aspect of transference also had to be understood by the therapist to prevent disastrous enactments that could obscure the therapist's ability to work clinically with the client's transferences and precipitate a premature termination of the therapy. The therapist's transference feelings were those of helplessness in the face of a challenging enemy. Whereas some may argue that these were realistic feelings, the important point here is that the case manager became the logical repository of the therapist's transference feelings of "dealing with the enemy." In this situation the therapist was dealing with a conscious dislike of the managed care situation and associated conscious and unconscious transference meanings.

At some point in the therapy, the client sensed the therapist's negative feelings toward managed care. This enactment on the therapist's part was only understood, contained, and rectified when the unconscious transference underpinnings became clear. The therapist had unconsciously responded to her own feelings of helplessness and anger toward the transference object of managed care by inserting her own feelings and desires about managed care into the treatment situation. The therapist's subsequent necessary introspective work was initiated when the client material indicated a detrimental shift had occurred secondary to the therapist's indirect communication of negative feelings about managed care. The prior feeling of alliance and teamwork with the client had vanished, and the therapist found herself feeling on the outside of the client's alliance with the case manager.

The therapist had inadvertently done two things. First, she had threatened the client's defensive need of the managed care company. If the managed care company was looked upon as negative, then the client might lose the protective cover of this supposed voice for her needs, thus running the risk of feeling her own separate feelings and needs. As is well known, when any defense is threatened instead of interpreted, the result is a heightening of the defense (Glover, 1931). This could be seen in the client "taking the side of" managed care against the "intruder" therapist. The client increased her insistence that managed care represented her interests and that she could not continue to come to therapy without it. Second, the therapist functionally served as an obstacle to the client's ability to have her own experience of managed care. This opportunity was circumvented by the therapist's actions in that the therapist then became the container for affect, including the projected affects of the client. Clearly, when the therapist could stop responding from unconscious transference pressure for fight or flight, her actions could come under conscious control. This allowed for containment of transference anxiety, which then allowed the therapist to resume interpretive interventions.

MS. B.: "NOT-ENOUGH-TIME" TRANSFERENCE

Ms. B. came to therapy with managed care insurance; her therapist was a panel provider of the managed care company. This client presented to therapy suffering with depression. Her history involved a pivotal experience of her parents being intolerant of her feelings and needs. Talking about feelings was discouraged as babyish, selfish, and unnecessary. Apparently overwhelmed, her parents retreated when she tried to do so. As a result, Ms. B.'s experience of feelings and needs became conflicted, imbued with the sense of there having been no time for her and with the fear that her feelings and needs were too great and had a hurtful potential. She had terminated an earlier therapy when she felt the therapist had found her unreasonable.

When she began the current treatment, Ms. B. spoke of her managed care company and her case manager in a positive light. She viewed the case manager's opinion as the statement of what she needed and did not need. The managed care company had initially authorized four sessions. The client and therapist jointly filled out a request for additional sessions on a twice-weekly basis. The case manager's response was that two sessions a week were not warranted and that the therapist would have to justify the request for this frequency of appointments. Twelve sessions over a three-month period were authorized. The therapist brought this information into the next session with the client. The client's unconscious associations to the information were to childhood examples of never being believed, listened to, or tolerated for her feelings. She related how she had protected herself by keeping her feelings to herself and dampening them inside of herself. She then referred back to the case manager's input and talked about cutting her twice-a-week sessions back to once a week. However, she made a slip when she said this and actually said that she should cut her sessions back to once a month. She caught herself and laughed. It became clear that she was offering a plan that she felt would not be sensitive to her needs, as she continued to feel that twice-weekly sessions were helpful.

It was the therapist's interpretation that the client was experiencing feelings about the case manager's response to the request for authorization that were similar to those she had about her parents when she had tried to express her feelings and needs to them and was not heard. Instead of experiencing the painful feelings of not being understood and listened to, which had significant meaning and history, she was doing what she had also done in childhood: She was protecting herself from those feelings by trying to erase them inside herself. This resulted in her passive agreement to a plan that did not address the extent of her need. She responded affirmatively to the therapist's interpretation and dropped the notion of reducing her session frequency from the already established two times a week. There also occurred an elaboration of her feeling bad and guilty about herself in childhood when she would be criticized for expressing herself. When she would try to tell her parents something that they found upsetting, unkind and hurtful motivations were ascribed to her.

Ms. B. had a parental transference reaction to the case manager that was dealt with interpretively in the treatment. There were also a positive transference and a negative transference toward the therapist, but those were not the prominent features or issues at that juncture. The client was clearly responding to the case manager as if she were responding to her parents, subsequent to her request for them to be sensitive to her emotional needs. As such, she was also experiencing her need for twice-weekly therapy as the infantile version of need, one that felt wrong to have and that made her feel helpless and frightened. As the unconscious transference meanings were separated out and detached from the client's reactions to the actual case manager, the client could act more appropriately with her own needs in mind. That is, there was less of a necessity to defend against her needful feelings when their frightening aspects could be analyzed. She no longer had to maintain the unconscious belief that all needs would be experienced in the childhood context of needing someone who was intolerant of those needs. In short, Ms. B. could experience her needs in a more mature form and feel the freedom to decide how she wanted to apply her insurance coverage to her treatment, instead of having it direct her treatment.

At that point in the therapy, the client began to hesitate in leaving at the end of the hour. After that hesitation had occurred twice, the therapist interpreted the hesitation as an expression of her "not-enough-time" feeling in the transference. The client went home from the session and telephoned her case manager to say that once-a-week sessions were not sufficient. Although the case manager had previously stated that she would not cover sessions more frequent than once a week, she responded to the client by authorizing three more sessions for that month of therapy.

It can be seen that the interpretive work resulted in further modifications in the client's use of her managed care benefit and in the meaning she attached to the case manager's recommendations. The therapist had brought to the surface the client's negative transference to the therapist. Although the client was feeling there was not as much time as she would have liked with the therapist, there was an unconscious component in this that linked her infantile experience of similar kinds of feelings to her current experience with the therapist. This made the therapist appear, unconsciously, to the client as the "not-enough-time-parent" therapist and that, in turn, made her feelings of need for the therapy dangerous. When the transference was elucidated and interpreted, the client was able to feel a less-conflicted resolve about her own feelings, and her reliance upon the therapist felt less dangerous. The client's experience of the transference interpretation allowed her to take a more active stance in the service of her needs and resulted in her call to the case manager to request more sessions.

The not-enough-time-parent transference was pervasive in this client's life. Since childhood, it was a feeling she had experienced both consciously and unconsciously in her relationships with others. When the therapist interpreted this client's transferential and defensive relationship to the case manager, this dynamic was able to come more clearly into view in the transference to the therapist. Each time the feeling of need—and, therefore, unmet need in the infantile sense—surfaced in this client, she tried to institute primitive defenses to protect herself. Those defenses ranged from more-direct forms, like leaving or reducing her therapy, to less-direct forms, such as involving other simultaneous avenues of help during her early period in therapy. Her transference relationship to the case manager was seen as no different from her relationships to others, including the therapist, in which she unconsciously enacted the unresponsive relationship she had felt with her parents in a repetitious way, as well as for defensive purposes. Interpretation of these issues allowed the client to see how the externally imposed managed care restrictions resonated with her internal need to restrict her needful feelings. What was first seen as an externally imposed issue could now be understood as having important inner sources.

Discussion

This chapter has illustrated the idea that the inclusion of managed care in psychodynamic psychotherapy can be understood not only as an external reality alone, but also as a transference object for both the client and the therapist. For therapy to work effectively and comprehensively, it must include working with the client's unconscious conflicts and issues. The two cases presented situations in which the client's transference to the case manager became an important focus of clinical attention. Both the client's defensive perception of managed care and the transferential nature of her reaction to the case manager were worked through, thus enabling each client to experience a more realistic and less unconsciously laden perception of the managed care insurance component of the therapy. Only after this therapeutic work could each therapy be more immune to the intrusions of managed care.

If therapists work with their clients' transferences to managed care and defensive use of managed care, they must be prepared to handle clinically their clients' negative transferences to the therapist and accompanying resistances to the therapy. As illustrated in the case reports, transference to the therapist is no longer defended against when these clinical issues in managed care are addressed.

The "wear and tear" of transference work is difficult on the client and the therapist (Bird,1972). The analytic stance facilitates the full spectrum of emotions involved in the transference. The client, naturally, wants to retreat from those emotions that are painful and experienced in the treatment. In addition, the therapist may wish to retreat from the transference relationship's "as-if" position in which difficult projections must be contained by the therapist. Each may seek refuge in the solace provided by the structure and rules of managed care. The client can feel more removed from the depth and immediacy of transference feelings when the intensity of the therapy is diminished, either through managed care restrictions on number of sessions authorized or through the ready-made opportunity to split off negative transference feelings from the therapy and onto managed care. On the other hand, the therapist can move away from the role of container of the client's negative transference feelings and feel more approved of when sessions receive authorization from managed care. It is important to be alert to transference, countertransference, and resistance possibilities. The suspension of immediate action in response to the demands of managed care is necessary if unconscious material is to be understood. This applies equally to requests from managed care companies and to requests for managed care actions from clients. When our own anxieties do not interfere, our actions can be guided by our clinical judgments. At that point the distinction between clinicians who are managed care providers and clinicians who are not on managed care panels becomes indistinguishable.

One further comment is warranted. As therapists, we must remain cautious in our conclusions about managed care treatment outcomes. Managed care introduces a parameter into therapy that intrudes upon the client–therapist transference relationship and that cannot be ignored or neutralized with good technique. Therapists sometimes participate in real intrusions into therapy when their activity and involvement in response to requests for authorization of sessions run counter to the rule of abstinence. The risk there is that the therapist's involvement creates a collegial dynamic in which aspects of the negative transference are covered over and rendered unavailable to being worked through. In Ms. A.'s treatment we saw how her maternal transference to the therapist involved feeling attached to a self-involved and unattuned mother–therapist. She held the transference fantasy that I would only have my own ideas about her and would not want to be involved with her ideas and feelings. She expressed relief that I would be involved in the authorization process. We are left with the question of whether there was a change in the transferential nature of Ms. A.'s relationship to me, or merely a shift in her conscious perception of me as a result of my involvement with her in the managed care authorization process.

We need the help of our own therapy and supervision to keep us clinically focused in our work. We should be continually exploring the problems posed by managed care in our own therapies and in our supervision hours. Our professional development should continue to be supported and facilitated by training that helps us focus on and understand our clients' clinical needs. We need to be able to discuss our clients' transference problems and our countertransferences to managed care in settings that facilitate our abilities to work effectively with these issues.

Managed care offers a challenge to clients and therapists alike not to abandon the treatment of unconscious issues. We are wise to remember Inderbitzin and Levy's (1994) warning about the compelling nature of reality as so easily visible when compared with the inferential nature of inner life.

References

Alperin, R. (1994). Managed care versus psychoanalytic psychotherapy: Conflicting ideologies. *Clinical Social Work Journal, 22,* 137–148.

Bird, B. (1972). Notes on transference: Universal phenomenon and hardest part of analysis. *Journal of the American Psychoanalytic Association, 20,* 267–301.

Bollas, C., & Sundelson, D. (1995). *The new informants: The betrayal of confidentiality in psychoanalysis and psychotherapy.* New York: Jason Aronson.

Busch, F. N. (1994). The impact of managed care on the psychotherapeutic process: Transference and countertransference. *Psychoanalysis and Psychotherapy, 11,* 200–206.

Davidson, T., & Davidson, J. R. (1995). Cost-containment, computers and confidentiality. *Clinical Social Work Journal, 23,* 453–464.

Freud, S. (1953a). *Fragment of an analysis of a case of hysteria* (standard ed., pp. 3–122). London: Hogarth Press. Originally published 1905

Freud, S. (1953b). *The unconscious* (standard ed., pp. 166–171). London: Hogarth Press. Originally published 1915

Gill, M. (1979). The analysis of the transference. *Journal of the American Psychoanalytic Association, 27*(Suppl.), 263–288.

Glover, E. (1931). The therapeutic effect of inexact interpretation: A contribution to the theory of suggestion. *International Journal of Psychoanalysis, 12,* 397–411.

Gray, S. H. (1992). *Quality assurance and utilization review of individual medical psychotherapies* (American Psychiatric Association Committee on Quality Assurance: A Report of the Committee on Quality Assurance). Washington, DC: American Psychiatric Association.

Higuchi, S. A., & Newman, R. (1994). Legal issues for psychotherapy in a managed care environment. *Psychoanalysis and Psychotherapy, 11,* 138–153.

Inderbitzin, L., & Levy, S. (1994). On grist for the mill: External reality as defense. *Journal of the American Psychoanalytic Association, 42,* 763–788.

Langs, R. (1973). *The technique of psychoanalytic psychotherapy* (Vol. I). New York: Jason Aronson.

Meehan, B. (1994). The impact of managed care on the psychotherapeutic process: Transference and countertransference. *Psychoanalysis and Psychotherapy, 11,* 212–228.

Miller, I. (1994). *What managed care is doing to outpatient mental health: A look behind the veil of secrecy.* Boulder, CO: Boulder Psychotherapists' Press.

Raney, J. (1993). Truth and context: Problems with reporting psychotherapy information to third parties. *Psychoanalytic Psychotherapy Review, 4,* 33–37.

Saakvitne, K. W., & Abrahamson, D. J. (1994). The impact of managed care on the therapeutic relationship. *Psychoanalysis and Psychotherapy, 11,* 181–199.

Sandler, J. (1976). Countertransference and role responsiveness. *International Review of Psychoanalysis, 3,* 43–47.

Shapiro, J. (1995). The downside of managed mental health care. *Clinical Social Work Journal, 23,* 441–451.

Waelder, R. (1936). Principle of multiple function: Observations on over-determination. *Psychoanalytic Quarterly, 5,* 45–62.

Zuckerman, R. (1989). Iatrogenic factors in "managed" psychotherapy. *American Journal of Psychotherapy, 43,* 118–131.

The author thanks Robert J. Campbell, MD, Jon R. Conte, PhD, Jo Hollingsworth, EdD, and R. Keith Myers, MSW, for their helpful input in the preparation of this chapter.

PART **THREE**

Notes from the Field

C. Clients with Severe and Persistent Mental Illness

CHAPTER 23

Editor's Commentary on "Losing Innocents" and "Notes from a Sinking Ship"

Gerald Schamess

Chapters 24 and 25 present a cross-section of clinical social work practice under managed care with people with serious and persistent mental illness. Braverman's chapter focuses on services for chronically ill people brought to a large city emergency room, mostly against their wishes. Edelstein's chapter presents the unfolding story of a community mental health center with a history of offering effective community-based support services to chronically ill clients as it comes under managed care control.

Patients with chronic mental illness present serious financial problems for managed care providers. When such patients are covered by an insurer who authorizes treatment of any kind, the insurer experiences a net financial loss, regardless of how the services are managed. In that situation, the only relevant financial question is how much money it will cost to serve the patient. As we all know, medication is less costly than ongoing relationships with professional caregivers in the community, and those relationships are less costly than hospitalization. Accordingly, the least-costly and "least-restrictive" alternative treatment is to medicate patients while drastically reducing the length of or eliminating entirely inpatient hospitalization (see chapter 18).

A number of questions follow from these general guidelines. Is medication alone the most cost-effective treatment? Is it more cost effective even if it leads to periodic brief rehospitalizations? Does community-based support reduce the frequency or duration of brief rehospitalizations? Do brief rehospitalizations cost more or less than ongoing community-based support? If rehospitalization costs more, how much support is sufficient to reduce its frequency, and for which patients? None of those financially driven questions consider the best interests of affected individuals, their families, or the community as a whole. In discussing medical care for serious physical conditions, Glasser (1998) commented that although "those of us who have fallen seriously ill know for a fact that the purveyors of managed care often wish we would go away or die—as quietly and quickly as possible—we're reluctant to draw the commercial moral of the tale. The system wasn't meant to care for sick people; it was meant to make and manage money" (p. 36). The comment is equally apt in describing the hidden, unarticulated relationship between patients with chronic mental illnesses and their insurers.

Among the many striking practice observations implicitly contained in Braverman's chapter is the amount of autonomy and power she is authorized to exercise in the emergency room, even though she is a recent MSW graduate. Although psychiatric consultation is available, at least from a resident, no mention is made of social work supervision or consultation. Nonetheless, Braverman takes psychosocial histories; makes diagnoses; and provides palliative, stabilizing care within the emergency room setting. Her power is limited in one regard, however, and the power denied her is even more striking than the powers she is granted: She cannot authorize continued treatment of any kind without approval from an insurance company case manager. In the vignettes she presents, having successfully convinced case managers to authorize brief inpatient care for two of the three patients she saw that day, she comments, "If I ever quit working in the emergency room I'm going to sell cars" (p. 245). In essence, then, the hospital views her as competent to authorize a patient's discharge from the emergency room but not to authorize ongoing treatment of any kind, anywhere in the hospital. What effect does the authorization process have on practitioners whose clinical judgment tells them to advocate for further care? To what extent do these universally applied procedures wear down practitioner judgment and ethical principles?

Quite in passing, Braverman makes a second striking observation when she comments on Ms. Darnell's medical record. Since Ms. Darnell has been a patient of the managed care company that currently insures her for at least five years (there having been a previous hospitalization), one would expect some relevant data about her condition in the insurer's record. When Braverman requests information, the response is "No diagnosis. No outpatient ever. No record of meds." Munson (1996) emphasized that, generally speaking, managed care mental health records are afforded little or no protection in terms of confidentiality, but here we have another, equally alarming phenomenon. Ms. Darnell's record contains no relevant information of any kind about her mental condition although she had previously been hospitalized, and (her daughter-in-law tells Braverman) Prolixin had been prescribed. What responsible insurer would tolerate an empty record of this kind? Is this an isolated instance? In the absence of formal research on the topic, it is worth noting that a great many anecdotal reports describe similarly empty or inaccurate records.

Even more significantly, Braverman's careful psychosocial evaluation reveals that Ms. Darnell's depressive symptoms started after her son was murdered five years earlier. Did any of her treators recommend outpatient psychotherapy for a complicated grief reaction? Or for ongoing relationship-based community support? Will the current inpatient stay produce either recommendation? Not if the insurer is attending to the bottom line.

Ms. Darnell's case brings us to the community-based program that Edelstein describes. In chapter 25 we read about a previously well-functioning staff of community-based care providers who, over time, effectively supported community-based living for a regional population of clients with severe and persistent mental illness. That is precisely the kind of program the idealistic proponents of "least-restrictive treatment alternatives" envisioned when they persuaded the Massachusetts legislature to close almost all of the state's mental hospitals and replace them with community-based services. Moreover, it is the kind of program that announces both to its clients and to the community at large that people with mental illness, troubled as they may be, difficult to manage in the community as they are, are *not* disposable. They have value as human beings.

Both because of internal financial difficulties and the ongoing process of consolidation taking place throughout the mental health care "industry," the program came under the control of a large mental health entity a few years ago. In its effort to contain costs, the entity curtailed outreach services for clients, leaving a significant number of them with less support than the program had previously deemed adequate. As a result, relationships with caregivers have been disrupted, and long-standing feelings of rejection or abandonment have been revived in clients whose overall functioning in the community is precarious at best. At present, it is still difficult to determine whether a suicide or other catastrophic consequence will result from these policies. Equally problematic, however, is the staff's belief that only a catastrophe will allow them to regain some measure of professional control over the program's clinical policies.

In addition to the vignettes that describe individual clients and their relationships with caregivers, chapters 24 and 25 present an important subtext that illuminates how staff members are increasingly faced with intolerable ethical dilemmas and how they are being exploited. What responsibilities does a social worker have to a distressed and vulnerable client with whom she has worked for more than a decade but who currently has been removed from her caseload because contact with that client is no longer "billable"? What responsibility does she have to advocate for that client's care with the program managers? What should her response be when her supervisor tells her she is free to volunteer her time on the client's behalf, but that if she does so, even though her wages have already been reduced significantly to control costs, her workload expectations will remain the same? What is the profession's responsibility to the client, to the therapist, and to the agency? Is unionization a possible answer? Or, as Edelstein writes, is the only reasonable solution flight "to those other jobs that still look good, perhaps because their problems haven't yet become familiar"? And finally, is even that a viable solution for the profession?

The clinical practices described and the ethical dilemmas revealed in chapters 24 and 25 are central to social work practice under managed care. Most of us prefer to think the profession is struggling with new theoretical and practice issues. Although that is true to a degree, at a much more fundamental level we are faced with a profound ethical and philosophical question: Do human beings have intrinsic value in and of themselves, beyond and above what they contribute to the economy? If not, managed care is and will continue to be the way to go. If so, fundamental change is necessary—sooner rather than later.

References

Glasser, R. J. (1998, February). The doctor is not in. *Harper's Magazine,* pp. 35–41.

Munson, C. E. (1996). Autonomy and managed care in clinical social work practice. *Smith College Studies in Social Work, 66,* 241–260.

CHAPTER 24

Losing Innocents

Amy Braverman

"I don't want to watch that guy die." I follow his eyes to the open double doors of the trauma room. On the bed a man is stripped of his clothes, which lay in a bloodied heap on the floor. The motions of the code team are frantic. A police officer is shouting over the instructions of the doctors as they stick a tube down the man's throat, shove an intravenous tube in his arm, and start counting bullet holes: "Black guy or white guy?! Black guy or white guy?!" Now they are pounding on his chest. I pull a chair to the doors and try to block them from opening. The lock is broken and the weight pushes the chair back into the room. I wheel a bed against the door. It stays for the moment, but the shouting can be heard clearly, along with the pounding and the flat line of the heart monitor.

"Leonard? Can I call you Leonard?"

He nods with his eyes still fixed on the doors. "Lennie," he whispers.

"Okay, Lennie. My name is Amy. I'm a psychiatric social worker. Can I ask you a few questions?" He nods again. "Look at me, Lennie," I say. "Don't watch the doors."

He looks at me with the blank, fixed stare of a schizophrenic. He is thin and his hair is matted. His skin is the ashen gray of a body left out in the cold, dry and cracked by wind and the raw winter.

"There's an address here, 536 Wyalusing—do you live there?" He shakes his head no. "Are you homeless?" He nods. "How long have you been homeless, Lennie?"

"A long time," he says.

"Longer than a month?" He nods. "A few months?" He nods again. "Longer than a few months?"

"I don't remember," he says. "A long time."

I write "homeless" on my consult sheet and when I look up Lennie is making his way toward the side door. "Lennie," I ask, "where are you going?"

"To get a glass of water."

"You have a glass of water," I say.

"You have a glass of water, Lennie," he repeats. A paper cup sits in front of him on the bed tray. He sits down. "Can I have a cigarette?"

NOTE: Originally published as Braverman, A. (1996). Losing innocents. *Smith College Studies in Social Work, 66,* 349–357

"You can smoke when we're done, okay?" He stares at me. "Did someone tell you to get a glass of water?"

"Yeah," he says.

"You hear a voice in your head, Lennie?"

"Yes," he says.

"Do the voices tell you to hurt yourself?" He shakes his head no. "Do they tell you to hurt anyone else?"

"No," he says.

"Is anyone trying to hurt you?" He looks frightened for a minute, then blank again. "Can you tell me more about that?"

"People on the other team," he whispers.

"Which team is that, Lennie?"

He inspects me for the first time. "The other team," he says.

"How many teams are there?"

"Two," he says. "God's team and the other team."

"Is the voice telling you who's trying to hurt you?" I ask.

"It says they gonna kill you. They watching me."

"Do you know whose voice it is?" I ask.

"It's God's voice," he says.

"Which team am I on, Lennie?"

He looks at me and says, "I don't know."

"I'm on your team, Lennie." I raise my hand in an oath. "I promise. I'm on your team." He gets up again. "Lennie, can you sit down until we're finished?" He sits down.

Lennie has already been here for several hours. Behind the trauma room, in the back of the emergency room, are my patients. "Pitchforks" they call them, because on the board they are identified by the Greek letter psi (ψ). Sometimes they are just called the "nuts," "wackos," "junkies," and "ODs." Sometimes they are just referred to as "mine" as in "You have three in 23." The emergency room staff doesn't like "my patients." They are listed as "priority three," which means their charts slide back in line every time a new patient who isn't a pitchfork arrives. A psychiatric patient may wait up to eight hours in the emergency room. Priority one is the man whose bullet holes are being counted in the trauma room. Priority two is anyone who isn't dying. A cold is priority two. Mental illness is priority three. I am not even allowed to give my patients the boxed lunches that are kept in the refrigerator for "the real" patients. But I have never been very good with rules; for me, anyone who is hungry gets a sandwich. Anyone who is in pain is a "real patient."

Lennie has paranoid schizophrenia. He is homeless, and the blisters on his lips and his hand tell me he is also abusing crack cocaine. He is a typical patient for me. Homeless, off medication, with more hospitalizations than he can remember. He is just one of the city's invisibles. He is the man on the corner talking to himself in the cold, asking you for a dollar for a sandwich, asleep in an alley under a paper bag with his head resting on an empty bottle of malt liquor. He will panhandle for drug money before food, and if he appears at the hospital it is usually cuffed to a police officer. He will get help when he becomes an annoyance. Asleep under the snow he is invisible. When his illness brings him to the point of being dangerous—that is, of danger to someone who matters—he is brought to me. As they tell me, it is not against the law to be crazy. You must show clear and present danger. If Lennie is a danger to himself, a slow suicide, he will be ignored. During the blizzard they counted the bodies of people like Lennie who froze in the snow. Seven were counted in three days the week before. Lennie will probably die on the street. Most of my patients will die on the street, alone, cold, mentally ill, and invisible. When I walk him to the bathroom he hobbles. He has been crippled by frostbite.

I fill out transfer forms for Lennie to go to a shelter. He isn't suicidal, so the managed care company won't authorize a stay. I bring him a sandwich and a blanket and we watch "Entertainment Tonight" as we wait for the ambulance. Lennie doesn't object to the plan; he says nothing. Occasionally he responds to the private nightmare in his head, waving away imaginary demons. He asks me twice if he has been followed to the hospital. He rests his swollen feet on the bed and closes his eyes. He just waits. The ambulance might take several hours to pick him up; again, he is priority three. His passivity is so filled with hopelessness it makes my chest ache. Finally, six hours after his arrival, he hobbles down the hall to the gurney that has come for him. He has no belongings except the clothes on his back. I give him some graham crackers and juice to take with him in case they don't feed him when he gets to his destination. I erase his name from the board, make copies of his forms, and stick the copies in the discharge bin.

My next patient is in room 11, still hooked to a heart monitor after an overdose. She is 21 years old, and her lips are covered with the charcoal they used to empty her stomach. It looks like soot. I can see the scars on her arms from what looks like a prior attempt. Dark lines up and down both wrists etched into bony skin. "Sharon?" I ask.

"Sharone," she says.

"Okay, Sharone. My name is Amy, I'm a psychiatric social worker. Can I ask you a couple of questions about what happened today?"

She makes a "tsk" noise with her tongue. "What you need to know? What does it look like happened?"

"It looks like you did a pretty good job of trying to kill yourself today," I say. "I'll tell you what it says on your chart. You were brought to the hospital today by fire rescue in respiratory distress, not breathing, with your blood pressure and your pulse dropping out. They stuck a tube down your throat, gave you a bunch of charcoal to make you vomit up the pills you took, and when you woke up you ripped your IV out and hit one of the nurses when she tried to put it back in."

"I hit her because she was a bitch," she says defensively. "There she is! Bitch!" she calls across the room.

"Sharone, come on. The nurses are only trying to help you."

"Well, I don't want help," she says.

"What happened today?" I ask.

"I tried to put myself out of my fucking misery," she says.

"What is so awful?" I ask.

"What do you care?" she says.

"I care. You must be in a lot of pain to do this. I wish you could tell me about it."

She scowls. I wipe her lips with a moist washcloth to clear off the soot and fix her blanket. Her gown is untied in the back, and it falls off her shoulders. "Lean forward," I say, and as she does, I fix her gown and then tuck her back in the bed. "Are you warm enough?" I ask.

She nods. "You wouldn't understand," she says as she starts to cry.

"Try me," I say.

"I just wish somebody loved me. I just had a baby, you know. She's six months old. I never seen her. She was born with cocaine and reefer in her, so they took her away. I never even seen her. She was sick." She looks at me before continuing. "I got four other kids, too. All a them got fetal alcohol syndrome. I got five sick kids. I'm only 21 years old."

"Do they live with you?" I ask.

"My mother's got 'em." She looks at me again. "See! Now see how you look at me, like I'm dirt. Leave me alone. I'm tired of answering fucking questions. Just let me die."

"Sharone, I'm not judging you. I'm trying to understand you. Do you feel like I'm judging you?"

Now she pulls the blanket up over her face and starts to sob. "I just want someone to love me. That's all I want. I'm not a bad person. They gonna give me visitation starting in two weeks of the baby. But I already have four kids, and I got nobody to help me. I just don't want her. They took her away, and I don't want her. I know this ain't the right thing to do, but I just don't want her. I don't want her."

Suddenly she sits up and starts tearing the patches off her chest that connect her to the heart monitor. Her hand grasps the intravenous tube in her wrist and she pulls, leaving a stream of blood floating into her hand.

"Let me out of here!" she screams. Two nurses and the director of the emergency room rush to the bed and hold her down. The doctor puts his hand across her throat, each nurse on one arm. I hold one leg as the security guard rushes in to put her in four-point restraints. "Leave me alone!" she screams. Finally, their work done, they leave her, and I go to call her insurance company to give them the clinical information.

When I come back she is quieted but still crying. "I'm sorry," she says. "I'm sorry."

"That's all right, Sharone. Just try to rest now. We're gonna take care of you."

"Don't be mad," she says. "Oh, God, don't be mad at me. I'm so sorry."

I sit on the edge of her bed and fix her gown again, tuck the blankets around her and stroke her head.

"I promise I'll be good if you take these off."

"No," I say. "You need to stay the way you are until you're calm. These are on not to punish you but to protect you. Will you do me a favor?" I ask.

"I do anything for you, Angel," she says.

I bring her a voluntary commitment form, and she signs it, still in restraints. "This is just for you, Angel" she says. "Just for you." Then she closes her eyes and lays back on the bed. For the next two hours she calls for me intermittently to sit with her and stroke her head. I tell her my name is Amy, but she still calls me Angel.

"I'm gonna be okay, Angel?"

"Yes, Sharone, you'll be okay. We're gonna take care of you."

The managed care company still sends one of their own evaluators to determine if Sharone needs a psychiatric admission when she's medically cleared. I call the supervisor and explain that she is too agitated for another interview, that her overdose was potentially lethal, and that she is still actively suicidal. Another interview, I say, would not only be unnecessary but, in her condition, cruel. They want to see for themselves before authorizing an admission. I explain this all to Sharone, who rises to the occasion by screaming at the evaluator and demanding a lethal injection if they don't admit her. The evaluator is in the room less than two minutes before authorizing Sharone's admission; she doesn't even sit down. But I have my five-digit number, and that's all I want from her right now. So far, I'm one up, one down for the day.

I don't think about how many children in this city are born addicted to crack cocaine and heroin or how many 21-year-old girls would rather be dead than face the lives they have been given. I don't know what it's like to think there isn't a person in the world who cares if I live through the night or what it's like to need to numb myself with drugs so desperately that my children are born with my disease. Sharone's hell didn't start this morning. As she tells me, she was in six foster care homes before she was 10 years old. She's been beaten and raped. Born to drug addicts and now herself an addict, she passes a legacy of neglect and abuse to her own children. There are so many "Sharones" out there in this cramped city that the thought of helping even a few of them is overwhelming. Their needs are so great and the resources to help them are scarce. According to the National Alliance for Research on Schizophrenia and Depression, nearly one-third of the nation's estimated 600,000 homeless people are believed to be adults with severe mental illnesses, primarily suffering from schizophrenia or depression. The statistics are staggering. To do a job, any job in this field, you have to keep a tight focus. Forget the numbers. I see one at a time.

Back in room 23 is an older African American woman wearing large wraparound sun glasses, a big black hat with plastic flowers, wool pants, and a hospital gown. She's a big woman; not fat, but strong. And she sits up straight in the bed with a scowl on her lips, ready for anything. She has a large suitcase propped next to her on the bed, and she clutches an overstuffed purse in her hand. She is here with her granddaughter's mother Denise. Her son, the baby's father, was murdered five years ago, but the woman and Denise are still close.

"Ms. Darnell? My name is Amy. I'm a psychiatric social worker. Can I ask you a few questions?"

She starts rambling in a loud, hostile voice. "I left my house this morning with that damn coat, with the snow into the garage there was nothing but my nails to do. Now, I lost that coat back in '78, but here it is today so don't you go telling me otherwise. I know a Doctor Fisher, damnit, and he'll tell you that not a day goes by that I don't know the songs of the righteous in the church I was born. Spell it." I look at her. "Spell . . . Fisher! Don't look at the sheet; spell Fisher!"

"F-I-S-H-E-R. Ms. Darnell, what brought you to the emergency room?"

"I'll be asking the questions around here, and you have a few more questions to answer yourself. I'm older than you, and I demand some R-E-S-P-E-C-T for my black ass!" She's off rambling again about the coat. Something about her granddaughter and the snow.

"Are you on any medication?" The daughter-in-law hands me three bottles of pills, none of them psychotropics: Procardia, Synthroid, Premarin. "Ms. Darnell, do you take these medications as they're prescribed?"

"Spell them, don't look at the sheet."

I start spelling. "P-R-O-C-A-R-D-I-A."

"Keep going," she shouts. "Don't look at the sheet. What are you, a cheater? Let's see how good you can spell, then we'll get onto the questions."

"Ms. Darnell, do you know where you are?"

"I got all the paperwork I need right here in this purse." She holds out a piece of paper to me, but when I reach for it she snatches it back. "Don't touch it! Didn't I tell you to touch nothing?" The paper says "d/c catapress."

"Ms. Darnell, have you ever been on lithium?" She rambles on. "Haldol?" The daughter-in-law sighs, "Prolixin?"

"Don't you dare give me a shot!"

Bingo. "You used to take Prolixin?"

"Spell it!"

I spell it, "P-R-O-L-I-X-I-N. When was the last time you had Prolixin?" I've lost her again. I lean over to the daughter-in-law and say, "See if you can get her to sign this. It's a 201 voluntary commitment form."

As I walk out I hear Ms. Darnell saying, "I ain't signing nothing that doesn't guarantee me $50,000."

"That's exactly what this is," the daughter-in-law says.

"Then damnit, Denise, hand me a pen!"

I call the managed care company and give clinical information on Ms. Darnell. Do they have anything else? She's only been with them since 1990, and there is one hospitalization on record. No diagnosis. No outpatient ever. No record of meds. I relay my interview with Ms. Darnell, careful to include the spelling bee and the shouting and give her a Global Assessment of Functioning score of about 20. They authorize an admission without sending an evaluator. If I ever quit working in the emergency room I'm going to sell cars. I'm two up, one down, and I have less than an hour to go.

I go back and talk to Denise. She's a nutritionist, a single mother raising her seven-year-old daughter. She gives me a little history. She doesn't know about medications or hospitalizations, but she knows this started when the woman's son was murdered five years ago. Every year around this time she gets "like this" but not this bad. This time it started during the big snowfall. She didn't get out of bed one day, spent the whole day in bed, and the next she was rambling like she is now. She only had one son; "he was her whole life." She used to be on medication, but Denise doesn't know what it was called. She looks tired.

"Go home," I say. "We'll take care of her now. You've been a great help." She sighs. She seems hesitant to leave before Ms. Darnell is on the unit. "It's okay," I say. "Go home and see your daughter. I'll keep my eyes on her. She'll be fine. You look like you need a rest." She nods and goes to say good-bye to Ms. Darnell.

Later I bring Ms. Darnell a sandwich, and she says, "Cheese on toast, two diet Pepsis." I've brought her turkey and some orange juice and try to help her prop the bed up into a sitting position. "I know how to eat lying down, believe me!" she shouts.

"We don't have diet Pepsi," I say.

"Then I'll take regular Pepsi."

"We don't have regular Pepsi."

She snarls at me, "Get away from me then. You've taken enough of my time today."

I walk outside for a cigarette. As I stand on the street corner a neatly dressed woman with a smile on her face rushes toward me calling my name.

"Keisha!" she says, "Remember?" I don't. I search my brain. Does this woman work here? Was she a patient? "You said to come by and let you see me when I was clean. Look!" She smiles broadly.

"Well, you look great," I say. "I'm really happy for you." She does look good, but I have no memory of her face at all, or her story. We talk for a while, and I go back into the emergency room to hand off the beeper to the night-shift psychiatrist on call.

The psychiatrist on call tonight is young, only three years out of school. She looks tired already. "How many are back there?" she says.

"Six?" I say. Really, I don't know. "You can start writing orders on Hill, Tylon is still being cleared, Darnell is up on five, Morris is gone, Linetta is in the waiting room."

She consults her own list. "I just saw that woman in 12." Her eyes fill with tears. "What a sad life!"

"Who, Sharone?" I ask.

"Yes! What a horrible life for such a young girl!"

I cock my head at her and am surprised she is so sad for Sharone. Or, I am surprised that I no longer register sadness the same way and wonder when I changed. I used to say that when people's stories stopped making me cry I would leave social work. Every once in awhile somebody really touches me, and I cry with them, or later in the car going home. But it is rare. Now the night just settles on me like the stink of the emergency room. It's an ache more than a slap.

I chose to work in an emergency room because I was tired of the intensity of the relationships you forge in one-to-one therapy. I didn't want to be in the position of straightening out all those tangled lives; I just wanted to put people in a place where someone could help them. What I didn't count on is that in one-to-one therapy you may have a caseload of 20 horror stories. In an emergency room, you hear five a night, 30 in the six-day week I work, over 1,000 in a year. I spit them out in my sleep like broken teeth. I come home smelling like sickness, with blood on the soles of my shoes. I ride down the elevator with my bag resting on a corpse under a blue plastic sheet. Still, I wouldn't change what I do. It's a war we're fighting, and this is the trenches.

An hour past the time I am supposed to leave I am done with my paperwork. I have a code number I write on five separate sheets of paper. I speak longer with managed care representatives than I speak with my patients. There is a vast and complicated system to attempt to find help through, and it is my patients who fall through the cracks. They do not make it to outpatient aftercare; they do not go to the pharmacy to fill prescriptions. The mental health service they use is psychiatric emergency services. When they come back they will not be better. Then they just don't come back at all. You can place blame where your sense of truth allows you. For me, it's been a good night. An admission means someone has a safe place to sleep tonight. I give my report to the nursing station, write all known dispositions on the board, and head to the back.

At 11 o'clock the trauma room is silent. The floor is littered with tubes and papers, and the gurney has been wheeled behind a curtain where the dead man will wait for his family to identify him. His bloody clothes are now stuffed in a bag beside his bed. There is a blanket over him, and he looks as if he were sleeping. He looks peaceful. I lean over him and look at his face. An orderly we call "Preacher" comes in to clean up the room as I am standing there, and I ask him to say a blessing for the man who died. While I hold the dead man's hand, Preacher prays aloud for his safe passage home.

> Blessed are the poor in spirit, for theirs is the kingdom of heaven.
> Blessed are those who mourn, for they shall be comforted.
> Blessed are the meek, for they shall inherit the earth.
> Blessed are those who hunger and thirst for righteousness, for they shall be satisfied.
> Blessed are the merciful, for they shall obtain mercy.
> Blessed are the pure in heart, for they shall see God.

CHAPTER 25

Notes from a Sinking Ship

Carol Edelstein

The community mental health center where I work has more than 100 employees in seven sites. The site where I work specializes in treating adults diagnosed with chronic mental illnesses, such as schizophrenia, affective and dissociative disorders, and personality disorders. Many of those adults also have substance abuse problems, and almost all receive state or federal assistance for food, shelter, and medical care. Clients are referred to us primarily by their social workers at the department of mental health or by the local crisis intervention team.

Arnold,[1] a handsome, disheveled, quiet man, age 44, has come to our agency (and we have gone to him at the various apartments and at the family home where he's lived) for more than 20 years. Diagnosed with chronic schizophrenia at age 19 and having a history of drug and alcohol abuse since adolescence, in the past several years Arnold has become sober and employed. He holds a part-time job in a retail store and lives independently (although, to ensure that his household bills are paid, his case manager from the state's department of mental health still disburses the monthly check he receives from the government). He lives in a poorly furnished walk-up apartment with few amenities. He struggles to have clean clothes and enough food. His main social contacts are his father (who is elderly and has recently moved into a subsidized-housing complex in a neighboring town), the nurse at our agency, his cohorts at a support group for people with both mental health and substance abuse issues, a vocational counselor, and me. He also has siblings who live in the area.

When Arnold discontinues his medications, he is at higher risk for using street drugs and alcohol. In the past, in that condition, he has committed crimes against people and property to support his addictions. Because Arnold has been relatively stable for several years, his insurance now will cover fewer contacts with professionals. As a result of so-called "managed care" decisions, he is forced to chose which services he'll go without because his insurance will now cover only one therapeutic contact per week, not three.

I predict that in the near future Arnold will require more intensive (and therefore ultimately more expensive) care, such as an inpatient hospitalization, a day rehabilitation program, or visiting nurses. Already, after only a few months with the

[1] Names and other identifying information have been disguised to protect the confidentiality of clients.

new limitations on service frequency, Arnold has become more distant and angry; he increasingly engages in "splitting" behaviors, neglects his hygiene, and reports some sleep disturbance. On one occasion recently, his landlord complained that Arnold had disconnected his smoke alarm and was using it as an ashtray.

Four years ago—the last time Arnold discontinued his medications and began using nonprescribed substances—he was receiving many residential and outpatient services, so I cannot assert that having a large number of therapeutic contacts necessarily prevents a relapse. I believe, however, that it is unwise to intentionally diminish our contacts with Arnold at this juncture in his recovery, especially because he is living in isolation from his main companion, his father. About a year ago the board of public health declared the house he and his father shared to be unfit for habitation after a storm severely damaged their roof. They have been unsuccessful in obtaining state or federal funding to assist in making the necessary repairs. The only public transportation available between Arnold's apartment and his father's apartment is cumbersome (a series of bus rides that take four hours each way), so the two now are in touch mainly by telephone. That drastic change in Arnold's living situation, resulting in his increased emotional dependence on professionals rather than his father and siblings, doesn't seem to be given proper consideration by those making decisions about the mental health care to which he is entitled.

* * *

That is one of the hundreds of half-stories I know.

I have been a social worker for the past 16 years in a mental health facility in the center of a western Massachusetts city. This once-flourishing mill town was a place of economic opportunity for the successive arrivals of various ethnic groups—Irish, Polish, French Canadians, Puerto Ricans. For most of those 16 years, I have loved my work here, despite our location in a neighborhood of tenements where drug and alcohol abuse, prostitution, domestic violence—problems arising from poverty and alienation—abound. I have loved it despite many obstacles standing in the way of our agency's mission—to provide comprehensive care to one of the most difficult-to-engage populations, people with severe, chronic mental illnesses.

In the past several years, a combination of internal fiscal mismanagement of funds and external pressure from the managed care system that took control of the center's administration has undermined the sense of community among our staff. My optimism is weathered but still strong. Our agency has a new and politically savvy director who understands the clinical needs of our particular clientele. The employees are becoming more insistent on having a strong voice within the organization and are discussing the possible advantages of unionizing. Ironically, the best chance that clinicians have to be vested with the authority to rebuild the energetic, resourceful treatment teams we once had will come about only if the latest series of changes imposed by the managed care system prove ineffective (at best) or dangerous (at worst).

In Massachusetts in the early 1970s, when I was a social work student and brand new in my job, changes in state law ensured the deinstitutionalization of people with mental illness and the creation of community-based residential and day treatment programs as alternatives to incarceration in locked hospitals. State policy mandated the "least-restrictive" form of treatment. Also, within our profession and within the larger society, we were learning more about the psychobiology of mental illnesses and finding newer, more-effective medications to offer clients.

At that time, state funding sources were not amorphous bodies but were actual people whose names we knew—people who seemed to recognize the particular needs of our clientele. Our agency had policies and the money to support active outreach on the part of clinical staff and a range of what would be considered case management duties—that is, liaisons with other services providers as well as practical assistance such as help with transportation, managing money, and keeping households clean and well stocked. We were encouraged to seek connections with our clients, many of whom had developed an expertise at avoiding other people and who had little insight into the nature of their illnesses. We also worked in teams with medical personnel to educate our clients and their families. Our own continuing education was an agency priority, and practitioners in various aspects of our work frequently were hired to come to us to consult and advise.

If, indeed, "small is beautiful," we as an organization have grown ugly. Under recent political pressures, our clinic merged with a larger organization and later affiliated with an even larger one whose administration is not committed to our original mission. I have no idea what role managed care has played in the extreme debt our agency has accrued over the past three years—debt that has resulted in recent layoffs of employees, increased expectations of clinical staff productivity (as measured in higher expected percentages of reimbursable services), decreased pay and benefits, and a pervasive mood of distrust between clinical and administrative staff. Admittedly, the leadership of our agency has been poor in recent years, but the pressures of the managed care health system have surely exacerbated the severity of our current fiscal problems.

The purported goal of managed care seems sensible—timely delivery of appropriate services. Yet even putting aside our agency's internal management problems, how could there be anything but a basic mismatch between for-profit efficiency and the notion of compassionate service?

* * *

Joanne, age 54, is of below-average intelligence and has a seizure disorder. As a young woman she was hospitalized numerous times, diagnosed variously with schizophrenia, chronic depression, and borderline personality disorder. She left Ohio as a teenager, fleeing her alcoholic father who physically and sexually abused her. Much of her early history is unknown. She lived for 13 years on a locked ward at Northampton State Hospital, Massachusetts, and for several years after that she did whatever was required of her (usually threats of suicide) to regain entrance there as frequently as possible. When the hospital finally closed its doors, Joanne was forced to center her life outside its walls. She became a vocal advocate for the empowerment of consumers of mental health services, finding fault with all offerings, yet gradually developing a tolerance and even some affection for some of the professionals and peers with whom she became familiar.

Six years ago, I became the latest in a string of 14 social workers who have worked with her. Last February, Joanne did not open her mail and so missed an appointment to be re-evaluated for continued eligibility for social security benefits. Eventually she was denied those benefits. She never appealed the decision and rejected my help in straightening out the situation. She lost her medical coverage, and when the bill-collecting hand of our agency learned the news, she was denied medications and counseling services.

If that had been the situation even as recently as three years ago, my supervisor would have advised me to persist in reaching Joanne and in helping her get her insurance reinstated. This year, such activities are not considered "cost effective." We are no longer subsidized by the state to do what it takes to re-engage Joanne in treatment with us. I'll wait (but with her case officially "closed," of course, in the event the unthinkable should happen), and with luck she'll come back through our doors, having paid the admission fee and gotten back her "ticket"—by decompensating to the point of having a relapse accompanied by a return of her psychiatric or medical symptoms and requiring hospitalization that is costly in more ways than one—but not costly to our agency.

Meanwhile, she calls me on the telephone, angry, isolated, and confused by my unavailability, and I fight off my feelings of annoyance and guilt because I am no longer being paid to speak with her. I do speak with her, briefly, and I imagine I sound to her like a broken record, urging her to do the things I know she can't really do on her own to get back her health insurance, secretly hoping she'll get "just worse enough" to get the help she needs. To do for Joanne what I know is truly the right thing, I'd have to decide to volunteer more of my time.

Meanwhile, there is Millie, age 35, an unusually tall and heavy black woman, diagnosed with acromegaly ("Abraham Lincoln's disease") and numerous other somatic problems, including asthma; a congenital heart valve defect; quite debilitating foot and toenail problems; and a history since early childhood of severe losses, depression, and difficulty in interpersonal relationships. A fraternal twin herself, Millie bore two sets of twins, four years apart. She lost custody of all four boys to adoptive homes because of her poor mental health and drug problems.

Millie had heart surgery and is in rehabilitation for the next six weeks or more. Because the rehabilitation unit has a social worker (with a caseload of 26 clients, many of them new to her), my visits to Millie, whom I have known for 15 years, won't be covered by insurance because that would be considered duplication of services. Under the old system, my supervisor, knowing how anxious and depressed Millie has been, would have said "Go ahead and visit Millie, just remember not to bill for it." He still says "Go ahead and visit Millie," but "you can't bill for it." Now, because I'm paid by the reimbursable hour rather than on a salaried basis, he is reminding me that when I see Millie, I'm seeing her "on my own time." When Millie wants to know why I'll be visiting her only once or twice (she remembers I visited weekly the last time she recuperated from surgery), I tell her that the rules have changed and that while she's in rehabilitation, my visits are not paid for by her insurance. I know that's a simplification and, partly, a lie because my visits when she was an inpatient before weren't covered either—but at that time our program was amply funded, and I was receiving a salary.

Most likely, nothing terrible will result for Millie—she'll have the company of family, professional staff at the rehabilitation unit; perhaps some friends will be resourceful enough to find their way out there. Nonetheless, I'm aware that this is a setback in my relationship with Millie, that I've disappointed her just at a point when she is particularly weak, both physically and emotionally. There is, by definition, a mercenary aspect to what I do—I am a paid professional—but this seems not to be the best time to confront Millie with that fact. I believe that what is "cost effective" for managed care will be, for Millie, another emotional abandonment that she'll add to her already large stack. What is "cost effective" will reinforce her sense of herself as unimportant and unloved.

"I'm really sorry," I tell her, but I know that the pragmatic part of me, the part that has begun thinking in managed care terms, is not sorry at all—I'm already thinking of this as the solution (albeit a temporary one) to a different problem: Because I'm expected to take on new clients at the rate of one per week (notice my language; it is language I would ordinarily use to describe not human beings but inanimate objects), there's already one to take Millie's place.

* * *

The pressure to do more, faster, has negative effects on our clients and on our own sense of competency. Proponents of managed care say, "See two clients for a half-hour each, instead of one for an hour." Yet there are only so many stories any of us can hold clearly in our minds. Were it possible to neatly quantify and compare the energy expenditure under these different circumstances and prove the results with figures, hard science would likely confirm what common sense tells us: To meet with two clients for two half-hour appointments represents more than twice the expenditure of emotional energy and certainly generates more administrative and liaison work than does seeing one person for one hour. Often, too, a half-hour is simply inadequate for making an effective connection with our clients.

Employee burnout was a recognized job hazard in many professions, including in the social services, well before the advent of managed care. However, in the past several years, the decisive trend within our agency has been toward replacing full-time, salaried employees with part-time or fee-for-service employees whose job benefits are prorated or nonexistent. The demands of a managed care system have set the stage for this change. As a senior staff member, I am paid 60 percent of a salary with prorated benefits, as long as I have 14 or more billable, face-to-face interviews each week. If I have fewer billable interviews, my salary and benefits are adjusted downward. In this piecework system, visiting Millie at the "rehab" or working more purposefully and intensively with Joanne to help her regain her social security benefits would lengthen my workweek without either reducing my productivity requirements or increasing my pay; that is, it would become volunteer work. And I am better off than the staff members employed on a strict fee-for-service basis. Certainly, in this less-stable environment we are seeing a higher rate of employee turnover. Thus, we are less likely to know one another, to do collaborative work, or to be drawn to celebrate or to grieve together.

One way to measure the strength of a given community is to examine what happens in response to the death of one of its members. In the past, when we learned of a death among us, a variety of rituals might be observed that marked business *not* as usual. The rituals could include closing our agency for part or all of a day; giving time away from usual responsibilities to attend funeral services or calling hours; gathering together within the agency to process thoughts and feelings about the loss of the person from our midst (particularly if the circumstances of death were sudden or violent); and, always, holding much informal discussion.

At the recent funeral of a client, Owen, I had a flash of resentment I am not proud to acknowledge. I realized I was attending without the support of my agency—that I had not been given the time, the money, or the invitation to grieve. Although Owen, diagnosed with bipolar disorder, was well known and well liked by many staff and clients for almost half his 36 years, the only formal event to mark his passing within the agency was the posting of his obituary on a bulletin board.

Some might consider this a frivolous concern, might think this use of time and money to be prime examples of the type of wastefulness that the managed care system is justified in discouraging. I hold that we must slow our pace. I believe that our collective inability these days to notice who or what is missing from our midst is a glaring symptom of an unwell body.

Because I've been in one place long enough to see a number of bad ideas arise, do their damage, and be wiped out, I'm still hopeful this body, our agency, will find ways to correct itself. There is a limit to what I or any one person in a large organization can effect. I believe that because we're no longer a small-scale business, we will need a professional organization, such as a union, with authority and leverage to help us bargain on our own behalf and on behalf of our disenfranchised clientele. We will need a union to help us correct the imbalances in the larger health system and those that have developed within the agency in the advent of "managed care." But there is much fear and weariness among the employees, and successful unionizing is a long shot. Perhaps even without a union, we can still have a meaningful influence on what develops from here. If that is not possible, some of us will stay and fight for that, and some of us will flee to those other jobs that still look good, perhaps because their problems haven't yet become familiar.

Afterword

In the weeks since I completed this chapter, I have become less hopeful. Four of the agency's top managers have left or announced their intentions to do so, including our chief executive officer (CEO). During her first week on the job, the new CEO was dismayed to learn of fiscal problems facing the agency that had not been made known to her during her hiring process. Nevertheless, she committed herself to staying on to help resolve them. But less than six months later, when an audit of fiscal matters predating her tenure with us revealed additional debts, she announced her resignation. A consultation team hired by the hospital with which we are affiliated has been designated as the managing entity for now. A longer-range plan has not been presented, and most employees I have queried are unable or unwilling to initiate questions or concerns or to speculate in any way about our collective future.

PART **FOUR**

Challenges for the Profession

CHAPTER 26

How Social Workers Can Manage Managed Care

Rita Vandivort-Warren

The success of managed care has shocked many social workers. Most currently practicing social workers have been trained under thoroughly different models of human services and find the insurance business orientation of managed care quite foreign. Yet it is a revolution affecting almost all segments of care, and social workers need to be versed in its tools and effects.

It is almost a cliché to say that managed care has transformed health care, but it is a fact. Yet, defining this phenomenon succinctly becomes harder every day, as managed care companies redesign agreements to each new purchaser to gain the contract. This increasingly pivotal role of the purchaser should not be forgotten when we seek to influence the shape of managed care. Especially for the large employer or state purchaser, managed care companies are willing to enter into various relationships—from administrative-services-only contracts to full-risk-bearing contracts—just to retain market share in this competitive business. Therefore, advocacy efforts to enhance services should not forget the employer's benefits managers or the Medicaid officials setting requests for proposals that lead to managed care contracts.

Managed care can be defined as the private regulation of services with the goals of controlling cost while ensuring quality. In the balance of quality with cost, there are those who say that managed care is only managed cost. Indeed, to the extent that providers resist measurement tools, we further the use of cost-based assessments of services. Outcome measurement has been a much greater focus of interest and some use since the emergence of managed care. Some managed care companies have invested substantial dollars into developing outcome measures, but the state of the art is still in its infancy, especially for mental health and substance abuse services.

This definition of managed care also underscores that managed care is, in fact, regulating health care, albeit as a private business enterprise. Such locus of control can be disconcerting to social workers, because we often prefer government regulation, which we may believe is more objective and has fewer commercial concerns. In fact, the invasion of human services by insurance and business terminology is a portent of managed care, as I examine later in this chapter. It is the underlying philosophical preference either for public or private control of health and human services that is at the core of the legislative battles about state regulation of the managed care industry.

Managed care includes three levels of action: (1) managed access, (2) managed benefits, and (3) managed systems (Substance Abuse and Mental Health Services

Administration, 1994). Managed access to care was one of the first tools used by managed care firms to lower utilization. Familiar forms include prior authorization, requiring second opinions, and denials of continued stays for inpatient care—jokingly referred to as "1-800-Just-Say-No." Managed benefits tools were then added, such as primary care gatekeepers and creating provider networks paid discounted fees. The managed care companies directed patients to such networks, as they directed care to less-expensive outpatient alternatives to hospitalization. Last, managed care companies have developed into managed systems of care, integrating providers and utilizing powerful computer-based information systems to measure performance. Computerized patient records (CPR) will complete this integration, as managed care companies of the future may require providers to log onto computers to chart client progress. CPR offers great potential to further continuity of care and provides decision support, such as access to the latest literature relevant to the consumer's condition. But first, fundamental threats to confidentiality must be addressed.

Application of these managed care tools has had its effects. Miller and Luft (1994) cited documented results: lower hospitalization rates, shorter hospital stays, reduced use of subspecialties, and decreased use of expensive technology. The overall effect has been lowered utilization and cost reduction. The first patrons of managed care were employers who saw its potential as they suffered under ever-escalating health care costs in the late 1980s and early 1990s. In the first half of the 1990s, managed care grew to be the predominant form of employer-sponsored health care in the United States.

This chapter gives basic information about what managed care has been and is becoming, especially in mental health services. It looks at managed care experiences in the employer market and in the public care systems. Public reaction and state regulatory legislation are discussed. Finally, responses to managed care by social workers are considered, with a focus on advocacy, adjusting practice, and affiliating with others.

Characteristics of Managed Care

Since the early 1990s, managed care has been characterized by rapid growth with massive consolidation. Figure 26-1 shows the tremendous growth of managed care in the employer market during the early 1990s (Foster, Higgins cited in Myerson, 1996). "Behavioral health"—the managed care term for both mental health and substance abuse—has shown great consolidation, with the top 10 firms accounting together for a 79.5 percent market share ("Proprietary MBH Companies at a Crossroad," 1997). Magellan, already the owner of Green Springs, accelerated this trend in 1997, with the acquisition of Merit, after Merit had acquired CMG. Magellan is now the largest single player, with an estimated market share of 25 percent, and the dominant carrier of large state Medicaid contracts ("Magellan Acquires Merit," 1997). The National Association of Social Workers (NASW) and others have raised antitrust questions about such concentration of market power.

Downsizing of provider networks is common with managed care, especially in mature markets, in which the high penetration of managed care products has lowered utilization of services. Downsizing can be done directly using techniques such as provider profiling, wherein all those on the network panel are compared on such variables as average length of stay or average cost per case. Using such analyses, the managed care companies then drop the "bottom" 10 percent, or those with the highest costs. In a more subtle form, the managed care companies identify 20

FIGURE **26-1**

Percentage of Insured Workers Covered by Employer-Sponsored Managed Care and Fee-for-Service Programs

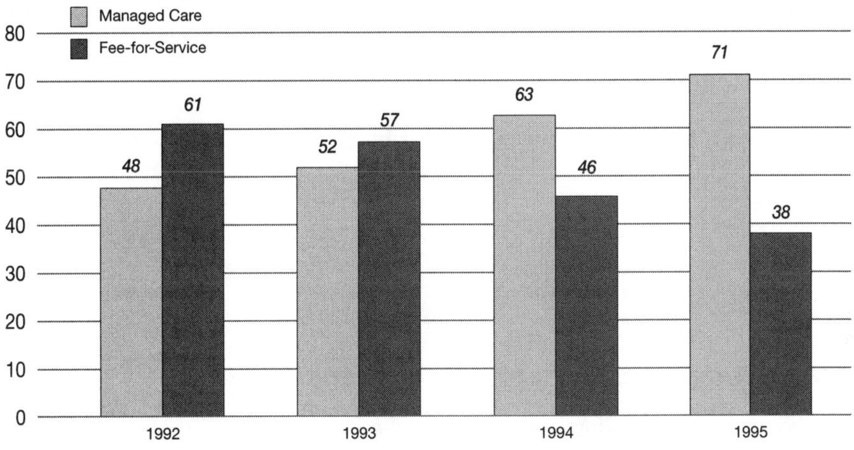

SOURCE: Foster, Higgins, cited in Myerson, A. R. (1996, March 17). A double standard in health coverage. *New York Times*, p. 1.

percent of their "best" providers and send them 90 percent of the patient volume. A provider not in this prime network may not be terminated but seldom receives a case. Again, provider profiling techniques highlight the need to develop better tools to assess quality of service so that such judgments on providers are driven by quality as well as cost measures. This is one area that managed care firms are eager to develop so they can promote their quality assurance as well as cost.

Managed care companies tend to prefer the large provider groups to many small private practices. Larger group practices can take over some of the utilization management functions of the managed care firm and may even have the resources to engage in at-risk contracts. Managed care companies have fewer providers to track and service. As a result, many providers have formed groups for managed care contracting, although the extent of the integration varies widely. That trend is expected to accelerate as lowering utilization decreases the need for providers.

Managed care is a diverse geographical phenomenon that varies by region in benefits, market penetration, and quality. A recent study by the National Committee on Quality Assurance (1997) showed that managed care organizations vary significantly in quality. The disparate levels of managed care penetration of markets are still evident ("Markets with HMO Penetration Greater Than 25%," 1995), as the movement—first supported by employers in California, Minnesota, and some places along the Atlantic seaboard—spreads throughout the country. Public managed care contracts under Medicaid have brought managed care to different areas, as many of the earliest states in managed care under Medicaid, such as Tennessee and Oklahoma, had little prior experience with managed care in their private markets. The organizational tactics of managed care also depend on whether the company derived from the 1960s–70s health maintenance organization (HMO) movement or from the 1980s behavioral health utilization management firms that later evolved into managed care companies. In either case, the development of managed care evolved through stages that respond to different operating strategies. Generally, the earlier a provider establishes relationships with managed care, the better. Once managed care is well entrenched, the need and opportunities for providers become more limited.

Another characteristic of managed care is a negative impact on professional training and research across many disciplines. Managed care companies have tended to refuse payment for services rendered by a student, even if that student is under the supervision of a licensed professional. The community mental health centers that once trained many social workers often are no longer receiving payment for such trainees—a critical factor in the managed care era, when those centers are struggling to survive financially. In addition, social workers in many organizations no longer have time to devote to supervision in downsized departments. Hospitals that once trained large numbers of social workers may no longer have a social work department or a social work supervisor.

Managed Care in Public Programs

Much like employers before them, Medicaid administrators in the early 1990s were looking for a way out of spiraling costs, and they latched onto managed care as the solution. Between 1985 and 1994, Medicaid costs more than tripled (Liska, Marlo, & Shah, 1996). By 1993 Medicaid took, on average, 20 percent of states' budgets, exceeding education expenditures for many of them. By using Medicaid waivers to support nonvoluntary enrollment, the percentage of Medicaid enrollees under managed care has increased from 10 percent in 1991 to 40 percent in 1996, as can be seen in Figure 26-2 (Kaiser Commission, 1997b). Medicare, in contrast, has only slightly grown in numbers under managed care. Much of this growth is attributable to large state programs with mandatory enrollment in managed care. By June 1996, more than 36 states had more than one-quarter of their Medicaid population

FIGURE **26-2**

Percentage of Medicaid and Medicare Enrollees Covered by Managed Care Arrangements

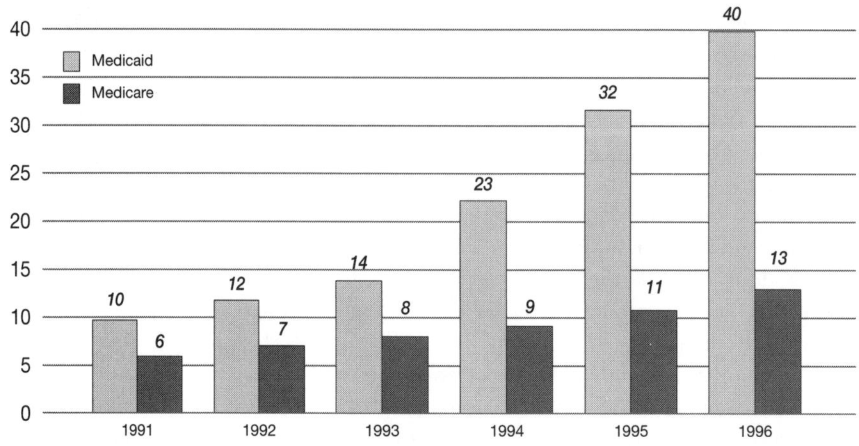

SOURCE: Health Care Financing Administration. (1998). *Managed care in Medicare and Medicaid.* Baltimore: Author.

enrolled in managed care (Kaiser Commission, 1997a). Of these, eight states have more than 75 percent of Medicaid enrollees under Medicaid managed care enrollment. By August 1997, 48 states had at least one managed care plan serving Medicaid enrollees (Health Care Financing Administration [HCFA], 1998).

An analysis of Medicaid clients under managed care coverage shows that almost all the programs have begun by enrolling the mothers and children from Aid to Families with Dependent Children/Temporary Assistance to Needy Families (AFDC/TANF) programs. It is interesting that these enrollees are the least costly (Figure 26-3) (Kaiser Commission, 1997b). Although the AFDC mothers and children constitute almost 73 percent of the enrollees, they account for only about 28 percent of the cost. Elderly men and women and people with disabilities account for 27 percent of the enrollees and generate 72 percent of the cost. Perhaps this fact is not surprising because managed care firms arose in the relatively healthy employer market and have little experience with elderly and disabled populations. Yet without careful contracting by the state, this population selection "creams off" low-risk populations to make better profit margins.

Numerous problems have surfaced as managed care implementation under Medicaid has progressed. Many states have not had the sophistication in bidding and contracting processes, resulting in much litigation and many contracts that are difficult to enforce for quality service. Some states, frustrated by long delays in HCFA waiver approval, have implemented managed care without sufficient planning and consumer implementation. Some managed care companies have used questionable door-to-door marketing, giving away prizes to get enrollees to join without an explanation of the plan's benefits or the need to change providers. Other states have used automatic assignment of Medicaid enrollees to providers, which ignores issues of ethnic and cultural heritage or past relationships. Some managed

FIGURE **26-3**

Percentage Comparison of Number of Enrollees and Associated Costs in Fiscal Year 1996

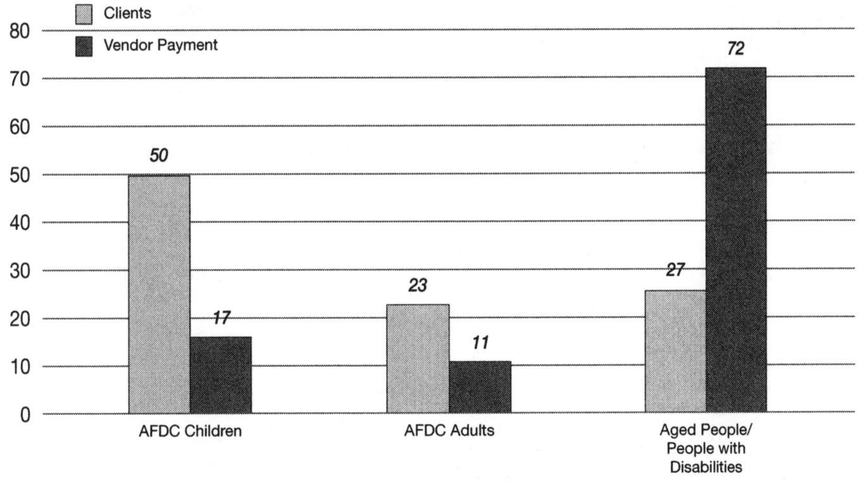

SOURCE: Kaiser Commission on the Future of Medicaid. (1997b, November). *Medicaid facts: The Medicaid program at a glance.* Washington, DC: Author.

TABLE **26-1**

Public-Sector Shifts in Health Care Terminology

FROM	TO
Catchment area	Covered lives
Program grants	Insurance premiums
Service planning	Benefit design
Single provider	Integrated systems
Public versus private	Public and private
Case management	Benefits management
Process evaluation	Outcomes measurement
Data inaccessible	Data manipulation

SOURCE: Crose, C. (1995, August). *Presentation to Federal Center for Mental Health Services,* Rockville, MD.

care programs have been fined for excessive denials of care at emergency rooms. The inclusion of health clinics and community mental health centers having expertise with special populations has been spotty.

Even beyond implementation concerns, there are fundamental questions in the current resource restrictions whether managed care systems can serve the more vulnerable and special-needs populations. Ware, Bayles, Rogers, Kosinski, and Tarlov (1996) conducted a study that found that elderly and disabled populations are two and one-half times more likely to decline in health status under managed care, compared with fee-for-service arrangements. Managed care's reliance on medical necessity as the criterion for treatment, consonant with the employers' rehabilitation model, often fits poorly with more vulnerable and chronic populations that have psychosocial needs impinging on medical treatment. There also continues to be evidence that primary care sites, so prominent in managed care, overlook depression, substance abuse, and other mental health problems.

Meanwhile, managed care technology increasingly defines the delivery of public services. Table 26-1 illustrates the sea change in the vocabulary of financing public mental health programs, essentially reflecting a paradigm shift from government funding to insurance funding. "Catchment area" becomes "covered lives," "program grants" become "insurance premiums," "service planning" is now "benefit design," and "case management" is now "benefits management." Managed care circles have touted how managed care industrialized mental health and substance abuse services, taking them from a cottage industry to a real business industry. Yet the place of the professional also has shifted from being an artisan in the cottage to being a factory worker, with all the associated loss of control. It seems no accident that managed care most often calls social workers "providers" rather than "professionals."

Public and Legislative Reaction

A recent study by the Kaiser Family Foundation (1997) documented a sense of public distrust of managed care. A majority of people (55 percent) in managed care plans, compared with 34 percent in traditional insurance, expressed concern that if they were sick their "health plan would be more concerned about saving money than about what is the best medical treatment." Sixty-one percent believed that the amount of time a physician spends with patients has decreased under managed care, and 59 percent believed that managed care plans have made it harder for people who are sick to see medical specialists.

Many of the increasingly empowered consumers have teamed up with frustrated professionals to spearhead legislation regulating managed care. Originally piecemeal, more and more comprehensive regulations on managed care have passed in state legislatures. In 1997, 17 states passed comprehensive legislation, often renditions of the American Medical Association's Patient Protection Act, which adds to the 13 states that already passed such legislation. Forty-one states now have banned "gag clauses," which were once commonly included in provider contracts to restrict a provider's ability to discuss plan benefits or treatment denial by the managed care company Provider choice has also been a locus of legislation, with 11 states passing point-of-service options for consumers to go outside of networks and 20 states passing Freedom of Choice legislation, although many of these legislated freedoms pertain only to pharmacies.

Once rarely addressed in statehouses, mandated benefits actions are now common. Twenty states have passed legislation mandating that insurance must pay for emergency room services if any "prudent layman" would have thought their condition was an emergency (Health Policy Tracking Services, 1998). Forty-one states have extended stays for mothers and newborns to address so-called "drive-through deliveries," and 13 states now have extended hospital stays for mastectomies. The trend continues as legislatures address benefits for diabetes (23 states) and bone marrow transplantation (11 states).

The fact that treatment guidelines must now come before the legislatures is a measure of how far we have strayed from private decisions between clinician and consumer. As managed care companies make decisions controlling whether there is coverage, some people increasingly seek to hold managed care companies liable for malpractice claims. Currently, most insurance companies are exempt under "no corporate practice of medicine" rules, but Texas and Missouri have removed this protection ("Managed Care and Malpractice," 1997). Recent court rulings in Arizona and Wisconsin have also pointed to holding managed care companies liable for some decisions they make in patient care ("Managed Care and Malpractice," 1997). The Employee Retirement Insurance Security Act (ERISA) protects self-insured plans, but there are those in Congress who would like to reverse that clause. The contracts with providers that commonly require the provider to "hold harmless" the managed care company are increasingly objectionable, and 13 states now bar such clauses in provider contracts (Health Policy Tracking Services, 1998).

The confluence of all these factors can be reduced to the following few defining trends:

- Purchasers—both public and private—are less willing to spend money on health care, particularly behavioral health care (National Alliance for the Mentally Ill, National Association of Psychiatric Health Systems, & Association of Behavioral Group Practices, 1998). Medicaid officials often expect 15 percent to 25 percent reductions in the first few years of managed care plans under Medicaid. Employer average per-member-per-month costs have decreased by 50 percent in many markets, more in others.
- Mergers are creating a field dominated by a few players, especially in behavioral health care.
- Public systems are struggling to survive.

- Medicaid managed care may have improved access to primary care for many AFDC women and children who previously had difficulties finding providers willing to accept the low rates under fee-for-service Medicaid, but there are serious concerns for specialty care and special populations under managed care, with some evidence of a lack of adequate services (Hall, Edgar, & Flynn, 1997).

There is a backlash against managed care in the press, courts, and legislatures. The insurance industry remains vocal about government regulations only increasing cost and lessening care, but they are clearly on the defensive.

What Managed Care Means for Social Work

There is good news and bad news for social workers under managed care. For social workers in private and group practices, managed care has included social workers to a far greater extent than previous fee-for-service plans. Few fee-for-service insurance programs routinely reimbursed social workers in independent mental health practice—only federally dictated programs like the Civilian Health and Medical Program of the Uniformed Services, the Federal Employee Health Benefits Program, and later Medicare. But in the era of managed care, the majority of behavioral health care companies include some social workers as independent providers. In fee-for-service Medicaid, only Montana and Minnesota included social work as independent mental health providers, although Medicaid often paid for care in clinics that employed social workers.

The analysis of a large employer who went from fee-for-service to a managed care arrangement is thought to reflect on the trends in the industry ("Behavioral Health Costs Vary Widely with Plan Design," 1996). As shown in Figure 26-4, social

FIGURE **26-4**

Percentage of Outpatient Visits by Discipline

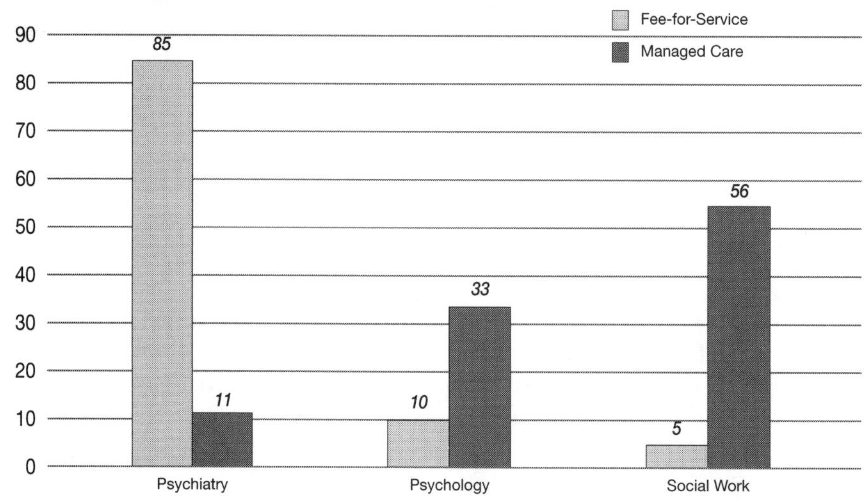

SOURCE: Behavioral health costs vary widely with plan design. (1996, February). *Open Minds, 10*(11), 12. Reprinted with permission.

FIGURE **26-5**

Comparing Fee-for-Service and Managed Care Per Visit Reimbursement by Discipline, in Dollars

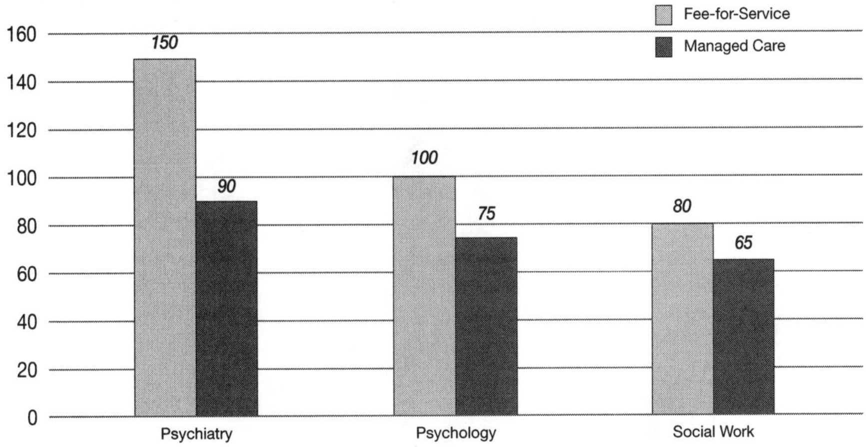

SOURCE: Behavioral health costs vary widely with plan design. (1996, February). *Open Minds, 10*(11), 12. Reprinted with permission.

worker visits accounted for only 5 percent of fee-for-service visits but for 56 percent of managed care visits. In contrast, psychiatrists accounted for 85 percent of fee-for-service visits but only 11 percent of managed care behavioral health care visits.

Yet the same evaluation portrays the bad news of managed care for social workers: The per visit reimbursement rate falls, and utilization is reduced. As seen in Figure 26-5, per visit average cost went from $80 to $65 for social workers. Psychiatry and psychology had even greater per visit reductions but still resulted in higher average reimbursement per visit. This decline in reimbursement is despite the greater burdens in paperwork and requirements for treatment authorizations—the so-called "high hassle factor" of managed care. Figure 26-6, also drawn from this study, shows the shrinking pie of utilization under managed care arrangements: lowered inpatient services, outpatient services, and per-member-per-month costs. Also in line with current thinking, HMOs show greater cost reductions than do preferred provider organizations or point-of-service plans that offer more choice in providers.

The Social Work Response

There are three desired professional responses to managed care. First, social workers must continue to advocate for better services systems and the inclusion of social work services. Second, social workers must make adjustments in their practices of social work. Third, social workers should affiliate with others in this increasingly integrated services system.

Advocacy forms the root of this profession and is needed now more than ever to infuse social work values into insurance-dominated interests. The office insulation of clinical practice can no longer preclude advocacy efforts. As always with social work, this advocacy entails promoting both social good for vulnerable consumers and social work services and skills. Social work's skills and capacities must be documented

FIGURE **26-6**

Comparison of Average Cost Per Service between Fee-for-Service, PPOs, and HMOs

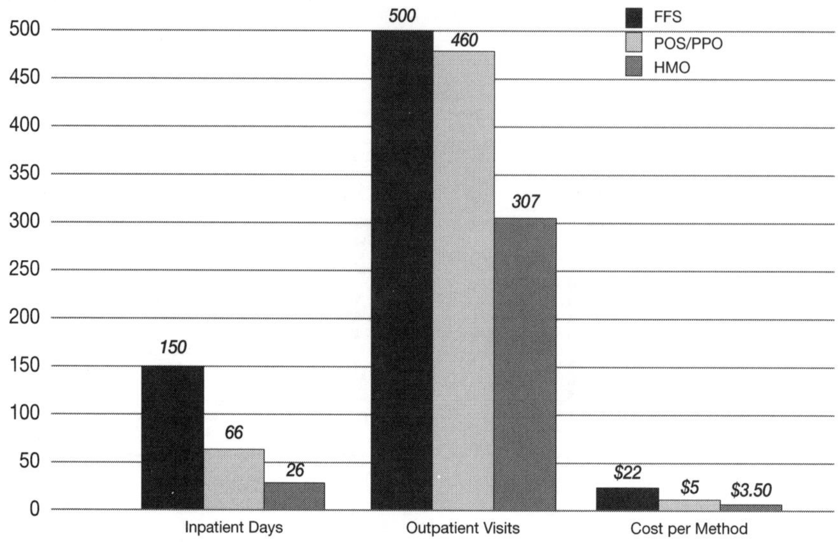

NOTES: FFS = fee-for-service; HMO = health maintenance organization; POS = point of service; PPO = preferred provider organization.
SOURCE: Behavioral health costs vary widely with plan design. (1996, February). *Open Minds, 10*(11), 12. Reprinted with permission.

and promoted because they are still not well understood by employers, insurance companies, or legislators.

A number of critical issues must be addressed to further improve health and other human services systems in the face of business interests. For one, systems must receive adequate funding. Managed care technologies have had the effect of squeezing dollars out of services, sometimes by competitive bidding practices, sometimes by diverting funds to dividend or debt load from mergers. To protect state resources, Iowa's managed Medicaid contract has set a cap on profits by the managed care firm beyond which monies saved must be predominantly reinvested in new services. But purchasers need to be convinced of the value of spending money on behavioral health services. Employers' lack of appreciation for mental health services is evident in their opposition to parity efforts that would treat mental health with the same benefits and caps as exist for medical services.

There are a number of other factors that should be included in the managed care system for public systems. One, the state must be actively involved in evaluating the services provided under managed care rather than delegating quality concerns to managed care firms. There should be meaningful consumer involvement throughout the entire process, from developing requests for proposals to evaluating the services given. A full continuum of services should be stipulated clearly in contracts, from prevention services to wraparound services. Safety-net providers may need special accommodations to have time to adjust to the new managed care environment. For instance, Hawaii and Rhode Island have given special payments to federally qualified health centers.

Social workers must also press for better criteria for treatment than "medical necessity." As the profession grounded in person-in-environment, social work needs to further the understanding by purchasers and managed care firms that strict "medical necessity" precludes needed treatment for those with more long-term disabilities and may result in more long-term costs. We can lead in defining treatment standards such as "psychosocial necessity," which is more applicable for meeting the treatment needs of those with serious mental illness and relapsing addictions.

Finally, social workers can advocate for better fraud mechanisms. Previous fraud efforts focused on overbilling by providers. The new managed care paradigm has built-in incentives to underserve, not overserve. Different tools are needed to detect such lack of services under managed care.

A concurrent response of the social work profession must be to adjust practice. Previously mentioned is the need to show consumers outcomes, both to demonstrate social work's expertise as well as to have managed care companies' provider decisions be based on quality as well as cost. Social workers can promote our expertise in cultural competencies, systems thinking, outreach, and use of community services. Skills in case management can provide a modality to promote in addition to clinical expertise. Group work is a cost-effective treatment modality that social workers can offer. Social workers can hone marketing and contracting skills in continuing education; they also can upgrade their skills with telecommunication technology to prepare for the increasing use of computers and the Internet for clinical services.

A recent survey of clinical managers working for managed care companies reinforces those needs (Shueman & Shore, 1997). Although the small sample size was questioned, a significant majority identified critical skills for practice in managed care that made clinical practice more transparent for the reviewer: problem-oriented, goal-focused treatment; developing realistic treatment plans; documenting care; and understanding the meaning or implication of medical necessity. In addition, skills were identified as critical that linked patient care to other systems: coordination of care and knowledge or appropriate use of community-based service alternatives.

Organizations face many challenges in adjusting to managed care and have little time in which to do so. Thinking should be oriented to the client as consumer, which may be quite a change for public agencies more accustomed to handling walk-ins and wait lists rather than marketing their services. Powerful management information systems typically have been lacking but are essential to managing risk contracts. In-house quality assurance mechanisms are needed to document outcomes and to evaluate utilization. Staff and board must seriously commit to becoming efficient and competitive. Marketing should focus on matching core competencies to purchaser needs.

The third social work response to managed care must be to create strategic alliances and build teams. Managed care creates integrated systems wherein one part feeds the other. The solo-practice person can end up being outside the flow of consumers of services. Certain considerations make for wise affiliates. First is to see how one fits in the geographic range that managed care companies seek. Also, solo practitioners should consider the niche in which he or she fits and how to associate with others unlike himself or herself to offer a continuum of care to managed care firms. Solo practitioners should be open to tailoring their practices to enhance participation opportunities. One of those opportunities is to market mental health and substance abuse services to primary care providers who do not have the time to deal with such issues.

NASW has mirrored this three-pronged approach at the professional level. First, NASW has advocated for the profession, our consumers, and better systems. Second, NASW has invested considerable energy at both the chapter and national levels to provide continuing education that will help give social workers competitive skills. Third, NASW has promoted practice standards, credentials, and interdisciplinary collaboration to enhance professional input into practice wisdom.

Does social work need to change for the new managed care environment? Yes and no. No because our core values remain the same. Indeed, systems thinking and person-in-environment perspective can be valuable to integrated managed care systems seeking greater continuity of care. The best managed care systems are committed to long-term, population-based health care and quality measures, as are social workers. Indeed, social workers are currently working for managed care firms at a variety of levels and, I hope, carrying social work values into the boardrooms.

But yes, social workers need to change in response to the new managed care paradigm. We can be activists for human services, advocating for minimum floors of managed care regulation to ensure that quality care is given even to the most vulnerable consumers. We can speak up for the value of care and, therefore, the need for more funding by both employers and public programs. For employers and those reimbursing for services, we also need to better describe and define what we do. Finally, we can be proactive in taking advantage of new practice opportunities.

References

Behavioral health costs vary widely with plan design. (1996, February). *Open Minds, 10*(11), 12. (Available from Open Minds, 44 South Franklin Street, Gettysburg, PA 17325)

Crose, C. (1995, August). *Presentation to Federal Center for Mental Health Services,* Rockville, MD.

Hall, L. L., Edgar, E., & Flynn, L. (1997). *The NAMI managed care report card.* Washington, DC: National Alliance for the Mentally Ill.

Health Care Financing Administration. (1998). *Managed care in Medicare and Medicaid.* Baltimore: Author.

Health Policy Tracking Services. (1998). *Major state health care policies: Fifty state profile, 1997.* Washington, DC: Author.

Kaiser Commission on the Future of Medicaid. (1997a, November). *Medicaid facts: Medicaid and managed care.* Washington, DC: Author.

Kaiser Commission on the Future of Medicaid. (1997b, November). *Medicaid facts: The Medicaid program at a glance.* Washington, DC: Author.

Kaiser Family Foundation. (1997, November). *Harvard/Kaiser Family Foundation survey: Most Americans give their own health plan a good grade, but have concerns about key aspects of managed care.* Menlo Park, CA: Author. Available online at www.kff.org/kff/library.html.

Liska, D., Marlo, K. O., & Shah, A. (1996). *Medicaid expenditures and beneficiaries, state profiles and trends, 1984–1994.* Washington, DC: Kaiser Commission on the Future of Medicaid.

Magellan acquires Merit: Consolidation of ownership grows. (1997). *Open Minds, 11*(10), 1. (Available from Open Minds, 44 South Franklin Street, Gettysburg, PA 17325)

Managed care and malpractice: States sort out liability issues. (1997, October 13). *State Health Care Notes Weekly,* p. 1.

Markets with HMO penetration greater than 25%, ranked by HMO enrollment. (1995, July 2). *Managed Care Outlook,* p. 4.

Miller, R., & Luft, H. (1994). Managed care plan performance since 1980: A literature analysis. *JAMA, 271,* 925–930.

Myerson, A. R. (1996, March 17). A double standard in health coverage. *New York Times,* p. 1.

National Alliance for the Mentally Ill, National Association of Psychiatric Health Systems, & Association of Behavioral Group Practices. (1998, June 25). *Behavioral health benefit dollars have plummeted, new study finds* [Press release]. Available online at http://www.naphs.org/news/hay/group%20newsrelease.html.

National Committee on Quality Assurance. (1997). *State of managed care quality.* Washington, DC: Author.

Proprietary MBH companies at a crossroad. (1997). *Open Minds, 11*(8), 5. (Available from Open Minds, 44 South Franklin Street, Gettysburg, PA 17325)

Rowland, D., & Rosenbaum, S. E. (1995, March). *Medicaid and managed care: Lessons from the literature.* Washington, DC: Kaiser Commission on the Future of Medicaid.

Shueman, S., & Shore, M. (1997). A survey of what clinicians should know. *Administration and Policy in Mental Health, 25*(1), 71–81.

Substance Abuse and Mental Health Services Administration. (1994). *Managed healthcare organizational readiness guide and checklist: Special report.* Rockville, MD: Author.

Ware, J., Bayles, S., Rogers, W., Kosinski, M. A., & Tarlov, A. (1996, October). Differences in 4-year health outcomes for elderly and poor. Chronically ill patients treated in HMOs and fee-for-services systems. *JAMA, 276,* 1039–1047.

"Wisconsin residents can sue HMOs for bad faith denials." (1997, December 12). *Mental Health Report.*

CHAPTER 27

Social Work Leadership in Hospitals: Handling Obstacles and Creating Opportunities in a Changing Health Care Environment

Terry Mizrahi and Candyce S. Berger

The health care system is undergoing dramatic changes in auspices, structure, and services delivery in response to an emphasis on market-driven, cost-containment strategies. Most health care organizations are restructuring to achieve flatter organizational structures by moving away from functionally defined structures (that is, departmental structures by disciplines such as departments of social work, nursing, medicine, and so forth) to more integrative structures. In this process, discipline-specific organizations are eliminated or reduced to allow greater focus on collaborative and more matrixed models of organization characterized by shared resources and better integration (Globerman & Bogo, 1995; Rosenberg & Weissman, 1995a). The consequences of those changes are that many social work directors are losing some or all of their administrative responsibilities or are expanding their span of control beyond social work services. These changes are having significant impact on the operations of social work services within the hospital setting (Berger et al., 1996).

How have hospital social work administrators fared in these turbulent times? What mechanisms and strategies have they used to respond to actual and anticipated changes? Are they optimistic or pessimistic about opportunities for hospital-based social work in the future? This chapter explores the role of hospital social work leadership in the current uncertain environment. Whereas conditions external to social work are driving drastic changes in health care delivery, the social work profession has promoted the role of social work in effecting change at the micro and macro levels. Indeed, the *NASW Code of Ethics* (National Association of Social Workers, 1996) insists that social workers work toward improving conditions in their agencies. We present here the attitudes and actions of social work directors in hospital settings, based on their perceived experiences in the field.

The Society of Social Work Administrators in Health Care and the National Association of Social Workers commissioned a national study to examine the impact of changes in the health care arena on hospital social work structure and practice (Berger et al., 1996). The primary focus of the study was to examine hospital social work directors' perspectives on the changes occurring in the hospital in general and the social work department in particular; the impact of these changes on social work roles, functions, and practices; and the strategies being used to influence the direction of hospital social work in reconfigured health care delivery systems.

This chapter specifically examines the responses to the following six open-ended questions:

1. Describe the breadth of changes occurring throughout your hospital, with specific examples of other departments or programs that have been affected.
2. Describe the major accomplishments of social work services within your facility.
3. Describe the failures, frustrations, and obstacles in the delivery of social work services.
4. Describe what changes you anticipate within your organization or social work department in the next two years that will affect the delivery of social work services within your institution?
5. Describe the major opportunities for social work created as a result of organizational changes within your hospital.
6. Describe the major threats and challenges for social work created as a result of organizational changes within your hospital.

Literature Review

For years, the topic of social work leadership has been neglected in the literature. To the extent leadership was considered, it was embedded in the context of social work administration or advanced primarily in regard to community organization practice in which social workers were viewed as change agents (Brilliant, 1986). It is important to clarify the distinction between management and leadership. Management is about getting the work done; it involves the technical and operational components of the job. Leadership is about establishing the direction, standards, and vision for an organization. The personal orientation of the leader, as well as his or her assessment of the internal and external environment and evaluation of the political economic climate, is likely to shape the organizational vision. In 1987 Rosenberg and Clark, the editors for a special volume of *Social Work in Health Care,* devoted an entire issue to the transition to leadership for social work directors in hospitals. It is this vision that shapes the organizational priorities that guide resource allocation, ultimately influencing the quality of services delivered (Ezell, Menefee, & Patti, 1997). Mayer (1995) stated, "Many of us were selected not necessarily because we had demonstrated superb management skills prior to our new jobs, but rather because we were politically savvy or well known within our institutions for being highly responsible" (p. 70). Dimond and Markowitz (1995) added that many people are capable of managing, but few people actually lead. In today's environment, leadership is the limited commodity needed to guide programs through these turbulent times of change.

In recent years, a small body of literature on social work leadership focusing on hospitals has developed (Berger, 1990; Irizarry, Gambeau, & Walter, 1993; Rosenberg & Weissman, 1995b). Most presentations have been anecdotal or have used a case study method. These have been useful in identifying a range of knowledge, skills, values, and attributes that successful social work directors need to survive and thrive in the increasing difficult times that began in the Reagan–Bush years (Bixby, 1995; Dimond & Markowitz, 1995; Mayer, 1995; Patti, 1984; Spitzer, 1995).

The major factors include an ability to balance the needs of the patient, the institution, and the staff, recognizing the tensions involved in meeting often competing or conflicting demands. The literature focuses more on describing what has been accomplished than on explaining how it has been accomplished. Much less has been written about failures or about strategies for managing the inherent pressures. Leadership involves unleashing the creative energy within organizations to create innovative approaches to service delivery. It involves helping staff to streamline processes by driving out redundancy and unnecessary work rather than merely "doing more with less" (Hammer & Champy, 1993; Rosenberg & Weissman, 1995b). Additionally, there are no recent, published, large-scale, comparative studies of social work directors across settings and communities. This chapter addresses that gap.

Methodology

An exploratory/descriptive survey design was used (see Berger et al., 1996, for more details on the methodology). A stratified random sample of 750 (of 3,700) hospitals was drawn from the member list of the American Hospital Association. Stratification was determined by the stage of managed care development, geographic location, and number of available beds. A standardized, self-administered survey instrument was developed, and questionnaires were sent to the 750 hospital social services directors. A total of 340 usable questionnaires were returned—a 45.3 percent response rate.

The questions were analyzed qualitatively using a grounded theory methodology (Abramson & Mizrahi, 1993; Mizrahi & Abramson, 1994; Strauss & Corbin, 1990). Two researchers read a sample of responses to the discussion questions and identified a series of themes for each one. Additionally, several key words or concepts selected from the narratives were separately coded (for example, case management, psychosocial factors, nurses). Finally, all the questions were read as a whole and rated as to whether the respondent was generally optimistic or pessimistic about social work in hospital-based health care.

A sample of 40 questionnaires was then separately coded by four additional social workers using the identified themes. The results were compared and reconciled with the predominant selected code used. The agreement rate among the four reviewers was over 80 percent, which allowed the rest of the questions to be coded by the principal author. Additional coders were consulted for the few responses that she felt were ambiguous.

Findings

The findings are compelling. A majority of social work directors use strategies that positively position social workers for policy and practice roles in their institutions and in the community, notwithstanding the challenges and problems confronting them. Among the social work leaders' accomplishments and opportunities were

- system and structural reorganization (that is, social workers contributed to efficiency, productivity, reduced lengths of stay, and cost savings)
- creation of new programs, policies, and standards, as well as education and training opportunities
- increased influence over hospital or patient decision making beyond the department's established role (that is, social work leadership in quality assurance, strategic planning, and other committees)

- development or integration of new social work roles and functions (for example, in cross training and case management)
- acquisition of new or increased social work lines or expanded social work coverage
- development of new, increased, or reclaimed social work functions, settings, and patient populations (for example, community practice and utilization review)
- preservation or maintenance of core social work functions.

At the same time, several failures, threats or, at the very least, challenges to social work were also perceived by most administrators. These included

- elimination, merger, or deprofessionalization of social work, especially actual or threatened takeovers of social work functions by nursing
- devaluation, lack of appreciation, or misunderstanding of social work roles
- difficulties involved in practicing social work in hospitals today (for example, pressures to do more with less, low morale, and a reduced psychosocial role)
- negative changes in the larger health care system adversely affecting social work, for example, decreased lengths of stay, lack of external resources, and changing patient demographic and disease factors
- decreases in the perceived quality of social work care
- internal frustrations with the social work profession, including convincing social workers to change their own attitudes and behavior.

SOCIAL WORK ACCOMPLISHMENTS AND OPPORTUNITIES

In spite of and, in some instances, because of the changes in hospital-based social work, most respondents identified a range of accomplishments. The most interesting finding probably is the creativity with which directors defined accomplishments and opportunities as well as the scope and extensiveness of their efforts. Many directors reported that the social work role was deepened and expanded at the clinical, planning and development, and management levels.

Creating New Programs

The most frequently described accomplishments were in the area of new programs. Typically, these programs extended beyond existing or traditional arenas of service delivery. The social work role in planning and program development was prominent. Social workers were responsible for initiating programs (for example, rape crisis services, support groups, hospice care), for obtaining grants and contracts, for developing protocols and standards, for performing research, for involving students, and for consulting inside and outside the hospital. These programs involved collaboration with other disciplines or services outside the social work department.

> We wrote a grant for a homeless program; social work received three MSW social workers with this program.
>
> [We were involved in] helping to establish outreach clinics; implementing fee-basis adult day home care and homemaker/home health aide programs; establishing an intensive psychiatric community care program with case

> managers. (This is the primary reason for our FTE [full-time equivalent] increase.)

On the downside was the fact that fewer respondents anticipated creating new programs in the future.

Expanding Social Work Functions and Settings

Beyond the creation of new programs under social work sponsorship, social workers described a variety of places, processes, and people with whom they worked. Enhancements during this period ranged from increasing the number of social work positions to assuming new functions and reclaiming former ones. In a time of downsizing, many directors had been able to add new lines or expand social work coverage on medical services. Other social workers moved into new settings or began working with additional patient populations both inside and outside the hospital. Some assumed new clinical responsibilities; others moved or anticipated moving into physicians' offices, outpatient settings, and primary care. Related roles in community organizing, planning, and collaboration with other health and human service agencies were featured.

The arena of most promise was the identification of new and increasing social work practice opportunities in a reconfigured health care delivery position; that is, social workers were becoming case managers and integral members of interdisciplinary teams. They were also active in cross-training initiatives which, from their perspectives, enhanced social work's status. These new functions and new ambulatory settings were two areas in which social workers saw opportunities increasing.

> I feel the choice of the case management structure to include a nurse and social work dyad and the choice of a social worker to head the case management department indicate the strength and the respect for social work here.

> We are shifting more staff to our ambulatory areas, negotiating all of our community agency and extended-care facility contracts for our new Medicare HMOs [health maintenance organizations], and continuing to drop our length of stay.

> We increased MSW staff by four FTEs (75 percent); obtained individual offices for all social work staff. We have expanded our obstetrical and nursery service and continue to receive increasing referrals . . . we just continue to expand.

Preserving Social Work

Unexpectedly, many of the respondents recognized the importance of "holding our own." They said that survival, that is, to be able to continue doing what they had been doing in a time of turmoil and downsizing, was a remarkable achievement. This category could be interpreted as a default category in that "it could have been worse," but it was not merely a minimalist stance. Some directors specifically noted that they were retaining or recapturing the basic social work function. Several defined this as including the clinical or basic professional social work role.

> We still exist and have only experienced minor reductions and a shift from a centralized department to unit-based services.

> [Our accomplishments were] Staying strong and vital. . . . Keeping discharge planning on the front burner.

Reorganizing Systems

Social workers also identified their accomplishments in systems and outcome terms, and in so doing described active leadership in administration, management, and coordination. The expected area of discharge planning loomed large; also prominent were active roles in quality assurance. They contributed to the structural reorganization of the hospital and believed that they increased social work's value to the institution. Several identified how they decreased lengths of stay, participated in prescreening activities and, through their productivity and programs, saved money for their hospitals.

> As Director, I have been asked to lead/participate in numerous organizationwide initiatives (that is, CQI [continuous quality improvement] teams, CQI teaching, vertical integration task force, utilization management oversight committee, etc.).

> By recentralizing and improving quality and process, the department's image as capable, competent, and in charge has grown. The chief of medicine, a former critic, announced at a medical board that social work was doing a great job at discharge planning—a complete turnaround.

> We reorganized the department; redefined the mission of the department; wrote a policy and procedure manual to comply with JCAHO [Joint Commission on Accreditation of Healthcare Organizations] standards.

Increasing Social Work Influence

Although it can be inferred that the social work respondents exercised their influence in order to attain what is described above, some of them specifically described their ability to achieve more power and influence in their organizations as an accomplishment in its own right. They increased their visibility, effectiveness, and persuasiveness by assuming leadership positions and, in some cases, by taking risks. They clearly recognized the importance of being "at the table" where decisions were made, leading teams, collaborating with other professionals and administrators, and being proactive overall. Several directors used the word "leadership" in accounting for the successful outcomes, but many more were performing it.

> Participation in the top management quality steering team to launch process action teams, organizational improvement teams, and redesign teams. Social work was conceptual as a component of the primary care team as opposed to a support service. In this way social workers participate in the "port of entry" as well as "contract" programs.

> Higher visibility (for social work) through participation on hospital committees and staff; an active part of case management and discharge-planning teams (for example, AIDS team). Higher visibility and credibility through very little turnover and the expansion of services in emergency department, psychiatry, and rehabilitation.

As the following comments of a leader demonstrate, there is a connectedness of process and outcome that points to the relationship between competency and indispensability:

> [We attained the following:] Community recognition of the prenatal substance abuse program . . . ; strong, competent social work staff who have gained recognition and support from other departments, that is, nursing; positive recognition by [various social work schools] as a desired social work field agency and also desired by students; strong supervision program for staff and interns; sponsored a child life specialist in-hospital, a position well received by physicians and staff. Expansion of resources and greater role clarification; positive community relations.

A majority of the directors cited multiple areas of accomplishment, seeming to recognize that success in one area was related to achievements in another area:

> [We accomplished] truly excellent clinical services all around; highly respected social work staff in all areas; enhancement of interdisciplinary, collaborative approach to care in medicine/surgery; active involvement and responsibility for developing a partial psychiatric hospital program; excellent relationship with managed care folks has served the hospital well at contract time; starting new programs in collaboration with the volunteer department; ER [emergency room]/social work services launched and extremely successful.

> Maintaining a level of clinical presence on all services [is one accomplishment]; we forged a formal alliance with patient education/community outreach as we move services to offsite programs; inclusion in hospital's planning, and development particularly as managed care contracts and criteria were developed.

> [We were involved in] substantially improved labor productivity; beginning clinical practice guidelines; obtaining dedicated housing and equipment dollars; obtaining a department LAN [local area network] and 27 computers; increased institutional visibility.

SOCIAL WORK FAILURES AND CHALLENGES

These social work directors by no means painted a one-sided, rosy picture of the field, not even those who projected a positive, optimistic view of present and future circumstances. They also reflected on present and projected failures, frustrations, obstacles, challenges, and threats to social work. Whereas numerically they identified fewer problems than positive opportunities, nevertheless, they encountered and anticipated a range of significant difficulties emanating from myriad sources. The following response by one administrator encompasses the range of problems encountered by others:

> Problematic staff who were extremely time consuming; 22 contracts with the county for prenatal services—very time consuming and stressful for the director. Lack of space for our department. Director and supervisor share one office. All other staff share another office with no privacy from secretary. Loss of several community agencies and closure of county office on Fridays. Turf issues with physicians and nursing staff.

Putting Pressure on Social Workers

By far the most extensive frustrations, reported by many respondents, were difficulties in providing social work services and in fulfilling social work roles. These ranged from an inability to recruit or retain social workers, to increasing caseloads and responsibilities (often with fewer staff members), to low morale and burnout, to a diminishing psychosocial or clinical component in social work activities.

> Discharge planning [creates problems]. We are required to outplace patients who are to leave the hospital soon. Having to perform too many concrete services and spend less time on treatment and use of professional skills.
>
> Not enough staff. Because we are social workers, the expectation is that this department is to be involved in other areas of groups, meetings, continuous quality improvement, policies; but not enough staff to stretch. Staff is tired.
>
> Increasing inpatient volume while having to lay off inpatient social workers. Politics with our utilization review department and finance, who want to take over discharge planning.

Devaluing Social Work Status

Many social workers discussed a more subtle negative change, namely, devaluation, nonrecognition, or lack of appreciation by others for social work roles and functions. Although that perception had not necessarily manifested itself in any structural changes, it still seemed to have negative consequences for the directors' stated ability to influence the direction of social work in their institutions. The respondents pointed to resistance to growth by nurses and, to a lesser degree, by physicians and administrators. Many of the directors identified a climate of tension, confusion, or competition, influenced by what was perceived as a continuing lack of understanding of social work's contribution to the organization and to quality patient care.

> [There is] resistance by non-MSW social workers to accept MSWs onto the staff. Resistance by nursing department to accept MSW-trained social workers to provide a variety of psychosocial services.
>
> [Failures include] maintaining a social work niche as other disciplines also look for opportunities to redesign and realign services. Sometimes feeling isolated and undervalued; voices speaking alone.
>
> Historically, RNs have done inpatient social services for years; there's lots of resistance; real turf problems. One RN in cancer unit has directed MSWs for 20+ years. RNs in discharge planning resist change to social work leadership; other departments, for example, nursing and patient care, want to keep the psychosocial area.

Eliminating or Deprofessionalizing Social Work

Fewer social workers had actually experienced negative consequences from the perceived deprecation of social work, but a few reported that this had occurred. More telling, perhaps, is the fact that this threat was the largest anticipated future problem for social work. This category included the elimination of social work positions and reducing requirements from MSW to BSW degrees, along with the assumption of social work functions or departments by nurses.

> The major threat is the loss of autonomy for our professional values if merged. . . . Our challenge is to financially justify our services.

> The loss of discharge planning [by social work]. It was an important activity garnering respect from administration, physicians, and other professional groups. With this loss, budget cuts and loss of prestige have occurred.

> In psychiatry we are still viewed as ancillary and supplemental. It is very difficult to break into the inner circle with these folks. We are trying to reposition the [social work] department in psychiatry, and they keep trying to get control of social work lines.

Dealing with Threats from the External Environment

Beyond problems internal to the hospital or department, some respondents depicted a variety of external circumstances that adversely affected their departments and would, in their estimation, continue to do so. These problems appeared to emanate from changes in the larger health care sector and changes driven by the political and economic conservatism of national leadership, including pressures placed on them by JCAHO, ethical issues, changes in the demographics and diseases of patients, and economic factors such as increased competition from other hospitals and decreased lengths of stay.

> For all the years I have been here we have lacked community resources, that is, adult day care, providers of custodial care, meals outside the towns, etc. This continues to be an area of frustration and obstacles.

> Shrinking public resources to refer to; lack of accountability on the part of public agencies to support governmental mandated programs; lessening inpatient population; shrinking reimbursement for care; increased needs on the part of patients.

Decreasing Quality of Care

Related to pressures on social work performance were specific references to the negative impact on patient care of the lack of resources or lower priority given to certain patient populations. Here the respondents expressed explicit frustration or lamented their departments' inability to meet patients' needs and expectations and also to advocate for patients.

> Our failure is we have not developed a family support service as I would wish; day-to-day services, especially discharges, suffer. Frustrations include the failure of the hospital to plan for future trends in a timely way. It is becoming increasingly difficult to be cost effective and advocate for our patients at the same time.

Dealing with Threats Related to the Social Work Profession

An important set of negative responses was also directed at the social work profession or at individual social workers within the respondents' own institutions. The frustrations involved not being able to advocate effectively for social work to their hospital's decision makers. According to the respondents, social work was not viewed as able to articulate social work's benefits or contributions to the hospital, particularly in cost-savings or cost–benefit terms. Conversely, a few directors lamented their inability to adhere to social work values in this bottom-line climate. Additionally, the respondents expressed some frustration at their own staffs for unwillingness or inability to adapt and change.

> [One frustration] is the social work staff not understanding need for change; caseloads without sufficient system changes to improve efficiency.
>
> Failure of administration to view social work as a cost-saving and revenue-producing program in multiple ambulatory care settings.
>
> We have had to fight for our positions in managed care. Administration and other departments had to be convinced that social work is cost effective in this new health arena.

REVISITING SOCIAL WORK LEADERSHIP: IS THE GLASS HALF-EMPTY OR HALF-FULL?

Virtually all the directors responded to all the questions we posed, suggesting that they assessed both the strengths and limitations of the system in which they operated and the impact of larger systems and policies on the social work department and services. These social work leaders analyzed in some detail the obstacles and opportunities they faced. However, when asked about failures, a large group of social workers often reframed frustrations as challenges.

> I don't know that we've experienced failures. The challenges have been to provide the best possible quality patient care with shrinking resources. The frustration is that our customers (physicians, nurses, families) have the same expectations they have always had.
>
> The lack of job security during the '94 downsizing period made it very difficult to remain a creative and risk-taking style of practice. It fostered a bit of "let's keep things the way they are" and "if it's not broken, don't fix it." However, the staff, given the time and opportunity to grieve the changes, truly rose to the challenge. We've worked on renewed ideas for re-engineering our services.
>
> We were unable to obtain increase in funding/FTE for increasing care social work positions to assign to primary care integration effort. This was accomplished by creative reassignment of existing staff.
>
> A case management program was implemented at end of 1994. Case managers are RNs. They have primary discharge-planning responsibilities. They are primary contact for families. Social work role changed to counseling patient/family on adjustment issues, and complicated discharge planning is handled by social work. The social work department decreased in size. It had a Director with 50–60 percent of time designated to management, 30–40 percent time with patients/families. Now the social work supervisor carries a full caseload and does management when time allows.

Discussion

Managed care, with its emphasis on fiscal constraint, is creating extreme pressure for hospitals to adopt quickly more cost-effective strategies for services delivery. These pressures significantly affect the way services are delivered. Ongoing changes in service delivery include major re-engineering of processes and restructuring of organizational structures. Although overall social work services may not be experiencing change to the same degree that hospitals are (Berger et al., 1996), ongoing changes nonetheless are having a significant impact on social work's role and function. Of particular importance is the impact on social work leaders, both in terms of job security and advancement.

In these challenging times, change does not occur without significant pain and loss. Many departments are being downsized or eliminated, decentralized, or redefined. The pressures of the work environment lead to significant problems of morale for both staff and management, eroding the strengths that so fundamentally reside in both the profession of social work and the institution. A major concern is the ability of social work managers to find an effective balance between optimism and pessimism or activity and passivity (Berger, 1993) in relation to fulfilling their roles as managers and leaders. Blumenfield (1995) set the tone for leaders in the present environment: "Diminished resources, on a societal or personal scale, are serious and upsetting. . . . These crises necessarily harbor good luck or great opportunities, but they do demand active and creative leadership" (p. 37).

Turbulent times call for more leadership, not less. It is not enough to be a good manager; one must also be an exceptional leader, able to steer social work through the rapidly changing health care environment. Rosenberg and Weissman (1995b) made five skills recommendations for successful leadership:

1. Accurately read the environment.
2. Re-engineer your own department (or others will do it for you).
3. Focus on those programs that are highly valued, recognized, and effective to maintain your strengths within your environments.
4. Innovate, experiment, and create new, more effective and efficient programs, and fund these through new revenue sources such as grants.
5. Create community partnerships based on social epidemiologic information by building on social work's strong relationships within communities.

Many of the social work leaders in this study described such skills and activities. The sketches on accomplishments were not anomalies. Widespread, active, creative, committed, and competent social work leaders are active participants in shaping both health care and social work services for the future. The respondents emphasized the importance of influence and positioning within the hospital environment so administrators actively contribute to steering the change process rather than merely reacting to it. Future leaders will require even more political acumen, knowing when to resist as well as when to acquiesce, adapt, or cope. Leadership involves mobilizing power resources within both individuals and systems to obtain the resources necessary for goal accomplishment (Berger, 1990). Building on existing strengths, re-engineering, developing new programs, extending the boundaries of social work practice into new arenas of care, and mobilizing community partnerships all were reported as areas of accomplishment.

A key to success in this changing health care environment is to move beyond a management function to a leadership role. Leadership is more than doing the job right. It involves motivating and unleashing the creative energy of those with whom one interacts. In discussing leadership, several authors have spoken to the importance of passion, a sense of optimism, political acumen, an ability to look into the future in shaping priorities, tenacity, and a joy for adventure (Blumenfield, 1995; Drucker, 1996; Mayer, 1995; Peters & Austin, 1985; Rosenberg, 1987; Spitzer, 1995). Positive change needs to be guided rather than forced. A leader must develop a vision and position an organization for the future (Austin, 1989), which require skills in management of interpersonal conflict as well as continued support for an environment that promotes positive morale (Bixby, 1995; Dimond & Markowitz, 1995). Leaders also need to view failures or setbacks as necessary steps toward goal achievement (Bixby, 1995). Blumenfield (1995) captured the essence of leadership for the future in the following description:

> Leadership in today's health care social work may require the energy and strategic skills of an Attila [the Hun], but must be tempered with the vision of Jane Addams, the intellect of Gordon Hamilton, the know-how of a Harvard MBA, with a dash of Joan of Arc fortitude, and early Napoleonic luck. (p. 21)

Additional research is needed to understand the issues, attributes, and attitudes of successful leadership in the changing health care arena. To what degree are social work managers' attitudes and perceptions shaped by situations or events that specifically affect them or their departments? For example, is a director–manager more likely to have a positive attitude if his or her department is downsized or, conversely, if staffing is increased? What other factors may account for positive or negative perceptions, for example, professional training, scope of administrative responsibility, and external realities for the hospital or department?

Conclusion

In conclusion, this research demonstrates that social work leaders in hospitals understand the complexities and challenges of the world around them. Beyond that, the majority have exhibited commitment and competence as well as confidence that they can contribute to the direction of change. This augurs well both for the profession and for the clients we serve. However, it remains to be seen whether the necessary knowledge, skill, and values the directors identify are sufficient to shape the future direction of health care.

References

Abramson, J. A. & Mizrahi, T. (1993). Examining social work/physician collaboration: An application of grounded theory methodology. In C. Riessman (Ed.), *Qualitative studies in social work research* (pp. 28–48). Newbury Park, CA: Sage Publications.

Austin, M. J. (1989). Executive entry: Multiple perspectives on the process of muddling through. *Administration in Social Work, 13*(3/4), 55–71.

Berger, C. S. (1990). Enhancing social work influence in the hospital: Identifying sources of power. *Social Work in Health Care, 15*(2), 77–93.

Berger, C. S. (1993). *Restructuring and rightsizing: Strategies for social work and human resource administrators in health care settings.* Chicago: Society for Social Work Administrators in Health Care.

Berger, C. S., Cayner, J., Jensen, G., Mizrahi, T., Scesny, A., & Trachtenberg, J. (1996). The changing scene of social work in hospitals. *Health & Social Work, 21,* 167–177.

Bixby, N. B. (1995). Crisis or opportunity: A healthcare social work director's response to change. *Social Work in Health Care, 20*(4), 3–20.

Blumenfield, S. (1995). Reflections on effective leadership: Strains and successes, strategies and styles. *Social Work in Health Care, 20*(4), 21–37.

Brilliant, E. (1986). Social work leadership: A missing ingredient. *Social Work, 31,* 325–331.

Dimond, M., & Markowitz, M. (1995). The effective health care social work director. *Social Work in Health Care, 20*(4), 39–59.

Drucker, P. F. (1996). Forward/Preface. In F. Hesselbein, M. Goldsmith, & R. Beckhard (Eds.), *The leader of the future* (pp. xi–xxv). San Francisco: Jossey-Bass.

Ezell, M., Menefee, D., & Patti, R. J. (1997). Factors influencing priorities in hospital social work departments: A director's perspective. *Social Work in Health Care, 21*(1), 25–40.

Globerman, J., & Bogo, M. (1995). Social work and the new integrative hospital. *Social Work in Health Care, 21*(3), 1–21

Hammer, M., & Champy, J. (1993). *Reengineering the corporation.* New York: Harper Business.

Irizarry, C., Gambeau, B., & Walter, R. (1993). Social work leadership skills through an international exchange: The Mount Sinai experience. *Social Work in Health Care, 18*(3/4), 35–46.

Mayer, J. B. (1995). The effective health care social work director: Managing the social work department at Beth Israel Hospital. *Social Work in Health Care 20*(4), 61–72.

Mizrahi, T., & Abramson, J. A. (1994). Collaboration between social workers and physicians: An emerging typology. In E. Sherman & W. J. Reid (Eds.), *Qualitative methods in social work practice* (pp. 135–151). New York: Columbia University Press.

National Association of Social Workers. (1996). *NASW code of ethics.* Washington, DC: Author.

Patti, R. (1984). Who leads the human services? The prospects for social work leadership in an age of political conservatism. *Administration in Social Work, 8*(1), 17–29.

Peters, T., & Austin, N. (1985). *A passion for excellence: The leadership difference.* New York: Random House.

Rosenberg, G. (1987). The social worker as manager in health care settings: An experiential view. *Social Work in Health Care, 12*(3), 71–84.

Rosenberg, G., & Clark, S. S. (1987). Social workers in healthcare management: The move to leadership. *Social Work in Health Care, 12*(3).

Rosenberg, G., & Weissman, A. (1995a). Introduction. *Social Work in Health Care, 20*(4), 1–2.

Rosenberg, G., & Weissman, A. (1995b). Preliminary thoughts on sustaining central work departments. *Social Work in Health Care, 20*(4), 111–116.

Spitzer, W. J. (1995). Effective leadership: The healthcare social work director. *Social Work in Health Care, 20*(4), 89–109.

Strauss, A., & Corbin, J. (1990). *Basics of qualitative research: Grounded theory procedures and techniques.* Newbury Park, CA: Sage Publications.

The authors wish to thank Ann Rausch, CSW, for her insights and assistance, and the collaborators on the study: Jay Cayner, Greg Jenson, Alice Scesny, and Judith Trachtenberg.

CHAPTER 28

Confidentiality and Managed Care: Ethical and Legal Concerns

Jeanette R. Davidson and Tim Davidson

Before managed care, social work services in the field of mental health tended to be needs driven. Increasingly, these services are resource driven, and there is a profit motive for the managers whether the resource is the public or the private dollar. As managed care companies take over the allocation of funds, the monitoring of treatment, and the measurement of outcomes, social workers encounter an ethical and legal dilemma with the demise of confidentiality in the professional–client relationship. The dilemma appears to be rooted first in the essential difference in primary purpose between social workers and managed care companies and second in the heavy reliance of managed care companies on burgeoning information systems.

Specifically, many social workers providing services within managed care systems are concerned about the quantity of information sought about the client; the sensitive nature of that information (which if exposed leaves the client entirely vulnerable); the way in which the client is, for all intents and purposes, forced to permit the disclosure of the information to ensure third-party payments (unless able to pay directly for services); the potential use of the information to deny rather than provide needed services to the client; and the all-too-often suspect security of the information systems involved. Social workers are also uncomfortable when they consider the potential negative effect that the loss of confidentiality may have on the client–worker relationship as well as the possible liability issues that may ensue.

Given that the profession has long heralded the protection of client confidentiality, it is timely that social workers re-examine traditional guidelines within this new context of managed care. If safeguarding confidences is still valued, then social workers, individually and in consortium, need to negotiate with managed care policymakers and government regulators to develop new mechanisms to protect client information.

Clash of Essential Purposes

DIFFERENCE IN MISSION

Social workers need to be aware of the fundamental differences in mission between managed care personnel and themselves as providers and the effect of those

NOTE: Originally published as Davidson, J. R., & Davidson, T. (1996). Confidentiality and managed care: Ethical and legal concerns. *Health & Social Work, 21*, 208–215.

differences on the treatment of client data. Because managed care companies primarily serve the funding bodies, they have an essential disparity of purpose from social workers. They are concerned with capitated risk for groups of people, and therefore any individual's particular need is evaluated in the context of all the other covered lives. Thus, managed care companies have gatekeepers in place who examine intimate details about a person from a distance and who may use that information to deny rather than provide needed services. In contrast, social workers' general aim is to work with all who request and need services. With managed care, then, the mission is restrictive and generalized, whereas with social workers service delivery is inclusive and individualized.

DIFFERENCE IN REASONS FOR DOCUMENTATION

When care is managed, client data become determinative. Recordings undertaken for managed care companies are first and foremost meant to establish the saving of health care dollars for employers and insurance companies. A document containing highly confidential material, in the hands of a managed care administrator, will be used whatever way is most profitable from a business perspective. This contrasts with the traditional use of social work records, which has been to chronicle, in the context of trust, individuals' treatment and progress for the purpose of assisting recovery.

DIFFERENCE IN USE OF OUTCOME MEASURES

An impetus for adopting a managed care format in behavioral health care is to promote the measurement of treatment outcomes. This purpose, seemingly laudable at first, belies another agenda. Marketers of managed care companies stress that health professionals will be better prepared to deliver the optimum treatment for each disorder once reams of outcome data are analyzed. Although managed care research is often flawed because of inappropriate questions (Shapiro, 1995), simplistic and reductionistically defined variables, and economic controls over the process, it may in fact produce some interesting and helpful conclusions.

In practice, however, outcome measures for managed care have ultimately been used to determine which populations are healthy and which populations predictably could drain the profits of the managed care company. Chronic, heavy users of health care services are not usually recruited by managed care unless there is a guaranteed safety net provided by state or local governments. The legitimate clinical principle of "least-restrictive alternatives" has been transliterated by managed care to mean "severely restricted alternatives." "Stop-loss" and "hold harmless" are fundamental operating procedures written into managed care contracts. Stop-loss clauses require the government to step in when providing care for those who are needy proves too costly, and hold harmless clauses require providers to shoulder the burden of further treatment and liability when managed care companies discontinue payments because it does not appear that a positive treatment outcome is cheap and imminent.

Social workers have traditionally advocated for people who need services, and so it seems perverse to contribute client data to a system that takes that information and uses it to figure out who should not receive treatment. For clients who have been approved for some managed care payments, the social worker's report of positive treatment outcomes frequently inclines the case reviewer to stop payment for further services because the clients' needs are then determined to be not great enough. Outcome measures are used, then, both to disenfranchise those most in need and to limit funding for others. Social workers support efficacy studies, but not at clients' expense.

Problems with Managed Care's Reliance on Information Systems

Irrespective of the form of managed care, whether a health maintenance organization, an employee assistance program, a preferred provider network with horizontal or vertical layers, or a management service designed to manage these and other kinds of managed care, client information is now shared in a much less discriminate manner than traditionally occurred in fee-for-service delivery systems. Before managed care, even in agencies with several layers of bureaucracy, strict guidelines governed the release of information to the various levels of administration and accounting.

With the use of managed care information systems that include telephone reviews, voice mail, faxes, cellular telephones, and highly unregulated computerized databases, there are few guarantees, if any, that sensitive information is stored securely. Rather, it appears that information, once passed from the social worker to a managed care service and logged into the medical database of a third-party insurance payer, may be as accessible as credit card information or mortgage payment records to people who know how to proceed with the electronic inquiry. As noted by the Legal Action Center (LAC) (1995), "The potential for wrongful disclosure of confidential information has expanded right along with the expansion of the capability of computers to move information from location to location" (p. 104).

UNPROTECTED DATABASES

Press reports from a number of sources delineate various problems within the managed care industry with respect to information systems. In an article in the *New York Times*, concerns about unprotected databases were cited and clearly indicated a clinical predicament involving trust for both clinicians and clients (Henneberger, 1994). A scathing article in *The Wall Street Journal* noted how "open" all medical information is as "it lies unprotected in a patchwork of databases where it is so easy to see" and how people who file for managed care visits to psychotherapists "build up especially detailed records" (Schultz, 1994, p. A5) that are easy to access. One defense lawyer, representing insurance companies and employers on work-related cases, blatantly admitted that he examined confidential therapy notes within managed care files to see if he could get clients to "look like Charlie Manson" (Schultz, 1994, p. A5). Not surprisingly, the public's generally held belief that sensitive records are protected by doctor–patient confidentiality is considered by lawyers to be more myth than reality. Medical benefits experts report that once therapy files are in the possession of employers and insurance companies, "so are the temptations to tap it, for a variety of reasons that have nothing to do with keeping employees healthy" (Schultz, 1994, p. A1).

VIOLATION OF FEDERAL LAW

Federal law is in place to protect certain client rights, but managed care companies often do not adhere either to disclosure or to redisclosure regulations. Even in the area of alcohol and drug abuse treatment, for which by law confidentiality requirements are very strict (Confidentiality Law, 1992), private insurance carriers and managed care entities "routinely share information through vast computerized networks" (LAC, 1995, p. 19). For example, one insurer "placed information about claims for reimbursement for drug abuse treatment on recorded telephone messages easily retrievable by anyone who has access to the patient's social security number" (LAC, 1995, p. 19). Such a cavalier approach to sensitive information is reflected again by managed care personnel who "frequently redisclose to third parties (for example, insurance companies, other health care providers, or government agencies) information that identifies the client as having received alcohol or drug services" (LAC, 1995, p. 86), even though such a practice is prohibited by statute and tradition.

VIOLATION OF RESEARCH PROTOCOL

It is important to recognize that research conducted within managed care systems, based on client information submitted by providers, ostensibly may be helpful with regard to "practice guidelines" and "efficacious, effective and efficient" treatments (Landers, 1994, p. 3). However, reflecting managed care companies' general tendency to conduct business in an unregulated fashion, the collection of such data may well be out of compliance with accepted guidelines for scholarship and research as outlined in the *NASW Code of Ethics* (National Association of Social Workers, 1994) and federal guidelines about alcohol and drug abuse client records (*Regulations for Confidentiality of Alcohol and Drug Abuse Patient Records,* 1987). In drug and alcohol treatment, for example, when programs permit access to patient-identifying information without the client's specific consent for purposes of research, there must be compliance with a protocol that is independently reviewed and approved by a group of three or more people; with regulations about securing data, including electronically stored data; with procedures for locking and blocking protected information; and with rules about access to the data only by authorized and qualified researchers (*Regulations for Confidentiality of Alcohol and Drug Abuse Patient Records,* 1987, § 2.52). In the evolving managed care industry, it is evident that such protection of research data is frequently breached.

ABSENCE OF KNOWN BOUNDARIES FOR INFORMATION TRANSFER

Before managed care and the widespread use of information systems, social workers could more reasonably assume that those who were privy to client information were identifiable, occupied a role specific to the provision of client care, were relatively motivated by the best interests of the client, and were able to safeguard the information disclosed by the client. Similarly, the location of hard copies of client records, which were gathered and stored by the clinician or agency, was "more knowable and securable" (LAC, 1995, p. 103) than is presently the case with managed care systems. Now, with a revolving system of unidentified case reviewers, social workers may not know who knows what or who will have access in the future to client disclosures they divulge for the purposes of being included in a managed care network.

PRESSURES ON SOCIAL WORKERS AND CLIENTS TO COMPLY

Clients in managed care environments find themselves compelled to sign consent forms to release information from the social worker to the gatekeeper of managed care services in the hope that doing so will ensure that third-party payments are paid to the provider. Social workers find themselves prevailing on clients to sign these release forms, which in effect relinquish the client's right to privacy, for management purposes, without there being a valid clinical reason to do so.

Confidentiality as a Core Value and Ethical Standard

Confidentiality has traditionally been regarded as a core value of the social work profession (Lindenthal, Jordan, Lentz, & Thomas, 1988; Loewenberg & Dolgoff, 1992; McGowan, 1995). The importance of confidentiality has been emphasized by its inclusion as an ethical standard in the *NASW Code of Ethics,* adopted in 1979 and revised in 1990 and 1994, to "serve as a guide to the everyday conduct of members of the social work profession" (NASW, 1994, p. v).

The *NASW Code of Ethics* (NASW, 1994) exhorts practitioners to "respect the privacy of clients and hold in confidence all information obtained in the course of professional service" (p. 6) and guides social workers to "share with others confidences revealed by clients, without their consent, only for compelling professional reasons" (p. 6). Furthermore, social workers are directed to "inform clients fully about the limits of confidentiality in a given situation, the purposes for which information is obtained, and how it may be used" (p. 6) and "to obtain informed consent of clients before taping, recording, or permitting third-party observation of their activities" (p. 6).

A resource guide on managed care published by NASW specifies that "it is imperative that all clinicians continue to protect the confidential nature of the patient–therapist relationship" (Jackson, 1995, p. 8.5). The guide urges managed care managers and agency staff to develop clear protocols for communicating about clinical issues, and it states that these protocols should be comfortable to clinicians and in accord with state laws and statutes.

Legal Responsibilities to the Social Work Client

It is clear that the social worker's ethical responsibilities and legal duties converge. McGowan (1995) observed that confidentiality is protected legally by a number of case decisions and by statutes granting licensed or certified social workers privileged information status in many states. Schwarz (1989) stressed the legal rights of clients, pointing out that because the law was created for the protection of the client, technically the privilege belongs to the client, not the professional. He explained, "If a client authorizes the disclosure of a privileged communication for purposes of obtaining insurance, such a client is not deemed to have waived the privilege for other purposes," and "the client has the right to limit to whom and for how long the privileged communication will be disclosed" (p. 224).

Social workers have serious legal obligations to maintain confidentiality. Of the six primary legal duties listed by Cournoyer (1991), two refer directly to the obligation to uphold confidential relationships. Besharov and Besharov (1987), examining categories of lawsuits filed against social workers, found that two of the prominent causes for action included breach of confidentiality and violation of clients' civil rights. Kutchins (1991) emphasized that the social worker has a strict fiduciary responsibility to keep information confidential, to tell the client the truth, and to be loyal to the client. He added that the ethical principles outlined in the *NASW Code of Ethics* "are not just desirable conduct to which social workers aspire" but that "if they ignore these ethical mandates, the law governing fiduciary relationships can make them pay dearly" (p. 107), even if the professional's defense is that he or she acted in accordance with accepted practice. The dilemma facing social workers who practice within a managed care environment is that they have a fiduciary responsibility to clients (which by definition is one that is power laden, protective, based on trust, and without any conflict of allegiance) (Kutchins, 1991) and at the same time are asked to give primary loyalty to the managed care network.

Informed Consent to Release Information

Informed consent is much more than the simple matter of signing a piece of paper (Reamer, 1987; Torczyner, 1991). Torczyner and Reamer highlighted as essential standards for valid consent that the person making the decision be competent; that the decision be voluntary and not a result of coercion or captivity or undue influence; and that the client know all the necessary facts, choices, and risks.

With managed care, the technicalities of consent to release information forms, dutifully signed by the client, have been taken to a new level of complicity. A proper legal format for consent to release information about clients in drug or alcohol treatment as defined by the U.S. Department of Health and Human Services includes among other items the name of the individual or organization that will receive the disclosure, how much and what kind of information is to be disclosed, and a statement that the patient may revoke the consent at any time (*Regulations for Confidentiality of Alcohol and Drug Abuse Patient Records,* 1987, § 2.31). With managed care systems the reality is often that the name of the individual or organization receiving the disclosure may change without notice, the information to be disclosed may consist of a verbatim account of the client's most sensitive information given to persuade a gatekeeper to continue to authorize services, and the statement about the client's being able to revoke consent at any time is an illusory proposition given the virtual irretrievability of electronic transmissions of data that are stored in various locations.

Under the auspices of managed care, both the spirit and the letter of social work guidelines relating to confidentiality and informed consent are broken regularly. What the social worker may want to give the managed care company—a molehill of sufficient detail about the client—too often develops into a mountain of intimate detail on computer files, the access to which is outside of the social worker's control. And although some social workers may believe they are protected legally by formal consent agreements, it should be clear that technical permission to disclose information does not solve the ethical problem of clients losing their right to confidentiality, nor does it excuse the social worker from fiduciary responsibilities to the client.

Rather, when social workers prevail on clients to give consent to release information to obtain third-party payments, the ethical problems around the issue of confidentiality are compounded, either by the social workers' active role in soliciting the consent or by their passive role in not advising the client fully of the uncertainty of keeping the information private. Kutchins (1991) put it succinctly: "Informed consent is a time bomb ticking away for social workers and other mental health professionals" (p. 111).

Questions for the Profession

A number of ethical questions emerge with the demise of confidentiality in the context of managed care. Some of these questions concern ethical decision making by the social worker regarding participation in managed care systems, legal issues, social work purpose, fiscal matters, and professional status.

DECIDING TO PARTICIPATE

Social workers may find the following questions of importance as they decide whether, or how, to participate with managed care systems:

- With managed care, is more good extended to more people, and is the sacrifice of confidentiality necessary for this to occur?
- Do the ends justify the means (that is, cooperation with managed care)?
- If a utilitarian philosophy rules the day, how might the most vulnerable members of society be protected (see Rawls, 1971)?
- Is confidentiality fundamentally good, and to what degree should it be extended or limited in a health enterprise?
- Does managed care perpetuate a class distinction whereby poor and middle-class clients are expected to give up the right to a confidential relationship with social workers although wealthy people who can pay independently are not required to do so?
- How much should the client bear the responsibility for his or her own decision about trading the right to confidentiality for services, and how much responsibility should the social worker bear?

LEGAL ISSUES

Questions social workers may have related to legal issues include the following:

- Is a social worker's cooperation with a managed care company inherently in conflict with his or her fiduciary responsibilities related to confidentiality, truth telling, and loyalty to clients?
- Are social workers colluding with managed care personnel to violate clients' civil rights?
- Because it may not be possible to have a clear understanding or accurate knowledge of the accessibility and distribution potential of information released to a managed care entity, are the customary consent to release information forms valid?
- To what degree is the social worker liable should an unforeseen outcome occur about which the client was given no warning?
- Is it always in clients' best interests for social workers to attempt to explain the limits of confidentiality in a managed care environment (what about the very fragile client?), and if not, how will the social worker justify ignoring the duty to tell clients the truth?

SOCIAL WORK PURPOSE

Social workers may need to ponder some of the following questions about professional purpose when working with managed care companies:

- Does the social worker's primary duty shift from the client to the managed care company?

- In a bureaucracy in which individual rights have been supplanted by principles of group management, are social workers moving subtly into a role in which they will function as agents of social control?
- Is the relationship with managed care a slippery slope, wherein the social worker initially discloses benign information but may be called on later to reveal information that could be used to discriminate against vulnerable people (for instance, to identify clients in gay or lesbian relationships, who may be considered high risk for insurance purposes)?
- What are the ethical obligations of social workers to clients as a collective group who appear to have little freedom to challenge this loss of rights to confidentiality or otherwise influence their situation as an organized group?
- Does this situation with managed care constitute a social justice struggle (forecast by Reid & Billups, 1986) against disentitlement and the emphasis on "the minimal rights and statuses of individuals" (p. 14)?

FISCAL MATTERS

A number of questions arise related to social workers' fiscal concerns:

- Because of the need to be paid for services by third-party payers, are social workers and social services agencies forced to sacrifice clients' rights in order to be recompensed?
- How far does the social worker's duty to aid go when there is an "inconvenience" to the self (for example, "punishment" by exclusion from managed care provider lists if designated "uncooperative") (Shapiro, 1995)?

PROFESSIONAL STATUS

Social workers have been diligent in developing standards of practice and a professional image, both of which are now threatened by dictates of managed care organizations. Practitioners concerned about professional status may ask the following questions:

- Does the advent of managed care accelerate declassification (Meyer, 1983) of the profession, with social workers being compelled to adhere to the managed care companies' directives that breach confidentiality?
- Is it right for managed care companies to have external authority over traditional social work standards of ethics, hierarchical ethical guidelines developed within the profession (Loewenberg & Dolgoff, 1992; Reamer, 1987; Rhodes, 1991), and even the social worker's internal ethical judgments?
- What are the costs of turning back the clock on social workers' fight for privileged communication with their clients?
- By agreeing to an administrative plan that undermines confidentiality, have social workers and social services agencies allowed professional honor to give way to expedience?

Recommendations for Change

Managed care appears to be here to stay, and soon almost all social work services, whether public or private, will be influenced by managed care systems. It is hoped that because managed care is a new and developing industry, the profession can influence its various forms and levels of administration. Given that managed care originated from cost-containment efforts of insurance companies and employers, there now needs to be a strong countermovement from social workers intent on serving clients fairly and not simply managing organizations efficiently.

To regain some of the ground that has been lost with regard to confidential care, the following changes are proposed:

- A depersonalized coding system should eventually replace all permanent entries into the computer databases maintained by managed care companies, with the main objective being to camouflage client-identifying information. If managed care companies' genuine purpose in monitoring clients' progress is to improve treatment and to track effective interventions, then these depersonalized records can be used to achieve this end.
- In keeping with NASW guidelines (Jackson, 1995), the computer software used in the transfer of client data should be restricted to use by certain personnel and should block sensitive information that could lead to patient identification. At the same time, tight confidentiality protocols should be maintained by all employees.
- All contracts with managed care companies should state explicitly the expectation of confidentiality in writing (Corcoran & Vandiver, 1996).
- Providers should refuse managed care contracts that include nondisclosure clauses (which restrict clinicians' discussion with clients about limitations imposed by the managed care organization). Social workers and their professional organizations should give unequivocal support to members of the profession taking such a stance.
- Outpatient case notes or hospital files should not be copied in part or whole into the databases of managed care or insurance companies.
- Clients should have the opportunity to review records that have been given by the social worker to the managed care company. This review should be made easily and routinely, if desired.
- Any personal information that is put on the files of managed care companies should be destroyed after service is concluded, and managed care companies should comply with federal regulations requiring the elimination of all patient-identifying information on completion of an audit or evaluation.
- If one managed care company is purchased by another company, clients should be notified of the change and guaranteed access to their records.
- If a government body, agency, or person wishes to gain access to information in the database of a managed care company, clients should be notified before the access is made and given veto power over dissemination of the records. In the event this does not occur, managed care companies should be liable for any personal injury that may ensue, based on violations of disclosure or redisclosure laws.
- Gatekeepers and case reviewers for managed care companies should be identifiable and held to the same standards of keeping information confidential as the professionals providing services.
- Managed care companies should be required to have periodic reviews of their record handling and storage of client data by an independent, external examiner with the authority to establish penalties if confidentiality has not been safeguarded.

- Individual social workers, groups of social workers, and organizations such as NASW must recognize their obligation to refuse to comply with managed care directives that contravene clients' rights and should work collectively in this regard.

Implementing those recommendations would address some of the ethical and legal questions that have been raised. If those recommendations were put into effect, social workers could better work with managed care systems without abrogating their legal and ethical responsibilities to protect confidentiality.

Conclusion

Managed care, with its many facets, has developed with the political, economic, and moral changes in American culture. Health and mental health care costs are high, emphasis is shifting from the care of one to the management of many, and the economic climate is such that managed care personnel are positioned to limit services to clients and to limit the power of social work professionals to provide those services. It would be naive to assume that landmark achievements relating to ethical and legal protection of clients would remain unchallenged when economic determinants are so different.

Within this context, it is important for social workers to resist the temptation to "go along to get along" in an effort to survive alongside an industry that is apparently adjusting to a downsizing economy. Clients' rights and the social work ethical and legal commitment to confidentiality are worth fighting for, particularly given that the managed care approach to confidentiality is determined by business interests in controlling resources, not the scarcity of resources. Huge windfall profits, coupled with the understanding that private client information is essential to the cost-containment efforts of managed care, debunk claims to the contrary.

Like any other industry, however, managed care will seek to protect its consumer base to whatever degree is feasible, including safeguarding confidential information, if doing so retains high currency in the culture of providers and consumers. Social workers can defend the value of confidentiality rationally on the basis of good business practices in a free-enterprise system. Specifically, they can highlight to managers the business merits of pleasing the customer by honoring confidentiality and treating client data with respect and of removing the risks of legal action. Thus, social workers' ethical and altruistic endeavors to salvage confidentiality and protect clients can be framed as compatible with businesses' self-interested motives to avoid punitive damages in court and to keep customers satisfied. Alternatively, social workers can develop and support provider-run networks committed to managing data responsibly, maintaining high professional standards, and using sound management principles.

At the same time, social workers must engage in social action to lobby for changes in managed care organizations' approaches to confidentiality and for legislative restrictions on dissemination of private client data. Social work leaders, theorists, and researchers need to publicly address the problems around confidentiality that practitioners face on a daily basis. Sadly, members of the profession have been largely silent about these critical challenges to confidentiality or have tended to gloss over problems with euphemistic language or naive optimism.

Because of technological changes and new management initiatives, clients no longer have the right to confidential relationships with their social workers. Confidentiality used to be set within an environment of restrained disclosure but now is lost in a culture of information processing. Social workers need to be clear that client information passed on to managed care companies is data with a purpose beyond the health care needs of a particular individual. Social workers need to re-examine their ethical and legal responsibilities to clients and to challenge managed care personnel to protect the clients' right to confidentiality.

References

Besharov, D. J., & Besharov, S. H. (1987). Teaching about liability. *Social Work, 32,* 517–522.

Confidentiality Law, 42 U.S.C. § 290dd-2 (1992).

Corcoran, K., & Vandiver, V. (1996). *Maneuvering the maze of managed care: Skills for mental health practitioners.* New York: Free Press.

Cournoyer, B. (1991). *The social work skills workbook.* Belmont, CA: Wadsworth.

Henneberger, M. (1994, October 9). Managed care changing practice of psychotherapy. *New York Times,* pp. A1, A50.

Jackson, V. H. (Ed.). (1995). *Managed care resource guide for social workers in agency settings.* Washington, DC: NASW Press.

Kutchins, H. (1991). The fiduciary relationship: The legal basis for social workers' responsibilities to clients. *Social Work, 36,* 106–113.

Landers, S. (1994, September). Managed care's challenge: "Show me!" *NASW News,* p. 3.

Legal Action Center. (1995). *Confidentiality: A guide to the federal law and regulations* (3rd ed.). New York: Author.

Lindenthal, J. J., Jordan, T. J., Lentz, J. D., & Thomas, C. S. (1988). Social workers' management of confidentiality. *Social Work, 33,* 157–158.

Loewenberg, F. M., & Dolgoff, R. (1992). *Ethical decisions for social work practice* (4th ed.). Itasca, IL: F. E. Peacock.

McGowan, B. G. (1995). Values and ethics. In C. H. Meyer & M. A. Mattaini (Eds.), *The foundations of social work practice* (pp. 28–41). Washington, DC: NASW Press.

Meyer, C. H. (1983). Declassification: Assault on social workers and social services [Editorial]. *Social Work, 28,* 419.

National Association of Social Workers. (1994). *NASW code of ethics.* Washington, DC: Author.

Rawls, J. (1971). *A theory of justice.* Cambridge, MA: Harvard University Press.

Reamer, F. (1987). Informed consent in social work. *Social Work, 32,* 425–429.

Regulations for Confidentiality of Alcohol and Drug Abuse Patient Records, 42 C.F.R. Part 2, §§ 2.31, 2.52 (1987).

Reid, P. N., & Billups, J. O. (1986). Distributional ethics and social work education. *Journal of Social Work Education, 22*(1), 6–17.

Rhodes, M. L. (1991). *Ethical dilemmas in social work practice.* Milwaukee, WI: Family Service America.

Schultz, E. E. (1994, May 18). Open secrets: Medical data gathered by firms can prove less than confidential. *Wall Street Journal,* pp. A1, A5.

Schwarz, G. (1989). Confidentiality revisited. *Social Work, 34,* 223–226.

Shapiro, J. S. (1995). The downside of managed mental health care. *Clinical Social Work Journal, 23,* 441–451.

Torczyner, J. (1991). Discretion, judgment, and informed consent: Ethical and practice issues in social action. *Social Work, 36,* 122–128.

CHAPTER 29

Managed Care: Ethical Considerations

Frederic G. Reamer

Managed care offers, at once, both a sobering future for social workers and genuine opportunities for practitioners who are prepared to adjust to the exigencies of a rapidly changing health care landscape. The scholarly literature highlights the more glaring trends in managed health care, particularly in relation to the provision of acute, primary, and tertiary health care and mental health services (including institutional and community- or home-based settings) and to the shift away from independent providers reimbursed under a fee-for-service arrangement and toward provider networks, capitation, and managed competition and care (American Medical Association [AMA], 1995; Caughey & Sabin, 1995; Ross & Croze, 1997). If all goes according to plan, managed care's proponents argue, this drift—although some critics would say "frenzied rush"—toward managed care will result in more rather than less clinical freedom, fewer bureaucratic rules, more efficient use of health care resources, increased emphasis on health promotion and prevention, greater profit, lower rates of inflation in health care costs, and enhanced patient satisfaction. That is a tall order, of course. How accurate this ambitious prognostication is remains to be seen and, ultimately, is an empirical question. We will need time, perhaps lots of it, before we know whether managed care can deliver all of the promised goods.

In the meantime, social workers must be responsible observers and, where appropriate, constructive critics of managed care. All of us have heard horror stories and troubling anecdotes about managed care's "underbelly." These tales include sagas involving clients in desperate need of help who were not able to obtain authorization for additional assistance; clients who were required to obtain services from one provider when they and their social worker thought another was more appropriate; and clients whose privacy was compromised during the managed care dance (Gorden & Kline, 1997) (see also chapter 28). Some of these tales may be exaggerated and embellished for dramatic or political effect, but many are not. Some of these stories provide compelling evidence that those responsible for implementing

NOTE: Portions of this chapter are adapted from Reamer, F. G. (1997). Managing ethics under managed care. *Families in Society, 78,* 96–101. An earlier version of this work was presented at "The First Managed Care Behavioral Health Care Invitational Conference for New England Graduate Social Work Faculty," funded by the Robert Wood Johnson Foundation, the National Institute of Mental Health, and the Alcohol and Drug Institute at the Boston University School of Social Work, October 1997, Boston.

managed care need to be mindful of a wide range of ethical concerns (Reamer, 1997a). Here are several examples involving health and mental health issues:

> A 27-year-old man presented with symptoms of depression. He had a history of substance abuse and had just broken off a long-standing relationship. He was HIV-positive and made occasional, vague suicidal comments. The social worker obtained approval for six sessions and then sought approval for at least four more. The social worker's request was denied because, according to the managed care company representative, "the client appears to be stabilized and doesn't pose an imminent risk."
>
> * * *
>
> A 19-year-old woman presented with symptoms of low self-esteem and problems in her relationship with her parents. After the fifth session, the clinical social worker concluded that the woman also manifested symptoms of a serious eating disorder. The social worker arranged for a psychiatric consultation, which confirmed her suspicion. The social worker and psychiatrist tried to hospitalize the client at a nearby, well-known hospital with a highly regarded eating disorders clinic. The managed care representative informed the social worker and psychiatrist that the company would authorize hospitalization only at a psychiatric unit of a community hospital that is a 45-minute drive away, with which the insurance company had negotiated a lower daily rate.
>
> * * *
>
> A 47-year-old man and his 42-year-old wife saw a social worker for marriage counseling. The couple focused on their frequent fighting, the husband's alcohol problem, and the wife's allegations of domestic violence. The husband acknowledged his drinking problem and his tendency to lose his temper, particularly when he is under the influence of alcohol. Between the fourth and fifth counseling sessions, the wife called the social worker to report that her husband had gotten drunk and had threatened to beat her. During the next counseling session the husband admitted he made the threat. The social worker was concerned about the husband's explosive tendencies. The managed care company, however, did not authorize additional counseling sessions.
>
> * * *
>
> A North Carolina appeals court ruled that the estate of a patient who committed suicide two weeks after being released from a hospital against his treating physician's medical judgment stated a wrongful death action for willful and wanton misconduct because the release decision was based on the expiration of the patient's insurance coverage. ("Patient Commits Suicide after Release," 1995, p. 1)

If nothing else, these case illustrations should grab our collective attention. They highlight some of the potential clinical and ethical risks that accompany managed care. These anecdotes also lead to two overarching questions:

1. Can social workers consider costs, provide services under significant cost constraints, and still practice ethically?

2. Assuming it is appropriate for social workers to consider costs and provide services under significant cost constraints, how can they do so in an ethical fashion, in accord with prevailing ethical norms in social work and as stated in the *NASW Code of Ethics* (National Association of Social Workers, 1996), and in a manner that minimizes their legal vulnerability and exposure?

Before I explore these ethical issues in some modest depth, let me state the assumptions on which I will base my observations (AMA, 1995; Reamer, 1997c; Sabin, 1994; Schreter, Sharfstein, & Schreter, 1994; Simon & Sadoff, 1992):

- Managed care is shifting control for social services from the service provider to the payer. We are in the midst of a dramatic shift from what traditionally was a two-party relationship (involving the social worker and client, primarily) to a three-party relationship (involving the insurer) and often to a four-party relationship (involving managed care organizations).
- Managed care will continue to encourage the use of "lower," less expensive levels of care. Forms of care that are lower in the social services "food chain"—such as self-help groups, occasional outpatient treatment, and some types of home-based care—will be favored over forms of care such as residential programs, hospitals, and other institutional settings.
- When residential, hospital, or institutional care is required, lengths of stay will be relatively short.
- There will be pressure on social workers to demonstrate their cost effectiveness to justify their existence in health care settings.
- Fiscal management will become more important than clinical management.
- Definitions of what constitutes appropriate clinical outcome will change, with increased emphasis on "managing episodes" as opposed to providing continuous care.
- Financial risk for social services will continue to shift from the payer to the service provider as a result of increased use of capitation and prospective, rather than retrospective, payment.

I believe there are two ways to think about the ethical issues generated by these assumptions and trends. First, social workers need to think about the diverse ethical dilemmas that practitioners and administrators are facing and will face under managed care. Social workers need to pay particular attention to what ethicists call the problem of "divided loyalties," in this instance between their loyalty to their clients and the duties they owe their employers and third-party payers (Kutchins, 1991; Levy, 1972, 1973; Loewenberg & Dolgoff, 1996; Reamer, 1990, 1995b, 1995d, 1997a; Rhodes, 1986). Social workers operating in managed care environments sometimes will face a number of exceedingly daunting ethical challenges about providing inadequate or insufficient services to clients whose problems require greater assistance than managed care will authorize; terminating services to clients who appear to be in need of additional help; exposing clients to possible privacy and confidentiality invasions; and exaggerating clients' clinical symptoms, diagnoses, and prognoses to obtain authorization for services. Social work administrators will need to make some difficult judgments about allocating scarce resources, a form of administrative triage if you will, or what ethicists refer to as problems of "distributive justice" (Dworkin, 1981; Rae, 1981; Reamer, 1993; Spicker, 1988). When resources are limited, which programs will be cut or trimmed? Whose needs are most compelling? What criteria should be used to allocate limited resources? Should resources be distributed based on some form of equality—that is, by distributing equal slices of the budgetary pie, by virtue of a lottery, or on a first come–first served basis—or by some kind of rank-ordering reflecting clients' needs, affirmative action principles, clients' ability to pay, or clients' prognoses? Those are not purely administrative decisions; they have ethical implications as well.

In addition, social workers practicing in managed care environments need to be mindful of potential ethical misconduct and legal and liability risks ("Preventing Liability in the Managed Care Setting," 1994). Malpractice, a form of professional negligence, occurs when practitioners act in a manner inconsistent with the profession's standards of care (Austin, Moline, & Williams, 1990; Reamer, 1994, 1995c). Malpractice can occur as a result of acts of commission (such as misfeasance or malfeasance) or acts of omission (or nonfeasance). A standard of care is determined by what an ordinary, reasonable, and prudent practitioner would do under the same or similar circumstances (Cohen, 1979; Cohen & Mariano, 1982; Dickson, 1995).

With respect to managed care, social workers need to be concerned especially about several malpractice, negligence, and liability risks. First, social workers must comply with informed consent standards and ensure that clients fully understand and consent to the treatment made available to them, including any relevant risks that may be associated with limits to treatment imposed by third-party payers (Reamer, 1987; Rozovsky, 1984). Social workers can discharge their ethical responsibility and protect clients by informing clients that social workers' delivery of services may be influenced and constrained by policies of and restrictions imposed by third-party payers and care managers. Social workers should inform clients about their benefit limits, the authorization process required by the care manager, clients' right to appeal utilization decisions, the potential invasion of clients' privacy as a result of the review process, and any other service options clients may have (Annas, 1997; Corcoran & Vandiver, 1996; Strom-Gottfried & Corcoran, 1998). Such disclosure should be part of the contract between social workers and their clients.

Second, social workers should be familiar with prevailing standards concerning the handling of clients who are engaged in self-harming behaviors, pose a suicide risk, or threaten to harm a third party. This is particularly important in light of the possibility that under managed care social workers will not be authorized to provide as much service to such high-risk clients as they might prefer (Houston-Vega, Nuehring, & Daguio, 1997). Third, social workers should be clear about their obligations to consult with colleagues when faced with high-risk or ethically ambiguous situations (Fletcher, 1986; Fletcher, Quist ,& Jonsen, 1989; Reamer, 1995a). Fourth, social workers should understand their obligations to clients whose insurance benefits have run out. Social workers cannot simply "abandon" clients whose benefits have been exhausted; rather we are obligated to refer clients to other service providers or, if possible, continue serving clients at a reduced fee or pro bono. Finally, social work supervisors must be careful to monitor supervisees closely to protect clients, supervisees, and themselves (Reamer, 1989). Under the doctrine of *respondeat superior* ("let the master respond") or vicarious liability, social work supervisors can be found partly liable for negligent acts committed by supervisees if there is evidence that the supervision was flawed somehow (for example, with respect to frequency, duration, or content). In their efforts to manage ethical issues associated with managed care, social workers also should consult relevant standards in the *NASW Code of Ethics* (NASW, 1996), particularly those related to informed consent

(1.03a), conflicts of interest (1.06a), client confidentiality (1.07b–e), termination of services (1.16b,e), consultation (2.05), referral for services (2.06), and billing for services (3.05) (Reamer, 1997b, 1998).

Social workers are responding to the proliferation of managed care as though it were a given, a phenomenon carved in stone. This may be the case—to use a different metaphor, perhaps this is a tide that will not be turned. If that is so, we should all hope that this service delivery approach only enhances the quality of care made available to people in need and does not lead to wholesale (or even retail) compromises in clients' access to services. Social workers are obligated to monitor the implementation of managed care and challenge any efforts made in the name of managed care to limit or withhold social services to those who genuinely need them (Siporin, 1992). Social work cannot afford to abandon our long-standing commitment to meeting clients' needs, particularly the needs of those who are the least advantaged, the most vulnerable, and oppressed.

References

American Medical Association. (1995). Ethical issues in managed care. *JAMA, 273,* 330–335.

Annas, G. J. (1997). Patients' rights in managed care: Exit, voice, and choice. *New England Journal of Medicine, 337,* 210–215.

Austin, K. M., Moline, M. E., & Williams, G. T. (1990). *Confronting malpractice: Legal and ethical dilemmas in psychotherapy.* Newbury Park, CA: Sage Publications.

Caughey, A., & Sabin, J. (1995). Managed care. In D. Calkins, R. J. Fernandopulle, & B. S. Marino (Eds.), *Health care policy* (pp. 88–101). Cambridge, MA: Blackwell Science.

Cohen, R. J. (1979). *Malpractice: A guide for mental health professionals.* New York: Free Press.

Cohen, R. J., & Mariano, W. E. (1982). *Legal guidebook in mental health.* New York: Free Press.

Corcoran, K., & Vandiver, V. (1996). *Maneuvering the maze of managed care: Skills for mental health practitioners.* New York: Free Press.

Dickson, D. T. (1995). *Law in the health and human services.* New York: Free Press.

Dworkin, R. (1981). What is equality? Part 2: Equality of resources. *Philosophy and Public Affairs, 10,* 283–345.

Fletcher, J. (1986). The goals of ethics consultation. *Biolaw, 2,* 36–47.

Fletcher J. C., Quist, N., & Jonsen, A. R. (1989). *Ethics consultation in health care.* Ann Arbor, MI: Health Administration Press.

Gorden, R., & Kline, P. M. (1997). Should social workers enroll as preferred providers for for-profit managed care goups. In E. Gambrill & R. Pruger (Eds.), *Controversial issues in social work ethics, values, and obligations* (pp. 52–62). Boston: Allyn & Bacon.

Houston-Vega, M. K., Nuehring, E. M., & Daguio, E. R. (1997). *Prudent practice: A guide for managing malpractice risk.* Washington, DC: NASW Press.

Kutchins, H. (1991). The fiduciary relationship: The legal basis of social workers' responsibilities to clients. *Social Work, 36,* 106–113.

Levy, C. S. (1972). The context of social work ethics. *Social Work, 17,* 488–493.

Levy, C. S. (1973). The value base of social work. *Journal of Education for Social Work, 9*(1), 34–42.

Loewenberg, F., & Dolgoff, R. (1996). *Ethical decisions for social work practice* (5th ed.). Itasca, IL: F. E. Peacock.

National Association of Social Workers. (1996). *NASW code of ethics.* Washington, DC: Author.

Patient commits suicide after release. (1995). *Mental Health Law News, 10*(9), 1.

Preventing liability in the managed care setting. (1994, January). *Mental Health Legal Review,* 1–3.

Rae, D. (1981). *Equalities.* Cambridge, MA: Harvard University Press.

Reamer, F. G. (1987). Informed consent in social work. *Social Work, 32,* 425–429.

Reamer, F. G. (1989). Liability issues in social work supervision. *Social Work, 34,* 445–448.

Reamer, F. G. (1990). *Ethical dilemmas in social service* (2nd ed.). New York: Columbia University Press.

Reamer, F. G. (1993). *The philosophical foundations of social work.* New York: Columbia University Press.

Reamer, F. G. (1994). *Social work malpractice and liability.* New York: Columbia University Press.

Reamer, F. G. (1995a). Ethics consultation in social work. *Social Thought, 18,* 3–16.

Reamer, F. G. (1995b). Ethics and values. In R. L. Edwards (Ed.-in-Chief), *Encyclopedia of social work* (19th ed., Vol. 1, pp. 893–902). Washington, DC: NASW Press.

Reamer, F. G. (1995c). Malpractice claims against social workers: First facts. *Social Work, 40,* 595–601.

Reamer, F. G. (1995d). *Social work values and ethics.* New York: Columbia University Press.

Reamer, F. G. (1997a). Ethical issues for social work practice. In M. Reisch & E. Gambrill (Eds.), *Social work in the 21st century* (pp. 340–349). Thousand Oaks, CA: Pine Forge/Sage Publications.

Reamer, F. G. (1997b). Ethical standards in social work: NASW Code of Ethics. In R. L. Edwards (Ed.-in-Chief), *Encyclopedia of social work* (19th ed., Suppl., pp. 113–123). Washington, DC: NASW Press.

Reamer, F. G. (1997c). Managing ethics under managed care. *Families in Society, 78,* 96–101.

Reamer, F. G. (1998). *Ethical standards in social work: A critical review of the* NASW Code of Ethics. Washington, DC: NASW Press.

Rhodes, M. L. (1986). *Ethical dilemmas in social work practice.* London: Routledge & Kegan Paul.

Ross, E. C., & Croze, C. (1997). Mental health service delivery in the age of managed care. In T. R. Watkins & J. W. Callicutt (Eds.), *Mental health policy and practice today* (pp. 346–361). Thousand Oaks, CA: Sage Publications.

Rozovsky, F. A. (1984). *Consent to treatment: A practical guide.* Boston: Little, Brown.

Sabin, J. E. (1994). Caring about patients and caring about money. *Behavioral Sciences and the Law, 12,* 317–330.

Schreter, R. K., Sharfstein, S. S., & Schreter, C. A. (Eds.). (1994). *Allies and adversaries: The impact of managed care on mental health services.* Washington, DC: American Psychiatric Press.

Simon, R. I., & Sadoff, R. L. (1992). *Psychiatric malpractice: Cases and comments for clinicians.* Washington, DC: American Psychiatric Press.

Siporin, M. (1992). Strengthening the moral mission of social work. In P. N. Reid & P. R. Popple (Eds.), *The moral purposes of social work* (pp. 71–99). Chicago: Nelson-Hall.

Spicker, P. (1988). *Principles of social welfare.* London: Routledge & Kegan Paul.

Strom-Gottfried, K., & Corcoran, K. (1998). Confronting ethical dilemmas in managed care: Guidelines for students and faculty. *Journal of Social Work Education, 34,* 109–119.

CHAPTER 30

Documentation of Client Dangerousness in a Managed Care Environment

Jay Callahan

The increase in managed care organizations has engendered much closer scrutiny of many aspects of social work practice. The rapid establishment of a therapeutic alliance, thorough evaluation, cost-efficient treatment, limited numbers of hospital days or outpatient sessions, and adequacy of the clinical record are all aspects of care that are being closely examined. In this environment, the production of written records is one primary way in which practitioners justify the process of treatment. Over the past several decades, gradual changes have occurred in what is generally expected in the clinical record (Kagle, 1983, 1984, 1993; Reamer, 1994). Managed care has accelerated this process. Contemporary records have quite different goals and contents than earlier ones. This chapter outlines historical changes in and highlights current guidelines for record keeping, focusing on the documentation of information relating to client dangerousness such as suicide and violence directed at others.

Historical Trends

Traditionally, social work records were "broadly focused on understanding clients in the context of their history and current relationships and on describing and analyzing the process of treatment and change" (Kagle, 1993, p. 193). Client records were thought to serve a number of functions: administrative, treatment, teaching, and research (Hamilton, cited in Kagle, 1983). Other conceptions of record keeping have defined its functions as service continuity, peer review, supervision, and consultation (Kagle, 1984).

One of the early models of client records, primarily used for monitoring client progress, education, and supervision, was process recording (Dwyer & Urbanowski, 1965; Wilson, 1980). In process recording, the social worker attempts to document virtually everything that happens in a client session in chronological order, paying special attention to changes in topic or in affective style. Process notes were almost always conceived in a psychodynamic framework. From the 1950s through the 1970s, psychodynamic viewpoints often led social workers to write extremely long psychosocial histories and assessments in narrative style (personal communication

NOTE: Originally published as Callahan, J. (1996). Documentation of client dangerousness in a managed care environment. *Health & Social Work, 21,* 202–207.

with B. Lohr, chief social worker, Adolescent and Child Psychiatry, University of Michigan, Ann Arbor, October 13, 1995).

Over the past 15 years, however, standards and expectations have changed. There has been a gradual transition from narrative styles of documentation to brief, problem-oriented approaches written in behaviorally specific, concrete terms (Bertsche & Horejsi, 1980; Kane, 1974). The increasing emphasis on monitoring of services by insurance companies, licensing boards, and regulatory agencies has been an important influence.

Documentation and Accountability

By the 1990s, the goals and functions of record keeping had changed dramatically. The audience for the clinical record is no longer the social worker, supervisor, and colleagues. The new "wider audience" (Kagle, 1993) includes third-party payers, clients themselves, their families, and the courts. Increasingly, the central function of record keeping is monitoring and accountability. Accountability means that the record confirms that the social worker is providing the service claimed and that the service is done in a professional, competent manner.

Confirmation is a primary concern to third-party payers, managed care firms, and health maintenance organizations (HMOs). Particularly in a managed care environment, fiscal responsibility, the rational allocation of scarce treatment resources, and the "medical necessity" of treatment are emphasized. In these instances, the payer has a fiduciary responsibility to ensure that contracted services are provided. For example, Blue Cross and Blue Shield of Michigan (BCBSM) (1992) published the following guidelines: "High standards of record keeping are required to support professional claims. . . . Third party payers such as BCBSM must be sure they are paying for therapy and procedures that actually were provided and that were appropriate, reasonable and necessary" (pp. A1–A2). Case records are the social worker's primary means of documenting provision of services.

Demonstration that the treatment was consistent with professional standards of the field is targeted at an audience that includes the client, his or her family and attorney, and the courts. Behavior inconsistent with the standard of care is negligence, and when a client or another person is harmed in the process, negligence is an important component in a finding of malpractice (Cohen, 1979; Schutz, 1982). The clinical record is used to demonstrate that the social worker was not negligent.

Managed care has underscored the use of the clinical record for confirmation and defensive purposes. Many managed care contracts with clinicians include a provision for the indemnification of the managed care company: If a managed care firm denies reimbursement for a particular course of treatment and the social worker is sued because of this lack of treatment, the social worker is solely legally liable for any malpractice action (Appelbaum, 1993; Petrila, 1995).

Perhaps the most difficult and important clinical decisions occur in situations of potential danger in mental health, substance abuse, and family services agencies. In these settings situations arise in which clients present risks of physical danger to themselves or to others. Responding to these difficult situations in clinically appropriate ways is clearly a paramount responsibility. Careful documentation of this response is also important but is a topic rarely discussed in educational or practice settings. A recent survey of social work programs revealed that most paid only cursory attention to methods of risk assessment, intervention techniques, and documentation (personal communication with B. Bongar, professor, Pacific Graduate School of Psychology, Palo Alto, CA, May 25, 1995). Discussion of record keeping in multidisciplinary settings such as inpatient medical or psychiatric units is beyond the scope of this chapter.

Documentation of Potential Suicide

Potential suicide is an important example of the need for detailed documentation of services. A consensus appears to be developing across a number of disciplines regarding basic standards of care in potential suicide. These emerging standards appear to fulfill both fiduciary accountability and risk management requirements. Primary among these standards is the importance of documentation (Bongar, Maris, Berman, & Litman, 1992). Careful documentation, more than any other method, demonstrates that the social worker has fulfilled the obligations and demonstrated the accountability that managed care and legal risk management require. Verbal testimony in court that certain clinical activities have taken place is allowed, but in situations in which the social worker is defending his or her previous behavior, written records carry much more credibility. Lawyers often say, "If it isn't written, it didn't happen" (Bongar et al., 1992; Reamer, 1994; Schutz, 1982).

ASSESSMENT OF SUICIDE RISK

In addition to the basic requirement of documentation, it is important to include in the record explicit assessment of suicide risk at all levels of care, especially in the transition from inpatient to outpatient or from partial hospitalization or intensive outpatient to routine outpatient (Maris, Berman, Maltsberger, & Yufit, 1992). Especially after stressful life events, an explicit assessment that includes a brief listing of risk factors and protective factors and an overall risk estimation should be documented (Bongar et al., 1992; Gutheil, 1980). For example,

> The client states that she thinks about suicide occasionally and made a previous attempt in a similar situation six years ago. However, she has no explicit method in mind, denies intent, is not hopeless or highly agitated, has never known anyone who has died by suicide, and is cooperative and engaged in treatment. Overall risk is low. Will continue outpatient treatment on a weekly basis.

* * *

> The client states that he is preoccupied with suicide since he lost his job last week. He is highly agitated and depressed, feels ashamed about his situation, and states that he is considering killing himself by carbon monoxide poisoning in his garage. However, he is cooperative with treatment and is hopeful he will get another job in the long run. Nonetheless, his risk appears high at present, and hospitalization is recommended.

A global estimation of risk can normally only be as specific as high, moderate, or low. However, it is important that the summary of risk and protective factors and the plan to follow are congruent with the risk estimation. High risk implies a need for protection, usually hospitalization. Moderate risk implies the need for hospitalization or, at the very least, close monitoring on an outpatient basis (Bongar, 1991;

Bongar et al., 1992). Such close monitoring includes frequent visits; telephone calls between visits; an explicit alliance with a family member, spouse, or roommate; and the removal of lethal means (such as guns and medications) from the client's environment. Taken together, the number, strength, and salience of the protective factors should outweigh the number, strength, and salience of the risk factors when the global risk estimation is low or moderate.

It should be noted that there is no duty to warn in cases of potential suicide. It is not necessary, for example, to warn the family that a person might be suicidal (Bongar et al., 1992). Of course, when the client is a minor the legal consent is derived from the parents, and the usual legal standards of confidentiality do not apply. Protecting information that the client feels is personal while keeping the parents informed about the overall course of treatment is a difficult but necessary clinical task.

CONTRACTS

If the social worker has used a "no-suicide" contract with the client, its details should be documented. A no-suicide contract is a written or verbal agreement between client and social worker in which the client agrees to a certain course of action, other than suicide, should he or she become acutely suicidal. These alternative actions may include calling the social worker, going to a local hospital emergency room, calling a suicide prevention telephone service, or taking some other action. Use of such agreements, although common, is a controversial area among experts in suicide prevention. There is no empirical evidence that such agreements are effective, and some experts feel that they are carried out primarily to reduce the social worker's anxiety and have little effect in preventing suicide (Davidson, Wagner, & Range, 1995; Drye, Goulding, & Goulding, 1973; Holzman, Bongar, Clark, & Drye, 1993).

CLINICAL INTERVENTIONS

When an intervention is clinically indicated but nonetheless involves some risk, it is important to document factors considered in deciding on the intervention. The most common example is the decision not to hospitalize a client who is at moderate risk for suicide. In such a situation, which often involves a client with chronic (as opposed to acute) suicide risk (Fine & Sansone, 1990; Lewin, 1992; Pulakos, 1993; Rosenbluth, Kleinman, & Lowy, 1995), the social worker should "think out loud in the record": He or she should cite the reasons for not hospitalizing the client at present, the pros and cons of the decision, and criteria regarding when hospitalization would be pursued (Bongar et al., 1992; Gutheil, 1980; Reamer, 1994). For example,

> Although this client continues to talk frequently of suicide, has explicitly talked of cutting his wrists, and has made several previous attempts, hospitalization is not appropriate at this time. His previous attempts have all been of low lethality; he is experiencing no specific stresses at this time; and his risk of suicide is chronic, not acute. Previous hospitalizations have led to significant regression and to decreased coping for some time afterward. A main therapeutic focus is the need for the client to take responsibility for his own life, and in the past hospitalization has significantly undermined this process. If his ideation or threats substantially increase, or if his relationship with his girlfriend ends (which he fears), hospitalization may be needed.

RECORDS OF EARLIER TREATMENT

Other specific issues that should be documented include the social worker's attempts to obtain records of previous treatment. Obtaining these records appears to be a general standard of care (Bongar et al., 1992; Monahan, 1993). Because previous records may contain valuable information about the possibility of dangerous behavior, failure to try to obtain them may be considered a breach of duty. A copy of a letter requesting such records is adequate documentation of the request, even if the records themselves are never received, as is so often the case (Bongar et al., 1992; Monahan, 1993).

INCLUSIONS AND OMISSIONS

The preceding recommendations for documentation are not exhaustive. Other more routine elements of evaluation and treatment must also be carefully recorded, such as the diagnostic assessment, psychosocial history, adjunctive interviews, and treatment plan (Kagle, 1993; Reamer, 1994). The social worker should not include process notes in the record, and "intimate, gossipy, or other personal details that are not directly germane to intervention should be omitted" (Reamer, 1994, p. 181). Overall, the social worker should write the record as if the client, the client's family, and the client's attorney will read it (Gutheil, 1980). Provocative or inflammatory words, such as "manipulative," "faking," and "uncooperative," should be avoided. Similarly, the social worker's own subjective inferences, hunches, hypotheses, and guesses should not be included, unless they are carefully phrased and clearly labeled as such (Cohen, 1979; Kagle, 1984; Reamer, 1994). These documentation guidelines are germane in a variety of contexts, but managed care firms' close scrutiny of the behavior and the record keeping of social workers and other clinicians underscores their importance.

Documentation of Potential Violence toward Others

In many ways, potential suicide and potential violence toward others are quite parallel. One unique aspect of potential violence toward others is the well-known "duty to warn" standard (Fisher & Sorenson, 1991; Monahan, 1993). This standard originated in 1969 in *Tarasoff v. Regents of California* (1976) and mandates that in certain circumstances, social workers and other mental health professionals have a duty to protect potential victims from harm threatened by clients. This precedent in case law has been transformed into statutes in many states (Kopels & Kagle, 1993). Originally there was a variety of ways in which a therapist could discharge this duty (Appelbaum, 1985; Runck, 1984), but the usual contemporary practice has been through two primary interventions: (1) initiating voluntary or involuntary hospitalization and (2) warning the potential victim. Implicit in these interventions is the explicit assessment of the risk of violence (Appelbaum, 1985; Kopels & Kagle, 1993).

Assessment of Potential Violence

The social worker should record the results of the assessment of potential violence, including risk factors and protective factors. If the risk is thought to be high, specific action should be taken and documented. Frequently this action includes the consideration of hospitalization, but hospitalization is not appropriate for some clients.

In a managed care environment, hospitalization is ordinarily reserved for clients who are thought to have a condition that will respond to brief, crisis-oriented treatment, such as psychosis, which can be treated with neuroleptic medication. The absence of serious mental illness frequently precludes voluntary hospitalization and even civil commitment, because the legal requirements for commitment in virtually all states include mental illness.

Documentation in such situations would take the form of explanations in the record about why hospitalization is not appropriate or possible. Thorough documentation might include notes of a discussion with the admissions officer of a psychiatric hospital or unit or the utilization review representative of a managed care firm. Some social workers complete required legal paperwork for civil commitment even when the client does not meet legal criteria, providing additional documentation that all steps were taken to try to prevent the client from doing harm.

WARNINGS

High risk of violence by a client also implies the need for protection of potential victims. In many states, the statutes do not require a warning but provide protection from charges of violation of confidentiality implicit in warning a potential victim. Whether the client provides the warning (from the social worker's office) or the social worker provides the warning without the client's knowledge, a summary of the telephone call should be recorded. The person contacted, the exact date and time, and the telephone number called should also be noted. Many state statutes specify that a warning is appropriate when the client "has made a specific threat of violence" (Illinois Mental Health and Developmental Disabilities Confidentiality Act of 1979, 1990 amendments, ch. 91½, § 811) or "where the patient has communicated to the [social worker or mental health professional] a serious threat of physical violence against a reasonably identifiable victim or victims" (Illinois Mental Health and Developmental Disabilities Confidentiality Act of 1979, 1990 amendments, ch. 91½, § 6103).

Many states also provide legal protection for social workers who notify the police in cases of potential violence. The date, time, and name of the police officer who takes the call should be noted. Normally the police department with jurisdiction over the area in which the potential victim lives or works is the appropriate department to call.

RECORD KEEPING

With clients at risk of becoming violent against others, the social worker should document the details of what the client said, what was observed, information obtained from other sources (with a notation as to the source), and an explicit risk estimation. In situations of low or moderate risk, when hospitalization is not pursued or a warning is not given, the social worker should record the plan to be carried out and a justification for that plan. In addition, other possible plans should be noted and the reasons for rejecting them listed (Beck, 1988; Kopels & Kagle, 1993; Monahan, 1993), again, "thinking out loud in the record."

A note such as "client not homicidal" is not very helpful. It is unclear whether this conclusion was based on an overall explicit assessment, the social worker's global intuitive judgment, or a specific client statement. An explicit assessment is needed—a clinical judgment by the social worker. This clinical judgment should be supported by a weighing of risk factors and protective factors, a notation as to the source of the data (when not obvious), and a conclusion as to the overall estimation of risk. A client's denial is only one piece of information, albeit an important piece. A social worker might conclude that the risk of violence is moderate or high even though the client denies any intent. Conversely, a social worker might conclude that the risk of violence is low even though the client has made a threat. In the latter case, of course, other information that leads to this conclusion (such as frequent threats in the past with no associated action) should also be noted in the record. For example,

> This client is enraged at his ex-girlfriend for breaking up with him and has little emotional distance from his anger. He has stated he would like to hurt her in retaliation for the way she has hurt him; his records indicate that he did physically attack a previous girlfriend in an argument about five years ago, and he has a history of bar fights over the past few years. Although he denies any specific intent to harm her, he seems quite capable of being violent. I advised him that I was obligated to warn her that he could possibly harm her, and although he then denied he would do so, he grudgingly acknowledged my concern. I called her, Mary Smith, at 312-555-1234, at 3:15 p.m. on 10/10/97, and advised her of this danger. She thanked me and stated that she already knew of the possibility. At 5:05 p.m. on 10/10/97 I called the Chicago Police Department at 312-555-6789, and advised Officer Cornell of the situation. Although the potential for violence exists, hospitalization is not indicated. This client's violence potential is chronic and fluctuating, and he is not in crisis and does not demonstrate any acute symptomatology that hospitalization would address. I will see him twice per week for the next few weeks as he adjusts to the loss of his girlfriend. He is cooperative and in agreement with this plan.

* * *

> This client is agitated, upset, and angry about being fired. Although he has vaguely stated his desire to "get someone" for what they have done to him, he has never been violent before, does not own any weapons, and acknowledges that his "bark is worse than his bite." He specifically denies that he would ever harm anyone, and he has made no specific threats. Hospitalization is not indicated and no warning is necessary—he has not specifically threatened anyone and the probability that he would become violent is low.

Consultation

There are few areas in social work in which the need for consultation is more important than with potentially dangerous clients. When potential danger exists, it is essential that the social worker obtain outside consultation from an experienced person who is an expert on suicide or client violence. When available, a clinical supervisor is an appropriate consultant. If a supervisor is not present, an outside consultation should be obtained (Bongar, 1993).

This consultation should be recorded by both parties. The social worker should document the consultation in the case record, and the consultant should record a summary of the situation and the recommendations made. When the consultant is not on the staff of the agency in which the social worker is employed, such records should simply be kept indefinitely in the consultant's files (Appelbaum & Gutheil, 1991; Bongar, 1993).

Conclusion

Managed care has accelerated the process of change in many areas of social work. One such area is the clinical record and its increasing use as evidence of the social worker's accountability. Guidelines for documentation and related areas of practice will undoubtedly continue to evolve as health and mental health care undergo dramatic and rapid changes.

References

Appelbaum, P. S. (1985). *Tarasoff* and the clinician: Problems in fulfilling the duty to protect. *American Journal of Psychiatry, 142,* 425–429.

Appelbaum, P. S. (1993). Legal liability and managed care. *American Psychologist, 48,* 251–257.

Appelbaum, P. S., & Gutheil, T. G. (1991). *Clinical handbook of psychiatry and the law* (2nd ed.). Baltimore: Williams & Wilkins.

Beck, J. C. (1988). The therapist's legal duty when the patient may be violent. *Psychiatric Clinics of North America, 11,* 665–679.

Bertsche, A. V., & Horejsi, C. R. (1980). Coordination of client services. *Social Work, 25,* 94–98.

Blue Cross and Blue Shield of Michigan. (1992, March 1). Payment determinations are based on appropriate documentation. *Facility News,* pp. A1–A4.

Bongar, B. (1991). *The suicidal patient: Clinical and legal standards of care.* Washington, DC: American Psychological Association.

Bongar, B. (1993). Consultation and the suicidal patient. *Suicide and Life-Threatening Behavior, 23,* 299–306.

Bongar, B., Maris, R. W., Berman, A. L., & Litman, R. E. (1992). Outpatient standards of care and the suicidal patient. *Suicide and Life-Threatening Behavior, 22,* 453–478.

Cohen, R. J. (1979). *Malpractice: A guide for mental health professionals.* New York: Free Press.

Davidson, M. W., Wagner, W. G., & Range, L. M. (1995). Clinicians' attitudes toward no-suicide agreements. *Suicide and Life-Threatening Behavior, 25,* 410–414.

Drye, R. C., Goulding, R. L., & Goulding, M. E. (1973). No suicide decisions: Patient monitoring of suicide risk. *American Journal of Psychiatry, 130,* 171–174.

Dwyer, M., & Urbanowski, M. (1965). Student process recording: A plea for structure. *Social Casework, 46,* 283–286.

Fine, M. A., & Sansone, R. A. (1990). Dilemmas in the management of suicidal behavior in individuals with borderline personality disorder. *American Journal of Psychotherapy, 44,* 160–171.

Fisher, L., & Sorenson, G. P. (1991). Confidentiality and the duty to warn. In L. Fisher & G. P. Sorenson (Eds.), *School law for counselors, psychologists, and social workers* (2nd ed., pp. 11–31). New York: Longman.

Gutheil, T. G. (1980). Paranoia and progress notes: A guide to forensically informed psychiatric record keeping. *Hospital and Community Psychiatry, 31,* 479–482.

Holzman, A., Bongar, B., Clark, D. C., & Drye, R. (1993, April). *Anti-suicide contracts: Indications and contraindications.* Paper presented at the annual conference of the American Association of Suicidology, San Francisco.

Illinois Mental Health and Developmental Disabilities Confidentiality Act of 1979, as amended 1990, ch. 91 1/2, §§ 811, 6103.

Kagle, J. D. (1983). The contemporary social work record. *Social Work, 28,* 149–153.

Kagle, J. D. (1984). Restoring the clinical record. *Social Work, 29,* 46–50.

Kagle, J. D. (1993). Record keeping: Directions for the 1990s. *Social Work, 38,* 190–196.

Kane, R. A. (1974). Look to the record. *Social Work, 19,* 412–419.

Kopels, S., & Kagle, J. D. (1993). Do social workers have a duty to warn? *Social Service Review, 67,* 101–126.

Lewin, R. A. (1992). On chronic suicidality. *Psychiatry, 55,* 16–27.

Maris, R. W., Berman, A. L., Maltsberger, J. T., & Yufit, R. I. (Eds.). (1992). *Assessment and prediction of suicide.* New York: Guilford Press.

Monahan, J. (1993). Limiting therapist exposure to *Tarasoff* liability: Guidelines for risk containment. *American Psychologist, 48,* 242–250.

Petrila, J. (1995). Who will pay for involuntary civil commitment under capitated managed care? An emerging dilemma. *Psychiatric Services, 46,* 1045–1048.

Pulakos, J. (1993). Two models of suicide treatment: Evaluation and recommendations. *American Journal of Psychotherapy, 47,* 603–612.

Reamer, F. G. (1994). *Social work malpractice and liability.* New York: Columbia University Press.

Rosenbluth, M., Kleinman, I., & Lowy, F. (1995). Suicide: The interaction of clinical and ethical issues. *Psychiatric Services, 46,* 919–921.

Runck, B. (1984). NIMH report: Survey shows therapists misunderstand *Tarasoff* rule. *Hospital and Community Psychiatry, 35,* 429–430.

Schutz, B. M. (1982). *Legal liability in psychotherapy.* San Francisco: Jossey-Bass.

Tarasoff v. Regents of California, 131 Cal. Rptr. 14, 551 P.2d, 334 (1976).

Wilson, S. (1980). *Recording: Guidelines for social workers.* New York: Free Press.

C H A P T E R 31

Evolution and Trends in the Relationship between Clinical Social Work Practice and Managed Cost Organizations

Carlton E. Munson

In the past three decades, there has been an explosion of theory and knowledge about mental health. We have learned an enormous amount about the origin and nature of mental illness. Diagnosis and treatment have been refined, and medications that alleviate mental distress have improved significantly. Licensing and certification for mental health professionals have expanded, and administrative supports for clinicians have grown, especially in the area of computer technology (Munson, 1988). These significant changes have been accompanied by and partially offset by the emergence of an industry commonly referred to as "managed care" or "behavioral health organizations." These businesses have become the chief administrators of mental health services in the United States, and the mental health agencies evolved over the past 60 years largely have been dismantled (Schamess, 1996). Analysis of what has taken place leads to the conclusion that the term "managed care" is a misnomer. The more appropriate term is "managed cost" organizations (MCOs), and that terminology will be used throughout this chapter.

A number of books have been published in the past decade (Ackley, 1997; Alperin & Phillips, 1997; Aronson, 1996; Browning & Browning, 1996; Feldman & Fitzpatrick, 1992; Goodman, Brown, & Deitz, 1992) to assist mental health professionals in "adjusting" to the mandates of MCOs. This chapter focuses on the evolution of MCOs and their effects on social work practice.

Background

We live in a world that constantly threatens our individual autonomy. In our personal lives we are threatened by big government that is widely resented but seems unmanageable. Most people surrender to the forces of control. This is reflected in the constant chant that "change is coming whether you like it or not, so you better get used to it or get out of the way." It conveys a clear message that Americans must

NOTE: Originally published as Munson, C. E. (1996). Autonomy and managed care in clinical social work practice. *Smith College Studies in Social Work, 66,* 241–260. Portions of the chapter were published as Munson, C. E. (1997). The future of clinical social work and managed cost organizations. *Psychiatric Services Journal, 48,* 479–482. The material is reprinted with the permission of the American Psychiatric Association.

accommodate change, regardless of the form it takes or whether it is good or bad. Advocates of managed care use variations on this quote in giving advice to mental health professionals, and this theme serves as the background for this chapter.

Government passes laws to protect "our freedoms," and people then discover that these laws severely restrict their rights. People feel threatened and victimized by large, multinational corporations that reorganize to maximize prices and profits, regardless of the cost to employees and customers. People are increasingly at the mercy of the media and computers even while constantly being bombarded by the illusion that we have "more options." Lasch (1979) and Sullivan (1995) both argued that the loss of personal control is the result of a complex mixture of modern economic conditions, shifting family interaction and structures, and individual cognitive responses.

The loss of individual control in professional life is well documented by Sullivan (1995). As government and private industry downsize and reorganize to "cut costs," mental health practitioners and their clients are faced with a significant loss of autonomy. Not surprisingly, health and mental health care reflect the pervasive loss of autonomy taking place throughout society. The management, cost, and delivery of health and mental health care have become chaotic, but no one seems able to do anything to make the system even slightly more rational.

A mental health client illustrated how chaotic the system can be by describing his most recent experience in choosing a health plan (Goodman et al., 1992): His employer, a large state agency, decided to make the health care plan more cost effective by inviting several companies to offer competing plans. Over the following three years, the client's cost increased by 300 percent, and he remained unsure about what coverage he had. He went to a "health fair" sponsored by his employer at which nine competing companies had "information booths." He described the scene as "bedlam," an interesting term to use because it is derived from one of the earliest mental institutions, St. Mary of Bethlehem, in England. More than 150 people were shouting at the lone representative in each booth. Everyone was grabbing information packets, and supplies were soon exhausted. The employees were panicked because the employer had given them an enrollment deadline. If they did not choose a specific plan by the deadline, they would have no health or mental health coverage until enrollment reopened a year later. At the health fair this participant realized he had completely lost control of his health and mental health care destiny. Most would agree this is not a rational way for people to make major decisions about health care for themselves and their families. On an individual basis, it illustrates the larger view that the U.S. health and mental health care system is in serious crisis.

Restructuring Effects

Society has been undergoing major economic restructuring that has been in progress for the past three decades. Restructuring is driven by a long-term, slow decline in economic growth (Madrick, 1995) that has resulted in the return to a two-tiered social-class structure in the United States (Rose, 1997). Changing economic structures are not resulting from the effects of short-term government policies, as most individual professionals and professional organizations tend to believe. In fact, the focus on the short-term political rather than the long-term economic aspects of restructuring has led professional groups to ignore changes that have significant impact on professional relationships with clients. On an economic level, the rise of managed cost enterprises is simply a cost-containment phenomenon, a reaction to the rising demand for and use of mental health services (Dorwart & Schlesinger, 1988) that provided profitable opportunities for business investors (Rodenhauser & Greenblatt, 1989). At the sociocultural level, the rising demand for mental health services became a social-class issue (Cohen, 1997), and when the demand for treatment expanded from upper-class to middle- and lower-class people, a means had to be found to limit access to psychotherapy. MCOs have been a convenient tool through which upper-class business managers can limit access to mental health services for middle- and working-class employees. The strategy is advantageous for work organizations, because the work environment often gives rise to the stresses in people that produce the need for mental health intervention (Cushman, 1995; Schor, 1991).

There is evidence that privatization has increased options for wealthy people and decreased options for poor people with respect to psychiatric hospital care (Dorwart, Schlesinger, Davidson, Epstein, & Hoover, 1991). For the past four decades, psychotherapy has increasingly become a cognitive and emotional safe haven from the stresses of economic and personal life for many Americans. Psychotherapy was the one remaining place where people could find some comfort, reassurance, and relief, but that refuge has been nearly eliminated in the past seven years for all except wealthy people. It is no accident that increasingly, health and mental health benefits are determined by employing organizations. It is unlikely that governments will make any significant effort to regulate the reactionary policies of MCOs, because governments use MCO strategies to reduce spending (Perkey, 1989). Professional organizations are beginning to become aware of the changes taking place in the social, political, economic, and cultural life of the country, but there is a serious question about whether professional groups can significantly influence, let alone alter, the restructuring described above.

Revolutions in information technology and communication methods have affected power relationships in the private, employment, and social spheres and are redefining the rules of social life as well as concepts of freedom and justice (Altheide, 1995). Massive mainframe and small personal computers have made it possible to manage, control, manipulate, and predict in ways that present people with serious new challenges. Computers and other information technologies make it possible for large corporations to eliminate jobs and centralize functions, thereby increasing profits at the expense of employees and consumers. Technological change has speeded up the pace of institutional activity, thus increasing stress. Employees are expected to accomplish more in less time, for less money. Consumers find many products obsolete almost immediately after they are purchased.

Restructuring also is occurring in the social services and clinical social work sectors. In many states, public social and mental health services are being privatized or contracted to MCOs (Feldman & Fitzpatrick, 1992). No reliable data indicate that privatization cuts costs, but there is compelling evidence that it results in inadequate services for clients and hardships for professionals who work in the privatized environment (Motenko et al., 1995; Munson, 1993b).

At the organizational level, change and technology continue to produce even larger entities. MCOs are directly linked to the concentration of corporate activity in larger entities because corporations prefer to negotiate employee benefits packages with larger insurers whose rates reflect efficiencies of scale. Larger hospitals, chains of nursing homes, and large group psychotherapy practices can be cost efficient without providing efficient or efficacious care. Large organizations assure us of their "entrepreneurial compassion" in dealing with clients and consumers, but we observe that when financial strain occurs, profit becomes the ultimate criterion. In that climate, clients, practitioners, and supervisors receive little or no support and few resources. As corporate entities become larger and more powerful, government programs and private insurance provide people with little protection. The combination of technology and privatization has transformed mental health services from a humanitarian commitment to a private industry. Some argue that mental health has always been an industry, but historically this has not been true, especially in social work. Traditionally, social workers have viewed mental health and other areas of practice as "a calling" rather than an industrial endeavor, that is, manufacturing product units for profit. It is commonplace for managed care officials to refer to the mental health services they provide as "product lines" and to clients as "bodies or lives covered." In the coming years, social work will have to confront a market orientation to mental health services that challenges the most basic social commitments of our profession.

Social Work's Unique Contributions

Historically, social work has made many contributions to the constellation of primary mental health professions. Of these, the most notable are an emphasis on social reform, a powerful focus on client advocacy, and a distinct model of clinical supervision. In regard to social reform, social work's emphasis was short-lived. It peaked in the 1920s (Lundblad, 1995; Reeser & Epstein, 1990) and has been declining since, to the point where advocacy currently is not typically emphasized as a part of either individual or organizational (social agency) practice. Concurrently, the decline in emphasis on social reform has coincided with decreased concern about client advocacy. Both trends have paralleled the development of the managed care model for social work practice. Ironically, social work first developed the short-term therapy models that are hallmarks of managed care. The evolution of short-term treatment can be traced from Mary Richmond (1917) to Helen Harris Perlman's problem-solving approach (1957) to Reid and Epstein's task-centered model (1972). The effects of managed care on the third major contribution, social work supervision, will be discussed later in the chapter.

Effects on Social Work

In many ways, clinical social work reflects society in microcosm. A "speeded-up" society is mirrored in the profession's emphasis on brief therapy and in applications of technology to practice. Among the most important technological innovations with which clinical social workers increasingly must contend is the use of machines to support and supplement their practice. Computers generate social assessments and diagnostic reports. Telephone answering machines, pagers, and word processors are used for accounting and record keeping. The use of audio and video recorders to record sessions for subsequent use in treatment and supervision is becoming more common, and machines are often third parties in treatment sessions. In some settings in which videotaping is considered a valuable therapeutic agent, there are few, if any, guidelines for its use. When used properly, videotaping can enhance treatment, but its improper application can produce desultory and destructive intrusions into the treatment relationship (Munson, 1993a).

Other types of technology increasingly used by clinicians are communication devices such as paging instruments. These devices are commonly used in hospital and public welfare settings and among private practitioners. All of these technologies have implications for psychotherapy-related "high-tech/high-touch" (Naisbitt, 1982) practice. No studies have been done regarding the effects of these devices on practitioner functioning. In some cases they are used voluntarily and in others involuntarily. In addition, there have been no studies of whether these instruments actually improve practitioner response time or effectiveness. Supervisors need to be more cognizant of the effect such devices have on the therapeutic process. Over time, the increased use of machines for communication is likely to result in procedures that minimize or eliminate direct contact between client and therapist and between therapist and supervisor (Handy, 1995).

Advances in technology necessitate greater emphasis on values and ethics in graduate programs. Increased use of machines in practice brings practitioners into closer contact with machine operators, designers, and analysts who have a "machine mentality." In such contacts, practitioners may find that their own values have been compromised, especially in large agencies and medical settings where, increasingly, machines are used on a grand scale. Technology also has increased electronic transmission of sensitive client information over telephone lines and has facilitated long-term archiving of client information in computer storage systems. These changes challenge practitioner values regarding confidentiality and privileged information. Practitioners are losing control of information they generate about clients and often fail to inform clients adequately about the use that organizations such as managed care companies and employers may make of confidential information.

Many of the technological changes noted above are forced on social workers by MCOs. One company, in its efforts to increase the use of electronic claims submissions, found the "lack of automation" by therapists a major hindrance to its automation plans. The company discovered that small and solo practices were the most resistant to technology and that 70 percent of such providers had nothing more sophisticated than a telephone in their offices. In response to these findings, the company embarked on a strategy to increase the use of technology by providers ("Survey Results," 1995).

Managed Cost Organizations

In social work, restructuring has been connected to the growth of MCOs. In 1990, approximately 29 percent of people with health insurance were covered by managed cost contracts. In 1995, 51 percent were covered (Randal, 1995). MCOs are directly connected to corporate restructuring because health care is usually incorporated into overall benefits packages that employers negotiate with one or a number of MCOs. They also are increasingly used to cover client services insured by public social service systems, many of which are being privatized. In these contexts, MCOs play an increasingly significant role in the delivery of mental health services (Munson, 1995a).

The increased use of managed cost models parallels the increased philosophical and practical importance of technology. That is not a new phenomenon. Beliefs about mental functioning and intervention strategies have always been closely connected to scientific theories. For example, in the 19th century, new knowledge about electricity and magnetism generated the belief that mental illness was caused by an unbalanced distribution of magnetic currents in the body. As a result, Franz Mesmer developed a procedure in which magnets were passed over the body to redistribute magnetic energy (Davison & Neale, 1990). A modern example of applying scientific paradigms to therapeutic endeavors is seen in our obsession with technology, especially the ability to complete tasks with ever-increasing speed and efficiency. This obsession has shaped a mental health delivery system organized to deliver specific prepackaged procedures rapidly and without variation to large numbers of clients, resulting in a decrease in the number of sessions allocated to accomplish specific therapeutic goals. The common practice of forcing practitioners to join large group practices also reflects the speeding process, in this instance under the guise of increased efficiency. No documented research demonstrates that any of these actions result in more efficacious treatment or greater productivity. Clinicians should always look for more effective and efficient ways of delivering care, but the managed cost efficiency movement has produced a shift away from clinical process and relationship toward brief, fragmented therapeutic procedures. The problem is compounded by the fact that schools of social work continue to teach process and relationship models of intervention, whereas MCOs approve only mechanistic, task-oriented, linear models. As a result, MSW graduates enter a practice world in which they have not been trained to function effectively.

Change and Autonomy

MCOs and other payers control major aspects of mental health practice in the public and private sector. Payers routinely state that benefits programs and intervention strategies are "fluid." They remind practitioners that mental health care is changing or will change rapidly. Constant change and threats of change concentrate control in the hands of a small number of managers capable of effecting change. This strategy keeps clients and practitioners off balance and renders them incapable of rationally planning treatment or treatment programs. The unbalancing effect of restructuring can be seen when MCOs force solo practitioners to join group practices to better control their therapeutic activities. In some instances, MCOs even buy out group practices, the rationale being that group practices are more effective and cost efficient. No research justifies this claim. Unfortunately, practitioners and professional organizations cannot counter these claims either because they have no research studies that address effectiveness and outcome or because they fail to use the existing outcome research. MCOs have no such difficulty because they have accumulated significantly more outcome data on professional practitioners than any of the major mental health professional organizations. In fact, independent studies by *Consumer Reports* ("Mental Health: Does Therapy Help?" 1995), and the National Advisory Mental Health Council (1993) provide compelling statistics on the positive outcomes of longer-term mental health intervention, as reported by clients. The shortage of professionally sponsored outcome studies and the failure to marshal even readily available research data are key indicators of the degree to which the professions have surrendered authority and control to external entrepreneurs.

Professional Relationships and Autonomy

Client–practitioner relationships are altered significantly by managed cost policies. Increasingly, practitioners receive fewer client referrals because payers are closing provider lists to cut costs. Such policies also affect clients. "Payers," rather than clients, determine which therapist the client will see. By depriving clients of control over whom they see in treatment and over how long they wish to be treated, "payers" violate the social work ethic of self-determination. In some sense, these routine procedures go to the heart of the problem MCOs present: Corporate control replaces client and therapist control in almost every instance.

INITIAL INTERVENTION

Selecting a therapist can be a complex process (Amada, 1995), and the ultimate decision should remain with the client. There is an old rule that if a client starts treatment and does not develop a positive relationship with the therapist, the client should find another therapist. Clients are advised to repeat this process until they find a therapist with whom they feel comfortable working. That choice is no longer available except for wealthy people who can pay for treatment "out of pocket."

Many MCOs implement procedures that reverse the traditional process of a client initiating contact with a therapist. New procedures require clients to contact the insurance company first. In many instances, the company then chooses the therapist from its provider pool and "authorizes" that therapist to meet with the client for a pre-established time, typically one diagnostic and two treatment sessions. Upon receiving authorization, the practitioner contacts the client to initiate treatment. This procedure puts therapists in the position of pursuing clients at the beginning of treatment. After the initial "authorization" expires, the therapist must then contact the company for a second "authorization," which typically results in approval of three to six additional sessions. Often, decisions about additional sessions are made by nonprofessional technicians or case managers using a standardized protocol. Individual client needs and preferences play little or no role in the decision. As a result, the course of treatment is based on financial parameters rather than on a diagnostic assessment. There is no research on how this allocation system affects either the therapeutic relationship or treatment outcome.

FEES

Loss of control over billing by therapists and the use of electronic billing procedures usurp another therapeutic function. A long-standing principle affirms that negotiating fees and discussing payment expectations are essential parts of the therapeutic process. Under current procedures, fees are not negotiated as part of the treatment process but instead are determined by the MCO. In addition, the therapist is often placed at risk for nonpayment when payers "authorize" sessions before therapy begins but deny payment on the basis of some minor technicality when the first claim is submitted. The increased use of electronic billing takes control of the process and mechanics of billing out of the therapists' hands and places it totally under the control of the payer.

PRIVACY AND CONFIDENTIALITY

Clients and therapists also lose control over the right to privacy and confidentiality within managed cost systems. Moreover, record keeping required by government agencies and mandated by recent court decisions severely limits privacy. Increasingly, therapists are required to tell clients that there is *no* confidentiality when the legal system or MCOs are involved. Some MCOs have radically altered the conditions of confidentiality. They require therapists to inform clients of a "no-confidentiality" policy as part of the initial provider agreement. One legal interpretation of no-confidentiality policies is "that the patient has to be told either to give up the right to confidentiality or forgo treatment" (personal communication with W. N. Mathias, May 16, 1995). Informal surveys have found that when a client's care is handled by an MCO, at least 17 people have varying degrees of knowledge about the person's treatment—a conservative estimate according to some experts. In some settings clients must sign confidentiality statements that are three pages in length (Zuckerman & Guyett, 1992).

SUPERVISION

The role of supervision has changed drastically as the locus of control shifts from practitioners to MCOs. Historically, supervisory practices have reflected the degree of autonomous practice endorsed by each of the mental health professions. In social work, a decreased emphasis on practice supervision has paralleled a quest for professional status through autonomous practice. In many states, supervision has been replaced by multiple-choice licensing examinations that constitute the basic method of establishing professional competence. As a result, the monitoring function of supervision has been significantly downgraded. MCOs do not require supervision because their model of accountability is not based on supervisory oversight. Face-to-face individual and group supervision provided by a seasoned clinician has been replaced with telephone and written contacts with managed cost case mangers, many of whom have no clinical background. In this process clinicians not only lose control of treatment but also, in many instances, of reasonable access to the case managers, who make crucial decisions about the availability, duration, and goals of care.

The only times clinicians regain a measure of control is when something goes wrong or there is litigation. The majority of MCOs require clinicians to sign contracts stating they will hold the MCO harmless. This means that still another institution, the courts, becomes involved in controlling what clinicians do. The courts have ruled that under certain conditions, "hold harmless" clauses are invalid. In the process of making these rulings, however, courts have defined specific steps therapists must take to avoid being liable when care or its termination is dictated by an MCO. Court rulings directly affect what therapists can and cannot do in treatment. Decisions in the *Tarasoff* (Munson, 1993a), *Ramona,* and *Diane Franklin* cases (Terr, 1994) and other pending legal actions have direct impact not only on therapist activity, but also on the monitoring function supervisors traditionally perform. The implications of these decisions are slow to affect the average practitioner, but in coming years they will change practice in fundamental ways.

Ironically, the historical complaint that supervision stifles professional responsibility and creativity has not re-emerged, even though managed care practices have eroded professional autonomy far beyond the control functions supervisors previously exercised. In the past, if supervisors had tried to enforce even a small measure of the control MCOs now exercise routinely, professional organizations would have initiated massive negative sanctions against the offenders. It is not clear why, at this point in time, professional organizations are not resisting MCO intrusions on decision making that directly affect client care.

Professional Language

Some clinicians (Corpt & Reison, 1994) advocate that practitioners "behaviorize" the language they use in record keeping to please MCOs. These authors identify a list of professional words that should be replaced with MCO "preferred language." For example, they recommend that "dealing with depression" be replaced with "affect management." Ironically, the suggested language is less descriptive than the original. Such changes involve micromanagement at a level that until recently, most professions would not tolerate. It is difficult to imagine a situation in which a supervisor would dictate the language a practitioner could use in record keeping. And if a supervisor did suggest different wording, it would be to clarify, not obscure. The "prescribed language" of managed care goes to the essence of our professional identity as social workers because language is the most fundamental connection between individuals and society as well as the "ultimate social tool" (Allman, 1994). If a profession is stripped of its own language, not much core of professional humanity or individuality remains. The postmodernists' view of language is relevant here: They hold that language is neither innate nor about communication, but rather involves a series of word games (Flax, 1990). In regard to MCOs, the game is about control.

Corpt and Reison's (1994) recommendations about behaviorizing professional language can be viewed as a kind of supervision guide, with MCOs functioning as the supervisor and practitioners as the supervisees. Corpt and Reison (1994) recommended that practitioners "Conduct . . . evaluation interviews with managed care in mind," remembering "that you are being rated by them on a continual basis" (p. 3). There is an old adage in supervision that the supervisor's role is to be symbolically present, looking over the practitioner's shoulder as treatment occurs (Munson, 1979, 1993a). In contrast to the established practices that guide traditional social work supervision, MCOs never share the results of evaluations with practitioners, even though they constantly rate practitioners on their "ability to take new patients, the thoroughness of . . . assessment and the length and efficacy of the treatment" (Corpt & Reison, 1994, p. 3). Corpt and Reison argued that it is possible to satisfy MCO expectations "without changing your theoretical perspective or without making major alterations in your clinical practice" (p. 4). In their view the degree of control payers exercise has little or no effect on what practitioners do or say and no substantial effect on the outcome of treatment. These assertions are not supported by any substantial body of intervention outcome research.

Research (Munson, in press) on externally determined lengths of treatment illustrates some of the problems involved in predetermining treatment duration. Practitioners were given a written case to analyze and were asked to make a diagnosis and develop a treatment plan. Subjects were randomly assigned six, 12, or unlimited sessions to accomplish their treatment goals. The study found statistically significant differences in diagnosis, treatment plan formulation, and treatment techniques based on the number of "authorized" sessions. It thus appears that predetermining treatment duration has a very significant effect on various aspects of the treatment process, including anticipated outcome. Moreover, the largest treatment outcome survey ever done, consisting of voluntary reports from 4,000 people ("Mental Health," 1995), found that positive outcome was directly linked to length of treatment. People in therapy for six months or longer reported the most improvement. This finding directly contradicts the managed care philosophy that brief therapy is equally or more effective. It also suggests that the MCO strategy of limiting treatment duration may increase rather than reduce long-term costs. Because MCOs rarely authorize anything close to six months of treatment, poor outcomes that cause people to re-enter treatment repeatedly may significantly increase costs over time.

Ethical Issues

The actions of MCOs have produced for social work practitioners serious ethical conflicts that are not being addressed by the profession. It is not surprising that the dramatic increase in professional concern about risk management and legal liability has paralleled the rise of MCOs. There are many contradictory statements in the *NASW Code of Ethics* (National Association of Social Workers, 1990, 1996) that limit its usefulness. However, it is the profession's only ethical guide, and it does state that social workers who subscribe to it, including members of NASW, are required to abide by it. A number of the guiding principles included in the *NASW Code of Ethics* create conflict for clinicians involved with MCOs either as employees or as contract providers. The *Code* requires social workers to

- regard as primary the service obligation of the profession
- accept that their primary responsibility is to clients
- make every effort to foster self-determination for clients
- respect client privacy and hold in confidence information obtained in the course of professional service
- adhere to commitments made to employing organizations
- assist in making social services available to the general public
- retain ultimate responsibility for quality and extent of service
- act to prevent inhumane or discriminatory practices against individuals and groups
- resist influences that interfere with the exercise of professional discretion
- provide clients with accurate and complete information regarding the extent and nature of services available to them
- inform clients of risks and rights associated with services to them
- not share client confidences without their consent, and then only for compelling professional reasons
- not withdraw services precipitously, except under unusual circumstances
- work to improve agency policies, procedures, and effectiveness of service
- take action through appropriate channels against unethical conduct by any other member of the profession
- advocate policy and legislative changes to improve social conditions and promote social justice.

Each item raises unaddressed ethical and moral questions for social workers in relation to MCOs. For example, a significant question posed is whether a social worker who contracts to provide services is an employee of the MCO. In the traditional sense of employment this is not the case, but under current practices it could be argued that social workers are employees and, accordingly, are obligated to "improve the employing agency's policies and procedures." Although some state licensing boards are currently struggling with this as a supervisory and employee–employer issue, the ethical requirements of the social worker–MCO relationship have not yet been clarified.

It has been argued that professional ethics codes are outdated and should be altered to conform with managed cost policies and procedures (Phillips, 1995; Wolf,

1994). The *NASW Code of Ethics* has been revised and modified in ways that reflect aspects of the MCO view of ethics and the new emphasis on "applied ethics" (Reamer, 1992, 1993). A profession that reshapes its ethical principles to comply with corporate managed cost guidelines has lost its moral compass. For ethics codes to be effective they must be clear, consistent, and enduring (Munson, 1995b). Changing our code of ethics to address supervisor–clinician dilemmas related to managed cost policies violates the rules of consistency and endurance. As professionals, we are required to ask which of the *Code* items listed above would we *want* to change to accommodate MCOs? Would we change our responsibilities to clients? The right to privacy? The right to self-determination? The requirement that we work toward changing policies that harm clients? The expectation that practitioners take responsibility for services delivered?

Instead of changing ethical principles, the profession should develop a model of clinical advocacy that helps clients obtain competent, fair, just, and understandable intervention in the managed cost environment. That kind of advocacy evokes a great deal of resistance, because many MCOs have explicit policies that punish providers who advocate for clients. In some cases they do so by removing offending practitioners from their provider lists.

ETHICAL PRACTICE GUIDES

Psychiatry has taken initial steps to identify what is considered ethical practice in relation to MCOs (Macbeth, Wheeler, Sither, & Onek, 1995), and many of the items they identify are relevant to clinical social work. To practice ethically in connection with MCOs, clinicians should ensure that clients can make informed treatment decisions based on knowledge of

- their options
- benefit limitations
- authorization process
- rights to appeal utilization decisions
- limits on choice and copay requirements
- potential invasion of privacy by the review process.

In addition to clinicians ensuring those understandings,

- No exaggerated claims of excellence or quality should be made by the MCO.
- Treatment should be competent and meet client needs within benefit limits.
- The utilization review process should not invade the therapeutic relationship.
- Reviewers should not be financially rewarded for denying treatment or claims (Macbeth et al., 1995).

PROCESS AND TASK

MCOs have forced practitioners to shift from a focus on relationship to a focus on tasks and outcomes. This shift has ethical implications. When practice is based on tasks related to outcomes, ethics do not play a role. MCOs have no stake in how practitioners conduct tasks or how outcomes are achieved. Task outcome is the only judgment of value. In a relationship model, ethics are central to the process because in relationships people always have expectations about how one person should behave toward the other, regardless of the expected outcome. This is a basic and crucial point that clinicians and supervisors who work for MCOs constantly must keep in mind.

VALUES, ETHICS, AND ADVOCACY

The surrender of the mental health professions to MCOs is almost complete. Clinical social work continues to have conflicts about its role in relation to MCOs that will take decades to resolve. Ethics conflicts related to confidentiality (Sabin, 1997), self-determination, and rights to informed consent remain unresolved. It is difficult for clinicians to find a forum in which to resolve these differences because no formal or informal structures exist through which clinicians can communicate with MCOs about professional and practice issues. The professional literature is confusing on this issue. For example, in *How to Partner with Managed Care* (Browning & Browning, 1996), clinicians who make an error in working with an MCO case manager were advised to "point the finger at yourself and ask for mercy" (p. 30). Of course, equal partners do not have to ask for mercy. What makes the mental health industry unique at this point is that no other industry has contractual partners who are in a structurally adversarial relationship. This reflects a major flaw in the "partnership" between MCOs and providers that must be resolved for the system to work more effectively.

Professional Organizations

Professional organizations also undermine practitioner autonomy by establishing licensing standards, devising multiple layers of credentialing, and requiring continuing education credits. Licensing is directly linked to managed cost policies because companies use licensing to establish provider eligibility. Professional organizations currently compete with one another to control practitioner functions and activities. NASW vies for practice turf with the National Federation of Societies for Clinical Social Work, which vies with the American Association of Marriage and Family Therapists, which vies with the American Association of Guidance Counselors, which vies with the National Registry of Certified Group Therapists, which vies with the American Psychiatric Association, which vies with the American Psychological Association. The list could go on and on as overwhelmed supervisors, practitioners, and clients respond with confusion and frustration. Competition among disciplines constantly shifts and reshifts the balance among the different professional organizations and allows MCOs to maintain and extend their control of mental health practice.

In spite of widespread practitioner dissatisfaction with managed cost practices, professional organizations have not taken steps to confront the problem ("Special Report," 1995). A survey by the National Federation of Societies for Clinical Social Work ("Managed Care Notes," 1995) found that 90 percent of 428 respondents reported an overall negative response to MCO care.

Professional Status

Current trends threaten our status as a profession. Sullivan (1995) has reaffirmed the time-honored criteria necessary to establish professional status: (1) specialized training based on (2) codified knowledge used to (3) live out a commitment to public service that is (4) carried out with a certain degree of autonomy as perceived and accepted by the public. Given the current relationship between social workers and MCOs, the only tenet of professionalism that does not appear to be eroding is specialized training. In regard to the second criterion, there is compelling research (Randall & Thyer, 1994; Thyer & Vodde, 1994) that the theory base of social work is not sufficiently codified. For example, their research shows that graduate students can achieve high scores on licensing examinations by randomly selecting answers on the scoring sheets, even when they have not read the examination questions. In regard to the third criterion, it seems clear that social workers who practice through MCOs are not performing a public service as defined by Courtney and Specht (1994). And finally, in regard to the fourth criterion, the previous section of this chapter documented the profession's growing loss of autonomy. These threats to professional status present the social work profession with a dilemma similar to the ethical dilemmas discussed earlier. Given the erosion of professional values and prerogatives, our failure to address these issues proactively is significant. Social work has devoted decades to convincing the public that it is an autonomous profession (Munson, 1979), but managed cost practices could seriously damage the profession's public autonomous image if present trends continue.

Social Work Education

Social work education must be more responsive to the practice changes that have occurred if the profession is to remain a major provider of mental health services. Massive and rapid changes require new models and new theories of clinical intervention. Social work education and research have not produced new models relevant to the changes taking place. Schools must alter how clinical practice is taught. Values and ethics must be explored, and specific guidelines for ethical practice must be developed and taught in graduate programs. Social work faculty must engage in extensive research that measures practice activities and outcomes. This research must be communicated to students and become a routine part of daily practice activity.

For clinical social work, technology should translate into practice research, accountability, outcome measurement, billing methods, and generation of new information. Advances in scientific method, research design, and computer applications have yet to influence practice significantly, and the lack of influence can be traced directly to the failure of social work schools to teach this content. Most of the practice literature remains speculative. The theory, science, and technology of practice must be taken into account and integrated.

The clinical social work literature is slowly expanding as the knowledge base broadens. Because most practice texts are still based on individual practitioner accounts, much work remains to be done in regard to theory and research. Few traditional surveys; experimental, adapted, single-subject research designs; or follow-up studies applied to dysfunctional or effective adaptive behavior have been done. The lack of empirically based research also has left us with limited and inadequate diagnostic categories and classification systems. Improving the quality and extent of clinical social work research is the immediate developmental task, and advances in research design and computer technology should be used to speed the process of generating research-based practice knowledge.

Historically, social work education has developed models of clinical education that reflect changes in society. In the past 20 years, critics have argued that schools have failed to develop a model of practice education that meets the needs of the largest segment of the student population. This debate emerged initially as an argument about casework versus psychotherapy. During the 1970s it turned to the adequacy of training for clinical practice. At present it is reflected in Courtney and Specht's (1994) attack on the profession and on schools of social work for abandoning social work's historical mission by exclusively emphasizing clinical practice education. Organizations that represent clinical social workers argue against the position that social work education has been taken over by clinicians, pointing out that the Council on Social Work Education's *Curriculum Policy Statement* (Council on Social Work Education, 1992) does not address clinical issues. The debate has moved on to issues of curriculum design and the preparation of practice teachers. The problem in this debate is the lack of clear guidelines about what constitutes foundation knowledge for effective clinical practice. If the practice community hopes to influence clinical curricula in schools of social work, its recommendations will have to be rooted in empirically based research findings.

Conclusion

No one can predict the future. The ideas in this chapter are based on observations of historical and current trends in the literature. The systems in which we operate are so fragile, fragmented, and destabilized that events can change practices rapidly, and I am acutely aware of how difficult it is to make predictions under these conditions. If we are going to provide rational, effective solutions to the problems we face, we must create a vision of the future and develop diverse methods to respond to the problems evolution presents. It is difficult to innovate and create a vision when you do not control your own practice activity or destiny. It remains to be decided how professional practice will advance under present circumstances.

What direction the control trend will take is unclear. It is most likely to continue (Patterson & Sharfstein, 1992) and to worsen. It is possible that our 100-year quest for professional autonomy will be altered significantly if there is no professional response to these trends. Ironically, the emerging role of social workers in the MCO environment is strikingly similar to the role of social workers who were paid agents in the charity organization societies.

There is hope that comes from an unsuspected source: the philosopher Nietzsche. He stated that tyranny of any kind leads to servitude, but the danger of tyranny "acquaints us with our own resources, our virtues, our armor and weapons, our spirit, and forces us to be strong" (Kaufmann, 1954, p. 542). There are increasing indications that society has begun to view certain aspects of MCO practice as unfair and worthy of negative sanctions. The fact that the State of Rhode Island recently fined an MCO \$100,000 and placed it on probation for one year because of "unfair practices" ("Managed Care," 1995) is perhaps a harbinger of change. Historically, social work has been a profession concerned with social justice and the well-being of oppressed clients. This is our hallmark, and it has distinguished us from psychiatry, psychology, and counseling (Reamer, 1992). Many of the oppressive trends in mental health care have been fostered by MCOs and other social institutions that have a disproportional impact on the lives of relatively disempowered people. It remains to be seen whether the social work profession will recover its historical role and its unique strength as advocate for disempowered clients or whether it will continue its slide into the role of willing slave to MCO philosophies and practices. The words of Kenneth Pray in his 1946 presidential address to the National Conference of Social Work can serve as an enduring guide for addressing the challenges that now face our profession:

> If American social work can stand true to its own faith, in its daily practice and in its broader relations with the whole society. . . . it can reach in our time an achievement of incalculable value to mankind, by bravely and competently helping at least some parts of this sorely troubled world, caught in the turmoil of a social revolution, to discover and to fulfill their own permanent, positive values and their own truly creative purpose. (cited in Fink, 1949, p. vii)

References

Ackley, D. C. (1997). *Breaking free of managed care: A step-by-step guide to regaining control of your practice.* New York: Guilford.

Allman, W. F. (1994). *The stone age present: How evolution has shaped modern life—From sex, violence, and language to emotions, morals, and communities.* New York: Simon & Schuster.

Alperin, R. M., & Phillips, D. G. (1997). *The impact of managed care on the practice of psychotherapy: Innovation, implementation, and controversy.* New York: Brunner/Mazel.

Altheide, D. L. (1995). *An ecology of communication: Cultural formats of control.* New York: Aldine de Gruyter.

Amada, G. (1995). *A guide to psychotherapy.* New York: Ballantine Books.

Aronson, J. (1996). *Inside managed care: Family therapy in a changing environment.* New York: Brunner/Mazel.

Browning, C. H., & Browning, B. J. (1996). *How to partner with managed care.* New York: John Wiley & Sons.

Cohen, C. I. (1997). The political and moral economy of mental health. *Psychiatric Services, 48,* 768–774.

Corpt, E. A., & Reison, M. (1994). Behaviorizing your clinical language. *Managed Care News,* pp. 1–5. (Available from the Council on Social Work Education, Alexandria, VA)

Council on Social Work Education. (1992). *Curriculum policy statement.* Alexandria, VA: Author.

Courtney, M., & Specht, H. (1994). *Unfaithful angels: How social work has abandoned its mission.* New York: Free Press.

Cushman, P. (1995). *Constructing the self, constructing America: A cultural history of psychotherapy.* Reading, MA: Addison-Wesley Press.

Davison, G. C., & Neale, J. M. (1990). *Abnormal psychology.* New York: John Wiley & Sons.

Dorwart, R. A., & Schlesinger, M. (1988). Privatization of psychiatric services. *American Journal of Psychiatry, 145,* 543–553.

Dorwart, R. A., Schlesinger, M., Davidson, H., Epstein, S., & Hoover, C. (1991). A national study of psychiatric hospital care. *American Journal of Psychiatry, 148,* 204–210.

Feldman, J. L., & Fitzpatrick, R. J. (Eds.). (1992). *Managed mental health care: Administrative and clinical issues.* Washington, DC: American Psychiatric Press.

Fink, A. E. (1949). *The field of social work.* New York: Columbia University Press.

Flax, J. (1990). *Thinking fragments: Psychoanalysis, feminism, and postmodernism in the contemporary West.* Berkeley, CA: University of California Press.

Goodman, M., Brown, J., & Deitz, P. (1992). *Managing managed care.* Washington, DC: American Psychiatric Press.

Handy, C. (1995, May/June). Trust and the virtual organization. *Harvard Business Review,* pp. 40–50.

Kaufmann, W. (Ed.). (1954). *The portable Nietzsche.* New York: Penguin Books.

Lasch, C. (1979). *The culture of narcissism: American life in an age of diminishing expectations.* New York: W. W. Norton.

Lundblad, K. S. (1995). Jane Addams and social reform: A role model for the 1990s. *Social Work, 40,* 661–669.

Macbeth, J. E., Wheeler, A. M., Sither, J. W., & Onek, J. N. (1995). *Legal and risk management issues in the practice of psychiatry.* Washington, DC: Psychiatrists' Purchasing Group.

Madrick, J. (1995). *The end of affluence: The causes and consequences of America's economic dilemma.* New York: Random House.

Managed care: Consumer complaints lead to sanctions against a company. (1995). *Psychotherapy Finances, 21*(9), 1.

Managed care notes. (1995). *Psychotherapy Finances, 21*(10), 5.

Mental health: Does therapy help? (1995, November). *Consumer Reports,* pp. 734–739.

Motenko, A. K., Allen, E. A., Angelos, P., Block, L., DeVito, J., Duffy, A., Holton, L., Lambert, K., Parker, C., Ryan, J., Schraft, D., & Swindell, J. (1995). Privatization and cutbacks: Social work and client impressions of service delivery in Massachusetts. *Social Work, 40,* 456–463.

Munson, C. E. (Ed.). (1979). *Social work supervision: Classic statements and critical issues.* New York: Free Press.

Munson, C. E. (1988). Computers in social work education. *Computers in Human Services, 3,* 143–157.

Munson, C. E. (1993a). *Clinical social work supervision* (2nd ed.). New York: Haworth Press.

Munson, C. E. (1993b). The "P" word and mental health services. *Clinical Supervisor, 11*(2), 1–5.

Munson, C. E. (1995a, March/May). Control and authority in mental health services. *Managed Care News,* pp. 2–4.

Munson, C. E. (1995b, August). *Foundation concepts for survival of ethical social work practice in the health care environment.* Paper presented at National Institutes of Health, Bethesda, MD.

Munson, C. E. (in press). Length of treatment, diagnosis, and treatment planning. *Clinical Supervisor.*

Naisbitt, J. (1982). *Megatrends: Ten new directions transforming our lives.* New York: Warner Books.

National Advisory Mental Health Council. (1993). Health care reform for Americans with severe mental illness: Report of the National Advisory Mental Health Council. *American Journal of Psychiatry, 150,* 1447–1465.

National Association of Social Workers. (1990). *Code of ethics.* Silver Spring, MD: Author.

National Association of Social Workers. (1996). *NASW code of ethics.* Washington, DC: Author.

Patterson, D. Y., & Sharfstein, S. S. (1992). The future of mental health care. In J. L. Feldman & R. J. Fitzpatrick (Eds.), *Managed mental health care,* (pp. 335–343). Washington, DC: American Psychiatric Press.

Perkey, B. (1989). Public and private responsibility for mental health services: A report on the Tennessee task force. *American Psychologist, 44,* 1148–1150.

Perlman, H. H. (1957). *Social casework: A problem-solving process.* Chicago: University of Chicago Press.

Phillips, D. (1995). Professional standards and managed care. *National Federation of Societies for Clinical Social Work Progress Report, 13,* 11.

Randal, J. (1995). Managed care reshapes health care delivery. *SAMHSA News, 3*(3), 10–14.

Randall, E. J., & Thyer, B. A. (1994). A preliminary test of the validity of the LCSW examination. *Clinical Social Work Journal, 22,* 223–227.

Reamer, F. G. (1992). From the editor: The wheels of change in social work education. *Journal of Social Work Education, 28*(10), 3–5.

Reamer, F. G. (1993). *The philosophical foundations of social work.* New York: Columbia University Press.

Reeser, J. C., & Epstein, I. (1990). *Professionalization and activism in social work: The sixties, the eighties, and the future.* New York: Columbia University Press.

Reid, W. J., & Epstein, L. (1972). *Task-centered practice.* New York: Columbia University Press.

Richmond, M. (1917). *Social diagnosis.* New York: Russell Sage Foundation.

Rodenhauser, P., & Greenblatt, M. (1989). Transformations in mental health system management: An overview. *Mental Health Administration, 19,*408–411.

Rose, N. (1997). The future economic landscape: Implications for social work practice and education. In M. Reisch & E. Gambrill (Eds.), *Social work in the 21st century* (pp. 28–38). Thousand Oaks, CA: Pine Forge Press.

Sabin, J. E. (1997). Managed care: What confidentiality standards should we advocate for in mental health care, and how should we do it? *Psychiatric Services, 48,* 35–41.

Schamess, G. (1996). Introduction and editorial: Who profits and who benefits from managed mental health care. In G. Schamess (Ed.), *The corporate and human faces of managed health care: The interplay between mental health policy and practice* (pp. 209–220), Northampton, MA: Smith College Studies in Social Work.

Schor, J. B. (1991). *The overworked American: The unexpected decline of leisure.* New York: Basic Books.

Special report: What is your professional organization doing for your practice? (1995). *Psychotherapy Finances, 21*(7), 6.

Sullivan, W. M. (1995). *Work and integrity: The crisis and promise of professionalism in America.* New York: Harper Business.

Survey results: A snapshot of managed care company policies. (1995). *Psychotherapy Finances, 21*(8), 5.

Terr, L. (1994). *Unchained memories: True stories of traumatic memories, lost and found.* New York: Basic Books.

Thyer, B. A., & Vodde, R. (1994). Is the ACSW examination valid? *Clinical Social Work Journal, 22,* 105–111.

Wolf, S. (1994). Health care reform and the future of physician ethics. *Hastings Center Report, 24*(2), 28–41.

Zuckerman, E. I., & Guyett, I.P.R. (1992). *The paper office 1.* Pittsburgh: Clinician's ToolBox.

CHAPTER 32

Our Uncharted Journey: The Clinical Social Work Federation's Response to Managed Care

Elizabeth V. Phillips

Bertha Capen Reynolds, a pioneer in the field of psychiatric social work and one of its great teachers, spoke out in her autobiography, *An Uncharted Journey* (1963), on behalf of professional integrity in the face of powerful economic interests. In this case it was the Community Fund Movement, which she described as being "under the leadership of the oligarchy of wealth." She stated that this movement allowed business interests to alter the standards of the profession. She cited interference with practice, which the ethics of no established profession would tolerate: "Social caseworkers are increasingly being forced to choose between practicing their profession ethically (that is, refusing to use their clients for the interests of any other group) or becoming slavishly obedient to powerful forces which must in the end destroy every vestige of professional integrity" (p. 180). The situation she described clearly parallels our current situation with managed care. What would she offer as advice? Resist! But as she also said, "to resist alone is professional suicide" (p. 181).

This chapter focuses on the Clinical Social Work Federation's (CSWF) responses to the emergence of managed mental health care from the mid-1980s to the present day. In the beginning we had no map, no compass. As a specialty professional organization, the CSWF represents some 11,000 clinical social workers in 34 state clinical societies. The federation has a responsibility to protect professionals and clients. We kept this in mind as we began our "uncharted journey" into the alien realm of managed care.

Among the roles professional organizations undertake are defining the parameters of the profession (codified in state licensure laws), the academic requirements for entry, the scope of practice, the ethical standards, the mission, and the goals and strategies for accomplishing the mission. Professional organizations promote the highest quality of professional service.

CSWF Mission Statement

The mission of the CSWF is to promote excellence in clinical social work practice for the benefit of clients and the clinicians who serve them by developing and advancing the profession. The mission enhances the practice of clinical social work as

NOTE: Portions of this chapter were originally published as Phillips, E. V. (1998, April). Our uncharted journey. *Managed Care News*. (Available from E. V. Phillips, 13 Cooper Road, New Haven, CT 06473.)

an independent and economically viable profession. CSWF undertakes the following tasks in pursuing its mission:

- advocating on behalf of members of the state societies with the federal government and other national organizations
- assisting state societies with education, marketing, reimbursement, research, image building, promoting standards and competence, legislation and regulation, and related areas at the state and national levels
- providing the means for clinicians with common interests to work collectively on a national level
- providing information to and advocacy for client populations who need and can benefit from clinical social work services.

CSWF Goals and Strategies

The three goals and strategies listed below flow from the mission statement and apply specifically to managed care:

Goal 1: To continue national-level advocacy

Strategies

- to represent the interests of clinical social work and the national CSWF through a strong lobbying and advocacy presence
- to keep informed of and to monitor current legislative and organizational issues (on both the national and state levels)
- to identify issues for short- and long-term legislative and organizational actions
- to make recommendations (by the advocates) to the national CSWF and to the state societies.

Goal 2: To continue promotion of legal regulation and vendorship

Strategies

- to plan, implement, and broaden efforts to influence payers to include clinical social workers as autonomous providers of mental health and substance abuse services
- to offer consultation and training to states dealing with licensure and vendorship; to secure licensing for all states; to work with the National Association of Social Workers (NASW) in licensing efforts
- to maintain and disseminate information from a central databank on vendorship and licensure (to individual states across the country).

Goal 3: To promote marketing and public relations for the clinical social work profession

Strategies

- to expand clinical social work's share of mental health and chemical dependency markets
- to expand the mental health and chemical dependency markets in cooperation with other pertinent organizations and professions
- to establish guidelines for marketing
- to establish a centralized databank, clearinghouse, and resource center for marketing.

The Advent of Managed Care

The CSWF is a diverse group representing a wide range of points of view about managed care. Some think that managed care is inevitable and necessary in the face of what has been described as the "health care crisis." Others believe the crisis was magnified and that corporate profits made by withholding appropriate treatment are immoral. Across that range of views, a good deal of current thinking about managed care is based on certain widely accepted propositions. These propositions are not necessarily proven but reflect a mind-set and value set. They include but are not limited to the assertions identified below.

Big-Business Orientation

There is a health care crisis.

- Costs have been rising at a destructive rate. Insurance companies could no longer make a profit to offset the risks they were taking.
- Industry, through its benefits packages, could no longer afford the increasing rates for medical insurance.
- The remedy cannot be a single-payer plan because that would amount to socialized medicine, which is anathema. People could not then choose their own doctors, and medical services would be rationed.
- Doctors are bleeding the health care system.
- Big government through legislation and regulation is a negative force.
- Only by using big-business acumen can the problem be solved.
- The measure of success is profits.
- Big business cannot be held to a standard of morality because the laws that govern are economic and neutral—for example, the law of supply and demand, free-market competition.

Humanist Orientation

There is a second, more humanist set of assumptions that is equally strongly held and also unproved. That set of propositions includes but is not limited to the following:

- Health is a right of all Americans.
- The federal government is the necessary protector of all Americans, especially children, elderly men and women, and people who are ill, weak, or needy.
- Medical treatment and mental health treatment should be governed by standards and ethics of the professions. These principles are defined by the Hippocratic Oath and by the codes and standards of the professional organizations. These include but are not limited to humane treatment, "at least do no harm," confidentiality, complete treatment (not withholding efficacious treatment), and comprehensive treatment.
- Attention should be paid to the indices of national health, with an attempt to improve the national health picture, for example, infant mortality and morbidity; maternal mortality; tobacco, drug, and alcohol abuse; longevity; rates of mental illness; and suicide rates.
- Mental health treatment has an offset effect on physical symptoms and health.

- Poverty negatively affects both physical and mental health.
- The measure of success in health care is the health of individual Americans.

Social work has had to grapple with these polar positions. The business position, asserting that there is a health care crisis, began building the foundation for the managed health care industry's takeover of health and mental health care more than 20 years ago. The more humanist view was silenced by the media hype that emphasized the "crisis." Managed care solutions were put in place before most professionals knew what was happening.

CSWF Advocacy in the 1980s

Before 1988, the CSWF was focused on helping state societies craft licensure laws. Some of those laws focused on title protection only. As we became aware that the profession and the public were better protected by scope-of-practice acts, we helped states draft these laws. This legislation passed only after struggle and delay in most state legislatures. By 1995, however, all states had some form of regulation.

Next came vendorship. With vendorship, clinical social work entered the insurance industry's orbit. Many states mandated (limited) mental health benefits. At first, social workers found security in being paid by indemnity insurance. Insurance payments provided a dependable means of support as well as autonomy for private practitioners. Subsequently, managed care organizations (MCOs) began to appear on the horizon. MCOs gradually took over indemnity plans. Micromanagement began to replace professional autonomy.

The CSWF acknowledged the importance of managed care in 1988 when the president of the CSWF (then called the National Federation of Societies for Clinical Social Work) appointed an ad hoc committee to study managed care and report to the board on its development. Thus, the first phase of CSWF's response to managed care was formally started in the mandate to the committee "to inform and educate" the clinical societies. In 1991, the committee produced a videotape on managed care to present to the First National Conference of Clinical Social Work. That videotape chronicled the development of health maintenance organizations (HMOs), preferred provider organizations, and the "carved-out" MCOs in mental health.

In 1991, the CSWF began publishing *Managed Care News (MC News)*, a newsletter for clinicians, by clinicians. The health care picture was changing too rapidly to inform members through semiannual program reports, so the *MC News* was published six times a year. This widely read and respected newsletter is still in publication. In 1993, the CSWF's managed care policy was written. The CSWF policy advocates three goals for reform of the national health care system:

1. to improve the quality of health care
2. to provide access for all citizens
3. to manage health care costs.

CSWF believes in the right to universal health care coverage, the elimination of exclusion due to pre-existing conditions, and free access and choice (for instance, access to any qualified and willing provider). CSWF policy advocates for short- and long-term treatment, partial hospitalization, inpatient hospitalization, and residential treatment for mental health and substance abuse care. We support coverage for all recognized treatment modalities and theoretical orientations. We support benefit parity for mental health treatment by all mental health professionals who provide the same type of treatment. We recognize the right of managed care companies to determine benefits but not to determine treatment. Treatment plans should be made by licensed clinicians on the basis of clinical diagnostic assessments.

OPENING MANAGED CARE PANELS TO CLINICAL SOCIAL WORK

The second phase involved a rush for inclusion on managed care panels. The development of panels created competition among professionals for scarce places. Many panels favored psychologists and psychiatrists. During this era we saw the proliferation of "carve-outs." Insurance companies outsourced supervision and management to a mushrooming group of new companies. Fees were slashed, and contracts were generated with odious "gag" and "hold harmless" clauses. Written and telephone outpatient treatment reports raised ethical questions about the widespread dissemination of confidential information about clients.

Nevertheless, the CSWF worked to open panels to clinical social workers at both the national and state levels. The National Institute for Clinical Social Work Advancement hired a specialist to open opportunities in the Employee Retirement Income Security Act (ERISA) for clinical social workers. We hoped managed care could be influenced to change. Our diverse membership led us to pursue a wait-and-see policy.

RECOGNITION OF MANAGED CARE ABUSE

The third phase, beginning around 1995, was one in which we recognized managed care abuses. By this time, a majority of Americans were already enrolled in some form of managed care plan. There was growing concern as we experienced the loss of confidentiality, the rationing of services, the strict and often spurious definition of medical necessity, "panel drop" (removal from panels), "rightsizing" (panel downsizing), and fee reductions. All these changes were made unilaterally by managed care companies, without consultation with mental health professionals.

A federation hotline was initiated in 1995 to hear the concerns of clinicians about their clients or their own mistreatment at the hands of managed care. The message on the 800 number begins with "If you wish assistance with managed care or health care systems issues which restrict clinical social work utilization. . . ." The hotline has helped more than 400 clinical social workers with a wide range of problems.

The dilemma for clinical social workers was that, whereas the humanist set of propositions listed above is more compatible with their training and experience, the insurance community, the business community at large, and the media continued to insist that there is a health care crisis and that managed care is the necessary and inevitable remedy. The managed care industry, with its profit focus, moved in so quickly and became so entrenched in the mental health field that it became a reality that had to be dealt with. Some of our members are employed in managed care. Many are dependent on managed care reimbursements. Others wanted nothing to do with managed care. New professionals were particularly vulnerable because their entry into the profession was altered by managed care policies. Because the CSWF represents this diverse group, it has been slow to make negative public pronouncements about managed care in general and abuses in particular. Nevertheless, both in the state societies and at the national level, the debate about abuses continues.

Within the societies, concern grew about ethical violations and standards of practice. To conform to managed care contracts and rules, it became necessary to alter our ethical practices and even, to some extent, our codes of ethics. One of the main issues has been confidentiality. The ethical position we learned as clinical social workers was stated by the National Federation of Societies for Clinical Social Work (now CSWF) in its 1988 *Code of Ethics*:

> The safeguarding of the client's right to privacy is a basic responsibility of the clinical social worker. Clinical social workers have a primary obligation to maintain the confidentiality of material that has been transmitted to them in any of their professional roles, including the identity of the client. (p. 13)

In the revised *Code of Ethics* (CSWF, 1997), the lead statement on confidentiality reads

> Clinical social workers have a primary obligation to maintain the privacy of both current and former clients, whether living or deceased, and to maintain the confidentiality of material that has been transmitted to them in any of their professional roles. Exceptions to this responsibility will occur only when there are overriding legal or professional reasons and whenever possible with the *written informed consent of the clients* [emphasis added]. (p. 7)

Some people see this change as elevating informed consent to the level of confidentiality.

As managed care companies proliferated, they initiated buyouts, mergers, and acquisitions that in 1997 resulted in 12 companies controlling the health care market. The recent announcement that Magellan will buy Merit Behavioral Care Corporation means that four of the top 12 firms and three of the top four firms will be under one operation. This gives the Magellan conglomerate 60 million covered lives, more than half of all people with insurance (Taylor, 1997).

GOVERNMENT RELATIONS COMMITTEE EFFORTS

Although the CSWF managed care committee responded by informing and opening opportunities for social workers, the government relations committee focused on legislative efforts. In 1994 we were included in the Medicare Act. At first the field rejoiced at being included. Under Medicare, however, social work psychotherapy fees were downgraded to 75 percent of psychologists' fees, and psychologists' fees were downgraded to 75 percent of psychiatrists' fees. This has become a widespread model for private managed care companies. As a result, social work fees and status have both been ratcheted down. The CSWF is continuing to work to change this formula. We have just achieved a seat on one panel of the Health Care Financing Administration (Medicare). Much more needs to be done, however, to further the recognition of the parameters and quality of our work as clinical social workers at the HCFA level. Clinical social workers should be represented on all their committees. The government relations committee worked equally diligently at the state level to help states with legislation to correct some managed care abuses, for example, the Texas law that now allows patients to sue HMOs for malpractice and the legislative efforts in other states against "gag rules" and "hold harmless" clauses. The committee has also been active in the Mental Health Liaison Group, a large coalition based in Washington, DC, that monitors legislation at the federal level.

The government relations committee worked to stay on top of the many issues dealt with in the Clinton administration's health plan, which they encouraged the federation to support. Nevertheless, a vocal minority within the organization proposed that the CSWF endorse a single-payer plan. At the October 1995 board meeting a motion to this effect was defeated in a close vote. Later that year the Clinton health plan was defeated in Congress. That defeat further opened the door to managed care and insurance industry control of health care.

The erosion of principles in the face of managed care requirements has created conflict among clinical social workers. The polarizing conflict is between ethics and what is viewed by many as the immutable realities of our position in the health care arena. There is also personal conflict for professionals between making a living and adhering to a code of confidentiality. The powerlessness engendered by this dilemma has lowered morale and eroded our will to question, let alone to fight back.

Alternatives to Managed Care

It became clear that action was necessary to maintain our profession, to protect our ethical principles, and to secure the livelihood of professional clinical social work therapists. Divided as we were by our separate practices, we knew we must unite. We began a search for coalitions and for alternatives to managed care programs, and we joined some as individual practitioners, some as a federation. At our October 1996 board meeting, three organizations made presentations to educate the CSWF about managed care and remedies for abuses. Those three organizations are profiled below.

NATIONAL COALITION OF MENTAL HEALTH PROFESSIONALS AND CONSUMERS

Formed in 1992 on Long Island, New York, this interdisciplinary group of mental health professionals and consumers' sole purpose is to combat the abuses of managed care. Its mission statement reads "A grass-roots organization of mental health professionals from all disciplines, consumers of mental health service and consumer advocates. Our goals are to preserve the personal privacy and confidentiality of consumers, protect the integrity and quality of psychotherapy and mental health services through public and professional education and legal and legislative action." The coalition consists of 20 chapters and about 1,000 members.

The coalition emphasizes that clients experience three main losses as a result of managed care: (1) privacy, (2) choice of therapist, and (3) diagnostically based decisions regarding type and length of treatment. Clinicians lose their role in determining appropriate treatment when their professional opinions are overridden by recommendations for brief treatment dictated by cost-cutting directives. The confidentiality of the therapist–client relationship is basically altered. Clinicians face unemployment if they do not sign managed care contracts, which often force clinicians to take legal responsibility for insurers' decisions (hold harmless clauses), prohibit clinicians from telling patients about proper care (gag clauses), impede clinicians' ability to make the best referrals, provide incentives for undertreatment, and drop clinicians who do not undertreat or who advocate for patients. Fear and intimidation sometimes drive clinical decisions.

The Coalition suggests the following remedies: regulating the industry through both state and federal legislation and encouraging alternatives to managed care such as medical savings accounts, single-payer plans, and guilds.

MASSACHUSETTS ALLIANCE FOR MENTAL HEALTH

The second group that has been of interest to the CSWF as an alternative to managed care is the Massachusetts Alliance for Mental Health. Founded by Peter Gumpert, PhD, as a worker cooperative, this professional alliance seeks contracts with business and industry to provide comprehensive mental health services and is in direct competition with managed care. A nonprofit corporation composed of licensed mental health professionals, the alliance arranges for its members to provide mental health and substance abuse treatment services.

The alliance believes the highest quality services can be provided at reasonable rates if there are no distributions of profit. Its membership of 700 dedicated practitioners in Massachusetts is qualified to offer psychotherapy, medication, day treatment, inpatient treatment, and employee assistance programs at a fixed annual subscriber rate. Clinical decisions, including length of treatment, are made by the clinician or the clinical team. Each practitioner has invested $200–$400 in the alliance and is committed to accepting only the fees paid by the alliance, supplemented by structured copayments. There are no profit distributions. The limited capital is supplemented by personal investment on the part of the professionals. There are alliances in 17 states, all of which are members of the American Alliance of Mental Health Professionals.

CONNECTICUT PSYCHOTHERAPISTS' GUILD

A third alternative to managed care is the guild model. Several guilds currently exist in the United States. The Connecticut Psychotherapists' Guild was founded in 1995 by five therapists who had become concerned about the impact of managed care on psychotherapy. Initially, all belonged to managed care panels and hoped managed care might work well and make therapy available to more people. Their experiences convinced them, however, that the profit motive of managed care companies did not coincide with the essential values of psychotherapy. Accordingly, they formed an organization comprising independent therapists who shared their values and concerns. Since its inception, 73 independent psychotherapists in clinical social work, psychology, psychiatry, family therapy, and nursing have joined the guild. Each is committed to the guild's principles and each pays an application fee plus $80 per month to support the organization's program of public education and advertising. All active members are included in the membership directory. The guild makes no profits and no shareholders. The guild alternative to managed care offers total confidentiality and a choice of therapists from a membership directory that includes half-page professional vitae. Therapists have control over the type, length, and goals of treatment. They offer sliding-scale or discounted fees.

THE SUMMIT

The CSWF was not alone in its concern about managed care or in its diverse membership; all the mental health professional groups were facing the same dilemma. The presidents of the American Psychological Association and the American Psychiatric Association convened a meeting in the spring of 1996 in which they shared their distress about managed care. The CSWF joined with eight professional membership organizations in the mental health field to form the "Summit." The CSWF has actively participated in this group of nine presidents, whose organizations represent 600,000 professionals:

- American Association for Marriage and Family Therapy (25,000 members)
- American Counseling Association (56,000 members)
- American Family Therapy Academy (1,000 members)
- American Nurses Association (180,000 members)
- American Psychological Association (142,000 members)
- American Psychiatric Association (42,000 members)
- American Psychiatric Nurses Association (3,000 members)
- Clinical Social Work Federation (formerly the National Federation of Societies for Clinical Social Work) (11,000 members)
- National Association of Social Workers (155,000 members).

The meetings were organized in response to the current health care climate in which profitability, rather than standards of quality patient care, are driving the market. As a result, standards of care have been disregarded, and professionals have been renamed "providers," a change which harms the relationship between patients and professionals by diminishing its integrity. Parity between health and mental health services is essential to fairness in meeting mental health needs, thereby strengthening families, the work force and communities in America.

The Summit met to draft a patients' bill of rights and to plan action strategies related to the bill. The bill of rights was endorsed by all the professional organizations that crafted it. It represents the highest ethical standards of the professions in that it emphasizes self-determination and is a document that is the most protective of data from patient records. The Summit continues to meet to further the acceptance of the bill of rights. The work atmosphere in this coalition is one of mutual respect and real collaboration, despite the historical differences that have divided these professional organizations. The complete text of the bill of rights can be found in Appendix 1.

Additional Efforts to Influence Managed Care

The CSWF has been active in the Institute of Behavioral Health (IBH), an educational organization that is supported by the managed care industry and which attempts to influence managed health care by improving the quality and structure of the industry. By 1997 CSWF had been effective enough in advocating with IBH to include a strong clinical emphasis in that year's conference.

Ivan J. Miller, PhD, president of the Boulder (Colorado) Psychotherapists' Guild and executive director of the National Coalition of Mental Health Professionals and Consumers, has written extensively about the dangers and abuses of managed care. He challenges the studies and the interpretation of data on which managed care bases its preference for brief treatment. In a press release announcing this work, the presidents of the American Psychiatric Association, the American Psychological Association, and the CSWF supported his work. One clinical social work commentary stated that clinically determined treatment may be short or long term. The issue is that treatment should be based on clinical diagnosis. We are in practice to diagnose and treat mental and emotional problems. We cannot put our assessment tools aside. We cannot overlook our profession's *Code of Ethics.*

Miller's (1997) work shows that managed care companies' insistence on brief treatment is based on flawed studies and misinterpreted data. He examined and analyzed the studies that claim greater benefits from time-limited therapy and dispelled the myth that long-term therapy is inappropriate or harmful. In addition, he has exposed the invisible rationing that increases profits for MCOs (Miller, 1996a).

In an article titled "Committee for Quality Assurance (NCQA): Who Is the Watchdog's Master?" Miller (1996b) stated

> The NCQA appears to be structured as an independent nonprofit organization. A look at its funding and structure, however, reveals that it is an extension of the HMO industry. According to NCQA's accounting department, almost all of their funding comes from voluntary accreditation fees collected from HMOs. . . . This dog is guarding the industry's profits from the proponents of true accountability and effective regulation. (p. 133)

In another article, "Anti-competitive Dangers Resulting from the Managed Care Industry Cartel," Miller (1996a) dealt with the actuarial firm Milliman and Robertson, which was hired by the American Managed Behavior Health Care Association. Its product is a proprietary (secret) document, "Best Practice Guidelines," which it sells to managed health companies.

Two organizations are seeking remedy through the courts for the anticompetitive thrust of the Milliman and Robertson and NCQA guidelines. The Coalition for Universal Access to Psychotherapy, with the National Coalition of Mental Health Professionals and Consumers, has prepared a white paper that was presented to the U.S. Department of Justice. Their allegation is that the managed care industry has established a de facto regulation apparatus that obviates the need for government oversight. A memorandum explaining the suit is presented in Appendix 2.

All the coalitions cited above have worthwhile agendas that aim to curtail managed care abuses. Some do so by education, some by persuasion, some by legislative action, some by influencing regulations, and some by court action. However, despite all their efforts they so far have been powerless to stem the tide of both fee slashing and contractual terms that are abusive to patients and therapists alike.

Guild/Union—An Option for the CSWF

What would Bertha Capen Reynolds (1963) say to us now? She would repeat, "Resist!"

> To resist in a strong protective organization inclusive of all who are employed in a given social service and allied with thousands of others in organized labor and professional workers' unions is to have real effectiveness. (p. 181)

Following the announcement of the formation of a guild by the Podiatrists' Association, several state presidents expressed interest in exploring union affiliation as a way of joining forces with a larger and more powerful coalition that would increase our power and help us regain control of our profession. The CSWF contacted the AFL–CIO national headquarters and met with the chief organizer, who suggested several possible union affiliations. We then interviewed four unions, finally choosing and being chosen by OPEIU (Office and Professional Employees International Union).

Not all the unions wanted us because some clinical social workers are independent contractors and therefore do not fit the mold of the traditional bargaining unit. This, however, is a significant part of our problem. If we are independent contractors, we are not protected. In many ways those of us who are independent contractors have become employees of managed care. We accept their fees, but because of antitrust laws we cannot bargain collectively for fee changes. The antitrust laws were never intended to curtail the opportunities of small entrepreneurs and independent contractors to make a living. As written and interpreted, however, the laws do not protect independent contractors from the fee slashing and other restrictions that managed care companies impose. All of those decisions, which profoundly affect our practices, have been made unilaterally.

A *labor union* is an organization of workers formed for the purpose of improving working conditions and wages. A *guild* is an association of people with similar interests, formed for mutual aid and protection and to maintain standards. Social workers in private practice need protection from the unfair and arbitrary practices of managed care. If we affiliate, we will become a guild because we cannot often engage in collective bargaining. The antitrust laws need to be changed to acknowledge what many of us experience as de facto; that we are more like employees of managed care than not. If we join a guild or union, we will not be a bargaining unit, nor will we strike, but we will have the power of 16 million AFL–CIO members behind us at the national level.

In October 1997 the CSWF board voted to move toward unionization by drawing up an affiliation agreement to be voted on in May 1998. A union has the weight we need. For example, the New York State Society for Clinical Social Work has 2,000 clinical social workers. Add New York's union members, and we are united with a group of several million. At the national level, with a union, we will have added 16 million interested people, and when we approach regulators and legislators, we will have the strength of those millions behind us. The additional numbers will be beneficiaries of services, not "providers." Our interest in dealing with managed care goes well beyond fees to issues at the heart of our profession. It reflects our concern about managed care controls that undermine the quality of our therapeutic work and challenge our ethical standards. Unions will support our efforts because they are interested in establishing ethical and clinical standards that will generate the best health care services for their members.

We need legislative consultants at the national level who can help with two HCFA issues: (1) a change in the Medicare legislation to remove the discriminatory fees for clinical social workers, currently pegged at 75 percent of psychologists' fees, and (2) better representation on HCFA policy committees, such as the American Medical Association fee-setting committee. A union can help us get to that table.

At the state level we need help with writing and rewriting managed care contracts. A union could be a "third-party messenger" (an accepted role in the new antitrust guidelines) who could appear on our behalf. Also at the state level we need help with legislation. For example, the Connecticut Society for Clinical Social Work has organized a coalition that plans to introduce confidentiality legislation. If unions in Connecticut support us we would have a better chance of passing that legislation.

Unions can help us get industry and business support for clinical social workers. ERISA plans, heretofore unavailable to us, will become accessible through union efforts at the bargaining table when benefits packages are being considered. Labor unions understand our need for a voice in our contracts with managed care companies, and they understand the abuses in the health care industry. They are concerned about the health care plans of their members and want the best possible mental health policies for their worker–members. They understand our dilemma over confidentiality, as well as the broader ethical issues. We need their protection from unfair and arbitrary managed care practices. Forming a union is not a panacea, but it is one of the strategies the CSWF is considering to give us the power we need to combat the overwhelming control that managed care exercises over our professional lives and the lives of our clients.

The issue that unites us all, professionals and clients, is that health care and its important component, mental health care, should not be a source of corporate profit. Bertha Capen Reynolds (1963) "advocated union organization for social workers because there was not an alternative if one was to assume mature responsibility for the services one gave" (p. 256). Her message is that

> Social work today is standing at the crossroads. It may go on with its face toward the past, bolstering up the decaying profit system, having to defend what is indefensible for the sake of the money which pays for its services. On the other hand, it may envision a future in which professional social service and medical service shall be the unquestioned right of all. (p. 143)

Reynolds insists that people (not profits) come first. She exhorts us to resist.

Resistance on a Personal Level

One day I called to change an appointment with a woman whom I was treating who works at an HMO.

The receptionist said, "She's with a *provider*."

I said, "A what?"

She said, "She's with a doctor."

My response: "Oh a *doctor*."

I was furious. At a recent Yale Department of Psychiatry clinical faculty meeting, I spoke with a colleague–psychiatrist who told me that he has left managed care because his constant anger was spilling over into his therapeutic sessions.

Not all of us can opt out of managed care. A piece of my solution has been to change my vocabulary. At least I can afford to do that. My change is partly a result of my work on the Summit bill of rights. My view is that managed care is an industry. I am not part of a managed care industry. Managed care uses "providers." I am not a provider. I am a professional. I call the people who come to me for psychotherapy "individuals." I do not call them "patients" (medical model) or "clients" (nonmedical, but lawyerly), and certainly I do not call them "consumers." I use the vocabulary of the marketplace to describe the marketplace. The marketplace is totally profit driven; I offer a sliding scale. It is concerned with monitoring costs; I am concerned with the quality of care. It is concerned with control; I am concerned about access to services. It is concerned with outpatient treatment reports; I am concerned with confidentiality. It wants to limit treatment; I want to build therapeutic alliances with those I treat and to plan treatment and its termination on the basis of individual wishes and needs. Managed care's vocabulary tyrannizes. I want to break free of it and to free new professionals and the profession as a whole from its words. Some of their vocabulary is from the marketplace. Some is just doublespeak. We become subservient to others' ideas and yes, ethics, by permitting them to preempt our vocabulary and replace it with theirs. The marketplace may dominate health care but only if it dominates the minds of professionals. I do not want to speak their language, and I will not succumb to the tyranny of their words.

References

Clinical Social Work Federation. (1997). *Code of ethics.* Arlington, VA: Author.

Miller, I. (1996a). *Anti-competitive dangers resulting from the managed care industry cartel.* Comack, NY: National Coalition of Mental Health Professionals and Consumers.

Miller, I. (1996b). National Committee for Quality Assurance (NCQA): Who is the watchdog's master? *Independent Practitioner, 16,* 133–137.

Miller, I. (1997, May 21). *Managed care methods based on fictional research.* Boulder, CO: Boulder Psychotherapists Press.

National Coalition of Mental Health Professionals and Consumers. (1992). *Mission statement.* In Membership recruitment packet. Comack, NY: Author. (Available from Box 438, Comack, NY 11725)

National Federation of Societies for Clinical Social Work. (1988). *Code of ethics.* Arlington, VA: Author.

Reynolds, B. C. (1963). *An uncharted journey.* Silver Spring, MD: National Association of Social Workers.

Taylor, V. (Ed.). (1997). *Managed Care News,* p. 3.

Suggested Reading

Miller, I. (1994). *What managed care is doing to outpatient mental health: A manual for psychotherapists and patients.* Boulder, CO: Boulder Psychotherapists Press.

Miller, I. (1996). Ethical and liability issues concerning invisible rationing. *Professional Psychology Research and Practice, 27,* 583–587.

Miller, I. (1997, March 19). Beware the Trojan horse from managed care: Dangerous provisions in parity legislation. *Independent Practitioner, 17,* 138–142.

Miller, I. (1997, August 31). *Standards for constructing and criteria for evaluating mental health service guidelines.* Boulder, CO: Boulder Psychotherapists Press.

Appendix 1: Principles for the Provision of Mental Health and Substance Abuse Treatment Service

A BILL OF RIGHTS

Our commitment is to provide quality mental health and substance abuse services to all individuals without regard to race, color, religion, national origin, gender, age, sexual orientation, or disabilities.

RIGHT TO KNOW

Benefits

Individuals shall be provided information from the Purchasing entity (such as employer or union or public purchaser) and the insurance/third-party payer describing the nature and extent of their mental health and substance abuse treatment benefits. This information should include details on procedures to obtain access to services, on utilization management procedures, and on appeal rights. The information should be presented clearly in writing with language that the individual can understand.

Professional Expertise

Individuals shall be provided full information from the potential treating professional about that professional's knowledge, skills, preparation, experience, and credentials. Individuals shall be informed about the options available for treatment interventions and the effectiveness of the recommended treatment. Individuals shall be informed of appeal rights and grievance procedures regarding the care offered.

Contractual Limitations

Individuals shall be informed by the treating professional of any arrangements, restrictions, and/or covenants established between third-party payer and the treating professional that could interfere with or influence treatment recommendations. Individuals shall be informed of the nature of information that may be disclosed for the purposes of paying benefits.

CONFIDENTIALITY

Individuals shall be guaranteed the protection of confidentiality of their relationship with their mental health professional, except when laws or ethics dictate otherwise. Any disclosure to another party will be time limited and made with the full written, informed consent of the individuals.

Economic coercion can be limited by *only* disclosing the following information: diagnosis, prognosis, type of treatment, time and length of treatment, and cost.

Entities receiving information for the purposes of benefits determination, public agencies receiving information for health care planning, or any other organization with legitimate right to information will maintain clinical information in confidence with the same rigor and be subject to the same penalties for violation as is the direct provider of care.

Information technology will be used for transmission, storage or data management *only* with methodologies that remove individual identifying information and assure the protection of the individual's privacy. Information should not be transferred, sold, or otherwise utilized.

CHOICE

Individuals have the right to choose any duly licensed/certified professional for mental health services. Individuals have the right to receive full information regarding the education and training of professionals, treatment options (including risks and benefits), and cost implications to make an informed choice regarding the selection of care deemed appropriate by individual and professional.

DETERMINATION OF TREATMENT

Recommendations regarding mental health and substance abuse treatment shall be made only by a duly licensed/certified professional in conjunction with the individual and his or her family as appropriate. Treatment decisions should not be made by third-party payers. The individual shall make final decisions regarding treatment.

PARITY

Individuals shall receive benefits for mental health and substance abuse treatment on the same basis as they do for any other illness, with the same provisions, copayments, lifetime benefits, and catastrophic coverage in both insurance and self-funded/self-insured health plans.

DISCRIMINATION

Individuals who use mental health and substance abuse benefits shall not be penalized when seeking other health insurance or disability, life, or any other insurance benefit.

BENEFIT USAGE

The individual is entitled to the entire scope of the benefits with the benefit plan that will address his or her clinical needs. Whenever both federal and state law and/or regulations are applicable, the professional and all payers shall use whichever affords the individual the greatest level of protection.

TREATMENT REVIEW

To assure that treatment review processes are fair and valid, individuals shall be guaranteed that any review of their mental health treatment shall involve a professional of the same training, credentials, and licensure as the mental health professional providing the treatment. The reviewer should have no financial interest in the decision and is subject to the section on confidentiality.

APPEAL AND GRIEVANCES

Individuals shall be provided information about the methods they can use to submit complaints or grievances regarding provision of care by the treating professional to that profession's regulatory board and to the professional association.

Individuals shall be provided information about the procedures that can be used to appeal benefit utilization decisions to the third-party payer systems, to the employer and purchasing entity, and to external regulatory entities.

ACCOUNTABILITY

Treating professionals and/or payers and other third parties may be held accountable and liable to individuals for any injury caused by gross incompetence or negligence on the part of the professional or by clinically unjustified decisions of the payer. The treating professional has the obligation to advocate for and document necessity of care and to advise the individual of options if payment authorization is denied.

Appendix 2: White Paper Presented to the Department of Justice by the Coalition for Universal Access to Psychotherapy and the National Coalition of Mental Health Professionals and Consumers

Memo from the Law Office of Kenneth C. Anderson, Esq.[1]

The focus of the presentation to the Department of Justice and the Federal Trade Commission is upon the joint efforts among managed care entities, working under the cover of otherwise legitimate associations such as the National Committee for Quality Assurance (NCQA) and the American Managed Behavioral Healthcare Association (AMBHA) to establish de facto the definitive standards by which to measure the delivery of healthcare services in a managed care environment. Should the effort succeed—and the private and public sector employer groups who have invested heavily in managed care—then healthcare providers and patients will be in dire straits. The Achilles heel in this bold effort is that antitrust laws generally prohibit competitors from jointly establishing a private standard-setting mechanism where doing so will have anticompetitive consequences. A strong argument can be made that a uniform nationwide set of managed care standards—which is clearly where all this is headed—is little more than a conspiracy to standardize (or fix) the minimum terms for the delivery of healthcare services. Neither the Antitrust Division nor the Federal Trade Commission appreciate what is happening and the potential implications thereof, and the central purpose of our project is to educate them and stimulate them to act.

[1]Kenneth C. Anderson, Esq., is an antitrust lawyer, based in Washington, DC, who coauthored the white paper with Ivan Miller, PhD. Complete text of white paper is available c/o Linda Mead, MSW, 141 East 55th Street, Apartment 7C, New York, NY 10022.

CHAPTER 33

Psychodynamic Psychotherapy after Managed Care

Joyce Edward

A growing awareness and concern throughout the country about the devastating impact managed care has had on the treatment of Americans with physical and mental illnesses has begun to raise the hope that we may yet see corporate health care replaced with a more humane and effective system. Those who wish to ensure that psychodynamic psychotherapy[1] will be included in such a system, under conditions favorable to its practice, face a significant challenge. The end of managed care does not necessarily guarantee the availability of this form of mental health treatment. Even in certain single-payer nations, where profits do not drive the system, the place of dynamically oriented psychotherapy, a form of treatment that tends to involve longer time periods, is not necessarily secure. As health care costs rise, pressure by the corporate sector is mounting in several single-payer countries to reduce health benefits in general and mental health benefits in particular.

Judging from the American experience, this is likely to mean, among other things, reducing the number of outpatient psychotherapy sessions to the barest minimum, seriously compromising the patient's right to confidentiality and self-determination, and reducing if not eliminating opportunities for a reliable and constant relationship with a helping professional.

That corporations could so adversely affect all health care and take such a toll on the treatment of emotionally troubled people suggests the low priority this country assigns to the well-being of this group of citizens. The relative ease with which corporate America has turned treatment into behavioral management and clinicians into providers is not only a testimony to its expertise, wealth, and power, but also suggests a readiness on the nation's part, as well as a willingness on the part of certain members within our profession, to tolerate the changes that have taken place, if not to accept them.

NOTE: An earlier version of this chapter was presented at a conference sponsored by the National Coalition of Mental Health Professionals and Consumers, the Consortium for Psychotherapy, and the Boston Institute for Psychotherapy, in Boston, May 1997. Another version of that presentation was later excerpted and appeared in the newsletter *Coalition Report* (1997, March).

[1]The term "psychodynamic psychotherapy" in this chapter refers to all forms of mental health treatments that take into account the existence of unconscious phenomena in mental life and that view the use of the relationship between patient and therapist and the acquisition of self-understanding as important components, albeit to varying degrees, in the therapeutic action of treatment.

Why, we may ask ourselves, have so few grasped the difference between psychotherapy and managed mental health care? Why have so many patients and clinicians, as well as policy makers and legislators, been unable to appreciate the importance of confidentiality, the significance of the patient–therapist relationship or the value of other fundamental components of the psychotherapeutic process? How can we account for the ease with which the country accepted the notion that people with long-standing, severe emotional problems can be helped in one to three sessions? Why have so many of our own colleagues sought to accommodate a system that demands they cast aside their codes of ethics; compromise their hard-won clinical skills; watch their incomes decrease substantially; and allow themselves to be controlled, demeaned, and in many instances, abused by those who profit from their efforts? Finally, why has it taken so long for our professional organizations to fight to ensure that patients have the right to be treated ethically and effectively?

As a nation, we have yet to determine the full cost of managed care in terms of the country's well-being. Patients are clearly suffering from the severe limitations on treatment duration and the restrictions regarding choice of therapist and form of treatment. Constant surveillance of therapists and the assumption of responsibility for therapeutic decisions by company personnel has undermined both therapists' sense of self-value and patients' confidence in their clinicians. Patients need helping persons whom they can experience as trustworthy, strong, knowledgeable people. Moreover, therapists must devote vast amounts of time and energy to protecting their patients' treatment and their own survival—time and energy that once were devoted to improving their clinical capabilities. Training programs have been weakened, if not closed, throughout the country. Increasingly, clinicians are leaving the field, reducing the availability of experienced therapists.

If we are to ensure a future for psychoanalytic psychotherapy, we would do well to bear in mind some of the circumstances that have facilitated the rise of managed care, as well as the impact corporate mental health treatment has had on this modality. With this information in mind, we may be in a better position to ensure that history does not repeat itself. In this chapter, I will review some of what has happened and offer a few suggestions about how we may seek to ensure the development of a sounder therapeutic enterprise in years to come.

Managed care did not come about because of popular demand. According to Betty Leyerle, author of *The Private Regulation of American Health Care* (1994), managed care represents the outcome of a carefully planned and executed effort designed to ward off a national health plan. Seeing their power and profits diminished by the passage of social legislation such as the Medicaid and Medicare amendments to the Social Security Act (1965), corporate America, along with other interest groups, sought to convince the public that rising costs in health care arose from overutilization of services by health care providers. To reverse the progressive trend toward more-inclusive health care legislation, the country was persuaded that health care needed to be taken out of the hands of practitioners and placed under the control of business. Toward this end, a carefully planned campaign was launched on every aspect of the health care delivery system: its structure, economic and political arrangements, knowledge base, and legitimizing philosophy (Leyerle, 1994).

This campaign was facilitated by the passage of legislation that created the professional standards review organization. Although positive in intent, this and similar legislation had the effect of undermining the power of helping professionals. They made it possible to monitor health care personnel and organizations and to diminish their credibility by calling both their professional knowledge base and their ethics into question (Leyerle, 1994). The success of these endeavors is history. Competition, cost, profit, and accountability have become the dominant ideologies in health care delivery, overshadowing the professional service ethic. The move toward a national health plan was successfully thwarted, at least for a while.

In their efforts, corporate America has had the advantage of certain societal attitudes and fears that have been in ascendance since the early 1970s. In the face of increasing economic instability, the demand grew for lower taxes, less government, and fewer social and health services. This trend was accompanied by the emergence of considerable resentment toward health care professionals, a growing hostility toward those in need, a deepening mistrust of government, and a desire "to get government off our backs," which for the most part has meant keeping the government off *business's* backs.

Managed care thrives in a climate in which the social contract appears to have given way. The idea that the strongest people should flourish at the expense of the weakest has become increasingly acceptable. Dependency is being viewed as an evil. Increasingly, those in need are regarded as enemies who consign future generations to a burdensome national debt. Many, including some of our most vocal legislators, now see helping poor people as a crime committed by government against the poor themselves, a burden from which we must release them. As this outlook prevailed, it became possible to abolish the nation's 61-year commitment to providing a federal safety net for poor families with children and to make it seem as though the government were performing a noble act (Moynihan, 1996). No matter that the legislation contains little assurance of job-training programs, insufficient child care provisions, and no guarantee that jobs will be available when families are dropped from the welfare roles.

There was similar rejoicing when people with mental illness were deinstitutionalized in the 1980s. The nation was encouraged to feel that hospitalized patients would now see the end of their confinement and neglect and the start of a new age in their treatment. In fact, with the help of drugs and community facilities, the future of people with mental illness did indeed seem promising at the time. The Community Mental Health Centers Construction Act, which was passed in 1963, committed the country to developing 2,000 community mental health centers for those deinstitutionalized patients by 1980. Only 480 such centers, however, ever became operational (Moynihan, 1996). In New York State it took years of work on the part of the National Association for the Mentally Ill, in alliance with a coalition of other health advocacy organizations, to pass a law (the Community Mental Health Act of 1993) that sought to ensure that at least some of the money saved through deinstitutionalization would be made available for community programs to serve people with mental illness. Despite this landmark legislation, little has changed. Deinstitutionalization, which was to have been a great step forward, has left large numbers of people homeless, uncared for, and untreated—a problem to themselves, their families, and society.

Even today, when the nation has succeeded in passing the Mental Health Parity Act of 1996 that seeks to equalize annual and lifetime aggregate limits for treatment of mental illness and physical illness, true equality and fairness for people with mental illnesses seems beyond reach. Ivan Miller (1997), vice president of the National Coalition of Mental Health Professionals and Consumers, carefully studied the

Mental Health Parity Act of 1996 and concluded that it is likely to provide mental health patients with less rather than more treatment, in spite of its framers' and supporters' good intentions. The predictions are that full parity will lead most employers and health plans to manage benefits more rigorously to contain costs. This outcome means a continuation of the current situation in which, for the most part, mental health patients receive only crisis intervention, in contrast to people with physical illness for whom treatment is aimed at facilitating as much improvement as possible. We cannot speak of true parity as long as companies cover *only* those psychological conditions likely to show significant improvement with short-term treatment, while complicated and serious medical conditions that require intensive or long-term treatment are *fully* covered.

Those who require mental health services and those who seek to provide them have always faced a struggle. Seriously troubled people have been feared, marveled at, ridiculed, abused, and neglected but rarely treated adequately (Alexander & Selesnick, 1966). Before Freud, individuals who were less obviously troubled were often openly disdained as "malingerers" or "degenerates," and their treatment was limited to advice, persuasion, and sometimes coercion. Despite significant progress over time in our understanding and treatment of those with emotional disorders, these earlier attitudes have persisted—witness our attitudes toward those who seek public office with a history of mental problems. Even as recently as 1988, when U.S. presidential candidate Michael Dukakis revealed he had seen a psychiatrist after his brother's death, his ratings in the polls went down immediately. Ronald Reagan responded to this information by saying he was "not going to pick on an invalid," and George Bush's campaign spokeswoman later asserted that "Real men don't get on the couch" (Rich, 1997). Managed care, whether deliberately or not, has taken advantage of such prejudices.

Many people with serious mental illnesses, including patients suffering from character disorders and psychoses, are excluded from any form of treatment other than medication. At the other end of the spectrum are the neurotic patients whose problems are often less obvious and whose functioning is apt to be adequate or even better. These patients are now disparagingly called the "worried well." For them, treatment is a costly and unnecessary indulgence. One part of the patient population is now deemed "untreatable," and another large segment is deemed "self-indulgent," without significant outcry, as far as I can tell, from the public or our legislators.

To the extent psychotherapy has been influenced by psychodynamic theory, it also has been possible for managed care companies to exploit the deep antagonism to an analytic perspective among various groups and individuals. Attacks on Freud and the analytic establishment today have become highly popular for reasons too complex to address in this chapter. It has never been easy, however, for us humans to accept the notion of being motivated by unconscious forces, and the vehemence of current attacks suggests that the resistance that Freud's theories evoked from the start has retained its strength. Analysts also are well aware that not all of the criticism reflects unconscious resistance. There is validity in certain of the criticisms, especially those related to Freud's early views on women, the profession's failure to take the perspectives of various nondominant cultural groups more fully into account, the barriers that for many years prevented nonphysicians from practicing analysis, the high fees often associated with analytic treatments, and dissension among various groups within the analytic establishment. The tendency of some analysts to regard their theories as the truth, to act as if their access to unconscious content lent them some special status, also has antagonized many people within as well as outside of the analytic community. In fact, analytically oriented practitioners have long and, for the most part, successfully worked toward addressing and correcting these problems. Analysis has changed dramatically since Freud's time, and the attitudes and practices of today's analytically oriented practitioners are vastly different from the stereotype that opponents of analysis criticize. The climate of public opinion has not yet caught up with the alterations. Thus, it remains easy for insurance companies to disparage psychodynamically oriented treatments and eliminate them from their offerings in the service of cost reduction.

Although it is not difficult to comprehend the attitudes and practices of managed care companies who, after all, are "just doing business," how do we understand the responses of so many of our colleagues? Why have so many professionals of various disciplines more or less accommodated to arrangements that undermine their standards of clinical practice as well as their ethical values? Some, of course, have experienced the practice of managed care as satisfying, effective, and remunerative and have experienced little conflict about serving as "providers." Others who have struggled with the system see no alternative to participating if they are to serve those who seek help and if they themselves are to survive financially. There also are the clinicians who feel they are accepting the "inevitable" and who "give in," if you will, too discouraged or too depressed to do anything else.

Whatever each person's reasons have been for going along, at the start mental health professionals were in a poor position to take an effective stance against managed care. Initially, and for some time thereafter, professional organizations generally took the position that managed care was here to stay. Thus, they largely devoted themselves to ensuring that their members were included in the system and to helping them adapt to it. The task of mounting an effort to fight the corporate takeover of the profession was left to individual practitioners. Those who did fight frequently found not only that they were risking their careers, but also that they were in conflict with their own professional groups in addition to managed care organizations.

The state coalitions that exist today were initiated by a few clinicians from varying disciplines in alliance with a few consumers. For example, the National Coalition of Mental Health Professionals and Consumers, the umbrella organization for many of the state groups, was begun by only 10 or so concerned social workers, psychologists, nurses, and psychiatrists on Long Island, New York. With considerable effort, the group succeeded in engaging only one consumer at the start. After making a significant contribution, she withdrew out of fear that her benefits would be withdrawn. Currently, a growing number of groups are working to regulate managed care, and some are seeking to replace it with a fairer, more effective health care system. Fortunately, most of our professional organizations have by now actively entered into this effort.

Welcome as the efforts of our professional groups are, I do not believe we can look to them to ensure the future of dynamic psychotherapy. Psychotherapists are only a small part of the membership of our largest professional organization, the National Association of Social Workers (NASW), an organization that must address the needs of a highly diverse group of social workers, many of whom do not identify with or as therapists. Moreover, many members who offer treatment are satisfied with the managed care model. Some are employed by companies as reviewers. Some even own or direct companies. In addition, certain of our professional organizations, like those of other disciplines, even when they decry managed care publicly, continue to rely on corporate contributions to support conferences and other activities. In light of these and other factors, it is not so difficult to understand why no organization, to my knowledge, has actually publicly acknowledged that when its members follow managed care requirements, they are in violation of that profession's ethical code and thus do not meet the profession's highest standards of practice.

If we are to mount a strong, active campaign on behalf of psychotherapy we, as social workers, shall have to look to those organizations that have a special interest in preserving psychotherapy. Among these are the Clinical Social Work Federation, its affiliated National Membership Committee on Social Work and Psychoanalysis, and the newly formed Private Practice Section of NASW. At the same time, we must remain actively engaged with those organizations that represent other mental health disciplines and that share our interests and concerns, and with the interdisciplinary coalitions that are forming all over the country.

Whether we act as members of professional organizations, participants in interdisciplinary coalitions, individual practitioners or, I hope, all three, I suggest that our first task must be that of educating the public to what psychotherapy is. Although resistance to treatment is ubiquitous for a variety of psychological reasons, most people simply do not know what psychotherapy is or who psychotherapists are. We have left what education exists to the media, which all too often distort our endeavors. With the exception of those therapists who work in schools, courts, community-policing activities, or other communal efforts, therapists have, for the most part, been isolated in their offices, regardless of whether they practice privately or in clinics. Many have deliberately kept a low profile to preserve that degree of anonymity that has heretofore been thought to be in the best interests of our patients' treatments. Unfortunately, keeping a low profile has frequently led to a public view of therapists as mysterious, elitist people—a view that engenders a certain amount of fear of and prejudice against us.

Ironically, the fight against managed care has led clinicians of all disciplines and persuasions to emerge from their offices and speak out about what they do. We have begun to see an increasing number of user-friendly publications, written to acquaint the public with what psychotherapy is and who therapists are. Coalitions have begun to publish informational pamphlets, and by now there are a significant number of Web sites that extend the story of psychotherapy into cyberspace.

We continue, however, to need more dynamically oriented clinicians who will write for the popular media so that moviegoers, television watchers, and periodical readers can acquire a more accurate picture of our field. We also need to encourage those who have gained from treatment to share their experiences publicly. We have seen what can happen when patients, disadvantaged by managed mental health care, have spoken out. Now it is time for those who have benefited from treatment to speak out to help those who are unfamiliar with its ameliorative potential. One such example is singer Harry Bellafonte's televised account of the value of his analytic experience, an account that later appeared on the Web site of the American Psychoanalytic Association.

It is important that a public, educated by cinematographer/actor Woody Allen to view therapists as odd creatures unsuccessfully treating the overindulged rich and famous, learn what large numbers of clinicians actually do, whom they serve, and what the potential benefits of treatment under favorable circumstances can be. It is unlikely that many people think of analysts as practitioners who risk street violence to make home visits to a hyperactive borderline child (Rowe, 1994) or who try to contain their personal responses so they may successfully treat a deeply troubled mother who has killed her infant (Chernus & Livingston, 1996). These are but two of the many kinds of treatment challenges psychodynamically oriented therapists routinely address in today's world (Edward & Sanville, 1996). We must somehow interest the media in telling these stories.

We also must publicize the many outcome studies that show the efficacy of psychodynamically informed treatment—psychoanalysis as well as psychotherapy. Instead, we have focused on the need for more outcome research, as if there is none. Surely we need more, but there is some very impressive research we should be bringing to the public's attention. Doidge (1997) summarized the findings of a number of outcome studies and noted that, contrary to the arguments advanced by managed care companies, those investigations show that long-term psychoanalytic therapy is highly effective. This view accords with the 1995 *Consumer Reports* study (Seligman, 1995), which demonstrated that long-term treatments, including those influenced by psychoanalytic principles, "did considerably better than short-term treatment. . . . Patients whose length of therapy or choice of therapist was limited by insurance or managed care did worse" (p. 965). Moreover, an investigation being carried out by Fonagy and Target (1996) at the Anna Freud Center in England, in collaboration with Yale University's Child Study Center, demonstrates the effectiveness of child analysis for seriously disturbed children under age 12 suffering from a variety of psychiatric disorders—another example of an outcome study that should be of considerable interest to the public.

It also is important for us to begin to acquaint the public with psychotherapeutic activities that have implications for communities and, indeed, for society at large. I think here of such communal projects as the Yale Community Policing Program in New Haven (Marans et al., 1995). In this collaborative project, police and psychodynamically trained social workers ride together to the homes of children who have witnessed a violent crime in the hope that immediate intervention may limit the traumatic impact of such tragic occurrences on the lives of those who physically survive them. At a societal level we have the work of Volkan (1988), a psychoanalyst who has been using analytic concepts to shape the negotiating techniques used at peace talks among enemy nations. In describing his work, Volkan noted

> I discuss how the concept of the enemy is intertwined with the child's developmental process of discovering who he is, from whom he is separated, to whom he is related, and from whom he should withdraw. A common enemy appears before the group as its members try to form and maintain a cohesive sense of self and, later, the sense of a group self in ethnic or national terms. (p. 4)

There are many more such endeavors that we need to bring to the public's attention, and many more such projects we need to develop. If psychotherapy is to remain a viable enterprise, we must demonstrate its value in dealing with problems that so deeply concern the American people today: violence, teenage pregnancy, drug abuse, racial prejudice, war, and so on.

The task of teaching the public about treatment, however, is no longer simply that of providing people with new information. It has become one of re-educating people on the topic. Before managed care we faced people who were largely unfamiliar with psychotherapy. Now we must consider a public that has been carefully "educated" by managed care companies. As a result, there is much to "unlearn." For the most part, managed care companies have succeeded in convincing people that managing symptoms constitutes treatment for emotional disorders. Companies also have been actively promoting their own ideas about what constitutes pathology and what treatment goals and methods should be.

Corporate mental health treatment has placed great emphasis on the role of genetics and biology in the etiology of emotional disorders and has minimized the role of extrinsic factors. The impact of adverse childhood experience is frequently disregarded. Typically, utilization reviewers do not want to know about the patient's traumatic past. All that is important is the here and now. As Dumont (1992) pointed out, we rarely hear any more about the relationship among mental illnesses, poverty, and racism. As treatment is increasingly limited to medication only, such circumstances no longer appear to be relevant.

People also are becoming accustomed to equating psychotherapy with crisis intervention. As soon as even one symptom abates and a particular crisis subsides, companies are apt to regard further treatment as unnecessary. Patients are advised they can return when a new crisis arises. A revolving-door approach is becoming normative. The goal of psychological repair has given way to psychological first aid. Whereas the traditional goal of psychotherapy has been to enable people to develop capabilities that would render them less vulnerable to the vicissitudes of life and reduce the risk of recurrence, managed care patients are learning to expect and accept a form of treatment limited to getting them through recurring crises. Moreover, the measure of need is rarely determined today on the basis of personal suffering. If a person can go to work every day, complete his or her daily chores, and is neither suicidal nor homicidal, the likelihood is that treatment will be judged medically unnecessary.

Of great concern, too, is the way corporate mental health care has begun to influence attitudes about who should receive psychotherapy. As noted earlier, those suffering from psychoses or character disorders are often deemed untreatable by anything other than medication, and those suffering from neurosis are thought not to be in need of treatment. The exclusion of large numbers of troubled people who in the past have been helped by treatment is not only detrimental to the people involved but is costly to society itself. Psychotherapy may not "cure" the psychoses, but it can enable many psychotic people to cope better with the challenges of everyday life and live more satisfying lives, and it can free their families to live more fully and richly. Excluding character disorders from psychotherapy not only deprives these patients and prolongs their suffering, but also is likely to have serious social consequences. Frequently, these patients suffer from impulsivity that can lead them to act destructively toward themselves or others, sometimes to abuse their children or spouses, to move repeatedly from job to job, or to give up work entirely. And as many of us know, often at firsthand, a neurosis can be painful. In this society we are less aware of the fact that neurotics also may act contrary to their own and society's best interests.

Managed care is not only shaping the public's ideas about pathology and treatment; it has gone beyond that. Whether intentionally or not, it is an effective tool for promoting the development of certain kinds of characteristics and attitudes throughout society. It rewards compliance and punishes independence of thought and action. It disempowers rather than empowers. It denies the uniqueness of each person and minimizes the importance of human relatedness. It has moved us into what Lifton (1973) referred to as a "technicist model" of therapeutic activity, in which patients are viewed as machines that have broken down. In that model, a more "scientifically" knowledgeable machine called a "provider" is called in to "repair" the first machine. The treatment process itself, being technical in nature, has nothing to do with the time, place, or particularity of the people involved.

We have much work ahead of us. Societal conditions and attitudes toward people with mental illness do not provide a favorable context in which dynamic psychotherapy can flourish. Without changes in the values, goals, and structures of society, our best efforts to ensure that people receive good mental health treatment are unlikely to succeed. Thus, even as we focus our efforts on a specific goal, we must align ourselves politically with all of those endeavoring to develop a society organized around the common good. We must, at the same time, find a way to help the public better comprehend the connection between untreated emotional disturbances and the social problems that burden this country. Finally, the country needs to become aware of how our present health care system has become a vehicle for compromising our most fundamental rights as American citizens. Gag laws that attack our freedom to speak and the loss of privacy and confidentiality in relation to our personal records are only two examples of how corporate health care has eroded our individual rights.

In closing, let me say that although I have stressed here the difficulties we face, I regard this as a time of great opportunity. Like those countries that rebuild more splendid edifices and institutions after a war, we have the opportunity to construct a finer psychotherapeutic enterprise for the future. In fighting managed care we have already begun to help the nation focus on the importance of mental health treatment and the costs to people and the nation when it is not available. Therapists of all persuasions, legislators, health personnel of all types, the recipients of health care, and their advocates have all begun to come together in a common endeavor. As therapists, we have started to discover what can be accomplished when, in the words of Peter Gumpert (1996), a leader of the National Coalition, "we abandon turf wars and replace competition between disciplines with cooperation" (p. 1). I hope that if those of us who value psychotherapy join in an effort to deal with the major societal problems that confront us all; if we perform our own work sensitively, competently, and ethically to the advantage of those we serve; if we curb our tendencies toward dogma and elitism; if we make psychotherapy more easily available to those who need and seek it; if we make our understandings and offerings as relevant to the human condition as possible by serving outside of the consulting room as well as within it; if we share more openly and more widely what we do and who we are; and if we can join respectfully with our colleagues from other disciplines and perspectives in a common endeavor, then psychodynamically informed treatments will not so easily be eliminated from the spectrum of treatments available in the 21st century.

References

Alexander, F. G., & Selesnick, S. T. (1966). *The history of psychiatry.* New York: Harper & Row.

Chernus, L. A., & Livingston, P. G. (1996). Clinical supervision: Its role in containing countertransference responses to a filicidal patient. In J. Edward & J. Sanville (Eds.), *Fostering healing and growth: A psychoanalytic social work approach* (pp. 386–403). London: Jason Aronson.

Community Mental Health Centers Act, P.L. 88-164, 77 Stat. 290.

Doidge, N. (1997). Empirical evidence for the efficacy of psychoanalytic psychotherapies and psychoanalysis: An overview. In S. G. Lazer (Ed.), *Extended dynamic psychotherapy: Making the case in an era of managed care* (pp. 102–150). Supplement to *Psychoanalytic Inquiry*.

Dumont, M. P. (1992). *Treating the poor.* Belmont, MA: Dymphna Press.

Edward, J., & Sanville, J. (Eds.). (1996). *Fostering healing and growth: A psychoanalytic social work approach.* London: Jason Aronson.

Fonagy, P., & Target, M. (1996). Outcome predictions in child analysis. *Journal of the American Psychoanalytic Association, 44,* 27–73.

Gumpert, P. (1996, November/December). Restoring our psychotherapy practices: Analysis and recommendations to professionals. *Consortium for Psychotherapy Newsletter,* pp. 1–7. (Available from the Consortium for Psychotherapy, 150 Clark Road, Brookline, MA 02146)

Leyerle, B. (1994). *The private regulation of American health care.* Armonk, NY: M. E. Sharpe.

Lifton, R. J. (1973). *Home from the war.* New York: Simon & Schuster.

Marans, S., Adnopoz, J., Berkman, M., Esserman, D., MacDonald P., Nagler, S., Randall, R., Schafer, M., & Wearing, M. (1995). *The police–mental health partnership.* New Haven, CT: Yale Universities Press.

Miller, I. J. (1997). Beware of a Trojan horse from managed care: Dangerous provisions in parity legislation. *Independent Practitioner, 17,* 138–143.

Moynihan, D. P. (1996). *Miles to go.* Cambridge, MA: Harvard University Press.

Rich, F. (1997, December 23). The last taboo [Editorial]. *New York Times,* p. A19.

Rowe, C. E. (1994). Musings of an analyst on a house visit to a ghetto child. *Contemporary Psychotherapy Review, 9,* 82–90.

Seligman, M.E.P. (1995). The effectiveness of psychotherapy: The *Consumer Reports* study. *American Psychologist, 60,* 965–974.

Volkan, V. (1988). *The need to have enemies and allies.* London: Jason Aronson.

PART **FIVE**

New Opportunities

CHAPTER 34

Primary Care as a Context for Mental Health Practice

Gunnar Almgren

Since the early 1980s and the dramatic fiscal successes of the Medicare prospective payment system, the national march toward managed care has been relentless, albeit unpopular. Some see managed care as a sinister societal transformation aimed at the de facto abolishment of basic access to adequate health and mental health care (Keigher, 1995; Wooley, 1993). Others, most notably health care economist Victor Fuchs (1974, 1993), have long viewed the national evolvement of managed care organizations as a desirable and necessary cost-containment prerequisite to the eventual achievement of universal access to health care. Whether managed care is viewed through a positive or a negative lens, the managed care model is now the dominant paradigm of both health and mental health care delivery systems, and primary care group practices are at the heart of the emergent managed care system model.

Fortunately, there are precedents within various approaches to group primary care practice that promote a genuine and promising integration of health and mental health care in a manner consistent with both the aims and the interests of the social work profession. The premise of this chapter is that the renewed emphasis on primary care as the prime locus of health care delivery has created new opportunities for social workers to engage in collaborative health and mental health practice in settings consistent with the profession's support of holistic approaches to health care. Under the general context of managed care, primary care has been reconceptualized and reborn. It has become more interdisciplinary, more collaborative, more focused on the person and person-in-situation, more holistic, and less centered on disease. The term "health and mental health practice" is used because the historic separation of these two domains of social work practice has been driven by the organization of American medicine, which in turn created divisions and artificial dichotomies of organization within the health care institutions that fostered the contemporary structures of professional social work (Bracht, 1978; Lubove, 1965). Consequently, psychiatric social workers and medical social workers, like their counterparts in medicine, train in different settings, tend to favor different schools of social work, support different professional journals, and generally seek professional support and credentialing through different professional organizations.

NOTE: Originally published as Almgren, G. (1998). Primary care as a context for mental health practice. *Smith College Studies in Social Work, 68,* 233–253.

One positive outcome of the trend toward managed care is the evolution of group primary care practice settings that are large enough to support a professionally diverse staff. Moreover, primary care practice settings demand the integration of both the health and mental health aspects of patient care in ways that defy the fragmenting biases of specialized practice, whether within medicine or within social work. Thus, social workers in primary care settings confront issues of family violence, drug and alcohol abuse, depression, and psychosis, as well as the compendium of concerns that arise in the face of chronic illness, disability, and death. Social workers in primary care settings also are able to address these highly sensitive problems with individual patients and families in a context that is inherently less stigmatizing than even the best traditional mental health agencies. Finally, because social workers in primary care practice settings enjoy the ability to follow individuals and families over years rather than weeks and months, they can help individuals and families address predictable life course issues in a timely and "normalizing" manner. This chapter documents the market forces behind the development of multidisciplinary collaborative primary care practice within managed care systems, describes the related emergence of models of social work practice that integrate the historically dichotomous aspects of health and mental health social work practice, and then concludes with some general implications for professional social work education and organization.

Emergence of Multidisciplinary Collaborative Primary Care Medical Practice under Managed Care

In his highly regarded social history of the medical profession, Paul Starr (1982) identified professional autonomy and free enterprise as two critical value orientations that had a large role in determining the basic organization of American medicine. Another critical trend in American medicine has been the trend toward specialization, fostered by technological innovation, an ever more sophisticated knowledge base, pursuit of the prestige that specialization represents, and a health care financing system that for years has favored specialized intervention and the use of sophisticated technology over conservative management and preventive care (Weisbrod, 1991). Thus, the archetype of medical practice until the past few decades has been the single practitioner office or small partnership, operating within an informal network of referral relationships to other physicians. The typical medical practice functioned like a small and highly specialized business, financially if not philosophically biased toward medicalization of social distress, with only limited capability and incentives to support collaborative partnerships with other nonphysician professionals.

The 1970s concluded with a fundamental reappraisal of the organization of American medicine. Peer review forms of cost control had clearly failed to control rising health care costs, the prestige and financial rewards of specialty practice had created a shortage of primary care physicians, and health maintenance organizations (HMOs) began to emerge as the only form of health care delivery demonstrably capable of cost-efficient health care (Institute of Medicine, 1996). The more fiscally successful HMOs of the 1970s shared a similar, primary medicine–driven organizational structure that has since emerged as the dominant form of health care system organization. As a result of the lessons learned from the successful HMOs in the 1970s, as well as the emergence of genuine price-based (as opposed to technology-based) competition during the 1980s, formally independent and largely autonomous hospitals have been merging and forming new partnerships at a frenetic pace in health care markets all across the United States. These new "organized care delivery systems" consistently place group practice primary medicine clinics at the center of a comprehensive health care network with controlled access to all forms of health care, including hospital and mental health care. In concert with increasingly sophisticated clinical information management systems, group primary medicine practice clinics perform the critical gatekeeping functions that are essential to the fiscal viability and competitiveness of the system as a whole.

Stephan Shortell, perhaps the foremost contemporary scholar of health care organizations, has identified the critical shared features of organized care delivery systems: vertical integration of a comprehensive array of health services (including primary care, acute hospital care, home health care, hospice care, and long-term care), coordinated care to a defined population, clinical and fiscal accountability for health outcomes, and integration with a defined insurance product (Shortell, Gillies, & Anderson, 1994). Shortell and his colleagues also argued that the most successful systems will need to achieve a high degree of integration in clinical decision making, an outcome that is far more consistent with group practice models rather than with the more traditional solo and small partnership practices.

Several stable trends in the market-driven health care reform of today reinforce the conclusion that multidisciplinary collaborative primary care practice models will continue their vigorous ascent to become the dominant means of access to both health and mental health care for all Americans. A brief list of the most important of these trends includes the movement toward population-based health care, the consolidation of health care markets into a few dominant systems of health care delivery, the ascendance of prevention over intervention-based health care, a renewed emphasis on outcome-based standards of practice, consumer preferences for quasi-individualized primary care, and a shift in the direction of physician training toward multidisciplinary collaborative primary care practice. I will describe each of these major trends and their relevance to the future dominance of multidisciplinary collaborative primary care practice. The particular importance of population-based health care warrants a more elaborate explanation, because such plans virtually dictate the future dominance of collaborative primary care practice models.

POPULATION-BASED HEALTH CARE

Throughout the modern history of the U.S. health care system, the predominant form of health care financing and delivery has been the individually based fee-for-service model. Under this model of care, the risks for increased health care costs (whether driven by the financial interests of the provider or the increased morbidity of the patient) are largely absorbed by the patient's health care insurer. In addition, both the patient and the provider have powerful incentives to use health care. In the case of the insured patient, this is because the patient generally perceives that health care services are beneficial to his or her well-being and because he or she believes that the health care insurer largely bears the costs of high health care utilization. This has never been true in the strict economic sense, but perceptions are far more important to consumer behavior than is truth. For providers, fee-for-service reimbursement means that their revenue is directly proportional to the type and quantity of health care services provided. Within surprisingly limited boundaries, providers also define the type and amount of health care that is prudent and necessary. Regulatory cost-control efforts, whether introduced by a government insurance program or an employer-based insurance program, cannot overcome such powerful consumer and provider incentives to promote the use of health care. Although politically relevant recognition of this fact has been slow in coming because of decades of often disingenuous tactics by the health care industry, now both the government and employers have embarked on a national campaign to dismantle the traditional fee-for-service model in favor of health care financing models that both limit access to care and place the burden on providers to deliver cost-effective services at a competitive price (Shortell & Reinhardt, 1992).

The essential features of population-based health care are the delivery of health care services through an integrated network of providers to a defined population at a uniform per capita price. Additionally, all large-volume health care providers in a population-based health care system generally are either employed by the insurer or have entered into a contractual relationship with the insurer that places the provider at financial risk for the cost of health care services that exceed a given target amount. In the case of the more traditional, staff-model HMO, physicians who work in a primary care practice clinic often have salary incentives that are tied to the extent patients in their practice have modest levels of health care utilization. Alternatively, for independent practice associations of primary care providers contracting with insurance plans that are population based, the contract language may contain fee incentives tied to low utilization of expensive health care services and technologies. In some insurance products, the contracting independent practice association may simply be given a set per capita fee to provide all necessary primary care over a defined period to a defined population of patients.

Whether the relationship to the population-based insurance plan is through direct employment or through provider contract, the primary care provider group has significant incentives to limit access to care that is unlikely to clearly benefit the patient or unlikely to prevent a more significant financial risk to the insurer. In addition, the population-based insurance plans also set productivity targets to keep staffing at the minimum level necessary to retain staff, attract customers, and meet health care outcome goals.

Health care outcome goals fall into two broad types: those that directly measure patient health outcomes (for example, infant birth weight) and those that primarily measure health care utilization (for example, annual mean acute care hospital-days by age and gender). Both types are critical to the marketability and financial viability of particular health plans in that the major purchasers of health care (employers and the government) have become increasingly sophisticated and demanding with respect to demonstrable health outcomes as a defined insurance product. Although the balance of cost and quality has a long way to go in health care, there is a strong consensus among the government and employers that population-based health care plans are the preferred option as a matter of national interest and future health care policy.

There are several points of convergence between the demands of population-based health care and the specific competencies and philosophical perspective of the social work profession. These include a renewed interest in prevention; a greater emphasis on the role of community in individual health outcomes; and the information management infrastructure and financial motivation to recognize the role of such issues as domestic violence, personal life crises, substance abuse, and mental illness as explicit health care concerns.

CONSOLIDATION OF HEALTH CARE MARKETS

As a matter of historic health care policy, health care insurance coverage has been primarily tied to employment. For this reason, health care markets correspond both geographically and economically to labor markets. Until the early 1980s, employers within a given health care market purchased health care insurance products with an eye to benefits that would be attractive to their employees, largely because there was little genuine price competition between providers of health care and the health insurance providers.

The diffusion of price competition across health care markets since the mid-1980s has been uneven, but a common adaptive process is apparent. First, as employers seek less-costly health care plans, insurance companies begin to restrict their contracting to health care providers who will meet their reduced fee schedule. Hospitals soon begin to struggle financially, some close (typically those that serve a higher proportion of the poor population), and others seek partnerships with formerly competitive hospitals that they believe will complement their joint viability. Similarly, independent physicians begin to seek larger partnerships as they are required to accept insurance contracts with more limited fee schedules and higher administrative costs. At the next stage of consolidation, a highly price-competitive managed care insurance carrier enters the market, both driving other health care insurers out of the market and entering into partnerships with a restricted number of potentially cost-efficient providers. Those providers that are left out of this partnership then scramble to put together competitive insurer–provider merged systems of their own, again introducing another round of provider mergers and hospital closures. At the final stage of market consolidation, a health care market has only a few mega providers left, each of which is an organized delivery system representing the merger or partnership of a number of formerly independent health care providers under the flag of a common group of insurance products. At this final stage, solo primary care practices have disappeared in favor of group practices owned by or affiliated with an organized delivery system. Specialists fare less well, with many facing either a significant career change or migration to a less mature health care market.

The consolidation of health care markets to a few dominant organized delivery systems has both positive and negative implications for the social work profession. Such systems are highly effective at reducing hospital utilization and cutting back hospital services deemed "nonessential" to hospital care. In many hospitals, this has meant the elimination of social work departments, wholesale reductions in social work staffing, and the elimination of social work services not tied directly to discharge planning. On the other hand, such systems also have created innovative opportunities for social work practice in outpatient settings that are attempting to structure the services necessary to sustain a well-integrated continuum of care. Within the Puget Sound health care region, the Providence health care system, the Group Health Cooperative system, and the University of Washington health care system have all offset inpatient social work staffing reductions with expansions of outpatient social work services in primary practice clinics. In general, these shifts to outpatient practice represent fiscally pragmatic attempts to place social workers where they are effective in promoting desirable health outcomes and are demonstrably capable of lowering unnecessary use of other health care services. To the extent that the social work profession can market itself in terms of these kinds of outcomes, such huge organized care delivery systems will have incentives to employ social workers. Clearly, the burden is on the social work profession to make a case for clinical effectiveness in areas valued both by consumers and the health care delivery system.

PREVENTION VERSUS INTERVENTION-BASED HEALTH CARE

Despite years of rhetoric from the health care industry and literally billions of dollars in preventive health care research, preventive health care has received relatively little emphasis as a component of the U.S. health care system. In large part this is because the principle proponent of preventive health care, the public health system, has been politically weak and fragmented both in its mission and its organization (Stivers, 1991). A key contributing factor to the weak political position of public health has been the medical profession's financial interest in promoting private, fee-based medical intervention over publicly sponsored health care programs in any form—including prevention programs (Starr, 1982). However, even HMOs have had mixed success with health promotion and prevention programs, largely because prevention programs often require significant changes in health behavior as an outcome. Achieving stable changes in health behavior can be expensive, and such programs must offset those initial expenses with a tangible health care cost savings. Given the instability of the consumer–insurer relationship, HMOs historically have had to focus on illness-prevention programs that both are effective at changing health behavior and result in health care dollar cost savings within a relatively short period of time.

Until recently, those realities have narrowed the scope of prevention activities considerably, again despite rhetoric to the contrary. However, to the extent that health care markets consolidate to a few insurer–provider organizations with stable populations of consumers, prevention programs become a much more viable investment and their vigorous expansion can be expected. Here the implications for the social work profession are nothing but positive. Sustained changes in health care behavior, whether at the community or the individual level, are within both the science and historical traditions of the social work profession.

OUTCOME-BASED STANDARDIZATION OF PRACTICE

In many respects, information technology, if not the costs of medical malpractice claims, has long been promoting the growth of outcome-based standards of practice. However, the convergence of other conditions necessary to the widespread adoption of outcome-based standards of practice is recent. These other necessary conditions include the providers' direct and tangible financial stake in the clinical outcomes of their decisions; investment in the information technology infrastructure necessary to sustain cutting-edge, outcome-based standards of practice; shared philosophies of practice; and recognition that clinical outcomes can be a discernible and important competitive feature in the health care market. All of these conditions are consequent to the consolidation of health care markets into a relatively small number of organized, competitive, population-based delivery systems. In the emergent health care markets of today, not-for-profit and for-profit health care corporations are striving to be the best at achieving measurable health care outcomes at the lowest per capita coverage price and are investing heavily in the information technology infrastructures necessary to do so.

The emphasis on outcome-based standardization of practice has mixed implications for the social work profession. On the one hand, the trend toward developing empirically based practice methods within social work should favor our capacity to adapt to an outcome-based versus structure-and-process–based health care market. In fact, the social work profession has already benefited from the recognition by many large insurance carriers that for many mental health problems, MSW psychotherapists can achieve the same treatment outcomes as psychiatrists. On the other hand, outcome-based standards of practice often do not adapt well where latent individual traits are highly relevant. In addition, outcome-based standards of practice are prone to ethnic, racial, or gender biases to the extent that they are empirically derived from a homogeneous population (Pincus, Zarin, & West, 1996).

CONSUMER PREFERENCES FOR QUASI-INDIVIDUALIZED HEALTH CARE

To defeat the Clinton Health Plan, the conservative elements of the medical profession and their health care industry allies needed to paint the plan as a government incursion into the sacred patient–doctor relationship. In a successful multimillion-dollar media blitz, the public were convinced that they would lose their ability to retain a doctor who understood their needs and who would act as an advocate for their interests. The success of this campaign has not been lost on the emergent mega health care organizations competing for the health care consumer's dollar. Although employer- and government-driven emphasis on reducing health care expenditures remains the pre-eminent factor in health care reform, the most successful systems will be those that give their patients a sense of confidence that their interests are protected and that their providers are sensitive to their needs. This criterion suggests that primary care practice clinics will need to convey a sense of empathetic individualized care, while at the same time meeting clinical productivity targets that limit patient–doctor encounter times.

Social workers can play two critical roles in enabling an organization to balance the competing priorities of individualized care and constraints on physician resources. The first role concerns the ability of social workers to assist physicians and clinic managers in creating an organizational environment sensitive to the diverse needs of patients, particularly in the domain of patient–provider communication. The second role concerns the ability of social workers to fulfill the role of "physician extender" to patients having problems that demand high levels of interpersonal contact time, such as, frail elderly men and women, patients with chronic illness, and patients in transitional life crises. Physician extenders are allied health professionals who increase the productivity of physicians by assuming some tasks and professional responsibilities that physicians need not perform or are not the best trained to perform. Although physician extenders are more often described in the medical literature as licensed physician assistants and nurse practitioners (Institute of Medicine, 1996), social workers have fulfilled physician extender functions for decades under the auspices of traditional medical social work (Bracht, 1978).

SHIFT OF MEDICAL TRAINING TO MULTIDISCIPLINARY COLLABORATIVE PRACTICE PRIMARY CARE

In the 1930s, nearly all physicians in private practice were in general practice. As medicine became more technologically sophisticated and its knowledge base expanded, medical schools shifted their training emphasis to specialized areas of medical practice, and the division of labor within medicine became highly differentiated.

Currently, nearly two-thirds of physicians are in nonprimary medicine specializations, and there is a general perception that a nationwide shortage of primary care physicians exists, particularly within rural areas and poverty-stricken urban neighborhoods (Institute of Medicine, 1996). In addition, as insurance carriers compete to cut costs, we see an almost frantic market driven by medical care delivery systems restructuring toward an emphasis on primary care. This effort has resulted in a major recruitment and training shift toward training in primary care, as medical schools retool their recruitment criteria and curricula to meet the market demand for primary care physicians. Finally, in contrast to historical training models in primary practice, primary care training programs today place much greater emphasis on multidisciplinary collaborative primary care practice as the envisioned context of practice. That is, physicians are more likely to be trained in contexts where patient care involves collaborative power-sharing efforts among physicians, nurse practitioners, and social workers. In part, that approach has evolved as a response to primary care practices becoming the focal point for managing chronic as well as acute illnesses (Institute of Medicine, 1996).

Obviously, the increased emphasis on multidisciplinary collaborative practice in the training of physicians is positive for the viability of social work in health care. Scholars of social work in health care have long held that to the extent physicians are exposed to positive multidisciplinary practice experiences with social workers in their training, they are socialized to value the professional contributions of social workers (Hookey, 1979). In many ways, the fee-for-service model of health care delivery offers few incentives for primary care physicians to seek collaborative practices with social workers, despite what may have been positive experiences in training. Now that most newly trained primary care physicians will be entering some form of managed care practice with a totally different calculus of fiscal incentives, training experiences may more closely reflect the likelihood that physicians will be proponents of multidisciplinary practice with social workers in their career settings. In fact, the American Academy of Family Physicians (AAFP) has now adopted a formal position calling for the further development of collaborative models of primary care practice that integrate the services of social workers and clinical psychologists with those of primary care physicians (AAFP, 1995).

Convergence of Health and Mental Health Social Work Practice in Contemporary Primary Care Settings

Thus far, this chapter has focused on the market forces that promote the dominance of multidisciplinary primary care practice models that operate at the basic nexus of integrated health care systems. Attention now turns to an examination of the opportunities for progressive social work practice within these settings, in particular the opportunity to promote a more functional synthesis between health and mental health practice. Like the foregoing discussion, the perspective assumed is generally optimistic.

It has long been established from national ambulatory care survey data that nonpsychiatric physicians function as the de facto mental health care system for most psychiatric problems (Regier, Goldberg, & Taube, 1978; Schurman, Kramer, & Mitchell, 1985; Zimmerman & Wienckowski, 1991). In their analysis of data from the National Ambulatory Medical Care Survey, Schurman et al. found that roughly 50 percent of professional visits that result in a primary or secondary diagnosis of mental disorder occur in nonpsychiatric physician offices. Their findings also included two other notable observations. First, they found that two-thirds of patients diagnosed with a psychiatric disorder presented a physical complaint as the reason for seeking care. Second, fewer than 5 percent of patients with a psychiatric diagnosis were likely to be referred elsewhere for treatment.

Despite the fact that the medical profession has long recognized that a significant proportion of primary practice use occurs in response to mental health issues, physicians and health care insurance companies have been slow to adapt the structure of primary practice medicine in a way that promotes more effective mental health outcomes. This is now changing because of two critical factors. First, the elimination of fee-for-service payment mechanisms in favor of population-based financing means that physicians are not rewarded financially for providing de facto mental health services through office visits. Second, mega health care delivery systems are now aggressively seeking ways to provide mental health services in a cost-efficient manner because mental health benefits remain in demand by consumers (Simon, Von Korff, & Durham, 1994), and unmet mental health needs are empirically linked to high health care utilization (Smith, Monson, & Ray, 1986). Given these factors, how are organized delivery systems likely to provide mental health services, and what are the implications for the social work profession?

Pincus (1987) identified six basic models through which mental health services are provided: joint care, consultation, referral, the independent provider, the autonomous primary care provider, and the autonomous mental health provider. Under the joint care model, both the primary care physician and the mental health provider are directly and significantly involved in the care of the patient, whereas under the consultation model, the primary care physician is the principal care provider of face-to-face services with some provision for consultant contact. The referral model is basically the inverse of the consultation model, with the face-to-face contact supplied by the mental health provider. Under the independent model, both the mental health provider and the primary care physician offer face-to-face direct services to the patient, with no collateral contact and coordination of care. Both of the autonomous models involve total and exclusive care through either the primary care physician or the mental health provider. From the standpoint of optimal mental health treatment, the latter three models are the least desirable because health and mental health care issues are rigidly dichotomized and mental health care is inherently more stigmatized.

Although the AAFP (1995) has adopted a formal position in opposition to "carve-out" management approaches that transfer the mental health care of patients with psychiatric diagnoses to specialized physician or nonphysician mental health providers, it is far more likely that mega health care systems will vary their approaches to the provision of mental health service on the basis of regional context. Three general approaches seem most likely to incorporate all the models of mental health care identified by Pincus (1987). In a Model I approach, the primary care physician performs a rigid gatekeeping function, generally permitting highly limited access to specialized "carve-out mental health services" for only the most severely affected patients. In addition, less-than-severe mental health issues are treated, except as they emerge as somatic complaints and behavioral management issues. In a Model II approach, mental health issues are recognized aspects of health care, but referrals to carve-out mental health services are the norm for both moderately and severely affected patients. In a Model III approach, mental health services are an integral component of primary care practice, and referrals to carve-out mental health services are reserved for only the most severely affected patients, that is, patients with mental illnesses that are "nonresponsive to primary care-based treatment" (AAFP, 1995, p. 6). Obviously, the three models represent markedly different organizational contexts for social work and thus have different strategic and role implications.

SOCIAL WORK IN A MODEL I ORGANIZATIONAL ENVIRONMENT

The organizational environment characterized in this model represents the convergence of the worst of two worlds in contemporary medicine. On the one hand, mental health problems are denied and marginalized because, for the most part, primary care physicians are poorly trained or are working within organizational structures that are biased against the treatment of mental health problems as an integral component of primary health care. On the other hand, primary care physicians also are constrained by various managed care incentives to avoid referral to specialists except as a last resort. Social workers employed in these organizational environments are more likely to be employed on the basis of their ability to act as case managers; perform tasks associated with pre- and post-hospital discharge planning; or, by virtue of their employment, provide services to some special population (for example, a maternal–child health care grant).

Whatever the basis of their employment, social workers' strategic challenge is to use their formal role as a base to transform the organizational approach to mental health care. Effective transformational social workers first use their formal role to gain credibility with their medical colleagues and administrators and then incrementally enable them to recognize that interpersonal conflicts, psychological distress, physical symptomatology, and support seeking are resource-consuming issues that are inexorably intertwined elements of everyday primary health care (Eurelings-Bontekoe, Diekstra, & Verschuur, 1995; Sartorius, 1989). A particularly effective strategy is to target focused social work intervention to patients who present multiple somatic complaints and are high users of service. Aside from the direct cost issues, such patients also can be deeply frustrating to physicians on a personal level. The empirical basis of this strategy is the well-established linkage between unmet mental health needs and health care utilization (Sensky, MacLeod, & Rigby, 1996; Simon, 1992; Smith et al., 1986).

SOCIAL WORK IN A MODEL II ORGANIZATIONAL ENVIRONMENT

Two important social work issues arise where the basic organizational norm for moderate to severe mental health problems is out-referral to mental health services. The first concerns the extent to which adequate mechanisms exist for close collaboration between the primary care clinic and the mental health providers. Fragmentation of mental health care is a problem in many organized health care delivery systems, and social workers can play a critical role in ensuring close collaboration between the primary care clinic and the mental health services providers. Most primary care physicians appear able to recognize the presence of mental disorders, but it is unrealistic to expect them to accurately diagnose specific psychiatric conditions and identify the most effective forms of mental health intervention (Andersen & Harthorn, 1989). Adequate collaborative practice standards between primary care and mental health providers include, at a minimum, clear referral criteria, clear assignment of pharmaceutical management responsibilities, periodic communication from the mental health provider about the patient's mental health status, and notification of the primary care provider where hospitalization occurs (Lazarus, 1995).

The second issue concerns the provision of "on-site" mental health services. Even in contexts where primary care physicians have access to organizationally sanctioned external mental health resources, many if not most mental health issues encountered in primary care practice are not likely to result in a referral to an external mental health provider (Burns & Burke, 1985). In part, this reflects the stigma attached to mental health services not provided within the medicalized context of a primary care clinic. In addition, many of the mental health problems encountered in primary care practice (adjustment disorders, mild mood disorders, and situational crises) can be addressed competently by a primary care physician with adequate, available consultation (Lazarus, 1995). Finally, many patients with chronic and serious health problems require a quality of relationship with their primary care providers that mirrors the relationship with a nurturing psychotherapist. Out-referral for mental health issues under such circumstances may be viewed by the patient (often accurately) as a rejection of legitimate dependency needs rather than a benevolent attempt to provide appropriate care.

That latter point is particularly relevant given both the market-driven shift of chronic disease management to primary care and the fact that decades of medical advances have prolonged the life of people with chronic diseases. For example, as HIV has shifted from a purely terminal disease to a chronic disease with an uncertain prognosis, it is increasingly the case that management of HIV disease is performed by primary care physicians (Feingold & Slammon, 1993). Mental health issues common to HIV disease include depression, separation, grief and loss issues, stress and coping support, anger management and interpersonal conflict, adaptive sexuality, caregiver stress, and at the later stages of the disease, organic psychosis. In addition, primary care physicians often have a difficult time adapting to the role of primary care providers for people with HIV. Providers frequently resent the burdens imposed by chronic disease, and HIV disease is fraught with stigma and unrealistic fears concerning its potential for casual contact contagion. Social workers with a firm understanding of the biopsychosocial aspects of HIV can enable their primary medicine colleagues to identify and obviate their fears and resentments so they can exploit more fully their strengths as professional care providers.

Social workers practicing within Model II primary care settings, whether or not they are viewed formally as mental health service providers, are and should be a critical link to external mental health resources. When linkages between primary care and mental health care providers are weak, social workers who facilitate onsite mental health training, mental health case conferencing, and case-specific liaison functions can promote better collaboration. In the common situation in which primary care patients with mental health issues are not referred externally for mental health care, social workers can help the primary care clinic provide competent mental health care through consultation with the primary care physician, focused training in such areas as domestic violence, and limited onsite individual psychotherapy. Social workers in Model II settings also can facilitate support groups for clinic patients with common mental health issues such as moderate postpartum depression, loss and grieving, coping with chronic disease, and specific relationship problems common to everyday life.

SOCIAL WORK IN A MODEL III ORGANIZATIONAL CONTEXT

Model III, in which only the most severely affected and nonresponsive mental health patients are referred for nonprimary care management, represents the organizational context most in alignment with both the social work profession's holistic orientation and the official policy position of the dominant segment of primary care physicians (AAFP, 1995). In a Model III environment, on-site multidisciplinary collaborative treatment of mental illness is the norm. The primary care physician remains the overall coordinator of care, but in-depth or extensive psychotherapy is provided on-site by another mental health professional, typically a clinical psychologist or a social worker. Even severely affected patients who are initially nonresponsive to primary care management return to primary care for management of all health care issues when their mental health conditions are stabilized.

The key strategic challenge to social work in a Model III organizational environment is to avoid becoming marginalized as a mental health care provider. The surest road to marginalization is to narrowly define practice in either the stereotypical task-oriented medical social work domain or within the confines of individual and family psychotherapy. As previously mentioned, both alternatives mirror and reinforce the dichotomization of social work, a profession that grew out of a historic pragmatic response to organized medicine. Clinic administrators and their prime professional constituents primary care physicians will regard social work more favorably than other competitive providers of mental health services to the extent that social workers in primary care settings develop and sustain competencies that both extend primary care physicians' capability to coordinate care across a complex continuum of health care services and allow them to provide effective on-site mental health services. Although some social workers may argue that it is impossible to be competent within both domains of practice, such protestations are more reflective of personal career choices and perhaps the biases sustained by traditional professional socialization.

It is the case, however, that many social workers who aspire to practice in these settings will need to retool in areas in which competencies have been limited by former training and experience. Social workers with professional backgrounds limited to traditional mental health settings will need to develop a knowledge base in such critical areas as basic medical terminology, aging, chronic disease, health care policy, the sociology of multidisciplinary practice, and community health care resources. Social workers with a background limited to traditional health care settings will typically need to develop a deeper knowledge base in psychopathology, psychopharmacology, brief individual treatment, and family therapy. In both situations, the development of a preceptor relationship with advanced social work practitioners is highly recommended. Adequate retraining will often require a significant professional investment, in many cases the equivalent of a third year of graduate school. However, the intrinsic rewards of practice within a cutting-edge professional environment are significant.

Discussion: Toward a New, Convergent Model of Health and Mental Health Care Practice

The jury is out with respect to which of the three basic models of primary care practice will emerge as the more dominant as macro-integrated health care systems evolve. Although there is some empirical evidence suggesting that both the cost and quality goals of organized delivery systems would be better served by Model III (German, 1994), factors such as aggressive efforts by corporate mental health providers, variation among state mental health policies, and divisions within the medical profession are likely to play a role in shaping the final outcome. However, each context depicted suggests that the social work profession should re-examine internal professional structures that sustain the historic distinctions between health and mental health practice. Social workers in diverse primary care settings clearly engage in professional activities that fall within both traditional domains of social work practice (Greene & Kulper, 1990), therefore compelling the profession to consider more seriously a convergent model of health and mental health practice.

It is beyond the scope of this chapter to define all the prerequisites of a convergent health and mental health model of social work practice, but some theoretical and substantive elements are suggested, given both the dominance of individual mental health issues and the integrative nature of practice in population-based health care delivery systems: an ecological or systems perspective that incorporates the role of family, community, and society; a well-integrated theory of individual human development and adaptation; a knowledge base in cross-cultural theories of health and illness; a knowledge base in the psychosocial aspects of acute and chronic illness across the life course; and specific skills in multilevel intervention, including individual, group, and family psychotherapy, as well as multidisciplinary team practice (Brochstein, Adams, Tristan, & Cheney, 1978).

Implications for Professional Preparation and the Division of Labor among the Health Professions

Social work's ascendance to a significant presence in the health care labor force occurred during eras of tremendous health care resource expansion. The first era occurred between 1900 and 1930 as the nation expanded its hospital resources from roughly 1,400 to 4,700 hospitals (Commonwealth Fund, 1947). The second era of major expansion occurred between 1965 and the early 1980s, when the U.S. government both assumed a major share of health care financing and subsequently required hospitals and some other specialized providers to provide social services to patients as a condition of participating in federally sponsored health care programs. We are now in an era of health care resource containment,[1] and the social work profession is experiencing intensified levels of interprofessional competition from nurses and even paraprofessional human services workers as health care delivery systems strive to define the most cost-efficient division of labor at a marketable level of quality. Organized health care delivery systems, whether they are for-profit or

[1]I avoid the word "shrinkage" here because the proportion of the gross national product allocated to health care resources is unlikely to diminish significantly below the current level. Americans still demand high levels of health care, and the age distribution of the population will promote higher levels of health care utilization well into the next century.

not-for-profit systems, are already competing in the same markets according the same cost and quality criteria. The winners will be those organized health care delivery systems most able to inspire consumer confidence at the lowest price, primarily through a highly rational, outcome-driven division of labor between the competing professions.

The implications for professional preparation in social work are many, but three seem particularly critical. The first is that schools of social work that retain health care curricula with limited emphasis on mental health content risk training their graduates for unemployment. The evolving health care system will need fewer, not more, narrowly trained MSW hospital discharge planners. The second implication is a more positive one: Social workers prepared to practice with the convergent knowledge base and skills in health and mental health practice are likely to be highly marketable, particularly as evolving organized care delivery systems grapple with the reality that their populations will demand (directly or indirectly) what are de facto mental health services. From the perspective of competition among social work, psychology, and psychiatry, the strategy argued here is to let the latter two health professions compete to be the "carve-out" providers of mental health services. Both in terms of its curriculum structures and its efforts in the field, the social work profession should instead aggressively seek to enlarge its foothold in primary care. A third implication is that social work, like the nursing profession, will have to confront the reality that dominantly task-oriented professional roles will fall to paraprofessionals. That reality means that attempts by the profession to rationalize the practice distinctions among MSWs, BSWs, and human services paraprofessionals need to be more definitive and grounded in the outcome-driven labor demands of competitive organized care delivery systems. In particular, the social work profession should focus its political efforts on the protection of turf that is explicitly professional and has a promising future in the evolving price- and outcome-driven health care economy.

References

American Academy of Family Physicians. (1995). AAFP white paper on the provision of mental health care services by family physicians. *American Family Physician, 51,* 1405–1412.

Andersen, S. M., & Harthorn, B. H. (1989). The recognition, diagnosis, and treatment of mental disorders by primary care physicians. *Medical Care, 27,* 869–886.

Bracht, N. (1978). *Social work in health care: A guide to professional practice.* New York: Haworth Press.

Brochstein, J. R., Adams, G. L., Tristan, M. P., & Cheney, C. C. (1978). Social work and primary health care: An integrative approach. *Social Work in Health Care, 5,* 71–80.

Burns, B. J., & Burke, J. D. (1985). Improving mental health practices in primary care: Findings from recent research. *Public Health Reports, 100,* 294–300.

Commonwealth Fund, Commission on Hospital Care. (1947). *Hospital care in the United States.* New York: Author.

Eurelings-Bontekoe, H. M., Diekstra, R. F., & Verschuur, M. (1995). Psychological distress. Social support, and social support seeking: A prospective study among primary mental health care patients. *Social Science and Medicine, 40,* 1083–1089.

Feingold, A., & Slammon, W. R. (1993). A model integrating mental health and primary care services for families with HIV. *General Hospital Psychiatry, 15,* 290–300.

Fuchs, V. (1974). *Who shall live? Health, economics, and social choice.* New York: Basic Books.

Fuchs, V. (1993). *The future of health policy.* Cambridge, MA: Harvard University Press.

German, M. (1994). Effective case management in managed mental health care: Conditions, methods, and outcomes. *HMO Practice, 8,* 34–40.

Greene, G. J., & Kulper, T. (1990). Autonomy and professional activities of social workers in hospital and primary health care settings. *Health & Social Work, 15,* 38–44.

Hookey, P. (1979). Cost–benefit evaluations in primary health care. *Health & Social Work, 4,* 152–167.

Institute of Medicine, Committee on the Future of Primary Care. (1996). *Primary care: America's health in a new era.* Washington, DC: National Academy Press.

Keigher, S. M. (1995). Managed care's silent seduction of America and the new politics of choice [National Health Line]. *Health & Social Work, 20,* 146–151.

Lazarus, A. (1995). The role of primary physicians in managed mental health care. *Psychiatric Services, 46,* 343–345.

Lubove, R. (1965). *The professional altruist: The emergence of social work as a career.* Cambridge, MA: Harvard University Press.

Pincus, H. A. (1987). Patient oriented models for linking primary care and mental health care. *General Hospital Psychiatry, 9,* 95–101.

Pincus, H. A., Zarin, D. A., & West, J. C. (1996). Peering into the "Black Box": Measuring outcomes of managed care. *Archives of General Psychiatry, 53,* 870–877.

Regier, D. A., Goldberg, I. D., & Taube, C. A. (1978). The de facto U.S. mental health services system: A public health perspective. *Archives of General Psychiatry, 35,* 685–693.

Sartorius, N. (1989). Psychosomatic medicine and primary health care. *Psychotherapy and Psychosomatic Medicine, 52,* 5–9.

Schurman, R. A., Kramer, P. D., & Mitchell, J. B. (1985). The hidden mental health network: Treatment of mental illness by nonpsychiatric physicians. *Archives of General Psychiatry, 42,* 89–94.

Sensky, T., MacLeod, A. K., & Rigby, M. F. (1996). Causal attributions about common somatic sensations among frequent general practice attenders. *Psychological Medicine, 26,* 641–646.

Shortell, S. M., Gillies, R. R., & Anderson, D. A. (1994). The new world of managed care: Creating organized delivery systems. *Health Affairs, 13,* 44–64.

Shortell, S. M., & Reinhardt, U. E. (1992). Creating and executing health care policy in the 1990s. In S. M. Shortell & U. E. Reinhardt (Eds.), *Improving health policy and management: Nine critical research issues for the 1990s* (pp. 3–36). Ann Arbor, MI: Health Administration Press.

Simon, G. E. (1992). Psychiatric disorder and functional somatic symptoms as predictors of health care use. *Psychiatric Medicine, 10*(3), 49–59.

Simon, G. E., Von Korff, M., & Durham, M. L. (1994). Predictors of outpatient mental health utilization by primary care patients in a health maintenance organization. *American Journal of Psychiatry, 151,* 908–913.

Smith, G. R., Jr., Monson, R. A., & Ray, D. C. (1986). Patients with multiple unexplained symptoms, their characteristics, functional health, and health care utilization. *Archives of Internal Medicine, 146,* 69–72.

Starr, P. (1982). *The social transformation of American medicine.* New York: Basic Books.

Stivers, C. (1991). The politics of public health: The dilemma of a public profession. In T. J. Litman & L. S. Robins (Eds.), *Health politics and policy* (pp. 356–369). Albany, NY: Delmar Press.

Weisbrod, B. (1991). The health care quadrilemma: An essay on technical change, insurance, quality of care, and cost containment. *Journal of Economic Literature, 29,* 523–552.

Wooley, S. C. (1993). Managed care and mental health: The silencing of a profession. *International Journal of Eating Disorders, 14,* 387–401.

Zimmerman, M. A., & Wienckowski, L. A. (1991). Revisiting health and mental health linkages: A policy whose time has come . . . again. *Journal of Public Health Policy, 12,* 510–524.

CHAPTER 35

The Role of Multidisciplinary Community Clinics in Managed Care Systems

Cheryl Resnick and Ellen Gelhaus Tighe

Managed care, as a cost-containing system of health care administration, is here to stay. However, this system can leave the most vulnerable populations—poor people, people of color, women and children, and older people—on the periphery. The populations in greatest need are often selected out of managed care systems because their high-risk status (poor nutrition, inadequate income, lack of prenatal care, substandard housing, minimal preventive medical care, and so on) ensures increased costs of care (Sederer & St. Clair, 1989). Specific environments (particularly underserved rural and urban areas) are less likely to be served.

The biopsychosocial and ecological systems models of intervention emphasize the importance of the social and environmental aspects involved in providing health care. This perspective is critical in an era of managed care, where psychosocial and environmental factors are easily lost in a sea of economic diligence. These frameworks are particularly useful in examining the role of the social worker in the community clinic.

Social work's involvement in primary care is not new, as demonstrated by the Cincinnati Social Unit, which functioned from 1917 to 1920 (Betten & Austin, 1977); the New York State Charities Aid Association, which focused on public health issues from 1893 to 1948 (Kane, 1985); and the Henry Street Settlement House of New York, which assisted with the control of infectious diseases (Kane, 1985).

These forerunners of the 1960s neighborhood clinics promoted the recognition that poor people, people of color, and special populations deserve access to comprehensive health care (Gropper, 1987). In 1967 the Office of Economic Opportunity provided for the establishment of neighborhood health centers. Neighborhood clinics of the 1960s perceived disease as an interplay among physical, social, psychological, and environmental factors, forming the basis for the current biopsychosocial model. Their mission was to provide comprehensive care to poor people, people of color, and socially disenfranchised people (Bassoff, 1982). A community clinic provides a setting in which underprivileged people can receive primary health care services within their own communities.

NOTE: Originally published as Resnick, C., & Tighe, E. G. (1997). The role of multidisciplinary community clinics in managed care systems. *Social Work, 42*, 91–98.

Vine Hill Community Clinic Experience

The Vine Hill Community Clinic is a primary care clinic established by the Vanderbilt University School of Nursing and the Metropolitan Development and Housing Authority of Nashville. Kellogg Foundation funding enabled its inception in October 1990. The foundation initiative involved funding the clinic to facilitate the provision of health care to low-income families and to create a model for community empowerment. Simultaneously, the clinic served as a multidisciplinary learning laboratory.

The clinic, which is located in a public housing development in Nashville, is staffed by a multidisciplinary team of family nurse practitioners, mental health clinical specialists, a medical social worker, a community outreach nurse, a medical assistant, a business manager, a janitor, and a receptionist–secretary. Physician preceptors include an adult primary care specialist, a pediatrician, and a psychiatrist, all of whom are on call for consultation and review charts weekly.

The clinic provides primary health care for a medically underserved, low-income, urban neighborhood and serves as a training site for nursing, medical, and social work students. The type of patient seen in the clinic has changed since the project began. Initially, the people most frequently seen resided in the immediate high-rise housing complex (referred to as "the Tower") and the surrounding cottages, both of which make up the Vine Hill Homes. The Tower was originally constructed as senior citizen housing, but it has become home to an increasing number of people with mental and physical disabilities (including some residents with AIDS). The Tower also houses a shelter for homeless men and a branch of a large community mental health center that includes a geriatric day treatment program. These agencies refer clients to the clinic on a regular basis. The cottage population consists of small families, frequently households headed by single women. The racial makeup of the Vine Hill Homes is predominantly white; however, its African American population has grown in recent years. The surrounding community is composed of lower-middle-class families who own or rent small homes. The major draw to the area is the Tennessee State Fairgrounds, which provides part-time, seasonal employment for many Vine Hill inhabitants.

According to the annual progress report submitted to the W. K. Kellogg Foundation in 1992 (Busby, Green, Anness, & Taylor, 1992), the community's central issues include a high degree of clinical depression, family violence, and sexual abuse. The clinic has strengthened existing community organizations, increased teamwork for accomplishing community goals, assisted in conflict resolution, and influenced policymakers in their response to the community. Groups such as the Vine Hill Volunteers, the community advisory board, and the Vine Hill Children's Coalition have emerged to address the needs of the housing development's residents. In 1992 the Vine Hill Volunteers received grant funding for a Maternal–Infant Health Outreach Program. Plans to develop a community day care center have been initiated, and clinic staff as well as social services agency personnel are training community residents to become day care workers.

With the advent of managed care three years into the project, collaboration with the community became even more important to the viability of the clinic. In January 1994 the Vine Hill Community Clinic became one of the primary care provider sites for the Vanderbilt Health Plan (part of the managed care Medicaid project initiated by the State of Tennessee, called "Tenncare").

Interdisciplinary Model

The managed care environment has motivated health care professionals to seek alternative means of providing appropriate care for clients. A popular method for providing appropriate care has been to maximize the use of interdisciplinary staff. Hooker and Freeborn (1991) evaluated the use of physician assistants in managed care health systems and found that using nonphysicians improved access to primary care at a reduced cost.

Physician assistants and nurse practitioners are not the only interdisciplinary staff capable of providing services to patients at a reduced cost. An enhanced social work role can significantly reduce burdens on medical staff under managed care systems. This enhanced function enables staff to meet the needs of more patients at a lowered cost. Winegar (1993) recognized the challenge social work administrators meet in formulating new roles for social work professionals. Along with several useful suggestions for negotiating managed care systems, Winegar recommended the "utilization of a variety of mental health professionals in addition to psychiatrists" (p. 175). In addition, "unless the complex social and medical needs of patients are recognized and unless a comprehensive package of services is provided based on an interdisciplinary health care model (that includes social workers), a majority of Americans will be underinsured or forced to pay significant additional fees for uncovered services or supplemental insurance" (Mizrahi, 1993, p. 89).

Role of the Clinic Social Worker

Between 20 percent and 80 percent of primary care visits involve the medicalization of presenting problems that are frequently psychosocial in origin (Azzarto, 1993; Curiel, Brochstein, Cheney, & Adams, 1979; Ell & Morrison, 1981; Gropper, 1987; Mullaly, 1988). Physicians spend an inordinate amount of time dealing with psychological, social, and environmental patient concerns when their preference is to refer nonmedical issues to mental health practitioners (Gropper, 1987). Effective use of physician time can be achieved through referral of appropriate issues to social workers. According to Gross, Gross, and Eisenstein-Naveh (1983), concerns that can be addressed by a social worker include family issues; resource concerns; mental health issues; behavioral problems; medical noncompliance; and issues involving children, older adults, and people with mental retardation. In addition, social work activities can potentially generate income through fee-for-service billing, grants, and consultation (Hookey, 1979).

The social worker's role in the clinic evolved after the clinic's genesis. In the initial months of the clinic's operation, the social worker met with as many patients as possible to determine what concrete services community residents needed. The firm establishment of the medical social worker as a critical team member enabled her to gain the trust of both staff and residents, and her functions expanded to include involvement in brief, time-limited crisis intervention. Although the implementation of managed care curtails social work provision of long-term services, in the first month of Tenncare, the number of social work screenings tripled, and social work staff hours were increased. The social worker became more involved with mental health screenings, because Tenncare preapproval for social work services is not needed, as it is for mental health services.

Through specific questioning of clinic patients, the social worker investigated the social, emotional, and health care needs of the clinic population and the local community. These interviews, along with staff and community agency input, resulted in the development of a self-administered social work screening instrument with 26 yes–no questions that facilitate autonomous social work case finding (Figure 35-1).

New patients are instructed to complete the screening form and an initial admitting information sheet. The receptionist highlights screened cases for social work services, alerting the social worker to the need for client interviews, biopsychosocial assessments, and interventions. The social work screening process occurs before any primary care interdisciplinary team member's involvement. The initial social work

FIGURE **35-1**

Social Work Screening Instrument

Patient's Name: ____________________

Date: ____________________

Address: ____________________

Telephone: ____________________

Please answer the following by checking yes or no as the statements apply to you and your family. Please ask for assistance if you do not understand a question.

I am pregnant and not receiving prenatal care.	Yes ____	No ____
I am pregnant and have no health insurance.	Yes ____	No ____
I am homeless or living in a shelter.	Yes ____	No ____
I need help with housing.	Yes ____	No ____
I am unemployed and trying to find a job.	Yes ____	No ____
I have no food in my house.	Yes ____	No ____
I need to apply for food stamps or WIC [Supplemental Food Program for Women, Infants, and Children].	Yes ____	No ____
I cannot afford my medications.	Yes ____	No ____
I have medical bills I am unable to pay.	Yes ____	No ____
I am over age 65 and need help.	Yes ____	No ____
My spouse, who lives with me, is disabled.	Yes ____	No ____
My child, who lives with me, is disabled.	Yes ____	No ____
I am going to be hospitalized soon and will need help after I am discharged.	Yes ____	No ____
I have been diagnosed with a serious illness.	Yes ____	No ____
I am having trouble dealing with my illness.	Yes ____	No ____
My children are not up to date on immunizations.	Yes ____	No ____
I am under age 18 and not attending school.	Yes ____	No ____
I am concerned someone may be abusing my child.	Yes ____	No ____
I have received psychiatric treatment now or in the past.	Yes ____	No ____
I am involved with the court system.	Yes ____	No ____
I want information about substance abuse programs.	Yes ____	No ____
I want to learn more about birth control or condoms.	Yes ____	No ____
I want information about child day care.	Yes ____	No ____
I want help managing my child's behavior.	Yes ____	No ____
I want information about Head Start for my child.	Yes ____	No ____
I want to see the social worker to ask some questions.	Yes ____	No ____

interventions and findings are charted on the bottom of the screening report so subsequent primary care providers are aware of client concerns and can recognize the need for follow-up. The screening form has been used as a pilot project, and current statistical data are lacking. The authors encourage clinics to develop their own instruments and initiate further study.

Because the social worker has established relationships with community services, she directs clients to services and follows up to ensure timely responses to client needs. Client–worker relationships are established early, and client comfort in seeking social work intervention on future occasions is enhanced. Social work counseling and case management services are complemented by supervisory, administrative, and educational roles.

Social workers' comprehension of group process enables them to assist with the negotiation of team roles, responsibilities, and functions. Their comprehension and recognition of group development and process augment the interdisciplinary understanding of knowledge, values, training, language, and perspectives. The helping relationship is conceived of as a process that views the person within the context of his or her environment. Detailed case records are maintained so a systems perspective of care can involve appropriate professionals and referrals. Thus, the social worker becomes educator for staff, residents, and nursing students in the biopsychosocial model.

Case Example

D is a 24-year-old woman who came to the clinic complaining about infected lacerations on her face and hands that had occurred in a motor vehicle accident. The social work screening instrument indicated that D was homeless and that she was interested in mental health services. This information alerted the social worker to question D further. D revealed a history of cocaine use, two recent suicide attempts, and a failed drug rehabilitation hospitalization. D's mother refused to allow D to reside with her because D withdrew from the drug rehabilitation program prematurely. D expressed great frustration and indicated that she would attempt suicide if her only option was living on the street.

Through the ensuing interview, D acknowledged a desire to change her circumstances. She described a scant social network consisting mainly of other addicted people. The social worker's familiarity with community resources enabled her to recommend an appropriate program. Interdisciplinary clinic staff (physician and nurse) implemented an immediate preadmission physical examination and laboratory work, allowing an intake appointment with the rehabilitation program to be set for that morning. The social worker's screening instrument and knowledge of human behavior and resources, along with interventions by a cooperative interdisciplinary team, set in motion an appropriate and necessary plan for the client. The clinic's ability to meet the immediate medical needs of the client were crucial to the negotiation of a suitable solution.

Involving the Community in Its Own Care

Ongoing dialogue between the social worker and interdisciplinary staff creates networking responsibilities for the social worker. Interface between the clinic social worker and social agencies enhances provision of services to the Vine Hill Community. Together, the clinic social worker and community agencies address the need for food, transportation, prescription medications, and employment. This cooperative effort continuously expands, and networking now includes community religious organizations and community action groups. Patients, practitioners, and students are taught from a community-based, problem-solving focus. Thus, the clinic has become a partner in community health as opposed to a mechanism for the diagnosis of individual pathology. Creating and maintaining a continuing dialogue between the clinic and the community has been one of the outstanding features of the Vine Hill Community Clinic.

The use of questionnaires, student home visits, group focus meetings (of community clinic patients and nonclinic community residents), and dialogue with the established residents' association encourage frequent community needs assessments. The clinic, along with the Vanderbilt School of Nursing, facilitates communication between community service agencies and community residents. The clinic often functions as mediator and interpreter for community residents regarding both health and nonhealth issues.

The diversity of the community population presents a special challenge to interdisciplinary team members. The needs of households headed by single mothers, people who are mentally ill, and people who are physically disabled must be met in the daily struggle to survive in an unsupervised environment (Busby et al., 1992). Before the inception of the clinic, the housing authority provided the only available social work services, with a focus on people who were unable to pay their rent. Mental health services were provided off-site, and lack of adequate transportation prevented intervention except on a crisis-only basis.

Highlighting the community encourages residents' and professionals' regard for racial, ethnic, socioeconomic, and cultural sensitivity (especially necessary when working with people of color and underprivileged populations). Understanding patients within the context of the larger community, involving these parties in their own care, evaluating effectiveness on the basis of the community's health status, and working in communities to implement change are all crucial elements in providing services (Zayas & Dyche, 1992).

As Shannon (1989) indicated, "services should include not only medical but psychosocial care and preventive educational health programs through outreach into the community" (p. 35). Taken a step further, community clinics can help the citizenry organize to meet its needs and desires, as the Vine Hill Clinic has done.

Populations at Risk in the Managed Care Environment

The interdisciplinary team effort can create a positive organizational climate of cooperation in managed care. Interdisciplinary sharing, teaching, and communication assist in decreasing the "assembly line" nature of service distribution in this cost-containing age. This climate of cooperation may be critical for two major reasons: (1) Managed care systems create environments that may not be conducive to compassionate, responsive service delivery, and (2) managed care systems frequently select out high-risk populations from care to control costs (Sederer & St. Clair, 1989).

Snibbe, Radcliffe, and Weisberger's (1989) research delineated issues pertaining to managed care environments. Psychiatrists and social workers had significantly higher scores on depersonalization and emotional exhaustion than physicians or psychologists working in managed care. This study highlights that organizational climate is critical to professional performance. Having control over the working environment affects the professional's ability to cope with the demands of managed care. The Vine Hill Clinic's team approach integrates interdisciplinary staff support with a sharing of staff responsibilities. An environment of cooperation diminishes staff stress and simultaneously enhances quality of care to patients.

Second, "by attracting a pool of subscribers who are at lower risk, managed care systems omit high-risk, high-cost patients, thereby transferring these patients to separate systems of care, which then absorb greater costs" (Sederer & St. Clair, 1989, p. 1143). Mizrahi (1993) also observed that managed care plans often are not geographically or culturally accessible. The likelihood increases that populations in greatest need—poor people, people of color, and women—will be neglected.

With rising health care costs, many states have enrolled Medicaid recipients in managed health care plans, hoping to expand access to health services while controlling costs. Both Moore and Hepworth (1994), in their study of perinatal care for Mexican American women receiving Medicaid, and Krieger, Connell, and LoGerfo (1992), in their study of Medicaid prenatal care, demonstrated that health care insurance coverage alone is an insufficient condition to ensure use of medical services. Moore and Hepworth found that mothers reporting higher levels of social support were more likely to initiate prenatal care and that problems such as transportation difficulties were associated with decreased prenatal visits. Krieger et al. demonstrated late enrollment in Medicaid by pregnant women regardless of which system of care was used (fee-for-service versus managed health care). They suggested "case finding" and "enhanced social support services" (p. 188) as potential solutions. Both studies suggested the need for heightened efforts in helping Medicaid recipients gain access to health care services.

The Vine Hill Clinic screening devices provide a mechanism for early detection of needed services. Initiatives such as the Vine Hill Clinic can provide services to high-risk populations within managed care systems.

Conclusion

The biopsychosocial model enables the clinic social worker to integrate clinic services with community environmental needs. The Vine Hill Clinic views clients as members of a larger community, and the community is transformed into a client. Negotiation of efforts that incorporates the neighborhood as an interactive client in a mutual relationship allows for a focus on preventive care and the development of prevention programs within the community. Such a cooperative effort genuinely encompasses the World Health Organization's definition of "health as a state of complete physical, mental, and social well-being and not merely the absence of disease and infirmity" (Shannon, 1989). The movement toward the empowerment of communities through the creation and maintenance of self-care capabilities provides exciting, creative roles for social work professionals.

Kark fashioned the concept of community-oriented health centers in South Africa in the 1940s. The community health center has become "a life-line to people in poverty—those who are at greatest risk . . . those who bear the heaviest burdens of morbidity and mortality." He stated, "A central tenet is that primary care should be rooted in communities, for communities, and with communities" (quoted in Geiger, 1993, p. 946).

With the advent of managed health care, impoverished populations, which are costly for managed care systems, are at greater risk of receiving inadequate health care services. Community-oriented health care services can protect these populations from being ignored and neglected.

Clearly, social workers can play many vital roles as interdisciplinary team members working in community clinics under a managed health care system. Redirecting emotional, psychological, familial, and social concerns to social work professionals liberates other primary care staff from dealing with issues that may not best fit their areas of expertise. Social work screening and case finding lessen the inappropriate use of valuable interdisciplinary professional time, thus increasing patient satisfaction.

In the managed care era of health care delivery, the proposed model of the interdisciplinary community clinic can conceivably deliver greater services at a lower cost to a population in need. If this model is viable, low-income populations need not be precluded from the best health care services the United States has to offer. There is a need for further study and data collection before alternative approaches to traditional health care delivery can be realized.

References

Azzarto, J. (1993). The socioemotional needs of elderly family practice patients: Can social workers help? *Health & Social Work, 18,* 40–48.

Bassoff, B. Z. (1982). The community clinics: Will they survive? *Social Work in Health Care, 1,* 71–79.

Betten, N., & Austin, M. (1977). Organizing for neighborhood health care: An historical reflection. *Social Work in Health Care, 2,* 341–349.

Busby, L. C., Green, A. H., Anness, N., & Taylor, C. R. (1992). *Vanderbilt University nurse managed clinic and community care project: Annual progress report to the W. K. Kellogg Foundation.* Nashville, TN: W. K. Kellogg Foundation.

Curiel, H., Brochstein, J. R., Cheney, C. C., & Adams, G. L. (1979). Interdisciplinary team teaching in a barrio primary care mental health setting. *Journal of Education for Social Work, 15,* 44–50.

Ell, K., & Morrison, D. R. (1981). Primary care. *Health & Social Work, 6,* 355–435.

Geiger, H. J. (1993). Community oriented primary care: The legacy of Sidney Kark. *American Journal of Public Health, 83,* 946–947.

Gropper, M. (1987). A study of the preferences of family practitioners and other primary care physicians in treating patients' psychosocial problems. *Social Work in Health Care, 13,* 75–91.

Gross, A. M., Gross, J., & Eisenstein-Naveh, A. R. (1983). Defining the role of the social worker in primary health care. *Health & Social Work, 8,* 174–181.

Hooker, R. S., & Freeborn, D. K. (1991). Use of physician assistants in a managed health care system. *Public Health Reports, 106,* 90–94.

Hookey, P. (1979). Cost–benefit evaluations in primary health care. *Health & Social Work, 4,* 151–167.

Kane, R. A. (1985). Health policy and social workers in health: Past, present, and future. *Health & Social Work, 10,* 258–270.

Krieger, J., Connell, F., & LoGerfo, J. (1992). Medicaid prenatal care: A comparison of use and outcomes in fee-for-service and managed care. *American Journal of Public Health, 82,* 185–190.

Mizrahi, T. (1993). Unmanaged care and managed competition: A primer for social work [National Health Line]. *Health & Social Work, 18,* 86–91.

Moore, P., & Hepworth, J. (1994). Use of perinatal and infant health services by Mexican-American Medicaid enrollees. *JAMA, 272,* 297–304.

Mullaly, Z. (1988). The application of a social health perspective: A shared social worker–doctor responsibility. *Australian Social Work, 41,* 5–9.

Sederer, L., & St. Clair, L. (1989). Managed health care and the Massachusetts experience. *American Journal of Psychiatry, 146,* 1142–1148.

Shannon, M. T. (1989). Health promotion and illness prevention: A biopsychosocial perspective. *Health & Social Work, 14,* 32–40.

Snibbe, J. R., Radcliffe, T., & Weisberger, C. (1989). Burnout among primary care physicians and mental health professionals in a managed health care setting. *Psychological Reports, 65,* 775–780.

Winegar, N. (1993). Managed mental health care: Implications for administrators and managers of community-based agencies. *Families in Society, 74,* 171–177.

Zayas, L. H., & Dyche, L. A. (1992). Social workers training primary care physicians: Essential psychosocial principles. *Social Work, 37,* 247–252.

C H A P T E R **36**

Social Work Case Management: Challenges for Social Work Education and the Profession

Suzanne Sankar and Deanna Brooks

Case management is both a new concept and a new role that has emerged from the managed care model of health care. As a growing field of practice, it is increasingly the key service component of managed care networks in community- and hospital-based health and mental health programs. Although many master's-level social workers now work as case managers, case management is not the exclusive domain of social work. Other professional and paraprofessional groups have gained a strong and influential foothold in the field. Isn't case management just good old-fashioned social case work? In many respects traditional case work and case management are similar (National Association of Social Workers, 1992): Both serve people with complex needs, and both are characterized by interventions aimed at the interplay between the person and the environment.

Schools of social work and the social work profession need to better understand the work of MSW case managers so that as a profession, we can better articulate to others (managed care companies, agency administrators, and other professions) the valuable contributions of social work case managers. This exploratory study attempts to describe the roles, knowledge, and skills of master's-level social workers providing case management services in the Boston area and their attitudes toward case management. Findings support the unique fit between social work skills and values, and the case management models that combine brokering services with clinical interventions. Opportunities for schools of social work to collaborate with agencies to define and develop social work case management skills in an era of rapidly changing health care services will be discussed in this chapter.

History of Case Management

Case management, as opposed to case work, emerged in the late 1960s in response to the general shift of human services from the institution to the community. As mental hospitals and state schools closed down, an insufficient patchwork of community services developed, and vulnerable consumers were often left to fend for themselves (Raeff & Shore, 1993). By the late 1970s, the National Institute of

NOTE: Earlier versions of this study were presented at the Annual Program Meeting of the Council on Social Work Education, March 1987, Chicago, and the NASW Annual Meeting, November 1996, Cleveland.

Mental Health funded service integration projects to coordinate, link, and reduce barriers to community services for people with mental illness. An important component of the new community support system was the case manager (Rubin, 1992).

Concurrently, initiated by the federal government's efforts to find community alternatives to long-term institutional care for elderly men and women, case management developed as a priority service for geriatric patients (Raeff & Shore, 1993). By the 1980s, case managers were key to service delivery systems for abused children, people with developmental disabilities and homeless people (Vourlekis & Greene, 1992). In the early 1990s, AIDS service networks developed a central role for case managers (Brennan & Kaplan, 1993). The most recent trend in case management is in medical hospitals because care is shifting from inpatient to community-based services (Berkman, 1996) and from social work to nurse case managers or to social work–nurse case management teams (Hawkins, Veeder, & Pearce, 1997). With the growth of managed care in the 1990s, a new role for the case manager involved overseeing cost containment for individual clients. The new role for the case manager shifted to overseeing cost-containment efforts for individual clients by managing service plans that ensure quality and fiscal restraint (Raeff & Shore, 1993).

Social Work Case Management

Although several studies have examined the roles, functions, and skills of generic case managers (Rothman, 1991; Rife, 1992), only a few authors looked specifically at the work of the MSW case manager (Netting & Williams, 1996; Vourlekis & Greene, 1992). Some authors speculated that social workers have been ambivalent about case management, indecision which has cost social work a presence in the field (Johnson & Rubin, 1983). The ambivalence has many possible explanations, including doubts that case management requires advanced practice skills (Moore, 1990), reluctance to take on responsibility for fiscal containment (Austin, 1990), and confusion about which case management roles are actually appropriate for social workers versus nurses or other workers (Vourlekis & Greene, 1992).

In fact, case management incorporates a wide range of professional and paraprofessional roles. Some focus primarily on arranging concrete services and are appropriately paraprofessional roles. Others require specialized medical knowledge and thus are best performed by a medically trained worker. Still other case management positions require both a complex understanding of people, families, and larger systems and the skills to effect change in these systems. Many of the latter positions, in hospitals, community health and mental health programs, and child welfare agencies, are held by MSWs who often practice a clinically informed role referred to as "clinical case manager" (Donner, 1996; Morrow-Howell, 1992) or "clinical specialist" (Berkman, 1996).

Clinical case management has historically been associated with services to people with long-term mental illness (Harris & Bachrach, 1988; Harris & Bergman, 1987; Kanter, 1988, 1989). It is a case management model that draws extensively on social work skills, knowledge, and values and thus is well suited to social work practice. However, it is one of the more debated models because it emphasizes the importance of the relationship between the client and case manager (Bryan, 1990), in contrast to the brokering model that views the relationship between the client and the case manager as only administrative (Raeff & Shore, 1993). Because it is a model that pays attention to the interplay between psychological, biological, and social issues while also acknowledging the therapeutic aspects of the case management relationship, it can help the worker anticipate boundary issues, work with complicated caregiver systems and dynamics; and guide a worker in assessing a client's level of self-care (Kanter, 1996; Raeff & Shore, 1993).

Morrow-Howell (1992) made a cogent argument for adapting the clinical case management model to gerontological social work. She emphasized the need for advanced practice skills to accurately assess and provide for clients' needs. A comprehensive assessment must include a careful review of the interplay between physical health, emotional well-being, and social–environment factors. She was critical of the idea that services can just be "arranged" (brokering model) for an elderly case management client and stated that sound clinical thinking is necessary to "plan" services successfully for an elderly person who may be grappling with illness, diminished functioning, loss of important relationships, or family conflict.

Berkman's (1996) model of a clinical specialist combined clinical and case management functions to address the psychosocial issues presented by patients in the health care system. Social workers in this role provide consultation to primary care providers regarding psychosocial stressors and mental disorders that may affect a patient's recovery from physical illness. In addition, the clinical specialist assists in securing benefits, obtaining community resources, and advocating for the patient within the health care system. Clinical functions include crisis counseling for patients and families, psychoeducation regarding adaptation to illness and disability, and help for families with ethical decision-making dilemmas.

Methodology

This study was developed to describe the roles of MSW case managers in the Boston area. The study explored the clinical skills and knowledge MSW case managers use with clients, caregivers, and community system and the value they place on their work as case managers. A pilot study was initially conducted with 10 social work case managers. The social workers were interviewed by the authors using both structured and unstructured questions. Based on their responses, a survey instrument was developed and mailed to 97 Boston-area MSWs who either had a job title of case manager or who spent at least 25 percent of their time performing case management functions. Four general questions were developed to guide the survey:

1. To what extent do MSW case managers perform generic case management functions—for example, developing service plans, brokering or linking clients to services, and monitoring service delivery?
2. When providing case management services, to what extent do MSWs use clinical skills and knowledge—for example, relationship-building skills or knowledge of diagnosis or family dynamics?
3. Do MSWs consider case management a valuable role for social workers? Do they use their professional training? Do they feel it fits within the mission of social work?
4. What roles do social work case managers take when working with other professionals or treatment team members? Do they feel valued by coworkers, administrators, and clients? How do they use a social work perspective when collaborating with others?

Questions explored the frequency with which respondents perceived themselves as performing generic case management tasks, using clinical skills, and applying clinical knowledge to their work with clients and client systems. Social work case management functions, skills, and knowledge lists were developed from a review of the case management literature, the clinical social work literature, and the pilot study. Open-ended questions were designed to gain a deeper understanding of the respondent's use of self with the client and within the caregiver network, to explore whether respondents experienced their work as a valuable role for social workers, and to explore respondents' perceptions about how others valued their work. Case vignettes were elicited to help respondents describe their interventions.

Findings

Fifty-five MSWs responded to the survey, a 56.7 percent return rate. Respondents described themselves as spending some or all of their time doing case management: 60 percent spent the majority of their time (50 percent to 100 percent) on case management. Thirty-eight percent worked in mental health settings, including inpatient and community-based facilities. Sixty-two percent worked in health care settings that included hospitals, elder programs, AIDS services, and community health centers. The social work case managers represented a wide range of post-MSW experience: 27 percent had 10 to 20 years' experience, 29 percent had five to 10 years' experience, 29 percent had two to five years' experience, and 11 percent were recent graduates.

CASE MANAGEMENT FUNCTIONS

The respondents perceived themselves as performing the generic case management functions described by Rothman (1991) and Rubin (1992) and used by most case managers (Table 36-1). More than 90 percent of the respondents reported frequently developing service plans, identifying community resources, and linking clients to services. Greater than 85 percent of respondents reported frequently doing psychosocial assessments, creating treatment plans, and advocating for clients. More

TABLE **36-1**

Case Management Functions

FUNCTION	SOCIAL WORKERS PERFORMING THE FUNCTION (%)
Developing a service plan	94.5
Identifying community resources	94.5
Linking clients to services	92.7
Creating treatment goals	89.1
Assessments	87.3
Client advocacy	85.5
Consultation to caregivers	78.2
Interdisciplinary team work	72.7
Monitoring service delivery	58.2
Therapy	38.2
Client identification	36.7

NOTES: Based on a four-point Likert scale assessing frequency, the following functions were ranked from most frequently to least frequently used. *N* = 55.

than 70 percent of respondents reported frequently consulting with the network of caregivers and working on interdisciplinary teams.

Less frequently performed functions included monitoring service delivery (58.2 percent), providing therapy (38.2 percent), and identifying new clients (36.7 percent). The lower frequencies may reflect the extent to which the case management role is shaped by the setting. For example, monitoring service delivery is more likely to happen in community mental health settings, in which chronically ill clients are followed over the course of the illness, rather than in hospital units, where contact ends at discharge. Client identification tends to be a function of outreach workers rather than of those providing office- or home-based services. Therapy also is a function that can be specific to its setting. In many mental health programs, therapy is integrated into the case management role but is not generally considered to be a case management function.

These findings indicate that MSWs in a variety of treatment settings are performing basic, generic case management functions that also are performed by non-MSW case managers. Variation in frequency in case management functions appears related to job role. The differences do reflect the wide range of case management roles and functions reported in the literature, which may contribute to confusion in the definition of case management.

APPLYING CLINICAL PRACTICE SKILLS AND KNOWLEDGE

In both closed- and open-ended questions, the majority of respondents repeatedly focused on the importance of applying clinically informed thinking and advanced clinical practice skills in all case management interventions. In Likert-scaled questions self-assessing the frequency of use of clinical skills (Table 36-2, column A), 89.1 percent of respondents reported frequently establishing a working alliance; 89.1 percent frequently provided emotional support to clients; 81.8 percent frequently assessed the impact of larger systems on clients; 76.4 percent frequently provided crisis intervention; 76.4 percent frequently helped clients adapt to life events such as loss; 74.5 percent frequently helped clients identify patterns and anticipate problems; 70.9 percent frequently identified psychiatric symptoms; 67.3 percent frequently provided psychoeducation; 63.6 percent frequently helped clients deal with interpersonal problems; and 61.8 percent frequently helped clients deal with painful affect. Respondents were then compared by work setting. Although there were differences between the mental health and health care respondents and between those who did brief treatment, usually in hospital settings, and those who worked with clients over longer periods of time, none of the variations were statistically significant (Table 36-2, Columns B–F).

In addition to using clinical skills in performing case management tasks, respondents self-assessed the frequency of applying clinically informed knowledge to all case management interventions (Table 36-2, Column A). Frequently applied clinical considerations included the following: assessing client strengths (92.7 percent); maintaining an awareness of boundary issues in the use of self (87.3 percent); supporting client empowerment (87.3 percent); understanding when to explore and contain painful affect (80.0 percent); assessing the client's capacity to use the helping relationship (80.0 percent); and understanding the client's family dynamics (74.5 percent). In open-ended responses, many respondents also described family systems skills, a complex understanding of how to work with community service networks, and skill as supervisors or team leaders of other case managers.

TABLE **36-2**

Clinical Practice Skills and Clinical Knowledge

CLINICAL PRACTICE SKILLS	A	B	C	D	E	F
Providing emotional support	89.1	81.8	95.2	85.3	86.2	92.3
Establishing a working alliance	89.1	87.8	95.2	85.3	86.2	92.3
Facilitating client motivation	80.0	72.7	85.7	76.5	79.3	80.7
Providing crisis intervention	76.4	69.7	80.9	73.5	82.8	69.2
Helping to adapt to life events, loss	76.4	72.7	76.2	76.5	72.4	80.8
Leadership in collaborating with other agencies	70.9	69.7	61.9	76.5	75.9	65.4
Identifying psychiatric symptoms	70.9	63.6	90.5	58.8	65.5	76.9
Helping to deal with loss or trauma	69.1	63.6	66.7	70.6	72.4	65.4
Providing psychoeducation	67.3	54.6	76.2	61.8	72.4	61.5
Helping to deal with interpersonal issues	63.6	54.6	76.2	55.9	58.6	69.2
Helping clients deal with painful affect	61.8	63.6	61.9	61.8	62.1	61.5
Helping team members identify and work through feelings stimulated by clients	60.0	63.6	52.3	64.7	62.1	57.7
CLINICAL KNOWLEDGE						
Assessing the client's strengths	92.7	96.9	95.2	91.2	89.7	96.2
Supporting client empowerment	87.3	87.9	88.2	85.7	89.7	84.6
Awareness of boundary issues in the use of self	87.3	84.9	90.5	85.3	86.2	88.5
Assessing larger system's impact on client	81.8	81.8	80.9	82.4	82.8	80.8
Assessing the client's capability to use the helping relationship	80.0	72.7	85.7	76.5	79.3	80.8
Understanding when to explore or contain affect	80.0	76.8	76.2	82.4	82.8	76.9
Identifying patterns and anticipating problems	74.5	69.7	80.9	70.6	75.9	73.1
Understanding the client's family dynamics	74.5	78.8	76.2	73.5	72.4	76.9
Understanding a client's defense mechanisms	65.5	72.7	66.7	64.7	55.2	76.9
Assessing the impact of early experience on the client's personality or functioning	61.8	60.6	66.7	58.8	51.7	73.1
Understanding transference and countertransference issues in the helping relationship	60.0	63.6	57.1	61.8	58.6	61.5

NOTES: Column A represents the advanced practice skills and knowledge most social workers, in a variety of settings, reported performing with case management clients. The use of skills was then compared with those who do 50 percent or more case management as part of the job description (column B) and to those who have a mental health (C) versus health (D) role and then compared with those who do brief treatment (E) versus longer-term treatment (F). *N* = 55.

In the following case vignettes, respondents illustrated their application of clinical knowledge and skills to case management tasks to guide the worker–client relationship; to anticipate boundary issues; and to help the client, family, and team members process affect-laden issues.

> A social work case manager at an AIDS services organization reflected on her conscious use of self in work with a gay man who was facing the break up of an important relationship as his health deteriorated. While providing emotional support and facilitating referrals for additional resources, the worker was "balancing the need to take action with a concern about not disempowering the client."
>
> * * *
>
> A community-based social work case manager working in a publicly funded program for people with mental illness described her attention to complex family dynamics while working with a client with a history of multiple psychiatric hospitalizations. The client came from a family with several generations of enmeshment. While helping the family make decisions and access treatment for their daughter "I was also setting limits. I used my knowledge of family systems, diagnosis, and the dynamics of separation . . . to work with this girl."
>
> * * *
>
> A social work case manager working on an inpatient oncology service described her interventions with clients and staff members' painful affect: "With each repeat admission for a cancer patient I am providing emotional support and monitoring changes in affect. With each successive admission, when appropriate, I help process more feelings, hopefully providing a safe environment to process grieving of death and dying issues."
>
> * * *
>
> A social work case manager assessed a middle-aged gay client from Central America for supports and stressors and facilitated access to community services. She helped the client deal with disclosure to his family and facilitated a family meeting with the medical team regarding end-of-life decisions. "I needed good assessment skills, an understanding of the dynamics of grief work and a family's cultural norms, and advocacy skills in maneuvering the client and family through the system."

CASE MANAGEMENT AS A VALUED ROLE FOR SOCIAL WORKERS

In addition to better articulating the social work contribution to case management, this study also sought to understand how the social work case managers felt about a role that has been criticized as being without adequate professional status. A full 80 percent of respondents replied yes to the question, Do you see case management as a valuable social work role? They recognized their education and value base as a good fit for case management and often stated case management was a "return to social work roots."

Open-ended responses further supported this opinion. Examples of responses were categorized by three themes:

1. Case management is valuable because it fits with the historic mission of social work to work with both the person and the social environment. A medical social work case manager stated, "Absolutely. Case management is part of our training and history. We have the advantage of systems thinking, community access, resource knowledge, and the ability to tolerate affect and understand human behavior."
2. Case management is a valuable social work role because it allows social workers to practice in a holistic fashion, taking a comprehensive view of the client's needs while allowing for flexibility in the type and level of intervention. A social work case manager in an outpatient health clinic stated, "Yes. To me it represents the continuum that we often call 'generic' social work and can include casework, program planning and development, groups, and education."
3. Case management is a valuable social work role because social work training, with its emphasis on applying social work ethics and values such as client self-determination and empowerment to practice, provides an excellent preparation for the demands of the role. A hospital case manager said, "Absolutely. Good case management is not just doing; it is being with the client and helping them do as much as possible themselves. Social workers are uniquely trained for this role."

The respondents reported their value was more often recognized by their teams or departments than by their agency administration. Seventy-eight percent of social workers perceived their team as looking to them to handle more complex issues involving high-risk clients, complicated family issues, and substance abuse. They were valued for their skill in dealing with client, family, or team members' affect and for their knowledge of the larger system and its resources.

> A social worker in a medical hospital stated, "Team members turn to the social work case manager when a worn-out family member causes a crisis in the ER."
>
> * * *
>
> An AIDS social work case manager helps the team "process the helplessness and anxiety of a suicidal, violent, or substance-abusing client or a grieving family member."

By contrast, only 41 percent agreed that their role was supported by administration. They felt case manager job descriptions and salaries tend to focus on generic case manager functions rather than to recognize social work education or skill level—although nurses' medical knowledge was often recognized by administrators. A focus on briefer treatment and discharge was seen as the primary concern of some administrators, especially in hospital systems.

Discussion

The purpose of this study was to achieve a better understanding of the functions and skills used by the master's-level social work case manager. The finding that this group of MSW case managers frequently perform job functions considered generic case management responsibilities should come as no surprise. The social work case management literature emphasizes the overlap in role definitions between social work and case management, with some authors viewing social work as synonymous with case management (NASW, 1992; Raeff & Shore, 1993; Rose, 1992). The findings did not support the speculation that social workers with advanced training devalued "concrete" services. Most respondents, who work in a broad range of settings, frequently develop service plans, link clients to services, and identify community resources, suggesting that for this group, concrete service provision continues to anchor the role of social worker and is congruent with the demands of the case management role.

In addition to providing concrete services, the findings suggest that MSW case managers use a range of advanced clinical skills and knowledge in performing case management functions. Woven into direct service functions are judgments informed by a biopsychosocial, psychodynamic, and systemic knowledge base. The blending of concrete and therapeutic functions and knowledge described by the respondents is most similar to the clinical case management models described by Berkman (1996), Kanter (1988, 1989), and Morrow-Howell (1992).

There appear to be specific skills, knowledge, and values that social workers bring to their role, their clients, and their teams. The respondents repeatedly focused on the importance of the working alliance and attention to boundary issues. They included a strengths perspective and an understanding of family dynamics and larger systems in assessments. They viewed empowering the client, advocacy, emotional support, and attention to affect as key interventions. They valued their communication skills with team members and other caretakers, and they recognized the need to see the whole picture and balance the needs of the client with the demands of the system. However, conflicts between social work departments and administration remain problematic for many of the respondents.

Perhaps social workers choosing case management positions are more attuned to its effectiveness and less concerned about professional status or work in systems where their role is more valued by others. As managed care continues to set the standards for service delivery systems, case management may be more valued by social workers who wish to stay current with market realities.

Implications for Schools of Social Work and the Profession

Two challenges face social work. The first challenge is internal to the profession. Can we value the case management role? Can we see case management fitting within our professional mission? Can we appreciate how case management mandates the use of advanced practice skills? The second challenge is external to the profession: Can we articulate to other professions, consumers, managed care companies, and administrators the unique and necessary contribution social work makes to the practice of case management?

Paradigms of treatment for complex or long-term problems are changing, as are the funding sources for services. More case management jobs are being created as hospitals downsize social work departments, as the aging and chronically ill populations need more home-based treatment, and as old models for treating major mental illness become inadequate. Social work educators will need to prepare students for these shifts in service delivery and teach the skills needed for these major roles.

Historically, social workers have not been very good at articulating their strengths, and the same appears true about articulating the importance of social work values and skills in case management services. This situation may be partly because case management is a new and evolving role and partly because it has a perceived lower status in the profession. However, social workers need to reclaim this casework role and define its unique fit with clinical case management services in order to clarify case assignments, supervision needs, salaries, and remaining effective in today's health care system. Effectiveness also requires documentation; in today's practice environment, it entails learning to evaluate the outcomes of social work case management interventions.

Opportunities for Collaboration among Agencies and Schools of Social Work

As we witness the "deinstitutionalization" of hospital-based health care services and the increase in case management as a key mode of service delivery in health care, an immediate concern is the expanding use of nurses and other disciplines as case managers in health care networks and the downsizing or elimination of social work departments. Although the growth of case management provides opportunities to expand traditional social work practice, it also poses a threat to established patterns of service delivery for hospital social work departments and to the professional identity of social workers and administrators.

In the Boston area, collaboration has begun among faculty from Simmons College and Boston College schools of social work, hospital-based medical social work administrators, and representatives of NASW. The goal of the Boston area collaboration is to assist social work departments and workers in articulating social work's contribution to case management practice as well as to develop mechanisms to document social work interventions and outcomes. During the initial stage the group began a dialogue about case management and changing health care practice and then expanded the discussion to include the broader social work community in a series of articles in the NASW Massachusetts Chapter newsletter (1997). The collaborative then worked to develop and present a continuing education program on case management. Future efforts will include providing faculty resources to help formulate research questions and offering assistance in documenting outcomes of social work case management interventions.

Summary

Managed care presents many new challenges to the social work profession and to social work educators. A primary challenge is to understand the key role that case management plays in most managed care systems and to articulate a role for social work case managers. Findings from a survey of Boston area social work case managers demonstrate their use of advanced clinical practice knowledge and skills in their work with client systems. The next challenge for schools of social work and the profession is to document the valuable outcomes of social work case management interventions in client care.

References

Austin, C. D. (1990). Case management: Myths and realities. *Families in Society, 71,* 398–405.

Berkman, B. (1996). The emerging health care world: Implications for social work practice and education. *Social Work, 41,* 541–551.

Brennan, J. P., & Kaplan, C. (1993). Setting new standards for social work practice and education. *Hospital and Community Psychiatry, 44,* 219–222.

Bryan, C. M. (1990). The uses of therapy in case management. In T. A. Kupers (Ed.), *New directions for mental health services* (pp. 19–27). San Francisco: Jossey-Bass.

Donner, S. (1996). Field work crisis: Dilemmas, dangers and opportunities. *Smith College Studies in Social Work, 66,* 317–331.

Harris, M., & Bachrach, L. (Eds.). (1988). Clinical case management. In M. Harris & L. Bachrach (Eds.), *New directions for mental health services* (pp. 15–29). San Francisco: Jossey-Bass.

Harris, M., & Bergman, H. C. (1987). Case management with the chronically mentally ill: A clinical perspective. *American Journal of Orthopsychiatry, 57,* 296–302.

Hawkins, J., Veeder, N. W., & Pearce, C. (1997). *Nurse–social work collaboration in the community: A case management model.* New York: Springer.

Johnson, P. J., & Rubin, A. (1983). Case management in mental health: A social work domain? *Social Work, 28,* 49–55.

Kanter, J. (1988). Clinical issues in the clinical case management relationships. In M. Harris & L. Bachrach (Eds.), *New directions for mental health services* (pp. 1–3). San Francisco: Jossey-Bass.

Kanter, J. (1989). Clinical case management: Definitions, principles, components. *Hospital and Community Psychiatry, 40,* 361–368.

Kanter, J. (1996). Case management with long-term patients: A comprehensive approach. In S. Soreff (Ed.), *Handbook for treatment of the seriously mentally ill* (pp. 256–277). Toronto: Hogrefe & Huber.

Moore, S. T. (1990). A social work practice model for case management: The case management grid. *Social Work, 35,* 444–448.

Morrow-Howell, N. (1992). Clinical case management: The hallmark of gerontological social work. *Journal of Gerontological Social Work, 18* (3–4), 119–131.

National Association of Social Workers. (1992). *NASW standards for social work case management.* Washington, DC: Author.

National Association of Social Workers, Massachusetts Chapter. (1997, March–June). Case management series. *Focus,* pp. 3–6.

Netting, E., & Williams, F. E. (1996). Case manager–physician collaboration: Implication for professional identity, roles, and relationships. *Health & Social Work, 21,* 216–224.

Raeff, N. R., & Shore, B. K. (1993). *Advanced case management: New strategies for the nineties* (pp. 1–19). Newbury Park, CA: Sage Publications.

Rife, J. (1992). Case manager perceptions of case management practice: Implications for educational preparation. *Journal of Applied Social Sciences, 16,* 161–176.

Rose, S. M. (Ed.). (1992). *Case management and social work practice* (pp. v–ix). New York: Longman.

Rothman, J. (1991). A model of case management: Toward empirically based practice. *Social Work, 36,* 520–528.

Rubin, A. (1992). Case management. In S. M. Rose (Ed.), *Case management and social work practice* (pp. 5–21). New York: Longman.

Vourlekis, B. S., & Greene, R. (Eds.). (1992). *Social work case management* (pp. xi–xvi, 11–24). New York: Aldine de Gruyter.

CHAPTER 37

The Professional Affiliation Group: A Case Study in Behavioral Health Management

Jay M. Pomerantz, Benjamin Liptzin, Alfred Carter, and Michael S. Perlman

This chapter focuses on a novel clinical and administrative design for blending diverse mental health professionals into a de facto organization capable of delivering managed mental health care in a clinically responsible, cost-effective manner. For the most part, the chapter describes a professional affiliation group (PAG) model in which a psychiatrist monitors utilization related to medical insurance contracts. In PAGs developed for other settings, such as schools and social agencies, social workers or psychologists could undertake the monitoring role—possibilities that will be further outlined later in this chapter.

Our program is entering its seventh year and involves 100 privately practicing mental health clinicians in combination with three hospitals and eight outpatient clinics. All are woven into a cohesive clinical and administrative entity to self-manage the mental health and substance abuse program of an independent practice association form of health maintenance organization (IPA/HMO). The entity is not a corporation or other legal structure, nor even an independent organization. It is easy to manage and allows full collaboration among privately practicing clinicians and those on salary. In managed care terminology, the design is a "carve-in"—it allows meaningful at-risk contracting for behavioral health providers who are part of a larger medical delivery system.

To understand the entity and its management, it will be necessary to provide a bit of history, describe the clinical model, and explain its ability to meet a budgetary target. Our first published article about PAGs detailed the history and development of the model (Pomerantz, Liptzin, Carter, & Perlman, 1994). This chapter describes our experience in securing an adequate budget and controlling expenditures while maintaining clinical quality and patient satisfaction. It highlights the differences between a PAG system and alternative models for managing behavioral health care. For the first time, we speculate on extending the model beyond medical insurance to the larger biopsychosocial arena.

History

At an early morning meeting in the summer of 1991, the administration of a local IPA/HMO declared its intention to "carve-out" the mental health and substance abuse benefit. That meant hiring an outside, for-profit, behavioral health management company to control and lower the cost of providing services. Three days later, at a hastily called meeting of psychiatrists, we volunteered for and were subsequently elected to a steering committee. The charge was to pursue an alternative to an outside management company. After considerable negotiation with the HMO administration and the IPA, an agreement emerged to suspend negotiations with outside management companies for three weeks. The HMO administration agreed to consider a carve-in proposal rather than a carve-out if the psychiatrists could come up with a way to manage the existing mental health network at a reasonable price.

The Professional Affiliation Group

A quick literature search failed to identify any organizational structure that seemed appropriate to our needs. We wrote a proposal describing an entirely new arrangement—a professional affiliation group with both clinical and utilization control functions built into multidisciplinary teams. The first test was to see if the 20 independently practicing outpatient psychiatrists in the IPA would agree to assume the role of team leaders. Surprisingly, almost all of them were enthusiastic about the PAG concept, and 15 agreed to become PAG managers, a clear signal to the HMO that we were serious about change. As described previously, each PAG is a small group of four to eight fully licensed, independently practicing mental health professionals from different disciplines. Each PAG includes at least one psychiatrist, who serves as the manager, and varying combinations of psychologists, clinical social workers, and psychiatric nurses, all of whom maintain an office, autonomy, and full responsibility for their own patients. Each professional bills for services independently. The PAG meets regularly, approximately every two weeks, to discuss difficult cases, coordinate treatment, and clear up problems with the allocation of sessions. Because the PAG is only advisory, legal responsibility for the patient continues to reside with the treating professionals.

Consultation rather than supervision is the glue that holds the PAGs together. The steering committee was clear from the beginning about this point: "The failure to appreciate the power of consultation has kept mental health professionals apart. Each jealously guards autonomy and fears supervision, the predominant modality of training" (Pomerantz, Liptzin, Carter, & Perlman, 1996a, p. 20). Not only is supervision an infantilizing period for the supervisee, but it carries legal peril for the supervisor who becomes liable for a treatment he or she is not doing (Woodward, Duckworth, & Gutheil, 1993).

The coordinating psychiatrist is obligated to provide timely psychopharmacological evaluation and medication for patients in treatment with that PAG's professionals. Patients who may require psychiatric hospitalization or are otherwise judged unstable also require consultation. Furthermore, the psychiatrist reviews all outpatient treatment requests for sessions beyond the initial eight visits. Disputes between the psychiatrist and other team members come before the entire PAG for resolution. The entire panel of 100 outpatient mental health professionals is split into 15 teams, each clustered around a single PAG managing psychiatrist. Other psychiatrists, who for one reason or another chose not to head a PAG, became regular team members, and their treatment requests are monitored by the PAG psychiatrist.

Between PAG meetings there is considerable paperwork exchange and telephone discussion among the other professionals and the PAG managing psychiatrist. Meetings are used to discuss problem patients (not identified by name). The allocation of outpatient sessions according to systemwide, written criteria (applied to particular cases) is another ongoing topic of conversation. Various multiproblem families in treatment with different PAG professionals also receive attention.

The increasing collegiality among PAG professionals, especially as it takes place in a joint managed care effort, has had dramatic implications for patient care and therapist support (besides the cost control originally envisioned). Not only is the PAG a vehicle for easy referral and follow-up, but meetings serve an educational purpose. For example, patients avoid psychiatric hospitalization (and its budgetary costs) because of early referral for antidepressant, anxiolytic, mood stabilizing, and antipsychotic medications. Difficult cases are evaluated by both the referring psychotherapist and the psychiatrist. Treatment options are discussed between them, with disputes resolved at PAG meetings. At meetings, professionals from different backgrounds and different disciplines consider a variety of possible approaches for treatment-resistant patients. A more complete discussion of PAG cotreatment, including case examples, is available (Pomerantz, Liptzin, Carter, & Perlman, 1996b).

The Contracting Process

We started from scratch without a track record and proposed an entirely new and untested clinical delivery system. Consequently, there was little desire to become a formal entity separate from the HMO. We had no independent way to pay claims, accept actuarial risk, provide liability insurance, or generate the data required to monitor a capitated contract. At first, it was not clear that the steering committee spoke for anyone but the psychiatrists. Before we could finalize any contract, we had to find out whether the nonpsychiatrist mental health professionals already on the HMO's provider panel would agree to join PAGs. We scheduled two systemwide meetings during which we presented the idea to the total 100-provider panel. Faced with the choice between a national carve-out managed care company or local control, albeit with psychiatrists as the primary organizers, the entire provider panel chose the latter with virtually no opposition. In response to concerns about psychiatric hegemony, we incorporated many suggestions from the meetings. We established a multidisciplinary advisory committee, made up of two psychologists and two clinical social workers, to meet regularly with the four steering committee psychiatrists. Decisions about fees, medical necessity criteria, provider qualifications, patient complaints, and so forth would be handled by a newly developed, multidisciplinary patient care assessment subcommittee. Periodic systemwide meetings to discuss administrative issues would continue as a supplement to PAG meetings.

Similar coalition building went into the potential division between salaried hospital staff and private practitioners. The chairman of the department of psychiatry of the dominant hospital in the system was deliberately selected for the steering committee because he could speak for the interests of the hospitals (including their inpatient, day treatment, outpatient, and emergency facilities). All providers (private practitioners, hospitals, and clinics) continued billing on a fee-for-service basis, with the entire program joined by, and subject to, a common target budget. A 15 percent withhold was deducted from all payments and held in reserve against any potential cost overrun for the year.

This kind of arrangement might be summarized as modified group capitation. Each individual provider is paid on a fee-for-service basis, but each also knows that the return of the withheld 15 percent depends on meeting the target budget. Also, any management fees are contingent on total expenditures coming in under the target budget figure. In any year during which the program fully returns the withhold and still has available money (that is, money not spent on patient care), there is a limited amount of money available to pay the steering committee, PAG managing psychiatrists, and all PAG members for meeting time and administrative work. This management fee cannot exceed a total of 50 cents per member per month (PMPM) in any year, that is, it must be less than 10 percent of the total program cost, and it may be zero.

This complex arrangement balances the desire of individual providers to maximize their income by providing treatment services, with the constraints of an overall mental health and substance abuse budget limit. There is continuing oversight by peers and, in particular, the PAG psychiatrist. Each provider periodically gets a printout of his or her statistics compared with all other system providers. The number of patients seen, number of visits per patient, and average cost per patient are all listed. Every provider is at risk for cost overruns and, to a certain extent, is rewarded for cost-effective care. The net effect is a balance of forces.

Medical Necessity

With a careful balancing of economic forces, it is possible to approach the difficult issue of medical necessity. Our criteria for medical necessity, both for inpatient and outpatient services, are written down and available to all providers in the system. These criteria, unlike those of most behavioral health management companies, are meant only as guidelines. Diagnostically based guidelines attempt to ensure that our most vulnerable patients can access at least 20 psychotherapy sessions per year (insurance benefit limit). Other patients, especially those with adjustment reactions or situational crises, may require only the initial eight sessions (or less) to resolve their presenting complaints. That leaves a middle group of patients for whom therapists' themselves choose how many sessions to use. It is our feeling that therapists know which of their patients need and are best able to use psychotherapy. When the therapist is in doubt about the appropriate number of sessions for a particular patient, the PAG psychiatrist is available for discussion. In any event, the PAG managing psychiatrist must sign off on psychotherapy session allocation that exceeds eight per calendar year. The entire PAG is also available to discuss session allocation in specific or general terms.

De Facto Organization

The choice of a de facto organization rather than an independent corporation has advantages. The carve-in design allows mental health professionals to remain wedded to mainstream medicine. Mental health professionals have expertise in mental health treatment, not insurance, law, or finance; the best design may be to have no business entity of any kind. To that end, the HMO contracts individually with each provider in the network. PAG managing psychiatrists sign one standard contract, and all other mental health providers sign another.

Our feelings in 1991 (and now) were that even though a separate corporate entity might allow participating mental health professionals to make a profit (above that derived from fees for service), that road is problematic both ethically and practically. Historically, separate state hospitals for mental patients have been characterized by underfunding. Similarly, the behavioral carve-out phenomenon, featuring both fragmentation of service delivery and fierce price competition, drives down the percentage of the health care dollar devoted to behavioral health. Whereas 10 percent of the medical dollar went for behavioral health under indemnity insurance, managed care companies featuring behavioral carve-outs are currently competing with one another for only 1 percent to 4 percent of the total medical budget. That marked reduction of expenditures for behavioral health does not take into account that the small sum left for patient care is further reduced by 25 percent to 35 percent for carve-out company administrative expense and profit.

The PAG system has done better than most carve-outs in securing money for behavioral health, staying consistently above 4 percent of shrinking total medical expenditures. We think this budget share reflects the HMO's appreciation of the PAG's sensible clinical design. Furthermore, because behavioral health is not carved out, psychiatrists and other mental health professionals serve on multispecialty committees. Behavioral health remains an integral part of the total HMO team effort. In turn, all behavioral health financial and administrative data derive from the HMO's own payment system and are thus available for everyone's scrutiny.

It is further noteworthy that the PAG system has survived through changes in the HMO's ownership, chief executive officer, and medical director. The HMO's substantial growth in membership, from 30,000 to more than 80,000 covered lives, also has not been a problem. The PAG design easily handles increased membership and greater geographic coverage through its modular design and decentralized clinical decision making.

A more complete discussion of the concept of a de facto organization, or as we termed it at the time, a "virtual" organization, is available (Pomerantz, Liptzin, Carter, & Perlman, 1995).

Centralized Intake and the Mental Health Administrator

Managed mental health and substance abuse networks require a centralized telephone intake process to facilitate outpatient linkage. Data collection, inquiries, complaints, and other day-to-day operations cannot be accomplished by busy practicing clinicians. Someone has to watch over inpatient utilization and monitor the clinics. All these functions and others were incorporated into a job description for a mental health coordinator (and eventually three assistants) hired by the HMO. The steering committee negotiated the right to participate in the interview of the final candidate and signed off on his hiring. Because the providers represented by the steering committee were financially at risk, whereas the mental health coordinator was not, the steering committee established policy for the coordinator to implement. The program has been most fortunate in having a sensitive and knowledgeable master's-level clinician to handle this difficult job. In addition to dealing with the public, he has had to contend with two sets of bosses who have different agendas and styles.

Figure 37-1 outlines the accessible telephone central registration process. Referrals are then triaged to providers. The key functions of cotreatment, consultation, coordination, and cost control occur peripherally in the PAGs rather than centrally (as in most other managed systems). Although the PAG system uses a central telephone intake, central intake does not serve a gatekeeper function. Patients are merely registered and given approval for an initial eight sessions. This registration can be done over the telephone by patient, primary care physician (PCP), or therapist. In contrast, every carve-out builds in a gatekeeper function somewhere in its intake process, whether by PCP referral or central intake screening program.

FIGURE 37-1

PAG Telephone Central Registration Process

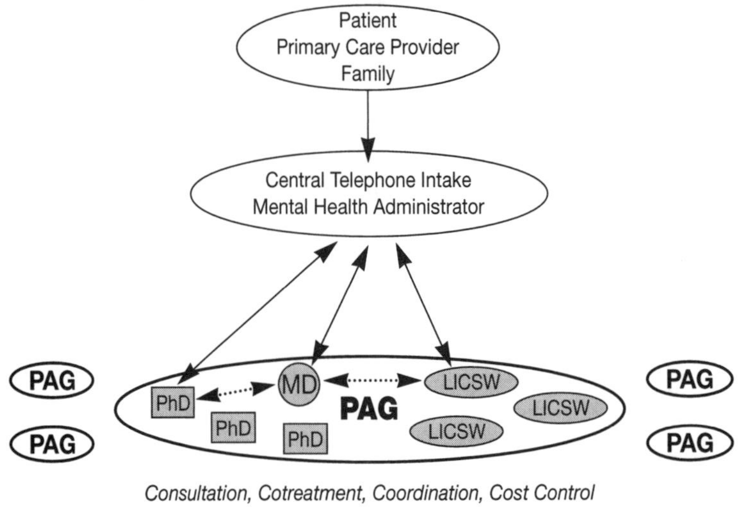

NOTE: PAG = professional affiliation group.

Ensuring Systemwide Fairness

Our unusual arrangement seemed to call for a unique management style. We could not be as trusting as a true group practice, in which profits and salaries are derived only from the corporation's income. Nor could we be as callous and distant as some managed care carve-out companies are, with their detailed requirements for case information and provider "profiling" and "pruning."

The method we use is a review and comparison of each provider's statistics. Each month, the HMO's computer system produces a report for the steering committee which lists, by provider, the number of patients seen, the number of visits, and the cost of care on a cumulative basis for the year. The report also tracks hospital utilization and provides an ongoing tally of the system's PMPM expenses. The steering committee then reformats the data into comprehensible data sets that are distributed to the PAG managing psychiatrists. The data are sorted by PAG, with each PAG member's utilization listed individually and also in comparison with all others in the PAG. Another table in the report shows each PAG's utilization compared with all other PAGs. The statistics are reviewed and discussed at a PAG managing psychiatrists' meeting and then taken to individual PAG meetings by that group's managing psychiatrist.

In the beginning, the data identified only the PAG member receiving them. As the system matured, all providers were identified by name. This openness now allows providers to discuss discrepancies in practice patterns with one another; sometimes these discussions become heated. More important, the discussions frequently lead to suggestions about how to handle difficult cases more efficiently.

As our management methods evolve, the next step will be to include the diagnostic category in the cost analysis. We are also beginning to track PAG and clinic referrals of patients for hospitalization. Data on the prescription of medication are available but await a comparison with accurate data from other care systems. Analyses of patient satisfaction and treatment outcome by provider are long-term goals. The purpose of all data is to improve overall patient outcome and cost effectiveness.

Personalizing the System

Just as we try to meet face-to-face with our patients for most of our work together, it is important to do the same with our colleagues. Each PAG requires a minimum number of meetings (16 to 24 per year) to remain a viable entity. Telephone, fax, and mail communications supplement the meetings. In addition, the 15 PAG psychiatrists get together three to four times per year to discuss administrative concerns and to discuss the differences in treatment patterns among the PAGs. Similarly, the coordinators of affiliated inpatient units have monthly meetings with the mental health administrator to review data about admissions (length of stay, readmissions, site of prior treatment, and reasons for admission). Finally, there are periodic meetings (two to three annually) for which the entire behavioral health provider system comes together. All meetings allow ample discussion time for provider opinion and suggestions.

Another innovation introduced by our mental health administrator is that all telephone calls to the central intake unit are answered immediately. There is no complex call routing, no queuing, and little recourse to message recording and calling back. This personal approach is important to providers who otherwise endure interrupted psychotherapy sessions or "telephone tag."

Results

The PAG arrangement and other managerial efforts have resulted in decreasing the HMO's expenditure for behavioral health from $7.75 PMPM to $5.25 PMPM this year. That is not as low a PMPM as might be offered by a carve-out. Cost shifting may account for some of the difference. For example, medication management in the PAG system is a behavioral health cost. A carve-out may delegate much of that service to a PCP. That cost would then disappear from the behavioral health budget, only to show up in the HMO's general medical budget. Nevertheless, carve-outs may spend less. Strict capitation invites undertreatment because the least care is the most profitable care for the providing organization.

It is also more difficult for providers to limit care for patients they know intimately than it is to make care-denying decisions impersonally while seated at a distant computer. So, too, it requires discipline to limit care for patients within what continues to be a fee-for-service system.

We believe the PAG system is appropriately balanced and has drawn a reasonable line between too much and too little care. Yet only when the whole field becomes more sophisticated about measuring clinical outcomes as a function of "dosages" of psychotherapy and pharmacotherapy will the true trade-offs between cost and clinical benefit become clear.

Our data show that all the cost savings in the PAG model have come from decreasing the expenditures of hospitalization for both inpatient psychiatric and inpatient substance abuse facilities. On the outpatient side, costs have remained constant, but the system is treating many more people (10 percent of the HMO total membership) for shorter treatment episodes. The system now averages between five and six outpatient visits per patient per year, but patients most in need of outpatient treatment can still use all 20 visits of the total behavioral health benefit. For high-risk patients, after extensive review, the program may pay for outpatient visits in excess of the 20-per-year limitation.

Although this kind of change is what carve-out organizations claim to deliver, we have implemented it within a provider-controlled, de facto organization with high provider and patient satisfaction. None of our providers has resigned except to leave the area for personal reasons. Our current waiting list consists of 275 providers who wish to join. Fees have increased slightly over the six years of the program's existence. Again, linkage to the HMO structure has helped; all cognitive medical areas (primary care and nonsurgical direct care, including behavioral health) benefited from a recent fee restructuring.

PAG Model Compared with Typical Behavioral Health Carve-Outs

The PAG system is designed, monitored, and updated by clinicians who continue to work within the system. The PAG system's most basic principle is to do what is right for both clinicians and patients rather than save money by confusing or hassling them. Instead of setting paperwork and approval hurdles for clinicians to overcome (at the risk of nonpayment for already performed legitimate services), the PAG system is willing to pay for any medically necessary service. That sometimes takes the form of overlooking administrative lapses if the service was performed in good faith by a network provider.

Our operating assumption that a satisfied clinician results in a satisfied patient is borne out by the HMO's yearly survey of patients: 94 percent to 95 percent of patients using behavioral health services report being satisfied with the services they receive. The level of patient satisfaction reported is the same for both therapists and the entire system. Patients are asked to rate their satisfaction with 14 item: eight about therapists and six about the system of obtaining care. On the system side, scores are asked for the following: ease of obtaining a referral, access to a clinician of one's choice, ease of setting up an initial assessment with a mental health provider, time to first appointment, financial coverage for the mental health care received, and the number of visits available for the patient's situation. The provider scale includes overall satisfaction with the mental health provider, maintenance of confidentiality, the provider's compassion and caring, amount of time the provider spent during each visit, comfort in talking with the provider, the provider's qualifications and competence, ability to reach the provider by telephone when needed, and the provider's knowledge about the problem that brought the patient to treatment. The overall satisfaction score is an average of the separate scores that are all above 90 percent except for the item dealing with the number of sessions available for treatment. That issue is a problem for all managed systems and results in only a 77 percent satisfaction score from our patients. Even including that item of built-in discontent, the overall percentage of satisfied patients averages 94 percent to 95 percent.

The PAG system is running a 10 percent penetration rate (percentage of total HMO enrollment using at least one behavioral health session in a given year), as opposed to half that or less in systems run by carve-out management companies. Community studies show high rates of mental health needs in the population (greater than 20 percent). Therefore, the issue is not that the PAGs are too welcoming. Instead, we believe that the commercial carve-outs are creating obstacles to access for potential patients. Carve-out company satisfaction data need careful scrutiny from that perspective. It is relevant to ask whether the scores that carve-outs achieve on patient satisfaction surveys should be halved to account for the 50 percent of potential patients who never make it to providers' offices.

Unlike the PAG system, which builds in locally coordinated care, most carve-out companies rely on care coordinators who attempt to hook up network psychiatrists with other therapists on an ad hoc, case-by-case basis, usually in an emergency. This leads to built-in disjointed care. Psychotherapists and psychiatrists who manage medication find it difficult to relate to one another when each has to relate to many cotreaters, each with only one to two patients in common. In addition, cost pressures result in psychopharmacology being thrust back onto PCPs; whatever is spent in care by PCPs does not come out of the mental health carve-out budget. That administrative arrangement results in many patients having less than optimal psychopharmacological management. In the PAG system, psychiatrists prescribe 51 percent of all psychopharmacological agents as opposed to the usual figures of 10 percent to 15 percent in carve-out arrangements.

Patient clinical data also are handled differently in a PAG system from in the typical carve-out company. With the PAG system, preserving patient confidentiality is a primary concern in the process for determining medical necessity. Only the diagnosis, date and type of session, short-term treatment goals, and Global Assessment of Functioning go to the HMO. The rest of the information used by clinicians and PAG managing psychiatrists to determine medical necessity for ongoing treatment never leaves the clinicians' offices.

In contrast, commercial carve-out companies require a frightening amount of personal data. That data also may be skewed toward increased pathology by therapists' attempts to obtain approvals for further treatment. Furthermore, these companies are constantly merging and becoming larger, for example, Value Behavioral Health currently belongs to HCA/Columbia (the for-profit hospital chain now under investigation for Medicare billing fraud and other illegal activities). Magellan Health Services, Inc., owns Green Springs Behavioral Health, Vista Behavioral Health, and Human Affairs International and has recently acquired Merit Behavioral Care. Magellan now earns $1.5 billion a year in revenues and is in charge of the behavioral health of 60 million people across the United States. Charter Behavioral Systems just bought Behavioral Healthcare Corporation, becoming a combined entity of 139 mental health care facilities in 36 states and Puerto Rico. It has revenues of $1.2 billion ("Industry Round Up," 1997). What will eventually happen to the enormous amount of obviously sensitive, not necessarily accurate, patient data these behemoth companies maintain in their files?

PAG Model Compared with Traditional Carve-Ins

A "carve-in" is the generic term for any large, all-inclusive health care organization's self-management of its covered population's mental health needs. A traditional carve-in would be the mental health unit of a staff-model HMO such as Kaiser Permanente. Full-time mental health clinicians on salary operate out of central or satellite sites, sometimes integrated with PCPs but usually off in their own quarters. These units typically feature central intake and coordinated, multidisciplinary care but control mental health expenses by limiting the number of clinicians. Waiting lists, limited choice of clinician, clinic-like facilities, and geographic accessibility problems have sharply limited this model's acceptance by patients. In response, many HMO staff models have merged with or developed IPA networks or point-of-service options.

This change to larger fee-for-service networks of mental health clinicians requires a different form of management for mental health expenditures and quality control. Most HMOs have abandoned self-management and contracted with behavioral carve-out companies. Others, such as Tufts and Harvard/Pilgrim, have developed their own internal management units that imitate carve-outs in managing care on a case-by-case basis, often using a more gentle approach.

PAGs versus Traditional Group Practice Models

The PAG system is quite different from traditional forms of group practice in that it is a virtual organization rather than a legal entity and thus is easy to establish. No lawyers, accountants, insurance agents, or pension plan experts absorb the virtual group members' time and money. Claim processing, provider profiling, patient satisfaction studies, and even central patient telephone intake and registration are functions that can be contracted for, or (as in our arrangement) obtained gratis from the host organization.

In contrast, the costs involved for setting up even small incorporated group practices quickly mount and limit the size of the practice—and the small size then becomes the group's major problem. The only contracts a small group can obtain are subcapitations from carve-out companies. These contracts inflict a heavy price on the group practice because of low capitation rates and regulation. In exchange for a subcapitation agreement, the carve-out organization stops micromanaging each case but demands documentation that all needs of the covered population are being met. In addition, the group practice still has to figure out how to manage utilization internally.

The only alternative to small mental health group practices is to merge with other mental health groups or become part of a large multispecialty medical group. This option may work well because large groups have sufficient market clout to secure all-inclusive capitation or insurance contracts. However, the costs involved in buying everyone's assets and then managing them require professional managers and outside capital. The new organization that emerges is more of a business entity than a professional one. The mental health clinician is tied up contractually and may not feel well used or in control of his or her work environment.

The Future

The PAG concept may have applicability outside the medical insurance area and may not have to be psychiatrist led in other domains. When a contract for referrals comes from a school system, a psychologist or social work member of the PAG might become the major intermediary with the referring system. With a social services agency, the clinical social worker member of the PAG would function in the role of contract negotiator and cost-effectiveness administrator.

This concept of particular disciplines leading the way in their natural arenas applies throughout the PAG system (multiple PAGs). Just as it is always the PAG psychiatrist who monitors utilization for medical insurance contracts, a clinical social worker or psychologist would function in that role if the contract were negotiated with a social welfare agency or school system. That arrangement allows the PAG system to compete in the biological, psychological, and social arenas for contracts and patients. The logic is really quite simple: Psychiatrists have a natural alliance and everyday interaction with other physicians. Physician hospital organizations and HMOs are built around physicians; when behavioral health leads with its nonmedical facets, it loses out to other medical specialty areas and to primary care. None of the above is meant to say that all behavioral care should be circumscribed by the medical model or that it should be entirely under the control of the biological team member (that is, the psychiatrist). Referrals can and should still go directly to the most appropriate PAG team member. In our system, 80 percent of the psychotherapy is done by psychologists and clinical social workers. Even when patients have split therapy with a nonpsychiatrist psychotherapist and a psychiatrist who prescribes medication, there is no supervisory relationship or monitoring of the psychotherapy. The biopsychosocial model of behavioral health care does not imply primacy of any one discipline over another.

Consultation

Each discipline should take the lead in obtaining contracts (capitated and otherwise) and referrals from their natural areas of interest and expertise. Usually, the budget available for behavioral health treatment is tight if not inadequate. One way around this dilemma is to educate and work with referring sources about the most efficient use of their in-house resources. That consultative process might result in fewer referrals for specialized mental health treatment. The original federal Community Mental Health Centers Act (cited in Levinson, 1972) of the 1960s made a large commitment to community consultation. Caplan (1970) wrote extensively about the different kinds of consultation possible among mental health professionals and other community caregivers. His pioneering work, which described consultation among mental health professionals and visiting nurses, clergy, funeral directors, and so forth, is just as relevant today as when it was first written. Indeed, the shift toward managed care (which implies a rationalization of resources) should eventually result in support for non–mental health community caregivers. Often, just saying "no" to a referral source is not appropriate. Consulting with that referral source about individual clients and even entire programs is preferable. This use of case and program consultation is a natural for PAG professionals who are already accustomed to using consultation and coordination within the PAG.

Conclusion

The PAG system allows providers in private practice to organize themselves for efficient clinical care. Furthermore, the PAG allows integration with either medical care systems or other funding sources. Leadership derives from the discipline in the biopsychosocial continuum best positioned to relate to the funding source. Consultation rather than supervision is the crucial concept. The alternatives are outside, for-profit, national behavioral carve-out management (which awaits any provider who wishes to go it alone); small group practices (which may not fare much better, given their bottom-dwelling position in a multilevel funding chain); and large, multispecialty group practices (which are viable but require outside capital and professional management). Within such large organizations, the choice again is between the PAG model and some variety of distant control.

References

Caplan, G. (1970). *The theory and practice of mental health consultation.* New York: Basic Books.

Community Mental Health Centers Act, P.L. 88-164, 77 Stat. 290.

Industry round up. (1997). *Behavioral Health Tomorrow, 6*(6), 29.

Levenson, A. I. (1972). The community mental health centers program. In S. Golann, & C. Eisdorfer (Eds.), *Handbook of community mental health* (pp. 687–698). New York: Appleton-Century-Crofts.

Pomerantz, J. M., Liptzin, B., Carter, A. H., & Perlman, M. S. (1994). The professional affiliation group: A new model for managed mental health care. *Hospital and Community Psychiatry, 45,* 308–310.

Pomerantz, J. M., Liptzin, B., Carter, A. H., & Perlman, M. S. (1995). Development and management of a "virtual" group practice. *Psychiatric Annals, 25,* 504–508.

Pomerantz, J. M., Liptzin, B., Carter, A. H., & Perlman, M. S. (1996a). Is private practice compatible with managed care? In A. Lazarus (Ed.), *Controversies in managed mental health* (pp. 19–27). Washington, DC: American Psychiatric Press.

Pomerantz, J. M., Liptzin, B., Carter, A. H., & Perlman, M. S. (1996b). The multidisciplinary team: Cotreatment in the professional affiliation group (PAG) model for private practice. *Journal of Practical Psychiatry and Behavioral Health 2,* 245–250.

Woodward B., Duckworth K. S., & Gutheil T. G. (1993). The pharmacotherapist–psychotherapist collaboration. In J. M. Oldham, M. B. Riba, & A. Tasman (Eds.), *American Psychiatric Press review of psychiatry* (Vol. 12, pp. 631–649). Washington, DC: American Psychiatric Press.

The authors acknowledge the contributions of Lee Walker, mental health administrator, and his staff for outstanding daily management of the PAG program.

CHAPTER 38

New Opportunities for Social Work with State Medicaid Managed Care Providers

Darleen M. Vernon

The goal of this chapter is to discuss the emerging role of social workers in helping state Medicaid contractors become more responsive to the unique needs of the Medicaid population. The Medicaid program is the focus because it is perhaps the most familiar to social workers, as it is the state-administered medical insurance program for the federal program known as Aid to Families with Dependent Children. It also may be the most visible, progressive, managed, and innovative of government-funded medical programs administered by the state, but experience has shown that its targeted population may be the least understood. This chapter highlights how social work staff can build on their unique skill sets and take a lead in strategy development and implementation while redefining their own roles as administrator, utilization manager, and health care provider.

Background

Because of the development of managed care, Medicaid program delivery is much different today from what it was 10 years ago. In the United States, there is an increasing trend for state and federal health and social services programs to contract with health insurance organizations (referred to as "plans"), prepaid health plans, health maintenance organizations, or physicians who are grouped together to form primary care case management systems to provide an array of managed care services to eligible clients. This is particularly true for Medicaid recipients enrolled in Medicaid-coordinated care programs, in which managed care delivery systems have proved to be an effective way to provide quality, cost-effective services to members. With most states in the United States operating under a Health Care Financing Administration (HCFA) 1915(b) waiver to enroll Medicaid recipients into capitated managed care entities, the United States was able to increase its base of eligible enrollees while controlling costs. From 1991 through 1996, the number of such enrollees quadrupled, from 2.3 million to 13.3 million; by June 1996, 40 percent of all Medicaid recipients were enrolled in coordinated Medicaid programs (American Association of Health Plans, 1997a).

The Balanced Budget Act (BBA) enacted in August 1997 has had significant implications for state Medicaid managed care programs and participating health plans. Whereas states still need a waiver to require special-needs children and certain

Medicaid-eligible Medicare beneficiaries to enroll in a managed care plan, the BBA now allows states to require that most Medicaid beneficiaries enroll in managed care programs. Furthermore, it has improved the enrollment process, expanded the array of organizations eligible for Medicaid contracts, and has set forth new enrollment and disenrollment requirements. The BBA now requires HCFA to develop national quality assurance standards and modify the current external quality review process. Additional provisions apply to maternal length of stay and to mental health parity requirements for Medicaid contractors enacted by the 104th Congress (American Association of Health Plans, 1997b).

I manage the Medicaid department for a health insurance organization, Regence BlueShield. As a leading health insurance organization in the State of Washington, Regence BlueShield arranges for delivery of capitated, comprehensive health services to approximately 50,000 Medicaid clients who reside throughout the state. Regence (formerly a group of county-based insurance "bureaus") initially became a Medicaid contractor for the Healthy Options program in 1993 by responding to a Healthy Options request for proposal (RFP) to provide services to this population. The process to qualify as a Medicaid contractor has undergone considerable change since that first year, but the RFP is still judged mainly on the cost of care per member per month, network adequacy, and quality of care. Once a contract is awarded, it is carefully monitored for compliance on a continuous basis, including member and provider satisfaction. Providers enter into a risk-based contract directly with the medical plan or subcontract with a medical service organization, which in turn contracts with Regence BlueShield. Like other eligible managed care entities, Regence BlueShield receives Medicaid member assignments through Washington's Department of Social and Health Services (DSHS), which has numerous customer service offices throughout the state to sign up and serve eligible members. Members can choose their providers and insurance plans; members who do not indicate a preference are assigned to a contractor that offers services in the member's area. DSHS pays their contractors monthly based on the number of assigned members and their age and gender; certain event-based services (such as deliveries and births) have enhanced payments and are paid by DSHS in response to the plan's billings.

Many aspects of this service delivery system may seem unusual to recipients of more traditional insurance coverage, but they have been instituted in response to the Medicaid member's needs and to provide Medicaid contractors with a way to manage the funds paid to them for the care of this population. The Medicaid product's contract requirements are unique among Regence BlueShield's various lines of business, including categories of care available, the care delivery system itself, and a variety of cost management parameters based on population-based differences. First among these population-based differences are a constellation of sociodemographic factors: Many Medicaid recipients lack telephones, adequate housing, good nutrition, and reliable transportation. A percentage of Medicaid recipients cannot read, and a large number are unable to read beyond the sixth-grade level. Cultural differences present problems in care delivery; many recipients do not speak English or understand how to use the health care available to them. What often appeared to be patient noncompliance was a major problem for Healthy Options providers and a barrier to achieving quality-of-care standards until program changes were instituted to help manage such population differences.

THE PROBLEM

As the program grew in Washington, the need to expand the depth and breadth of existing networks became a major issue along with the education of both the medical insurance plans and care providers. Plans new to Healthy Options (Medicaid) were often unprepared for the lack of health literacy among the Medicaid population and found the program difficult to administer. Plans with Healthy Options experience found that the sophistication of contractual requirements seemed to increase along with the DSHS knowledge base about the Medicaid population. It became more and more difficult to structure the care delivery system in response to mandated program requirements. From the time the program began in the early 1990s, the Medicaid definition of "at risk" has broadened and now seems to focus on the following five trends among its population base:

1. Members frequently initiate prenatal care at a later date than other insured populations.
2. Compliance with follow-up maternity care is less likely.
3. Care indicators for school-age children suffer because of the higher mobility of their parents.
4. Adolescent family members face a wider range of societal problems, and the method of service delivery becomes a critical component of meeting adolescent health care needs.
5. The responsibility for providing mental health care services is split between the plan and the regional support network (RSN), but there is a noticeable gap between the covered contract benefits and the array of services provided by the RSN.

The plan's contract with DSHS is specific in delineating what types of services are covered benefits and must be made available to members; it also indicates that the plan must provide and arrange for all necessary medical assistance at no cost to the Medicaid recipient. The provider network must have sufficient depth and breadth to provide a wide range of services and to have those services available to all members where appropriate. If an enrollee has a condition or disease that requires treatment by a specialist, a referral must be made to an available and accessible specialist. The contractor must ensure that the required care is provided with reasonable promptness and in a manner that ensures continuity of care. Medically necessary care must be both available and accessible 24 hours a day, seven days a week. Utilization is closely monitored, with underutilization representing more of a quality concern to DSHS than overutilization.

Meeting these standards would be virtually impossible without two critical programs in place: a utilization management program that monitors the amount, type, and outcome of client services, and a viable outreach program tailored to the population served and the communities in which they reside. In general, this would include at least care and case management, language translation services, transportation resources, and specialized maternal and pediatric services for at-risk members. Washington's 1998 RFP for the Medicaid (Healthy Options) program had already addressed some of these issues in the requirements for health care entities to follow for the 1998 contract year.

Reassessing Social Work Roles

In the past year or so, Regence BlueShield has begun to reassess the role of social workers within the realm of government program medical management. The apparent intent is both to increase the number of social workers and to enrich their involvement in member management. Three social work–related events have occurred within the past 18 months that may have had an impact on this decision:

1. The involvement of social workers in the successful management of several complex and high-profile Medicaid cases highlighted how poorly defined and underutilized their skills had been.
2. A social worker had been promoted from a line medical management role to a supervisory position in a community-based Supplemental Security Income (SSI) pilot program implementation and had guided the program and her staff to such a level of excellence that it became a "best practice" for SSI implementations in the rest of the state.
3. As Medicaid program manager, I was asked to work with a small team of DSHS leaders to develop innovative solutions to Medicaid program problems, with a particular emphasis on meeting the needs of hard-to-reach and hard-to-serve members who might fall through the Medicaid safety net.

The time appeared to be right for the Regence BlueShield social workers to come forward and lead the way in making their new role in the Medicaid program a central one in the care and management of the member population. There had been a long-standing debate within the medical management staff over whether social workers could be used much like nursing staff, who already did the majority of the medical management work. Traditionally, the most central role in the medical management sections companywide has been medical review—working with care providers to ensure an appropriate match between the patient's illness or medical needs and the intensity of service provided. Prospectively, inpatient care and a variety of treatments and procedures have to be reviewed for medical necessity and then preauthorized or precertified for payment. Once medical necessity is ascertained, nurses are often tapped for coordinating medical services for clients, primarily when either medical risk or care costs are—or are expected to be—high. Some nurses were doing specialized case management with special populations (for example, maternal and child) or were collaborating with case managers from medical groups who work directly with these populations to oversee care management and ensure contract compliance.

In contrast to this central and traditional role for nurses, social workers had been hired to work almost exclusively to help coordinate resources for individual clients or client groups. However, their roles both in the medical management section and outside in the community setting had been ill defined, and job satisfaction had been low. When the social work group got together to discuss their concerns, they wanted to talk primarily about the division of labor between nurses and social workers. The discussion also focused on the aspects of Medicaid program medical management that needed to be revised and how social workers could be involved. During the discussion, several trends were noted:

1. There was no focus on the behavioral aspects of health and illness, so problems such as noncompliance and the medical implications of certain lifestyle choices were rarely addressed—consequently, patients labeled as "difficult" often remained so.

2. Mental health care concerns regarding this population had been largely unexplored, and costs were not well managed because there was no medical management staff with interest in or needed expertise for this task.
3. Many nurses complained about working with multiproblem families and were unsure of how to manage them—but were unaware of social work expertise in this area.
4. Community outreach efforts needed to be expanded and reworked to better serve the needs of Medicaid clients, but social work staff felt they were not supported in their efforts to make this happen because senior-level management was unaware of the benefits of such outreach work.

The Challenge for Social Work

There was unanimous agreement that improving services to Medicaid clients could go together with enhancing the role of social work in the plan's Medicaid program. The issues were divided into two broad areas: (1) meeting the needs of the Medicaid client and (2) improving the effectiveness of the Medicaid program (Table 38-1). Already there has been substantial progress in moving toward those enhancements. Medical Management for Government Programs (a part of Regence's HealthCare Services division) has released a guideline for referrals to medical management care

TABLE **38-1**

Enhancements to the Role of Social Work to Improve Services to Medicaid Clients

	PURPOSE	
SOCIAL WORK ROLE ENHANCEMENT	MEETING NEEDS OF MEDICAID MEMBERS	IMPROVING EFFECTIVENESS OF MEDICAID PROGRAM
Develop education program for providers about unique needs of the Medicaid client	Member needs are not well understood, and providers are not prepared to deal with them	Develop education program for providers, evaluating extent of need and best focus
Case management with noncompliant and behaviorally high-risk clients	Focus has been on medical rather than psychosocial needs affecting health and illness behavior	Develop policy and procedures for social work referral and management of members
Oversee management of mental health care concerns	Covered benefits acknowledge incidence and severity, but care needs to be more available and accessible	Initiate thorough review of issues and progress to date; develop plan for resolution
Coordinate needs of multiproblem families	Overlap of medical concerns and problem resolution overlooked; need to refocus on social system	Develop policy and procedures for referral and management of members
Redefine community outreach program	Evaluate community resources and develop liaisons to meet needs outside medical necessity or covered benefits	Assess current program and do needs assessment; consider pilot programs in underserved communities
Develop outcome management program to monitor and evaluate enhancements	Evaluate effectiveness of changes on client population; include satisfaction measures	Initiate business case plan; develop interventions; monitor and evaluate

coordinators, and there is a long section devoted to social work interventions and reasons such referrals would be appropriate. Whereas access to resources is listed, other referral reasons are more prominently displayed: problems with loss and grief, social isolation, noncompliance issues, mental health concerns, vulnerability to abuse or neglect, legal concerns, exposed substance abuse, or anticipated changes in lifestyle or living arrangements.

There also have been other changes that speak to the versatility of social work skills. Since the beginning of 1998, several more social workers have been hired, and there has been a concerted effort to define more broadly the role of social work in managing the government program client. Three social workers are now in highly visible roles that have an effect on the Medicaid product: One coleads the process to revise a small-scale "best practice" maternity outreach program so it can be implemented in all the counties served by Regence BlueShield, and the other two work in the quality and education department with Medicaid provider groups that have been delegated to do their own utilization management and credentialing. Just a year ago these program development positions would have been filled with nurses rather than with social workers.

However, although community support for outreach enhancements is evident in county oversight meetings, specific community programming for the unique needs of Medicaid clients remains in development. A range of available community and public health indicators provide a close fit with the needs of this population. *Healthy Communities 2000* (American Public Health Association, 1991) provides a reliable source of community-focused interventions and can be evaluated against variables, incidence and prevalence rates, and expected outcomes being measured by other health entities. Many of the counties served by Regence BlueShield still have a local office, and at least three of the counties have sufficient medical management staff on-site to implement and oversee any intervention program. That is the direction in which social work may want to go to further improve programming for the Medicaid population and to enhance social work opportunities as well.

References

American Association of Health Plans. (1997a, June 6). *Coordinated care in the Medicaid program: Overview of enrollment trends and waiver implementation* [Policy Brief]. Washington, DC: Author.

American Association of Health Plans. (1997b, September 15). *The Balanced Budget Act Medicaid provisions: What do they mean for states and health plans?* [Policy Brief]. Washington, DC: Author.

American Public Health Association. (1991). *Healthy Communities 2000: Model standards* (3rd ed.). Washington, DC: Author.

PART SIX

Challenges for Professional Education

CHAPTER 39

Managed Health Care: Forcing Social Work to Make Choices and Changes

King Davis

Over the past decade, the social work profession may not have placed sufficient attention on the close relationship between health care services, costs, risks, human resources, and emerging health care policy. Nor was adequate attention paid to the increased impact of health care costs on corporate profits and the Medicaid budgets of state governments. As a result, the social work field did not forecast or prepare for the significant challenges to clinical practice brought about by the displacement of the fee-for-service system by managed health care policy between 1992 and 1998 (Cummings, 1996).

This chapter provides an operational definition of both fee-for-service and managed care within the shifting economic context in which managed care has emerged as the prevailing public policy. In addition, it identifies three areas of crisis in social work (human resources, clinical practice, and education) that resulted from the emergence of managed care. The chapter concludes with a discussion of the multiple opportunities for social work practice and education that have been precipitated by the effort to control the costs of health care in the United States.

Conceptualizing and Defining Fee-for-Service

The American health care system has used a variety of public and private insurance plans to indemnify financial risk for consumers and compensate physicians, hospitals, and other providers of health services (Freeman & Trabin, 1994; Mauer, Jarvis, Mockler, & Trabin, 1995; Starr, 1982). However, over the past 45 years, the fee-for-service payment plan emerged as the premier public strategy in American health care insurance (Starr, 1982). *Fee-for-service* is defined here as "the traditional health care payment system, under which physicians and other providers receive a payment that does not exceed their billed charge for each unit of service provided" (United Healthcare Corporation, 1994, p. 33). Under this payment plan the greater the number of discrete service units provided, the greater the potential income for the provider and the greater the financial risk to the third-party payer and employer

NOTE: An earlier version of this work was presented at "The First Managed Care Behavioral Health Care Invitational Conference for New England Graduate Social Work Faculty," funded by the Robert Wood Johnson Foundation, the National Institute of Mental Health, and the Alcohol and Drug Institute at the Boston University School of Social Work, October 1997, Boston.

(Berkman, 1996). In a fee-for-service environment, financial risk and loss are ultimately shared by the insurer, corporations, and governmental agencies that offer health care as a benefit of employment or as an entitlement (for example, Medicaid). Providers and consumers in fee-for-service have minimal financial risk associated with the consumption of services. In this health care cost-and-risk equation, the greatest interest in establishing processes and policies to control costs and share risks will come from those businesses and governments that subsidize health care for their employees, retirees, or recipients of public assistance under Medicaid or Medicare.

Efforts to control the cost of health care and spread its financial risks potentially develop considerable tension among purchasers of health care (government and business), providers (individuals and organizations), and consumers. Successful cost controls include changing key ingredients (autonomy, choice, relatively unlimited access to professional service, and relatively unlimited reimbursement) in the former indemnity fee-for-service payment plan favored by providers and consumers. In addition, successful external control of health care costs through managed care requires a series of major changes in the context and approach to professional clinical practice and subsequently in the programs or schools that provide preservice and continuing education. For social work or other professions that are relatively new entrants to competitive proprietary contracting and fee-for-service reimbursement, the changes stemming from external efforts to control costs bring about a crisis in human resources, clinical practice, and professional education (Brown, 1994; Freeman & Trabin, 1994). How each of these three crises is resolved may be an important determinant of the strength, competitive market position, and future of clinical social work. The future of social work education may be determined by its ability to identify and build on new educational and training opportunities in a rapidly changing health care environment in which managed care is but the most recent policy reconfiguration.

Defining Managed Health Care and Its Economic Background

Managed care, as defined here, is a series of traditional and nontraditional insurance processes designed (within the profit-making, corporate sector) to shift, control, and ultimately reduce the multiple economic risks (increase in total costs, annual increases above inflation, increased percentage of the gross domestic product [GDP]) in health care incurred heretofore almost exclusively by American corporations and government. Within the managed health care industry, *managed care* is defined "as a system of health care delivery that influences utilization and cost of services and measures performance. The goal is a system that delivers value by giving people access to quality, cost effective health care" (United Healthcare Corporation, 1994, p. 45). Bernier (1994) suggested that

> the term managed care is used to describe everything from traditional health maintenance organizations to hybrid, flexible healthcare delivery systems, to specialty programs integrated into a healthcare benefit plan. Managed care may therefore be defined more precisely as a highly structured health care delivery system which allows the payer to select and deselect providers based on the clinician's ability to assure effectiveness. (p. 2)

Managed health care systems use a variety of overlapping insurance processes and policies to change long-standing patterns of provider and consumer behavior related to access, utilization, costs, quality, and outcomes of health services (Kongstvedt, 1997; Mauer et al., 1995). Some of these processes include capitation of costs, preadmission certification, medical necessity criteria, closed access or gatekeeping, credentialing, field underwriting, utilization reviews, practice guidelines, and deductibles and copayments (United Healthcare Corporation, 1994). Within the past six years, these managed care insurance processes have increasingly dominated health care practice and, to a lesser extent, continuing professional education. Before exploring the crises developed in social work practice and education by managed health care processes, it is important to put managed care policy in the economic context that stimulated and supported its development and proliferation between 1992 and 1998.

Economic Background of Managed Health Care

Between 1950 and 1990, total annual expenditures for health care in the United States changed in dramatic ways. In 1950, Americans spent $12.7 billion for all health care. The annual figure (controlled for inflation) increased to $667 billion by the beginning of 1990, $840 billion by 1995, and to $1 trillion by early 1998 (Robert Wood Johnson Foundation, 1991; White House Domestic Policy Council, 1993). When looked at on a per capita basis or in relation to the GDP, the changes in figures are no less dramatic. In 1950, the United States spent $80 per capita, or 4.5 percent of the GDP, for health care (Robert Wood Johnson Foundation, 1991). By 1990, per capita costs had increased to $2,601 and 12 percent of the GDP. Forecasts for the year 2000 predict that per capita expenditures will reach $6,148, or 18 percent of the GDP, without congressional intervention to establish a global budget (White House Domestic Policy Council, 1993). Total spending for health care in the year 2000 is predicted to exceed $1.7 trillion. Additional forecasts suggest that health costs as a percentage of GDP will approximate 33 percent by the year 2030 unless policy action is taken by the federal government (Bureau of National Affairs, 1993; White House Domestic Policy Council, 1993).

Spending for health care between 1980 and 1988 exceeded the annual expenditures as well as the proportion of GDP of both national defense ($290 billion, or 6 percent of GDP in 1988) and education ($342 billion, or 7 percent of GDP in 1988) (Robert Wood Johnson Foundation, 1991; White House Domestic Policy Council, 1993). As the nation spends more of its resources on health care, American goods and services are at risk because the cost of health care is passed through to the consumer. Other essential goods and services may be put out of reach as a result of the growth in health care costs, and American products may be less competitive in a world market.

When compared with other highly industrialized nations, the United States spends more for health care in terms of overall funds, proportion of GDP, and per capita expenditures. The Robert Wood Johnson Foundation (Center for Health Economics Research, 1993) attributed the differences between the United States and other nations to a combination of three factors: (1) the limited extent to which health care costs are regulated successfully in the United States, (2) the relatively limited financial role that government plays in health care, and (3) the disproportionate amount (24 percent) that Americans expend on administration of the health care system.

Of importance in understanding the increasing costs of health care (and the current effort to manage costs) in the United States between 1950 and 1990 has been the relative failure of previous national policies to curb the growth in health care service costs or the cost of administration (Robert Wood Johnson Foundation, 1991). As new public policies have been implemented to reduce health care expenses, utilization of services, and unit costs, alterations have been made in other parts of the system that were unaffected, thus continuing the overall rise in costs (Robert Wood Johnson Foundation, 1991). Three areas (hospital utilization, administrative overhead, and physician fees) account for 82 percent of health care cost increases and total expenditures over the past three decades. Between 1960 and 1990, hospitals accounted for the largest share of health care expenditures and increases in the United States—although this share declined slightly between 1980 and 1988. Physician fees accounted for 22 percent of total personal health care expenditures in 1960, 19 percent in 1980, and 22 percent in 1988. Compared with other cost centers, physician fees increased more significantly between 1980 and 1988. By late 1996, it had been noted that managed care policies and processes had reduced the long-term trend in health care costs in the United States from an average growth rate of 10.1 percent to less than 2.5 percent per annum (Hilzenrath, 1997; Keigher, 1995). During this period, utilization of inpatient hospital services and unregulated access to physicians (particularly specialists) declined dramatically.

The combination of increased costs, overconsumption of services, maldistribution of services, limited risk sharing, and the failure of previous cost-containment policies led to the conclusion by the Clinton administration in 1992 (White House Domestic Policy Council, 1993) that the health care system was out of control, or unmanaged. Central to this conclusion was the perception that a major causative aspect of the crisis in health care cost was the unregulated behavior of providers (hospitals and physicians) and consumers. It was further concluded that the absence of financial risk by providers and consumers limited their interest in cutting costs or reducing unnecessary services. Thus, it is not surprising that managed care policy seeks to alter the rise in health care costs by designing and implementing processes to alter the inveterate behavior of providers and consumers and by shutting down the capacity of the health care system to continue its growth spiral by shifting volume and demand to other areas to maintain revenue and profit.

Growth in health care costs may be the result of what Manderscheid (1997) called the "commodification of health services" and what Geller (see chapter 3) calls the "industrialization of mental health care." In both of these schemata, the production and distribution of health services take on characteristics similar to other goods, services, or commodities in the economy, where markets, volume, pricing, and profit are the key motivating variables. Recent public exposure of the extent of fraudulent billings by large health care corporations and the inability of the federal government to oversee Medicare and Medicaid reimbursements may strengthen the public and legislative demand for strictly enforced managed care policies and processes to curb repetition of these dilemmas. In that scenario it seems unlikely that social work can escape the extensive public, legislative, and corporate outcry for effective measures to scrutinize the provision of health care by controlling its costs, access, quality, outcomes, the number of providers and the nature of their practices.

The successful effort to manage health care costs seems inevitably to require managing the delivery of professional services as well as the organizations and professionals that provide them. Managed care organizations and processes are designed to control the number of professionals eligible to practice in a market as well as affect the nature of professional practice in such a way as to stem the rise in unit costs, duplication of services and equipment, and the overutilization of inpatient care. Managed care achieves its costs savings as other industries have by making major reductions in human resources, by modifying the balance between the number of people in the labor market and the number of jobs available, and by altering how clinical practice is carried out. Changes in these three areas have important implications for the professional education and continuing education of social workers.

Crisis in Managed Care and Human Resources in Social Work

One key strategy in human resource management is to monitor the number, experience, productivity, and compensation of staff vis-à-vis the number of actual positions in a system. Several strategies can be considered here. A key strategy of managed care organizations is to limit the number of providers by linking service provision to membership in a network of providers under contract to the managed care organization. At the same time, consumers are provided fiscal incentives to encourage them to seek health care from members of the network. A second strategy is to contract with providers in the network at specified levels of compensation. Because large managed care organizations can control the health care market in certain geographic areas by contracting with large purchasers of services, managed care can monopolize both the type of services provided in a given market and the rate of compensation per unit of service, episode, or case. Providers who are not members of the managed care network or those members who do not abide by the managed care rules can be excluded from the market, resulting in their loss of revenue. Managed care organizations can establish any set of criteria for their network providers to solidify their market position. For example, managed care organizations can require board certification, licensure, specific clinical expertise, and knowledge of special populations as well as the number of postdegree years of experience. These latter requirements potentially place further limits on the number of providers who are accepted into the managed care network of human resources.

Part of the rationale for the emphasis on human resource policies by managed health care organizations is the belief that an oversupply of unregulated providers in the market drives up the overall cost of care. Data from Manderscheid and Sonnenschein (1996) supported the finding that there is an oversupply of health care providers. Those authors showed the distribution of clinically trained mental health professionals by state, total number, and rate per 100,000 population. Steenbarger (1997) added additional support for that argument by showing the distribution and rate per 100,000 for all clinically trained mental health professionals by state. In 1996, there were 94,128 clinically trained social workers, as reflected in National Association of Social Workers (NASW) membership figures. Close to 82,000 of those social workers are located in 25 states. (It is estimated that an additional 95,000 clinically trained social workers are in practice but are not members of NASW.) The rate of social workers per 100,000 population nationally was 35.9 in 1996 (Manderscheid & Sonnenschein, 1996). The rate of all clinically trained mental health professionals for 1996 was 113.4 (Steenbarger, 1997). In 39 states, the rate of social workers to 100,000 population is below the national mean. When the data are looked at by region, the highest rate of social workers per 100,000 population (76.4) is found in the New England states, and the lowest regional rate (17.6) occurs in the East South Central states (Manderscheid & Sonnenschein, 1996). However, when individual states are considered, a number had rates that were nearly twice the national rate, and some states were markedly below the national rate (Table 39-1).

TABLE **39-1**

Distribution of Social Workers by Selected State and Rate per 100,000

STATE	*N*	RATE PER 100,000	RATE FOR ALL MENTAL HEALTH PROFESSIONALS PER 100,000
Alabama	596	14.0	47.0
Alaska	596	98.8	141.5
Connecticut	2,326	71.4	143.8
Hawaii	747	62.9	106.5
Louisiana	453	18.2	76.3
Maryland	3,450	68.4	138.8
Massachusetts	5,469	90.0	228.8
Mississippi	306	11.3	32.1
New York	14,340	79.1	156.8
North Dakota	91	14.2	66.2
Rhode Island	750	75.8	121.3
Washington, DC	598	107.9	325.4
West Virginia	295	16.1	75.8
Nationally	94,128	35.9	113.4

It seems clear that in a number of markets (particularly the New England states) the rate of social workers per 100,000 population is significantly greater than the national rate and could easily be seen as an oversupply. It is equally important to examine and compare the rate of social workers per 100,000 to all clinically trained mental health professionals in a state. Because managed care seeks to lower costs of health care, the rate for all clinically trained mental health professionals in an area is of major importance. These data suggest not only that there appears to be a saturation of social workers in given states, but also that those same areas tend to have a high concentration of mental health professionals overall, thus saturating the areas to an even greater extent. Steenbarger's (1997) conclusions about the significance of such figures is valuable:

> To put these numbers in perspective, consider that 7 percent of a population may utilize mental health services in a year and that the average number of outpatient sessions across public and private sectors, for all ages, is about 10. A population of 100,000, therefore, could be expected to yield 70,000 sessions per year. If each clinician worked 50 weeks out of the year for 20 sessions per week, a clinician ratio of 70 would be appropriate. Note, however, that despite these generous figures, the national average is more than 50 percent higher than this ideal ratio—and the average in many eastern states is double the ideal. Clearly there is an oversupply of clinicians, even as managed care is reining in demand. (p. 5)

To counteract this oversupply and saturation of clinically trained mental health professionals, managed care organizations will need to make an effort to reduce the entry of new providers into the market, limit the production of new potential providers, or drive some existing providers out of the mental health marketplace (Cummings, 1996; Giles, 1993; see also chapter 3). The most recent effort by the federal government to provide incentives to medical schools to reduce the number of physicians is a case in point. An analysis of human resources in social work helps to illuminate the human resource issues and the question of oversupply in the era of managed health care. There seems to be a clear conflict between the policy direction and human resources needed in managed care and the increase in production of human resources by social work schools.

Crisis in Social Work Education

Although the market demand for clinically trained social workers (and other staff) is potentially narrowing under managed care, social work schools have increased the number of new enrollees as well as graduates prepared for careers in traditional clinical specialties over the past decade (Gibelman & Schervish, 1997; Manderscheid & Sonnenschein, 1996). These opposing trends could result in a severe aggravation of the problem of oversupply of clinically trained mental health professionals in managed care markets. The Council on Social Work Education (CSWE) (Vandivort-Warren, 1996) issued a report on the implications of managed care for social work practice and education. However, the strategic plan within the report did not address the human resource development issues and the dilemmas for the schools and the profession into the next decade precipitated by the expansion of managed health care policy as the basis for clinical practice.

Analysis of the actual number of degrees awarded in the field of social work helps clarify the potential human resources choices and dilemmas associated with managed care. When these figures are looked at by degree (BSW, MSW, and PhD/DSW) and by year, between 1984 and 1989, the number of social work graduates overall increased by 54 percent (Manderscheid & Sonnenschein, 1996). The most significant growth, however, was in the increase (66 percent) in the number of BSW degrees awarded over the past decade. The number of MSW degrees awarded during that same time period was 46 percent. Of particular interest regarding both the BSW and MSW degrees was the difference between the rate of increase in the first half of the decade and in the latter half. For example, the BSW awards increased by only 13 percent between 1984 and 1989, but their numbers increased by 45 percent between 1989 and 1994. If the number of undergraduate degrees in social work were to continue to accelerate at the same rate, there would be close to 17,400 graduates in the year 2004, compared with 10,500 noted in 1994. Overall growth in the number of MSW degrees awarded has not been as pronounced as the BSW. For example, between 1984 and 1989, the number of MSW degrees awarded in the United States increased by only 14 percent. However, the growth rate for the MSW degrees doubled between 1989 and 1994. For the full 10-year period, the number of MSW degrees awarded increased by 46 percent, compared with an increase of 66 percent for the BSW. If the growth pattern for the MSW degrees noted in the past 10 years were to continue until the year 2004, there would be a net increase of 6,000 MSW graduates for that year.

Growth over the past 10 years for doctoral degrees in social work has not been as consistent as that of the other two degrees. Major growth in the number of doctoral degrees awarded in social work occurred between 1984 and 1989—just the opposite of the growth pattern in the BSW and MSW degrees. In that time frame, the number of doctoral degrees awarded increased by 36 percent. However, in the past five years, doctoral degrees awarded increased by only 19 percent (Manderscheid & Sonnenschein, 1996). For the full 10-year period, the number of doctoral degrees awarded increased by 62 percent over the figure noted for 1984. If this trend were to continue for the next 10 years, the number of doctoral degrees awarded in 2004 would approximate 476.

In the period 1994 to 1995, almost 25,000 students were reported as enrolled in BSW programs throughout the United States (Manderscheid & Sonnenschein, 1996). Between 1984 and 1994, the number of BSW enrollees increased by approximately 68 percent, far greater than the expansion of jobs in the market. At the beginning of 1994, approximately 33,000 students were enrolled in MSW programs, with their numbers having increased by 51 percent over the total noted for 1984. The expansion of master's-level students also exceeded the growth in available positions within the market, where positions are shrinking from managed care. Enrollment in doctoral programs increased the least (47 percent) between 1984 and 1994. Total enrollment in social work programs increased by 57 percent between 1984 and 1994. If social work enrollment figures continue the patterns noted over the past 10 years, there will be close to 94,000 students enrolled in social work programs soon after the start of the new millennium. By 2004, assuming a constancy of demand, MSW enrollment would approximate 50,000 students; close to 41,000 students would be enrolled at the BSW level, and close to 3,000 would be in doctoral programs. As noted for 1994, about 40 percent of all students enrolled during the year actually graduate in that same year. If the proportion of graduating students remains at the 1994 level through the year 2004, social work schools will graduate close to 37,000 students into a saturated managed health care marketplace—contributing to the problem of oversupply and to the potential lowering of compensation.

It is vividly clear that social work education is expanding at a rapid pace, as shown by the number of individuals in training and the annual number of degrees awarded. However, mental health organizations operating under managed behavioral health care policies and processes may not be able to absorb the vast growth in graduates from these schools who will be looking for meaningful work. Between 1972 and 1992, professional positions within mental health organizations in the United States approximately doubled (Manderscheid & Sonnenschein, 1996). The most significant increases were in positions in nonfederal general hospital psychiatric services, Department of Veterans Affairs medical centers, and private psychiatric hospitals. The total number of mental health organizations increased from 3,005 to 5,498 between 1972 and 1992, but the number of inpatient beds per 100,000 population declined from 160.3 to 107.5. As a proportion of total staff in mental health organizations, social workers increased from 4.7 percent of the total work force in 1972 to 9.7 percent by 1992. The total number of social work positions increased by 40,000 during that same period. These figures show that the expansion in social work positions across all organizations, prior to managed care, was less than 4,000 per year nationally. With the onset of managed care in 1992, the demand for expansion of social work positions seems considerably less than the projections of graduates in the BSW and MSW programs noted here. Geller (chapter 3) indicated that master's-level social workers may be replaced by those with bachelor's degrees. CSWE (Vandivort-Warren, 1996) recognized this possibility in its report.

Social work education is highly dependent on the availability of unpaid field placements in local community agencies. However, newer credentialing and licensure standards under managed care may have a tendency to reduce these traditional placements because students will not be able to generate revenue. Of importance as well is the realization that hours devoted to supervision of social work students cannot be billed to a third-party payer. The inability to bill third-party payers for services provided by students and the potential loss of billable hours spent in supervision could result in a decline in the number of field placements (Vandivort-Warren, 1996). A severe reduction in field placements would threaten the existing model of social work education.

Clinical practice in managed care emphasizes a short-term, problem-focused, acute care model based in part on measurement scales designed to aid in diagnosis and outcome assessment. The acute care model of practice will require social work schools to modify existing clinical courses, models, and theoretical content and to add new courses to the curriculum. In its research, CSWE (Vandivort-Warren, 1996) conducted a series of focus groups to identify the type and range of skills needed by social workers in a managed health care environment. CSWE identified 23 skill areas that social workers need for successful practice in a managed care market and found that schools of social work and their faculty have not established the curriculum content to address these needs. To ensure that graduates are competitive in the managed care marketplace, schools of social work will find it necessary to increase faculty knowledge and preparation to teach new content. Currently, there are few courses in schools of social work that address managed care clinical or policy practice.

The key areas of opportunity for social work schools in the new managed care marketplace are in continuing education and retraining of social workers already in practice. The potential market demand for continuing education in social work exceeds 150,000 people currently in practice. These are people who were trained in more long-term practice models that did not rely on measurement scales, case management, and documentation of practice outcomes. Social workers in this everexpanding market will need training and retraining in new skills in intensive case management, utilization review, early intervention, short-term intervention, and collaborative teamwork as well as retraining to be consistent with the demands of managed care and, perhaps, licensure. Some of these social workers will be people who have been displaced and may need to change completely the course of their professional careers. Social work schools also could offer this training to other professionals. The demand for continuing education should exceed the demand for pre-service training.

In some states, maintenance of licensure status for social workers requires continuing education. Because licensure also is part of the required credentialing in most managed care plans, social work schools should advocate for states to require continuing education in social work environments as a part of maintaining licensure.

In response to the needs of practicing professionals for continuing education, coupled with a constancy of demand for admission, social work schools can decrease the size of their enrollments in the BSW and MSW programs over the next decade. A decline in enrollment as well as in the annual number of graduates of social work schools over the next decade would partially reduce the problem of oversupply while maintaining the revenue base of the schools. A decision to reduce enrollment would require specific attention to the differences by region in the number of social work schools, current enrollments, and annual number of graduates. To be most competitive over the next decade, schools of social work must increase the rigor and managed care emphasis within their curricula, reduce the size of their enrollments while increasing the standards for admission, and tie continuing education to licensure and credentialing. Without those changes in emphasis, social work schools will continue to burden an oversupplied field with far too many additional graduates who cannot be readily absorbed in traditional jobs.

Crisis in Clinical Practice

Managed care organizations attempt to reduce overall health care cost increases by focusing their policies and processes on the interrelated areas of access, unit costs, quality, and utilization (Mauer et al., 1995). However, the key hidden variable in each of those generic areas in the health care equation is the nature and extent of professional health and mental health practice. Although many health and mental health professionals may prefer the maintenance of autonomous practice models (Munson, 1996), successful implementation of the policy goals and economic aims of managed care seems inevitably to require changes in key areas of professional practice, not the least of which is compensation. Review of the social work literature from 1992 to 1997 confirms that practitioners see themselves affected by managed care in a vast number of ways (Alperin, 1994; Altman, 1995; Berkman, 1996; Brown, 1994; Corcoran & Gingrich, 1994; Cornelius, 1994; Davis, 1997; Gibelman & Schervish, 1996; Gorin & Moniz, 1992; Hudson & DeVito, 1994; Keigher, 1995; Mizrahi, 1993; Munson, 1996; Scuka, 1994; Shapiro, 1995; Shera, 1996; Strom, 1994; Vandivort-Warren, 1996; see also chapters 3 and 28).

Trends in Patient Care

LOCUS OF PRACTICE

One means of understanding the extent to which the health care environment has changed and is being influenced by managed care is through a brief examination of trends in patient care episodes. The number and locus of these episodes determines the locus and to some extent the nature of clinical practice. Between 1955 and 1992, the number of annual patient care episodes in the United States increased from 1.7 million to 8.8 million (Manderscheid & Sonnenschein, 1996). Interestingly, the growth in number of episodes per year parallels the annual growth in costs of health care and the growth in the number of mental health professionals in practice (Manderscheid & Sonnenschein, 1996). Under the unregulated fee-for-service payment methods, the greater the number of episodes of care, the greater the overall costs and potential for provider profits. As there is an increase in the number of providers entering such a market, the number of episodes and unit costs remain elastic to accommodate the increase in providers. In response to the increase in number of episodes, affiliated costs, and number of providers in the marketplace, managed care organizations can exercise several related strategies that directly affect clinical practice:

- Patient care episodes can be shifted away from costly inpatient services to outpatient services.
- The amount of compensation can be fixed at a specific amount per capita, per case, per diagnosis, or per episode.
- The number of actual visits can be fixed annually.
- Limitations can be applied to the length of services provided.

The number of providers in the market is therefore controlled, and total compensation for providers remains relatively constant. However, these strategies raise legal questions about restraint of trade and price fixing ("Suit Targets Managed Care," 1997).

The shift in locus of episodes occurred even before managed care. In 1955, for example, 77 percent of all patient care episodes were in inpatient settings; only 23 percent were in outpatient settings. (That 1955 distribution of patient care episodes is consistent with the distribution of social workers in practice before managed care [Manderscheid & Sonnenschein, 1996].) However, by 1992, the beginning of the spread of managed care, inpatient episodes had fallen to only 26 percent of the annual total, and outpatient care accounted for 68 percent of all patient care episodes (Manderscheid & Sonnenschein, 1996). However, close to 60 percent of social workers in 1992 continued to be employed in inpatient health and mental health settings. If the shift in locus of episodes continues over the next two to four decades, almost all patient care episodes will be on an outpatient basis. Partial care episodes that were not available in 1955 accounted for 6 percent of the total episodes for 1992. What is clear here is that the locus of health and mental health care practice will increasingly shift to outpatient care, a trend which is more congruent with the aims of managed care but incongruent with the long-term pattern in social work employment.

CREDENTIALING: LICENSURE, NETWORK ADMISSION, PRIVATE PRACTICE, AND AUTONOMY

Data on the oversupply of mental health professionals (Manderscheid & Sonnenschein, 1996; Steenbarger, 1997) establish a basis for managed care organizations and government to develop a series of processes to limit cost increases by limiting the number of professionals in practice. Although the government can influence the pool of providers by withdrawing support from pre-service academic training centers, managed care organizations have the capability to institute other measures after training takes place. The ability of a managed care organization to dominate a market through its contracting for covered lives has placed these organizations in a gatekeeper position of determining who qualifies for entry into or for continued practice. Managed care organizations determine who can practice social work in their plans by establishing a series of criteria, credentials, or experience required for a professional to be accepted into a managed care practice network. Chief among these processes is credentialing and recredentialing of providers on a regular schedule. Managed care organizations can base their credentialing on the verification of licensure, insurance claims history, professional and legal censure, board certification, loss of licensure, quality assurance feedback, cultural competency, continued education, and language skills, in addition to specific clinical experiences and skills (Mauer et al., 1995). To be considered for practice in a health care network or panel, social work providers must demonstrate the extent to which they meet the credentials required. Once accepted on a panel or network, the providers have a reasonable degree of financial and practice security because the responsibility for obtaining covered lives rests with the managed care organization. Long-term security, however, may be more elusive.

A number of professional organizations have combined their concerns about clinical practice in managed care in a legal challenge to the credentialing and compensation policies established by managed care organizations ("Suit Targets Managed Care," 1997). A lawsuit has been filed on behalf of social workers, psychologists, and psychiatrists to alter what is termed the "imbalance in power" between managed care organizations and mental health providers. These providers and their professional associations allege that managed care organizations restrain and control their practices, access to clients, and compensation through a conspiratorial process. The suit challenges the payment practices and credentialing processes that determine who has access to the managed care panels. Managed care organizations are seeking to dismiss the suit by proposing that they have public and perhaps legislative sanction to reduce the cost of health care. To meet these goals of managed care requires that they restrict the number of providers as well as the compensation they are able to demand ("Suit Targets Managed Care," 1997).

COMPENSATION

The essence of managed care processes is the intent to control and spread financial risk. Before 1992, the risk of financing health and mental health care was primarily assumed by insurance companies, employers, and government as third-party payers. However, managed care policy seeks to redistribute financial risk by shifting the reimbursement system away from fee-for-service toward more fixed fees. For example, managed care organizations may contract with social work providers to compensate them for care on an annual per capita or case rate basis, regardless of the number of episodes of care required by a client. If care exceeds the projected level, the social work provider is expected to provide the service at no additional compensation. Managed care organizations can also require that services provided by specialists be preauthorized by primary care gatekeepers. Primary care gatekeepers may thus determine the extent to which specialists such as social workers actually receive referrals. Managed care organizations can also affect access, cost, and quality of care through the use of utilization review of services as they are being provided or afterward. As a result of these utilization reviews, provider compensation may be reduced or denied, or efforts may be made to recover payments already made. Utilization review data can also be used to determine whether the provider remains part of the network or panel.

Because managed care organizations are rapidly increasing the number of lives covered under their plans, their penetration share of the available market is increasing significantly (Keigher, 1995). The number of Americans now covered by managed care plans in the private and public sectors is increasing at approximately 14,000 per day. In some states, 100 percent of the population is covered by a form of managed care plan (Steenbarger, 1997). As a result of the market share controlled by managed care organizations through their contracts with businesses and government, these organizations are in a position to negotiate levels of compensation with social work providers as well as cut the prices they are willing to offer providers. If managed care organizations in an area reach an agreement on the level of compensation that will be offered to all providers, the providers will be virtually locked out of the market and unable to compete. Here, too, issues of restraint of trade and monopolization seem relevant legal concerns for social work providers.

CLINICAL PRACTICE MODELS

The sine qua non of managed care policy is the provision of brief, cost-effective models of clinical services. Such models not only are congruent with the emphasis on lowering of costs but also are congruent with research findings showing that there is minimal difference between the outcomes of short- and long-term intervention. Although the profession of social work was among the first professions to develop short-term intervention models (Perlman, 1957), those models have been in less frequent use since the onset of fee-for-service payment plans. Under managed care policy, the clinical protocols and de-emphasis on pre-existing or chronic conditions seem to preclude maintenance of unlimited lengths of care, as was once the practice under fee-for-service. Social workers have an opportunity to increase their share of the managed care service market by redeveloping and strengthening the brief models of mental health care they established. The more that social work can demonstrate the efficacy of those models, the stronger the position social work will hold in this new environment.

As managed care captures larger shares of the health and mental health market, it may become more difficult for social work providers to maintain viable small private clinical practices. Increasingly, consumers will need to rely more on those providers who are part of integrated networks of services or pay additional premiums for point-of-service options. Managed care organizations express a preference for practices that are large enough to include an interface between health and mental health and to produce the desired economies of scale through the volume of services provided. Few small, independent practices are able to do this and are likely to be abandoned if managed care does not contract with them for specific units of services. Standards of service operations required by managed care are also likely to contribute to the dilemmas of private clinical practice.

Conclusion

In the past several months, mental health professions, including social work, have expressed the urgency of their concerns about managed care by pursuing a legal strategy. The court pleadings portray a group of professions who feel that managed health care organizations seriously interfere with their ability to practice, hamper the access to services by their clients, and manipulate the fee structure to the economic detriment of the professions. The response by the American Behavioral Health Care Association, the industry's voice, suggests that managed care organizations are doing what they were asked to do by the public and Congress: lower the cost of health care in the United States ("Suit Targets Managed Care," 1997). That the effort by managed care organizations to lower national health care costs reduces the income or the autonomy of mental health professionals or borders on the restraint of trade is a necessary by-product according to the industry. In part, the industry response reflects the general perspective that there are too many health care professionals, costs are rising too rapidly, access is far too open, and quality is questionable. The industry's economic argument is strengthened by the findings that total health care costs and the steep escalation in costs have been reduced by managed care processes in the past five years. The legal struggle and counterarguments are good reflections of the dilemmas that arise in the health care system as public expectations and demands for access increase, but there is no adequate congressional response to the need for national health care. Many of the financial problems that were associated with fee-for-service payment methods have been reduced by managed care but have been replaced by new questions about a decline in the quality of care, equity of benefits, consumer choice, an assault on the health professions, and excess profits by managed care organizations.

It seems important for social work and other health care disciplines to distinguish among managed health care policy and processes and the organizations that administer them. There should be little question of a need to manage the cost and quality of care in the American health care system. Fee-for-service health care was not a panacea that guaranteed access or quality of care for the American population. Fee-for-service health care was a weak safety net with numerous holes through which the working poor, unemployed, disabled, and minority populations found themselves falling (Davis, 1996). There is clearly a need for a change in policy direction in health care. The profession must recognize that, albeit fraught with problems, the current effort to change health care is but the most recent effort to do so. In the past 50 years, there have been numerous attempts to change the financing, organization, and functioning of the health care system. Managed health care is not likely to be the final effort to modify the system. There have been other efforts to change health care policy, and in the next millennium the probability is great that there will be others.

The profession of social work must turn the crisis of managed health care and the process by which it developed into opportunities for close introspection and strengthening itself (Altman, 1995; Keigher, 1995; Munson, 1996). Managed health care should force the profession to clarify and solve its inveterate identity issues ("Survey Takes the Membership's Pulse," 1997), develop a long-range vision, distinguish its specific skills and contributions to the marketplace, balance the needs of the marketplace with the capacities of its university programs, and determine how it will conduct ongoing evaluations of its outcomes. Managed care should stimulate the profession to examine its professional associations, the methods for increasing membership, and the trend toward splintering into specialized guilds within the profession. Managed care should stimulate the profession to examine carefully the human resource issues that are needed to avoid oversaturation of the field. The profession must also consider the national importance of first-rate continued education as a requirement for continuing practice. Foremost, from this crisis social work and other professions must address the issue of their involvement in the policy process at the local, state, and national levels, where the public debate over the direction of health care is taking place.

It seems clear that managed health care is affecting social work practice and education in a variety of ways. It could be argued that social work, psychiatry, nursing, and professional counselors are close to five years behind the trends in managed health, whereas psychology has been more proactive. The crisis in social work that is precipitated by this change in paradigm does, however, present social work with a series of opportunities to strengthen the profession's position in the health care market. Those opportunities center on brief methods of practice, involvement in case management, emphasis on prevention, focus on families, educative approaches to increase compliance, and quality assurance efforts that have been part of the history of social work. Social work services may also cost considerably less, without a loss of quality, when compared with some other professional groups. Failure to respond to the crisis precipitated by managed care could diminish the profession and lessen its opportunity to prepare for the next phase of health reform, in which managed care principles are likely to be in operation, but managed care organizations will have changed form, become fewer in number, and refined their processes and in which more direct contracting between payers and providers will be the zeitgeist.

What stands before the social work profession and others is the need for a new vision not only of how health care is to be packaged and delivered but also of our explicit knowledge, skills, and roles in such systems.

References

Alperin, R. M. (1994). Managed care versus psychoanalytic psychotherapy: Conflicting ideologies. *Clinical Social Work Journal, 22,* 137–148.

Altman, H. (1995). A response to Richard Alperin's article: "Managed care versus psychoanalytic psychotherapy: Conflicting ideologies." *Clinical Social Work Journal, 23,* 223–226.

Berkman, B. (1996). The emerging health care world: Implications for social work practice and education. *Social Work, 41,* 541–550.

Bernier, S. A. (1994). Managed care today. In A. D'Alessandro (Ed.), *Managed behavioral health care: Provider and training development manual* (pp. 1–15). Clearwater, FL: Of Course Publications.

Brown, F. (1994). Resisting the pull of the health insurance tarbaby: An organizational model for surviving managed care. *Clinical Social Work Journal, 22,* 59–71.

Bureau of National Affairs. (1993). *Description of the President's health care reform plan.* Washington, DC: Author.

Center for Health Economics Research, Brandeis University. (1993). *Access to health care: Key indicators for policy.* Princeton, NJ: Robert Wood Johnson Foundation.

Corcoran, K., & Gingrich, W. (1994). Practice evaluation in the context of managed care: Case-recording methods for quality assurance reviews. *Research on Social Work Practice, 4,* 326–337.

Cornelius, D. S. (1994). Managed care and social work: Constructing a context and a response. *Social Work in Health Care, 20,* 47–63.

Cummings, N. A. (1996). Foreword. In C. H. Browning & B. J. Browning (Eds.), *How to partner with managed care* (pp. v–ix). Los Angeles: Duncliff's International.

Davis, K. (1996). Primary health care and severe mental illness: The need for national and state policy. *Health & Social Work, 21,* 83–87.

Davis, K. (in press). Race, unemployment, managed care and cultural competency. In F. Brisbane (Ed.), *Cultural competency for health care professionals working with African American communities: Theory and practice* [Special Collaborative Edition No. 7]. Bethesda, MD: U.S. Department of Health and Human Services, Center for Substance Abuse Prevention.

Freeman, M., & Trabin, T. (1994). *Managed behavioral healthcare: History, models, key issues, and future course.* Tiburon, CA: Behavioral Health Care Alliance.

Gibelman, M., & Schervish, P. H. (1996). The private practice of social work: Current trends and projected scenarios in a managed care environment. *Clinical Social Work Journal, 24,* 323–338.

Gibelman, M., & Schervish, P. H. (1997). *Who we are: A second look.* Washington, DC: NASW Press.

Giles, T. R. (1993). *Managed mental health care: A guide for practitioners, employers, and hospital administrators.* Boston: Allyn & Bacon.

Gorin, S., & Moniz, C. (1992). The national health care crisis: An analysis of proposed solutions. *Health & Social Work, 17,* 37–44.

Hilzenrath, D. S. (1997, June 30). Backlash builds over managed care: Frustrated consumers push for tougher laws. *Washington Post,* p. 1.

Hudson, C. G., & DeVito, J. A. (1994). Mental health under national health care reform: The empirical foundations. *Health & Social Work, 19,* 279–287.

Keigher, S. M. (1995). Managed care's silent seduction of America and the new politics of choice [National Health Line]. *Health & Social Work, 20,* 146–151.

Kongstvedt, P. R. (1997). *Essentials of managed health care.* Gaithersburg, MD: Aspen.

Manderscheid, R. W. (1997). *Changes in managed care and the implications for cultural competency.* Unpublished presentation. Myrtle Beach, SC: Mental Health Policy Institute on Cultural Competency.

Manderscheid, R. W., & Sonnenschein, M. A. (1996). *Mental health, United States, 1995.* Rockville, MD: National Institute of Mental Health.

Mauer, B., Jarvis, D., Mockler, R., & Trabin, T. (1995). *How to respond to managed behavioral healthcare.* Tiburon, CA: CentraLink.

Mizrahi, T. (1993). Managed care and managed competition: A primer for social work. *Health & Social Work, 18,* 86–91.

Munson, C. E. (1996). Autonomy and managed care in clinical social work practice. *Smith College Studies in Social Work, 66,* 241–260.

Perlman, H. H. (1957). *Social casework: A problem-solving process.* Chicago: University of Chicago Press.

Robert Wood Johnson Foundation. (1991). *Challenges in health care: A chartbook perspective 1991.* Princeton, NJ: Author.

Scuka, R. F. (1994). Health care reform in the 1990s: An analysis of the problem and three proposals. *Social Work, 39,* 580–587.

Shapiro, J. (1995). The downside of managed mental health care. *Clinical Social Work Journal, 23,* 441–451.

Shera, W. (1996). Managed care and people with severe mental illness: Challenges and opportunities for social work. *Health & Social Work, 21,* 196–201.

Starr, P. (1982). *The social transformation of American medicine: The rise of a sovereign profession and the making of a vast industry.* New York: Basic Books.

Steenbarger, B. N. (1997). What's News. *Online, 1*(12), 1–7.

Strom, K. (1994). Social workers in private practice: An update. *Clinical Social Work Journal, 22,* 73–89.

Suit targets managed care. (1997, July). *NASW News.* Washington, DC: NASW Press.

Survey takes the membership's pulse. (1997, September). *NASW News.* Washington, DC: NASW Press.

United Healthcare Corporation. (1994). *A glossary of terms: The language of managed care and organized health care systems.* Minnetonka, MN: Author.

Vandivort-Warren, R. (1996). *CSWE/NASW Report on preparing social workers for a managed care environment.* Washington, DC: National Association of Social Workers.

White House Domestic Policy Council. (1993). *Health security: The President's report to the American people.* Washington, DC: Author.

CHAPTER 40

Educating Students for Social Work in Health Care Today

Kay Davidson

In the current managed health care environment, a much-reduced number of traditional social work positions remain in health care settings. The roles of social workers and potential new social work positions have moved to an outpatient and community arena in which services and care for all kinds of health concerns are now located (Berkman, 1996; Simmons, 1994). As a result, social workers are confronted with the need to find concrete ways to be included in the delivery of community-based health care services.

This shift in the location of care has happened together with the changes brought about by major reductions of hospital services and with the concomitant effects of deregulation and deprofessionalization (Cornelius, 1994).

A great challenge exists for social work to identify funding for the multiple psychosocial services that remain important for vulnerable populations needing health care, especially those experiencing debilitating and chronic illnesses. Those lacking resources and choice, notably chronically ill people and frail elderly men and women, constitute a majority of those with serious health problems, and do so at a time when we have extended longevity and turned fatal illnesses to chronicity yet have not arrived at widespread successful aging. Consequently, those with the greatest need and the least ability to negotiate systems for themselves receive inferior-quality care. Their family members also may be seriously depleted of the energy and resources needed to pursue quality care as they strive to care for patients over long periods.

The move toward health care becoming more "businesslike" by shifting to capitated care seems to result in only those who are well-informed consumers receiving better value for their money. For many users of managed care services, there is neither a choice of provider nor control over the type or extent of care.

Whereas capitation plans could offer extensive coverage, as they do in single-payer or national health systems elsewhere, when they are integrally linked to the concepts of industry and profit, as in the current climate and developments in the United States, they offer vulnerable populations the lowest level of care that can be justified to the public.

NOTE: An earlier version of this work was presented at "The First Managed Care Behavioral Health Care Invitational Conference for New England Graduate Social Work Faculty," funded by the Robert Wood Johnson Foundation, the National Institute of Mental Health, and the Alcohol and Drug Institute at the Boston University School of Social Work, October 1997, Boston.

It has been apparent for at least a decade that health care social work needs to move the core of its services into the community, but a base of funding for such services continues to elude us. Indeed, even home care—a vital place for social workers to help patients adjust to illness and disability, as well as to provide family support and health education, is not well covered by any insurance reimbursement. It has been very difficult to convince insurers, including the Health Care Financing Administration (HCFA), that people receiving their care at home have psychosocial needs that bear on their recovery or on the management of their physical illness. Likewise, the presence of social work services in long-term care is neither as strong nor as extensive as is needed to respond appropriately to the serious and complex psychosocial consequences of chronic illness.

Mental health managed care offers the opportunities for social work to provide the bulk of such services in aggregated agencies; can a similar model be applied to physical health and its profound and often traumatic effects on patients' lives? Can social work agencies develop contracts to provide health-related social services in the community, as they have at a few major medical centers? Possible sites could be in schools, senior citizen centers, community centers, and doctors' offices as well as in home care and long-term care facilities (Simmons, 1994). An example of this potential can be seen in the school-based health clinics of the Hartford Public Schools in Connecticut, where social workers are employed by the school system to work as part of a health team. Consideration of how social workers' services can be funded in the community raises the question of whether we have the data available to make a sufficient and clear case for the cost benefit of such work as well as its social imperative. It seems clear that the presence of social workers in the community, in places such as doctors' offices and group practices, would release many physicians from their attempts to manage psychosocial concerns that they find onerous and for which they lack appropriate knowledge and qualifications, but such programs are not yet common.

A good model of such presence is Community Practice Social Work at New Britain General Hospital in Connecticut. It offers social work services as a free service for physicians and their patients in their offices. Like the Health Outreach Program at the New York Hospital, which offers free education and counseling to people ages 65 and over in the community, this innovative service can prevent problems and keep costs of care from escalating. Despite such programs, the psychosocial arena is too often perceived as everyone's area of expertise. It remains imperative for social workers to demonstrate through research studies that the professional expertise that allows us to provide supportive services to families produces positive and welcome results, such as reduction of lost work or school days; decreased stress-induced illness; and fewer of the medical crises that are often related to lack of knowledge, noncompliance with treatment, and overburdened caretakers. Research findings can then be used to advocate for provision of psychosocial services throughout health care programs (Monkman, 1991; Ell, 1996).

In many areas of practice, social work has already moved away from the traditional, pathology-oriented, medical model that so influenced the early days of the profession. In educating students for practice today, we teach them to focus on strengths and capabilities as the building blocks of change and support for individuals, families, and communities (Saleebey, 1992; Lee, 1994; Rapp, 1998). As we prepare students for this practice, we need also to prepare them for varied and expanded roles if they are to find a place in managed health care that will allow meaningful and empowering services both to people and to communities. Such programs and roles for social workers may be in health promotion and education; in informing institutions about communities' needs, wants, and capacities; and in facilitating community relations (Simmons, 1994).

For example, at some major medical centers, such as Massachusetts General Hospital, social work knowledge and skills in communication are applied to the development and implementation of cancer and other education programs. Thus, social work graduates need to use their understanding of the implications of managed care for their clients to advocate for them and help them advocate for themselves. Our graduates also need knowledge of how organizations work and how communities' needs can be assessed as well as skills to influence and help institutions respond through provision of appropriate and adequate services.

In educating students for innovative roles, we must create field placement experiences in settings that are testing new approaches and programs. Although it is frequently supposed by practitioners that schools move too slowly from old models to new needs and realities, field instructors, even in new settings, may be tempted to use teaching models from their own earlier learning that are familiar and comfortable. Schools and practitioners in the field must find ways to work together to develop new models for practice and new ways of teaching that will encourage adult and autonomous learning. To expand potential teaching and learning opportunities in the field, traditional field instruction may be adapted and augmented by the addition of task instructors in different areas of practice, group supervision, student rotations through diverse settings, and other approaches. Schools must be open to and support such new models of teaching and the use of various forms of recording as teaching tools.

Such enhanced opportunities in field educaton must also include a focus on the short-term services that are supported by managed care financing within a continuum of care. Social workers have traditionally practiced and taught their students both short-term and long-term work; they also have a long tradition of using other models that may not have been labeled adequately or accurately. In the real experiences of many social workers in health care, especially in their work with the consequences of the increasingly chronic nature of most serious illnesses, episodic care is frequently practiced although not necessarily acknowledged.

Social workers have tended to consider their work a failure if clients leave before "completing" some work only to return with another aspect of the problem at a later date. Yet this very model may be highly effective for many clients in the health arena as they take what help they need and can use at a particular point in their adjustment to and acceptance of the reality of their illness (Miller & Rehr, 1983). Thus, we may already have in place an adaptable and useful model of brief, intermittent care that we need to recognize and teach our students to use and value. The current professional climate in health care calls for greater self-direction and autonomy of social work practitioners (Berkman, 1996).

The interest of educators in developing methods to teach increasingly autonomous practice (Livingston, Davidson, & Marshack, 1989) has been promoted further by the changes and reduction in supervisory structures for practitioners in greatly downsized organizations.

To bring new content to the curriculum and classrooms of the schools, further collaborative activities must bring practitioners in not only as occasional guest lecturers but also as teachers for courses that prepare graduates for new health careers—courses on health and mental health policy and practice, practice-based research, and administration. Faculty in schools and the field need to undertake joint research projects and work together in advocacy on health issues. Coalitions can be formed through collaborative work in professional committees and organizations, such as the National Association of Social Workers, the Council for Social Work Education, and specialized health groups such as the Society for Social Work Leadership in Health Care. Such groups provide rich opportunities for sharing knowledge of changes in health care practice and developing networks through their regular meetings and conferences. Traditional "town and gown" tensions can be greatly diminished by faculty from schools and agencies working together around common interests and collaborating on research projects, presentations, and publications that combine academic skills in analysis and teaching with practitioners' current knowledge.

To teach self-reflective and self-monitoring practice, educators must think about *how* to teach as well as *what* to teach. To produce graduates who can think critically and independently and to prepare social workers adequately for new and challenging professional roles, educators in the classroom and the field must model careful consideration and critical assessment of data. The basis for an approach to teaching that presents a model of autonomous practice assumes an adult-learning, andragogical model that encourages students to experience doubt, to raise criticism, and to keep questioning (Knowles, 1980). This can be a hard model to implement, because students, especially when new and anxious beginners in the field, would like answers in the form of a blueprint for practice. Even our more experienced students may seek similar certainty, and confirmation of what they already knew and were doing in their preprofessional work. It is also difficult for educators to respond to the students' desire for certainty by asking them to live with a level of uncertainty because we recognize that they are seeking to provide answers for their clients and to appear expert and prepared to their colleagues from other disciplines. Yet our task in preparing students for the new roles and challenges of the managed care practice world is to encourage them to be curious and critical, even as they build their body of knowledge and expertise. At the same time, we must help students to be responsible for identifying their own learning needs and to be self-reflective and self-monitoring in their practice, whatever their units of attention and whatever practice methods they are using.

As I have stated elsewhere, the "experience of doubt stimulates practitioners to reflect on their work and its observed results, introducing the possibility of reformulating theories and developing innovative programs and services" (Davidson, 1990). Even if they are open to reflection on their practice roles and functions, practitioners may still fail to produce innovative ways to help patients in the managed health care arena unless they have been educated to become graduates who understand organizational behavior and who can analyze social policy as a basis for influencing changes. Nothing could seem more pertinent for our curriculum today as we strive to find a place in the managed health care arena and new pathways to provide health care social work services to vulnerable clients and communities.

References

Berkman, B. (1996). The emerging health care world: Implications for social work practice and education. *Social Work, 41,* 541–551.

Cornelius, D. (1994). Managed care and social work: Constructing a context and a response. *Social Work in Health Care, 20,* 47–63.

Davidson, K. (1990). Doubt as a source of innovation in developing effective services to families. *Families in Society, 71,* 296–302.

Ell, K. (1996). Social work and health care practice and policy: A psychosocial research agenda. *Social Work, 41,* 583–592.

Knowles, M. (1980). *The modern practice of adult education: From pedagogy to andragogy.* Chicago: Follett.

Lee, J. (1994). *The empowerment approach to social work practice.* New York: Columbia University Press.

Livingston, D., Davidson, K., & Marshack, E. (1989). Education for autonomous practice: A challenge for field instructors. *Journal of Independent Social Work, 4,* 1.

Miller, R., & Rehr, H. (1983). *Social work issues in health care.* Englewood Cliffs, NJ: Prentice Hall.

Monkman, M. (1991). Outcome objectives in social work practice: Person and environment. *Social Work, 36,* 253–258.

Rapp, C. (1998). *The strengths model.* New York: Oxford University Press.

Saleebey, D. (1992). *The strengths perspective in social work practice.* New York: Longman.

Simmons, J. (1994). Community based care: The new health social work paradigm. *Social Work in Health Care, 20,* 35–46.

CHAPTER 41

Postmodern Approaches:
Education for a Managed Care Environment

Patricia Kelley

In this chapter I discuss two main trends in clinical social work that seem at odds with each other: (1) managed care and (2) an emergence of more constructivist forms of practice. Managed care pushes clinical social workers toward more time-limited treatment, DSM-IV diagnoses of clients, concrete problem definitions, and very specific goals and preapproved treatment plans based on empirically proven treatment methods. The emphasis on a medical model implies a more expert role for the social worker. Meanwhile, the constructivist therapies are based on a view of the world that is nonlinear, denies the possibility of objectivity, and holds multiple views of reality with no fixed truths. Furthermore, the treatment, as well as reality, is co-constructed by client and therapist with the emphasis in therapy on constructing new meanings through dialogue rather than problem-solving activities directed by the therapist. Can these two seemingly polar opposites be practiced together? Here that question will be addressed by looking at one form of constructivist therapy—the narrative approach—and assessing which parts of it are and are not compatible with managed care practice.

Educators need to address these issues as they prepare students for the reality of today's practice. In fact, there are many realities in today's practice: the needs to educate for practice in managed care systems, to prepare students for culturally competent practice, to teach ethical practice built on individualized client service, to help students to planfully evaluate their own practices, and to increase their understanding of the theoretical and empirical bases underlying interventions.

Managed Care

As noted by Sederer and Bennett (1996), managed care had its formative years in the 1970s and evolved by the 1990s into a whole system of health care reform that has radically altered and shaped mental health care. They also noted that education for and research regarding mental health care are affected because some contracts do not allow trainees to treat people who are insured and most education and research for the mental health professions come from university and community training

NOTE: This chapter was presented at the Annual Program Meeting of the Council on Social Work Education, March 1998, Orlando, Florida. An earlier version, "Narrative Therapy in a Managed Care World," is in press for the journal *Crisis Intervention and Time-Limited Treatment.*

centers. Managed care no longer affects only people who are privately insured but has now reached out to public service delivery systems, including community clinics, and can leave the most vulnerable populations—those in high-risk groups—underserved (Resnick & Tighe, 1997).

Managed care has also been influential in pushing clinicians toward more outcome research regarding their practice. As noted by Dornelas, Correll, Lothstein, Wilbur, and Goethe (1996), clinicians need to produce quantifiable data for nonclinicians, although it may seem reductionistic. Managed care programs are looking to findings from outcome research to set policy regarding what practice will be funded (Beutler, Davison, Kim, Karno, & Fisher, 1996). This practice could be useful as clinicians make closer examinations of their work. Concerns have been raised, however, that such policies will exclude many practice methods that may be useful and will not value those clinicians who favor more qualitative and naturalistic methods of inquiry (Beutler et al., 1996). Strupp (1997) noted problems in measurement in the strictly quantitative designs as applied to treatment in which relationships are a chief factor and in which there is more to measure than symptom reduction, and Seligman (1996) noted the importance of both observational and empirical data in getting the full picture.

Winegar (1992) outlined strategies for successful practice in the managed care environment, and his list included the following recommendations: using the DSM-IV codes and terminology; developing a written treatment plan with clear goals; establishing specific outcome measures for the treatment goals; using time-limited treatment; and maintaining clear written treatment notes with a specific format (such as the subjective–objective assessment plan [SOAP]) for documentation. These recommendations are the basis for the comparative analysis presented in this chapter.

Paradigm Shifts

Just as the systemic family therapy movement of the 1960s and 1970s was a major paradigm shift from emphasis on intrapsychic factors and uncovering root causes for problems to emphasis on interpersonal processes and current behavior, so is the current constructivist movement a paradigm shift back to more emphasis on feelings, meanings, and myths. Whereas systems approaches are based on cybernetic theory—a mechanistic theory of control that Hoffman (1985), as early as the mid-1980s, declared had lost its usefulness—constructivist approaches are based on second-order cybernetics, in which the observer and the observed mutually affect one another. The systems theories, like several of the behavioral and cognitive approaches that emerged at about the same time, are based on the modernist view of objectivity, rationality, and knowing through observation. The postmodern view, of which constructivism is a part, recognizes the many realities and truths that coexist and sees reality as being socially constructed rather than a given (Laird, 1993; Neimeyer, 1993).

Neimeyer (1993) characterized constructivism as a "meta-theory that emphasizes the self-organizing and proactive features of human knowing" (p. 221) and a view of humans as "meaning making agents" (p. 222). Its roots can be traced to George Kelly's Personal Construct Theory, first articulated in the 1950s (Kelly, 1955). Kelly himself cited semanticist Korzybski (1933), who also influenced cognitive (Ellis, 1967) and systems (Watzlawick, Weakland, & Jackson, 1967) therapists, and Moreno (1937), who developed psychodrama. Although there are historical roots, constructivist approaches to therapy have risen to prominence in the past decade as the postmodern perspective has crossed many academic disciplines to become a major force in the popular culture as well.

As noted by Friedman (1993), postmodernism comprises many diverse elements. A number of therapeutic approaches fall under the general rubric of postmodernism, including the strengths-based approach (Saleebey, 1996), the solution-focused approach (de Shazer, 1991; O'Hanlon & Weiner-Davis, 1989), the collaborative language systems approach (Anderson & Goolishian, 1988), and the narrative approaches (White & Epston, 1990). Those approaches have been found useful in feminist practice (Sands & Nuccio, 1992), multicultural practice (Holland & Kilpatrick, 1993; Waldegrave, 1990), stepfamilies (Kelley, 1996), lesbian and gay families (Laird, 1996), people facing adversity (Borden, 1992), abuse victims (Dolan, 1991), family violence offenders (Jenkins, 1991), and health care practice (Kelley & Clifford, 1997; Wynne, Shields, & Sirkin, 1992). In addition, postmodernism's usefulness in social work education has been noted (Kelley, 1995; Laird, 1993), and books have summarized the various approaches (Friedman, 1993; Hoyt, 1994).

With this proliferation of literature in the 1990s on the postmodern approaches, it is important to assess the approaches' usefulness in the managed care environment. Because the postmodern approaches are philosophical in nature, it might be asked how they can be time limited. Some, such as the solution-focused approaches (Berg, 1994; de Shazer, 1991; Dolan, 1991), are clearly brief in nature and quite interventive and planful, whereas others, such as the collaborative language systems approach (Anderson & Goolishian, 1988), have little planning and no set goals or time frame. The narrative approaches offer a midrange view between the two, and it is this approach that I have chosen to assess in terms of managed care.

Narrative Therapy

The narrative approach discussed here is based on the work of White and Epston (1990) of Australia and New Zealand, respectively. Their approach has developed in relation to the postmodern influence that has been permeating thinking in many fields and in relation to the constructivist and constructionist therapy approaches developing in North America (Anderson & Goolishian, 1988; de Shazer, 1991; Tomm, 1987) and Europe (Andersen, 1987; Boscolo, Cecchin, Hoffman, & Penn, 1987). As these approaches codeveloped at about the same time, they took different forms. White and Epston (1990) drew on the works of French philosopher and historian Michael Foucault (1980) as well as the works of Jerome Bruner (1986) and Gregory Bateson (1972). It is interesting to note that the systems thinkers also drew heavily on Bateson, demonstrating overlap in theory development and suggesting that paradigm shifts are rarely complete.

The narrative approach draws on both the deconstructivist theory of literary criticism, in which narratives are taken apart and analyzed for meaning, and the social constructionism in social psychology, in which reality is believed to be coconstructed in the minds of people in interaction with each other and with societal beliefs. We all "story" our lives to make sense of our experiences, and the narrative therapist listens carefully to the client's story to understand the meanings ascribed to events, as well as to understand the events themselves. The therapeutic process consists of a dialogue in which new realities are developed. While carefully attending to and understanding the client's problem story, other aspects of the story are also sought—aspects that may have been overlooked in the focus on the problem. Negative experiences and their effects are never denied or minimized, but the meanings attached to them and the power they are given over the client's life may be challenged.

This treatment model offered by White and Epston (1990) names specific practices and outlines stages of treatment without being too prescriptive or technique driven. As noted, their approach would fall midrange on a continuum on several variables, such as role of therapist, degree of intervention and planning, and focus on problems. In the systems' approaches, the therapist is the expert who stays in charge, and interventions are planned and prescribed. Specific problem sequences are mapped and interrupted, problematic family structures are modified, and presenting problems are specified and solutions are sought. Those approaches tend to be short term and lend themselves well to managed care (Greene, 1996), with the emphasis on specificity being especially useful there. Solution-focused therapy (de Shazer, 1991) can be seen as a direct outgrowth of its problem-solving predecessor, but the emphasis is put on strengths and what is already working rather than on problems. In other strengths-based approaches (Saleebey, 1996), there is a similar shift from the client's problems to the client's strengths.

Some of the social constructionist views (Anderson & Goolishian, 1988; Tomm, 1987), in contrast, put little emphasis on therapist expertise, intervention, or problem-solving or solution-seeking activities. Likewise, they outline no specific stages of treatment because assessment is ongoing and all sessions are seen as therapeutic. It is hoped that the client's view of reality may be expanded through dialogue. These approaches are more difficult to put into a managed care environment.

Falling between those approaches on a continuum of specificity, White and Epston (1990) spent time and effort understanding the problem, realizing that clients come in to talk about problems that oppress them. They also outlined broad stages of the therapeutic process, recognizing that some activities are more appropriate at earlier or later stages of treatment. Their first stage is deconstruction, in which the clients' stories are heard and specified and then gradually deconstructed for meaning. In an approach that is different from some constructivist therapies, the problem stories are carefully attended to by the therapist. How is the problem defined? How is the client experiencing it? What meaning is ascribed to it? How does this problem fit into the overall life story? Who else is involved in the problem, and what historical events have played a part in its development?

From the beginning, the problem is externalized through the language used by the therapist. Through this process, the person is separated from the problem so that it is viewed as something not intrinsic to the client but as something that has interfered with his or her life and has been oppressive. Clients are encouraged to challenge and stand up to these problems. At this point the client and therapist join together to fight the effects of the problem, and new meanings begin to take shape for the client.

As the therapeutic conversation continues, the problem story is more fully deconstructed through summary and questioning. The dominant story is not questioned or disputed, for the client would not feel understood or respected, but gradually other interpretations and meanings of events can be assessed to bring out alternative truths, which are also valid. The client is helped to assess the relative influence of the problem over the life story: past, present, and anticipated future. That influence is assessed over several spheres of clients' lives: social, personal, interpersonal, and intellectual. The problem is "historicized" as the clients are invited to explore the problem's development over time, further assessing the people and events that were part of its development. This discussion further helps the client feel control over the problem instead of feeling controlled by it.

In the second stage, reconstruction, other truths are discovered—truths that have been subjugated because they did not fit into the dominant problem-saturated story—and these other truths may involve strengths and coping. This subjugated knowledge is brought out through careful listening for unique outcomes: those behaviors, events, or outcomes that cannot be explained by the dominant problem story. For example, the therapist may wonder how the client was able to go to work and manage the children in spite of the problem she was facing.

Here, the similarity to de Shazer's (1991) solution-focused therapy can be seen, but instead of asking for "exceptions" that the client may not see, the therapist carefully sorts through the conversation in a detectivelike manner to find the evidence of things that fall outside of the problem-saturated story. Just as the client had been asked to think about who else was involved in the construction of the problem story, now the client is asked to think about who else was involved in helping him or her develop these other attributes and strengths. Social and cultural forces are explored, as are interpersonal forces. As clients find other views, their reality becomes broader, offering more options than previously recognized. Furthermore, mobilizing their strengths helps clients fight the problems rather than deny them or be oppressed by them.

In this restorying, White and Epston (1990) found that certain activities help move the process along. They made extensive use of writing: clients writing their own stories and ideas as well as the therapist writing to the client to summarize ideas and to elaborate on ideas discussed. Furthermore, they used certificates, awards, and ceremonies to mark certain events or progress. Those latter activities were used in a playful way and were especially useful when working with families with children. In addition, White and Epston used reflecting teams to explore further and look for unique outcomes. They borrowed that idea from Andersen (1987), but they used the teams in a special way to fit their approach. Those ideas will be explored in relation to managed care in another section of this chapter.

Good Fit with Managed Care

There are ways in which narrative approaches fit in well with managed care. First is the question of length of treatment. In spite of its philosophical basis and its emphasis on storytelling and developing new realities, narrative treatment is usually conducted in a few sessions. Several things make this possible. First, although the number of sessions is small, the sessions may be spread over a longer time period instead of every week, giving the family time to think about and try new things. Related to this idea is the fact that unlike some constructivist therapists, White and Epston (1990) often asked clients to try certain activities between sessions. Although not as intervention oriented as the systemic therapists, they were not restricted by an "overbelief in noninstrumentality" (Cecchin, Lane, & Ray, 1993) and were willing to try different things that will help clients develop new stories. Furthermore, the aim of such therapy is focused on helping the client with a specific request, which helps keep therapy brief.

Next, unlike some strengths-based therapists, White and Epston were not hesitant about identifying, discussing, and labeling the problem. Instead of reframing all problems as strengths, they validated the client's concern about the problem and then externalized it so that the client could feel some control over it. Strengths were mobilized, but the client's problem story was heard. The labeling of the problem may not be in psychiatric nomenclature—rather something like "temper" or "sadness" or "fighting"—but it is specific enough to write a treatment plan for a managed care company.

This identification of specific problems makes it possible to set up the treatment goals and outcome measures required by managed care companies. Even if such measurement is not consistent with the theoretical or philosophical base of the postmodern approaches, it is possible to go with a specific treatment plan to help the client receive treatment without altering the spirit of the approach. In addition, clients often like to see this progress themselves. Browning and Browning (1997) outlined a scaling procedure useful with managed care companies that keeps the clients in charge of the problem definition. The clients write down the specific problem or complaint that brought them in; rate its severity on a seven-point scale, comparing now and a few months ago; and then note the circumstances that increase or decrease it. Those questions are similar to those of solution-focused therapy (de Shazer, 1991), but the autographic form makes for a visual that managed care companies like, and that is helpful for clients as they see progress over time using these forms. The goal of narrative therapists is to help the family stop, control, or alleviate the specific problem that has oppressed them and that they have identified. Such goals are easily noted in outcome terms.

The use of DSM-IV diagnoses is not part of the narrative approach, but with problem specification such terminology may not be required by some insurers for some services. When they are required, or when there are major mental illnesses, there is nothing in the narrative approach that would deny the use of the DSM labels. Generally, a narrative therapist would leave such labeling up to a physician, who would be in charge of medical treatment but would leave the psychological and social aspects for the therapy sessions. For example, if a client were diagnosed with schizophrenia or with an affective disorder, the narrative therapist would not deny that view of reality but would help the client view it as only one aspect of himself or herself. The client would then be encouraged to find other aspects of himself or herself that are also true, including strengths that could be mobilized to fight the effects of the condition. Similar to narrative work with people with a medical disorder (Kelley & Clifford, 1997; Wynne et al., 1992), in which a disease is seen as "afflicting but not constituting the self" (Wynne et al., 1992, p. 12), a psychiatric affliction can be a problem to manage and it can be seen as only a part of one's entire life.

In some situations the narrative therapist may work with the client's physician in establishing a DSM diagnosis and developing a conjoint treatment plan involving the client, physician, and therapist that would satisfy the managed care company. In these cases the therapist helps the client to become an active consumer making choices about the treatment rather than a passive recipient of services. In these situations it is also helpful to use outside resources, such as homework assignments and to recommend support groups or workshops for the client. As noted by Browning and Browning (1997), such activities can be listed as "other interventions" and are generally appreciated as creative by managed care companies.

In many situations, however, there is not a major mental illness but a situational or interpersonal problem. Most managed care companies will not accept a DSM-IV–V code, the "non-nervous or mental" disorders, as a diagnosis. Therapists need to work with clients to discuss whether they wish a diagnosis in order to obtain treatment. If so, a discussion with them about the nature of the diagnosis and its ramifications is needed. Now that managed care has reached into the public sector and even community clinics, these discussions are more problematic, for these clients may have no other means of treatment or of payment. Often, the Adjustment Disorder category is appropriate, for clients often are feeling anxious or depressed about the presenting problematic situation or are acting out because of it. In addition, the request for a limited number of sessions helps secure approval.

The language that narrative therapists use with clients and the way they think about problems do not conform with DSM-IV terminology. However, it is possible to transform the language for the reports and still keep the narrative language and thinking for working with clients. For example, "mobilizing client's strengths so he or she can search for a job" would be understood better than "creating new views of reality." Good practitioners often need to go back and forth between different worldviews to keep discussion open with other professionals in the community. Those same skills are important for relationships with managed care companies.

In summary, there are some ways in which narrative therapy can be compatible with the managed care environment. Brevity is the most obvious factor, but there are other elements that make brief therapy work that fit the managed care model. Fisch (1994) outlined the basic elements of brief therapy as narrowing the database, using interactional versus intrapsychic concepts, using task versus insight orientation, and knowing when to stop. Those basically strategic therapy concepts from the systems approach also apply to narrative work. Like systems therapists, narrative therapists keep the focus on what clients bring in as goals and do not aim to uncover root causes or intrapsychic conflicts. Such a focus keeps both the therapist and the client from going on longer than needed. Different from the systems therapist is the nonexpert collaborative stance between therapist and client and the emphasis on meaning and stories. In spite of these differences, narrative therapists do keep to a few sessions, usually spread out over time (Combs & Freedman, 1994; Dickerson & Zimmerman, 1993; White & Epston, 1990), keeping the focus on the client's goal, which also aids in assessment of outcome.

Poor Fit with Managed Care

There are some aspects of narrative work that are more difficult to fit into the contemporary managed care world. Ironically, the aspects of narrative therapy that are most problematic for managed care contracts are those elements that reduce the number of sessions needed. The practice of writing letters to clients has been found useful for reducing the number of sessions—such letters potentiate the effect of therapy sessions and, thus, allow for more time between sessions (Freeman & Lobovitz, 1993; Friedman, 1993; White & Epston, 1990). These "therapeutic letters" to clients summarize the therapist's notes regarding how he or she heard the client describe the problem as well as any solution knowledge obtained in the session. Clients are requested to make corrections, deletions, and additions to make the letters more accurate. Clients have reported that each letter is worth about four sessions (White, 1992). Although these activities reduce the number of sessions needed, they take considerable time for the therapist—time that is not covered as therapy time. This is problematic when agencies are pushing for more billable hours. If the letters can double as therapy notes, time can be saved.

The other activity that White (1992) said reduces the number of sessions significantly is the use of reflecting teams. Clients also rated this activity as worth several sessions, adding potency to each session. Friedman, Brecher, and Mittelmeier (1995) also noted that reflecting teams use therapy time effectively and should be useful in managed care settings. Reflecting teams, a concept borrowed from Andersen (1987, 1990), differ from teams behind one-way mirrors used by systems therapists. In the use of systemic teams, members helped to devise strategies, offered suggestions to clients, noted interaction patterns, and sometimes devised a paradoxical injunction. Reflecting teams do not engage in any of those activities. In addition, narrative therapists, different from the Milan group (Boscolo et al., 1987), do not develop hypotheses or give positive connotations. Here, the reflecting team members observe the clients from behind the one-way mirror or even by sitting in the same room. Partway through the session the team trades places with the clients, and the team discusses its observations and ideas about the session, focusing especially on unique outcomes to the problem story and wondering about how the stories developed. Team members also give their personal reactions and ask others to discuss theirs. There are no corrections or suggestions, nor do the members point out individual or interactional behavior patterns. The discussion about their observations is designed to bring about deeper discussion and new ideas and meanings. After this discussion, the team and clients change places again, and the clients respond to the team's observations with their own ideas about the subject. In other words, they reflect on the team's reflections.

From the point of view of deconstructing and reconstructing life stories and finding new meanings, it can be seen how helpful these discussions would be. However, the cost of using reflecting teams consisting of several therapists is expensive. These teams are generally used only in training centers or agencies that serve as practicum sites for universities, with trainees or students as team members. With some managed care companies now refusing to accept services provided by students, some agencies are unable to take students for training. This is an unfortunate outcome of managed care, because social workers and other mental health professionals learn the practice part of their work through supervised practicum or internships. Having students on reflecting teams may be one allowable way to have students involved in professional activities, but it can never be the only way. Because it takes longer than the usual 50-minute session to have the entire reflecting process, it would make sense to have (and charge for) double sessions and schedule them less frequently.

Other potential problems of trying to fit narrative therapy into the managed care world include the differing uses of language, differing beliefs about the power and validity of empiricism as the only basis for choice of treatment, and the practice of managed care firms' prescribing certain treatment for certain problems. The first problem has been discussed here, and the need to talk in two voices has been noted. The latter two problems are related: Managed care contracts often include prescribing the treatment based on the empirical evidence from a particular study of many people with a specific diagnosis. For example, a situational depression might bring six sessions of cognitive therapy, regardless of the individual nature of the depression or of the therapist's specialized skills. Large-scale empirical studies can never take into account a person's need, nor are they designed to do so.

In addition, because narrative therapy is new, there is not much empirical evidence regarding its effectiveness, so it is not likely to be in a managed care guidebook. Another reason that there is little empirical research testing narrative approaches is that postmodernism denies the possibility of objectivity, which is at the heart of empiricism. Constructivists do not assume the linear relationships among variables required for most statistical procedures. Neimeyer (1993) suggested several research methodologies that are appropriate for assessing constructivist therapies, including repertory grids, transcript analysis of developmental levels, task analysis of change events, stochastic modeling, and time series studies. He stresses the need for diverse approaches to research to show a fuller understanding of complex phenomena. Ethnographic qualitative research has also been found useful for assessing the effectiveness of constructivist approaches (Charmaz, 1990; Kelley & Clifford, 1997; Sells, Smith, & Moon, 1996). White and Epston (1990) and Besa (1994) found client satisfaction and symptom improvement using case study approaches and single-subject designs.

On the one hand, then, it is important to educate managed care companies about the importance of using a broader range of research methodologies to answer difficult questions that cannot be properly addressed using only one method. On the other hand, however, narrative therapists need to see the relationship of their work to other approaches. All human change theories have some underlying commonalities that can be highlighted and used. As already noted here, there are elements of narrative therapy that are related to systems approaches and to solution-focused therapy, both of which are better known to managed care providers. In addition, narrative theory has many similarities to cognitive theory (Neimeyer, 1993), as both theories aim to expand worldviews and see things differently. Cognitive therapy is especially favored by managed care companies because its effectiveness has been well documented, but it can bridge a wide range of approaches and does not have to be as specific as some think (Matheny, McCarthy, Brack, & Penick, 1996). Bridging approaches can be helpful not only in the language we use, but also in the way we practice.

Conclusion

Because narrative approaches are generally brief in nature and focus on the client's goal, as opposed to curing underlying problems, it should be valued by managed care companies. However, it will have to be explained to them in understandable terms and put into "treatment" language. In addition, bridging the approach with more-known approaches, such as cognitive therapy, is important. Continuing problems include the use of reflecting teams and letter writing as important parts of narrative therapy, which are difficult to justify to managed care companies. Those companies do approve of outside activities, however, and perhaps such activities could also be noted as "other interventions." We need to demonstrate how the use of reflecting teams and letters can minimize the number and frequency of sessions, and ways to reduce the amount of time spent on the activities that cannot be billed also needs to be explored. Last, it would be helpful for the field of psychotherapy in general to recognize the need for using a broader range of research methods in evaluating effectiveness.

References

Andersen, T. C. (1987). The reflecting team: Dialogue and metadialogue in clinical work. *Family Process, 26,* 415–428.

Andersen, T. C. (Ed.). (1990). *The reflecting team: Dialogues and dialogues about the dialogues.* Kent, England: Borgmann.

Anderson, H., & Goolishian, H. A. (1988). Human systems as linguistic systems: Preliminary and evolving ideas about the implications for clinical theory. *Family Process, 27,* 371–393.

Bateson, G. (1972). *Steps to an ecology of mind.* New York: Ballantine Books.

Berg, I. K. (1994). *Family based services: A solution-focused approach.* New York: W. W. Norton.

Besa, D. (1994). Evaluating narrative family therapy using single-system research designs. *Research on Social Work Practice, 4,* 309–325.

Beutler, L. E., Davison, E., Kim, E. J., Karno, M., & Fisher, D. (1996). Research contributions to improving managed health care outcomes. *Psychotherapy, 33,* 197–206.

Borden, W. (1992). Narrative perspectives in psychosocial intervention following adverse life events. *Social Work, 37,* 135–141.

Boscolo, L., Cecchin, G., Hoffman, L., & Penn, P. (1987). *Milan systemic family therapy.* New York: Basic Books.

Browning, C. H., & Browning, B. J. (1997). *How to partner with managed care: A "do it yourself kit" for building working relationships and getting steady referrals.* Los Alamitos, CA: Duncliff's International.

Bruner, J. (1986). *Actual minds, possible worlds.* Cambridge, MA: Harvard University Press.

Cecchin, G., Lane, G., & Ray, W. (1993). From strategizing to nonintervention: Towards irreverence in systemic practice. *Journal of Marital and Family Therapy, 19,* 125–135.

Charmaz, K. (1990). "Discovering" chronic illness: Using grounded theory. *Social Science and Medicine, 30,* 1161–1172.

Combs, G., & Freedman, J. (1994). Narrative interventions. In M. F. Hoyt (Ed.), *Constructivist therapies* (pp. 67–91). New York: Guilford Press.

de Shazer, S. (1991). *Putting difference to work.* New York: W. W. Norton.

Dickerson, V. C., & Zimmerman, J. L. (1993). A narrative approach to families with adolescents. In S. Friedman (Ed.), *The new language of change* (pp. 226–250). New York: Guilford Press.

Dolan, Y. M. (1991). *Resolving sexual abuse: Solution focused therapy and Ericksonian hypnosis for adult survivors.* New York: W. W. Norton.

Dornelas, E. A., Correll, R. E., Lothstein, L., Wilber, C., & Goethe, J. W. (1996). Designing and implementing outcome evaluations: Some guidelines for practitioners. *Psychotherapy, 33,* 237–245.

Ellis, A. (1967). *Reason and emotion in psychotherapy* (4th ed.). New York: Lyle Stuart Press.

Fisch, R. (1994). Basic elements in the brief therapies. In M. F. Hoyt (Ed.), *Constructivist therapies* (pp. 126–139). New York: Guilford Press.

Foucault, M. (1980). *Power/knowledge: Selected interviews and other writings.* New York: Pantheon Books.

Freeman, J. C., & Lobovitz, D. (1993). The turtle with wings. In S. Friedman (Ed.), *The new language of change* (pp. 188–225). New York: Guilford Press.

Friedman, S. (Ed.). (1993). *The new language of change.* New York: Guilford Press.

Friedman, S., Brecher, S., & Mittelmeier, C. (1995). Widening the lens, sharpening the focus: The reflecting process in managed care. In S. Friedman (Ed.), *The reflecting team in action* (pp. 184–204). New York: Guilford Press.

Greene, G. J. (1996). A dialectical–pragmatic approach to time-limited treatment. *Crisis Intervention, 2,* 213–242.

Hoffman, L. (1985). Beyond power and control: Toward a "second-order" family systems therapy. *Family Systems Medicine, 3,* 381–396.

Holland, T., & Kilpatrick, A. (1993). Using narrative techniques to enhance multicultural practice. *Journal of Social Work Education, 29,* 1–12.

Hoyt, M. F. (Ed.). (1994). *Constructivist therapies.* New York: Guilford Press.

Jenkins, A. (1991). *Invitation to responsibility: The therapeutic engagement of men who are violent and abusive.* Adelaide, SA: Dulwich Centre.

Kelley, P. (1995). Integrating narrative approaches into clinical curricula: Addressing diversity through understanding. *Journal of Social Work Education, 31,* 347–357.

Kelley, P. (1996). Family-centered practice with stepfamilies. *Families in Society, 77,* 535–544.

Kelley, P., & Clifford, P. (1997). Coping with chronic pain: Assessing narrative group approaches. *Social Work, 42,* 266–279.

Kelly, G. A. (1955). *The psychology of personal constructs* (Vols. 1 and 2). New York: W. W. Norton.

Korzybski, A. (1933). *Science and sanity* (4th ed.). Lakeville, CT: International Non-Aristotelian Library.

Laird, J. (Ed.). (1993). *Revisioning social work education.* New York: Haworth Press.

Laird, J. (1996). Family-centered practice with lesbian and gay families. *Families in Society, 77,* 559–572.

Matheny, K. B., McCarthy, C. J., Brack, G. L., & Penick, J. M. (1996). The effectiveness of cognitively based approaches in treating stress-related symptoms. *Psychotherapy, 33,* 305–320.

Moreno, J. L. (1937). Inter-personal therapy and the psychopathology of interpersonal relationships. *Sociometry, 1,* 9–76.

Neimeyer, R. A. (1993). An appraisal of constructivist psychotherapies. *Journal of Consulting and Clinical Psychology, 61,* 221–234.

O'Hanlon, W. H., & Weiner-Davis, M. (1989). *In search of solutions: A new direction in psychotherapy.* New York: W. W. Norton.

Resnick, C., & Tighe, E. G. (1997). The role of multidisciplinary community clinics in managed care systems. *Social Work, 42,* 91–98.

Saleebey, D. (1996). The strengths perspective in social work practice: Extensions and cautions. *Social Work, 41,* 296–305.

Sands, R., & Nuccio, K. (1992). Postmodern feminist theory and social work. *Social Work, 37,* 489–494.

Sederer, L. I., & Bennett, M. J. (1996). Managed mental health care in the United States: A status report. *Administration and Policy in Mental Health, 23,* 289–306.

Seligman, M.E.P. (1996). Science as an ally of practice. *American Psychologist, 51,* 1072–1079.

Sells, S. P., Smith, T., & Moon, S. (1996). An ethnographic study of client and therapist perceptions of therapy effectiveness in a university based training clinic. *Journal of Marital and Family Therapy, 22,* 321–342.

Steenbarger, B. N., Smith, H. B., & Budman, S. H. (1996). Integrating science and practice in outcomes assessment: A bolder model for a managed era. *Psychotherapy, 33,* 246–253.

Strupp, H. H. (1997). Research, practice, and managed care. *Psychotherapy, 34,* 91–94.

Tomm, K. (1987). Interventive interviewing: Part II, Reflective question as a means to enable self-healing. *Family Process, 26,* 167–184.

Waldegrave, C. (1990). Social justice and family therapy. *Dulwich Centre Newsletter, 1,* 6–64.

Watzlawick, P., Weakland, J. H., & Jackson, D. D. (1967). *Pragmatics of human communication.* New York: W. W. Norton.

White, M. (1992, October). *The re-authoring of lives and relationships.* Workshop presented in Iowa City.

White, M., & Epston, D. (1990). *Narrative means to therapeutic ends.* New York: W. W. Norton.

Winegar, N. (1992). *The clinician's guide to managed mental health care.* New York: Haworth Press.

Wynne, L. C., Shields, C. G., & Sirkin, M. I. (1992). Illness, family theory, and family therapy: Conceptual issues. *Family Process, 31,* 3–18.

The author thanks University of Iowa student Mary Cerda for her invaluable assistance with this project.

C H A P T E R **42**

Fieldwork Crisis:
Dilemmas, Dangers, and Opportunities

Susan Donner

As social workers, it is essential that we participate actively in a response to the ongoing crisis in clinical social work field education. We must think creatively about new ways to respond to human need within the constraints of managed care and become involved in reshaping the service delivery system in ways that are not only responsive but also effective.

My contribution to this response stems from my experience as director of fieldwork at the Smith College School for Social Work (SSW) from 1985 to 1994. This uniquely structured fieldwork program afforded me direct exposure to national trends that affect both human services delivery systems and social work education. As an orientation, I will describe briefly the school's fieldwork structure and philosophy. The school, which specializes in clinical social work, operates within a "block plan." Coursework is offered on campus during three 10-week summer sessions (June–August); field placements involve eight-month full-time (35 hours per week) internships in agencies across the country from September through April. The relationship between the internships and the academic curriculum is recursive, with a back-and-forth flow of ideas concerning what is central in learning about clinical social work practice.

Smith College placements, located in 19 states, include mental health settings, inpatient and outpatient medical settings, schools, settlement houses, community centers, residences for people who were previously homeless, college counseling services, and programs for battered women. Our goals are to assist students in acquiring the complex knowledge and skills to help diverse client populations improve self-defined social, psychological, or environmental aspects of their lives. The school requires settings to offer students a minimum of two hours' weekly supervision in addition to other educational input. The students we place are able and energetic. They invest substantial time—35 hours a week—with additional study time after hours. Overseeing and nurturing this unique internship experience while responding to the mandates of the profession and of the academic curriculum are the primary responsibilities of the field director. These tasks have become increasingly more challenging as the ground for practice has shifted. Fewer practice settings are available that have stable staff, stable programming, or the ability to commit to the

NOTE: An earlier version of this chapter was originally published as Donner, S. (1996). Fieldwork crisis: Dilemmas, dangers, and opportunities. *Smith College Studies in Social Work, 66,* 317–331.

educational endeavor. How and where we will train tomorrow's social work students remain unanswered questions.

The magnitude of the changes in health and mental health care and the attendant problems in training are increasing. Although current solutions are fragmented and not adequate in view of the enormity of the changes, some new initiatives may return us to serving populations to which the social work profession has been historically committed but that it has often overlooked. Some initiatives taken by SSW are described here as possible models for other fieldwork departments. Other contexts for practice that we have contemplated as possibilities are also briefly explored. First, to set the context for these initiatives and ideas, there follows a brief definition of some of the more pervasive concerns and shifts in the field that provide the impetus for change.

The Training Crunch

What is the training crunch? Although the details vary from state to state and sometimes from agency to agency, there are several consistent themes.

DECREASE IN LONG-TERM MENTAL HEALTH SERVICES AND THE PRIMACY OF TIME-LIMITED TREATMENT

Long-term outpatient mental health services are disappearing. Short-term treatment is getting shorter. In most instances, traditional long-term psychotherapy is no longer a clinical option. It exists mostly in private practice, although it is also threatened there because of limits on benefits. Those who receive long-term treatment pay most costs directly. Similarly, long-term inpatient psychiatric care is limited. The average inpatient stay is now 10 days and shrinking. Traditionally, SSW students have learned long-term skills through clinical work in outpatient mental health settings, family services agencies, outpatient and inpatient psychiatric departments associated with training hospitals, or in college counseling settings. Almost none of these settings currently receive funding for long-term work. Therefore, finding opportunities to train students in long-term work has become extremely difficult. The skills necessary to practice this valuable treatment service eventually could disappear.

The loss of these training opportunities is a loss both to our clients and to the profession in several ways. The argument has been made that trainees can best reach a clinical appreciation of the complexity of the human psyche and situation by exposure to long-term work, although there is not agreement about whether the mastery of clinical skills learned in long-term clinical work provides the strongest foundation for learning brief and crisis-oriented modalities (Budman & Gurman, 1988). The appreciation of complexity that is gained through training in long-term work provides a foundation of understanding that can be used in more-focused, shorter-term interventions. Our educational approach assumes that some exposure to long-term work does provide an experience that can strengthen both assessment and intervention skills across the treatment continuum. Educationally, long-term exposure to a particular clinical course is seen as a necessary, although hardly sufficient, component of a clinical social work education.

There is also not a lot of agreement about who benefits most from long-term clinical interventions. Each case must be evaluated specifically in terms of what options best meet the client's needs. Nevertheless, I would suggest that there are some conditions or situations in which a purposeful, focused, long-term clinical relationship may be appropriate, either as the treatment of choice or in conjunction with additional supports. These situations include severe trauma, sexual or physical abuse, complicated grief reaction, some problems related to addiction, profound and ongoing difficulties with parenting, and severe and persistent mental illness. The modality may be individual, family, or group therapy.

I would like to illustrate, by example, work with people who are persistently mentally ill. In the summer of 1994, SSW sponsored a public managed care symposium. There was an interesting discussion between then–Commissioner of Mental Health in Massachusetts Eileen Elias, our featured speaker, and several faculty members. The commissioner presented articulately and passionately the virtues both of managed care and of consumer-oriented group programs as a substitute for one-on-one clinical work with people who are persistently mentally ill. She outlined the rationale for diverting monies from both inpatient and outpatient care and reinvesting them in clubhouse as well as other programs that build on community supports. A member of the clinical faculty countered with a poignant story about an elderly woman with schizophrenia whom he had seen or had telephone contact with for more than 12 years, not weekly but consistently. This was, of course, a story about a long-term clinical relationship. What his detailed and moving story about his relationship with this woman suggested is that a stable, long-term, clinically informed relationship may function as the only connection people with mental illness have to the outside world.

A continuing reliable individual relationship may also be the ingredient that makes it possible for a vulnerable person to participate in a consumer group or in a milieu setting. Vulnerable people have a lot to offer other vulnerable people, sometimes because of shared vulnerability and sometimes because of courageous accomplishments. They also can cause each other great consternation. In some situations, fluctuating interpersonal vicissitudes can result in disorganizing affective overload. Managing and putting that overload into perspective often require the assistance of a trusted, skilled, stable, and ongoing individual clinical relationship—not as a substitute for relationships with other consumers but as a support to them. More frequently, in contemporary practice, consumers are given a case manager rather than an assigned clinician. The troubling separation of case management from clinical skills has become another prevalent trend with this population, a concern to which I will return.

RESTRICTIONS ON PAYMENT FROM MEDICAID OR OTHER MANAGED CARE PROVIDERS

In many states, Medicaid and other managed care providers restrict reimbursement for services provided by students. This has several implications for our students and SSW. First, because agencies often cannot bill for services rendered by students, many can no longer afford to train students. This policy limits the pool of available field placements at a time when many schools, including Smith College, have increased their enrollments. Second, in many traditional agencies students no longer work with poor people because Medicaid managed care provisions will not reimburse a range of previously provided services. This is both a loss for poor would-be clients and for the development of social work professionals. Third, even in agencies that will accept students, new limitations are placed on student roles that often strain traditional school–agency relationships, for example, students are often assigned limited caseloads (Austin, 1997). Reimbursement issues limit case assignments as well as other case-related activities that can and should be carried out on behalf of clients. Home visits, for example, are rarely a viable option because no one will pay for the actual time that such visits take.

LACK OF INSTITUTIONAL SUPPORT FOR STUDENT SUPERVISION

The mandates of managed care, coupled with increased demand for productivity and the serious nature of the social and psychological problems that clients face, have resulted in overstressed staff members. Students are more often viewed as burdens than as assets. Ten years ago many agencies with which we were affiliated gave supervisors five hours of weekly workload credit for supervising each student in a 35-hours-a-week placement. There was often competition among staff members as to who would be chosen to supervise. Although there are still many excellent supervisors who take pleasure and care in supervising, they do so at their own expense. Now supervisors are given little time, work credit, or institutional support. This is a particular problem for new supervisors.

Increasingly, agency culture is significantly altered as staff are hired as contract fee-for-services workers without benefits. The pool of professionals who can act as mentors for students is diminished at a time when students appear to be entering graduate school with more complex learning needs. Students struggle with personal issues that often make the process of learning more arduous and complicated for them. A thoughtful educational approach is needed for students whose personal issues or histories initially present a barrier to clinical learning. The students with extra-educationally focused attention can learn to become able clinicians. In the context of increasing demands, this demanding educational work has become very difficult for many supervisors to provide. Although many supervisors are skilled at engaging students educationally with complicated learning issues, the increased demands for productivity and the decreased support for time allotted to training needs puts some agency needs and some student needs on a collision course.

Complicating the challenges within agencies, faculties at schools of social work are receiving less support for field advising. They are under increased pressure to publish and to undertake research. In and of itself, this is beneficial for the profession, particularly if the research enhances the quality of practice. However, the increased pressure to publish has often meant that field advising has been neglected. Some faculty give short shrift to fieldwork assignments, which are not viewed as advancing their careers. This is educationally indefensible. Certainly adjuncts can expertly carry out the field-advising function, but when institutions rely exclusively on adjuncts without participation from resident faculty, the relationship between the curriculum and the world of practice is weakened. The students in the field need more involvement and guidance from faculty, whether resident or adjunct, and practice settings need active partnerships within their educational liaisons.

Implications for Social Work: Micro and Macro

What does all this mean for clinical social work training? At a microlevel it means that directors of fieldwork need a great deal of support from their deans and from fellow faculty members. Too often, field practice has been considered secondary to the central mission of schools of social work. Too often, the academic curriculum is envisioned as providing its own context. It does not. The world of practice, *changing* practice, must be the context for curriculum development. Schools must be equally committed to coursework and fieldwork. Mutual problem solving between faculties and the field can be both generative and invigorating for all involved. The fundamental issues that require collaboration are the following: What constitutes responsive, effective practice and for whom? In what settings can practice be most effectively located? How can we best educate students to evaluate, rethink, and carry out effective practice? What are the feedback mechanisms between the field and the curriculum?

At a macrolevel, social work, in concert with other related professions, must bear witness and give voice to what changes in service delivery mean in the lives of clients. At every level of our profession—administrative, clinical, educational, and organizational—we must be willing to define and advocate for acceptable standards of service. Speaking out is necessary each time when we know that our clients need services but cannot get them or when our students need training that is not available. We must document urgent need and must demonstrate to the public and our legislators that we are able to address those needs effectively. We must document social and financial costs and costs in terms of human suffering. Students should also be trained in sophisticated advocacy skills as part of their professional responsibilities. There is some evidence that this is happening (Bogo, Michalski, Raphael, & Roberts, 1995). No solution to the crisis in clinical fieldwork training will be sufficient without policy change and without educating society about the meaning and consequences of choices we are presently making.

Useful Challenges to Limiting Assumptions

Our present crisis and an awareness of the limitations of some of our past assumptions about practice have given rise to creative rethinking. If we can distinguish between the development of new strategies and interventions that enhance human well-being and those that simply increase profits, our students and our clients will benefit. For example, managed care has forced practitioners committed to long-term clinical work to consider much more vigorously the potential of short-term and crisis interventions. It has forced us to rethink our concepts about how people change and grow. Although, as discussed previously, the total demise of long-term clinical work may be a loss for clients, clinicians, and students, the powerful challenges to the primacy of long-term work also bring with them needed change. The culture of clinical social work, particularly as influenced by dynamically oriented psychotherapy, has not traditionally explored the potential of short-term work. A much wider range of clients and problems than anticipated are proving themselves amenable to briefer modalities based on different theoretical orientations (Budman & Gurman, 1988). Research suggests that, even when long-term clinical work is available, the average number of client visits is still quite small (Duncan, Hubble, & Miller, 1997). Brief treatment closely approximates the reality of what clients want. Now, at least, brief treatment can be planful and intentional. There is also evidence that setting a reasonable goal, working toward it, and achieving reasonable success provides an experience that people can and do build on after they have ended treatment. Change continues in areas of functioning not directly connected with the client's original presenting problem (Budman & Gurman, 1988).

There is also evidence that short-term work can stimulate reality-based hope in clients as effectively as can long-term work. Achieving functional hope is a major accomplishment in any modality, and the fact that it is often possible to do so in a short-term intervention is significant. Intermittent brief therapy, both individual and family oriented (an increasingly valued modality that some plans will now finance), may also mesh well with the way in which many of us change. People tend to grow and change in spurts followed by periods of consolidation. To take advantage of what is now possible, all our efforts, both in the field and in the classroom, should examine, support, and when necessary, redesign brief intervention models for the richness they can yield. The movement to shorter hospital stays, the stabilization of people in acute distress, and the effort to return them as soon as possible to a more normal life has been of benefit to large numbers of people in acute psychiatric crisis. It has assisted them in uncovering buried strengths and has prevented many from becoming too identified with the patient role.

On the other hand, for some in psychiatric crisis, short-term stays have been disastrous. Schools of social work must train students to differentiate between interventions based on need versus those driven by cost reductions. Students need to be involved in evaluating the benefits of short- versus long-term work through research that also has implications for the research curriculum.

Rethinking Interventions and Valuing Diverse Skills

Cutbacks in traditional services provide us with another opportunity to think about the kinds of services and supports that contribute to positive mental health in different populations. Individual therapy is not the only route to enhanced well-being and, for many populations, it is useful only in the context of myriad other interventions (Hopps, Pinderhughes, & Shankar, 1995). In social work, part of our professional mission is to assist people toward a better sense of well-being, however they define it. Sometimes we become too invested in using the approaches we know best and value and do not develop new ways of helping that may better serve our clients' interests. Students as well as professionals need to look at what motivates them to overvalue some approaches and devalue others. There is, for example, growing evidence to support the claim that people with severe or persistent mental illness do well in group-oriented programs, particularly the clubhouse model. This and other similar models facilitate stabilizing support from ongoing relationships and shared activities with other clients. Although such programs usually employ professionals, staff members do not usually engage in individual clinical work with clients. Instead, they function as group workers and administrators. Monthly check-ins for medication, case management services, and participation in group- and consumer-oriented programs become crucial interventions.

Eileen Elias (1996) saw this approach as an appropriate support to consumers who would have previously been housed in state hospitals—a creative and effective response to the partial defunding of inpatient and outpatient mental health services for clients with mental illness. Training students in such programs and helping them understand how programs work from a clinical point of view is important, even though students are not learning what they view as traditional "therapeutic" skills. One of our most important jobs as educators is to help students appreciate that any intervention that builds on personal, social, cultural, or economic strengths and is based on an understanding of human behavior is clinical at its core.

Clinically Informed Case Management

Social work has made a mistake in trying to separate case management from ongoing clinical work. It is not possible to "manage" any case without some understanding of the person or without developing a relationship in which both worker and client are engaged (see chapter 19). At times, concrete services are removed entirely from a relational clinical context. Students and agencies often fail to see any connection between services and some form of relationship. Assisting a person with persistent mental illness in finding suitable employment is, in part, a concrete service, but if conceptualized only as that, in many instances there is a high risk that the employment will not last and that the person placed in a job will be labeled incorrectly as unmotivated. Similarly, participating in placing a person in a nursing home and working with available family ideally requires sophisticated clinical skills. The interventions may be brief, and the initial assigned task quite concrete in nature, but it may require much that is not so concrete. The ability to listen, to assist with loss, to understand crisis work, to appreciate the conditions that facilitate hope in the face of change, and to work with family dynamics may be what distinguishes finding a free and affordable bed from facilitating necessary change with dignity, respect, caring, and fundamental human understanding.

Institutional and agency support are necessary for integrating case management and clinical skill. Our educational processes, however, are responsible for conceptually linking case management and clinical understanding so our students appreciate the importance of clinically informed case management. Part of our present challenge is to rethink what constitutes effective intervention and to train our students to see the myriad clinical opportunities that traditionally have not been defined as such. Rethinking the context in which clinically informed services, including more sustained clinical relationships, can and should take place and assigning students to those types of internships may be one of the most important and creative shifts we can make.

Innovative Practice and Training Programs

Possibilities now exist for schools of social work to build educational components into the development of innovative services that address the most pressing client needs. Creative and aggressive efforts are needed to secure funds for pilot projects and to develop mutually beneficial relationships with organizations at which these projects may be located. Many of these organizations, such as community centers or schools, do not envision themselves as providers of clinical services or as social work training settings. Exploring the benefits of innovation and collaboration may be the necessary first step.

SSW has initiated several such collaborations. They have not solved all of our field problems, as they have accommodated a relatively small number of students at considerable financial and faculty investment. They are a start, however, and reflect one of the directions we need to go. Expanding such programs will require ongoing aggressive pursuit of grant monies. Nevertheless, we view this as a direction in which both fieldwork education and practice development should lead if clinical social work practice and training are to be responsive to our present context.

Part of the impetus for looking for new training contexts came from concern that our educational requirements for students were too frequently in conflict with the profession's mandate to serve those with the greatest social need. Because serving disenfranchised people is part of social work's commitment, the faculty at Smith College decided to rethink some of our training affiliations. Part of the problem was, and is, that many agencies or institutions that work with the neediest clients do not have the educational resources we require to support internship learning. We committed ourselves to investigating several local organizations that work with underserved populations to see if we could develop relationships with them and then build in the educational opportunities we need. Ironically, placements that we have called "innovative," because of the unusual nature of our relationship with them, have become sites where our students have been able to do the most sustained, traditional clinical work because reimbursement for services has not been an issue. These settings are where clinical services may be and should be offered. For the immediate future, however, schools of social work may have to pursue the monies that support the provision of services and provide such training supports as supervision and seminars, which traditional agencies used to provide.

Examples of SSW Innovative Training Settings

HOMELESS RESIDENCE

We are currently affiliated with a homeless residence for families that abuts the Smith College campus. This is a successful program run without professional social workers, and the personnel there were somewhat skeptical about the influence of professional social workers. Understandably, the staff and administration initially were reluctant to affiliate with us. The program did not provide any traditional clinical services, and staff feared that what our students might provide would either alienate staff or residents or be irrelevant to their needs. This is not what has occurred.

Students have provided services that this agency has come to value. Students work directly with children who have difficulties functioning within the residence and at school, meet weekly with parents who are adjusting to life in the residence, and run groups—one of which focuses on creative writing as a mode of communication and as a way of building self-esteem. In addition, students have offered more follow-up services to clients who have moved back into the community. Students' presence in the residence has also provided opportunities for those who live there to engage in conversations around issues of daily living that they might be reluctant to discuss in another context.

Students, in the main, have valued the placement and have found the clinical learning multidimensional and rich. This project has required an enormous amount of work on the part of several faculty, including providing supervision. It has been necessary to help students understand that clinical relationships in a homeless residence require a different kind of flexibility and boundary management than traditional clinical relationships in mental health centers. Beyond providing training for the students, it has also been a learning experience for faculty and has helped us think more constructively about the many contexts and modes of practice that have clinical value. Equally important, it has helped us expand our ideas about what can become a viable educational experience if the SSW builds in adequate educational support.

BATTERED WOMEN'S PROGRAM

We have also developed a relationship with a program for battered women in a nearby community. Although this program already delivered clinical services, it had no social workers on staff. Initially, we hired a social work supervisor, which made the program a viable educational experience for our students. Our students proved to be so helpful to clients that the program consequently hired a professional social worker who now provides supervision, and we have been able to increase the number of students we place there. Flexibility of role functioning has also been a key to educating students in this context. Students not only provide direct clinical services, but also spend time in the center's residence doing a variety of tasks.

PUBLIC SCHOOL SYSTEMS

On a larger scale, public schools are beginning to provide the institutional context for many mental health and health services. Some people now view schools as the organizations in our communities most likely to deal comprehensively with the needs of families and children. Schools are among the few public institutions that serve large segments of their communities and thus are a logical choice for delivering wide-reaching community services. School-linked services, wraparound services, and one-stop shopping presently combine the goals of education, clinical work, and community organization in services delivery programs within some school systems (Adelman & Taylor, 1997). Although the policies and resources are not yet available on a large scale, it is possible that in the not-too-distant future, many more schools will serve as locations for community health, mental health, recreational, and nutritional services. This possibility calls for thinking about services in more innovative ways and strengthening the ties between school systems and all aspects of community life (McDonald et al., 1997). Schools of social work ought to be part of this movement, expanding on the work many social workers already do in school systems. If we are actively involved and willing to pursue resources for training, school systems can become major training centers for our students. Certainly, schools of social work, in conjunction with other professional programs, can forge relationships with public schools in which they think together about the services that need to be delivered and creative ways of delivering them.

Defining our role, as we have with the Springfield, Massachusetts, public school system, has involved collaboration among students, principals, teachers, parents, community organizations, and administrators. This process, in and of itself, has provided an educational opportunity for students. It has required an understanding of interdisciplinary relationships; organizational structure; student–teacher dynamics; the relationship among learning, environmental factors, and emotional states; and the intricate interaction that develops among community and educational institutions. Roles for students and social work practitioners are multidimensional and comprehensive, requiring a great deal of flexibility. Documenting the needs of children and their parents plays a prominent part in modifying policy and in developing a rationale for establishing multiservice centers within the schools. SSW students in the Springfield schools are functioning in multiple roles: consulting with teachers on helping students with behavioral problems; assisting elementary school children with basic socialization skills; running anger management groups; advocating with and for parents; providing direct counseling for parents and children; working with school personnel on issues of violence in the community; leading activity groups;

and documenting the needs of teachers, families, and children as they work together for the well-being of a community's children and families. Learning in this setting is preparing students with skill and vision for how services can be delivered in a school setting.

Expanding Training Contexts

As is the case for any school of social work, efforts to create services and to build in the educational components are costly, both financially and in terms of faculty resources. The SSW projects consequently have been on a limited scale. The scale of our efforts only begins to address the scope of possibilities. There are, of course, many other contexts in which educational institutions can and have instituted clinical and educational programs. Consider the following settings.

FAMILY PRESERVATION PROGRAMS

Family preservation programs can also provide new training opportunities. The work they do is intensive and multifaceted, and they are good models for effective, time-limited interventions. Understanding how to assist a family so it can support its members and keep itself together requires a breadth and depth of clinical skills. Students do not always appreciate this learning opportunity, and it is our task then to engage them in discussions that help them reframe and honor the inherent possibilities for learning and for successful clinical work. In addition, there may be opportunities to do follow-up work with families, particularly with the kinds of families that research tells us cannot or do not sustain the progress they make after a brief, intensive intervention. We need to sponsor research that will help us decide which families do not need further assistance and which do. Here, too, we find clinical opportunities we can incorporate into field training programs.

PRISONS

With the closing of more state hospitals, the number of people with serious psychological difficulties who are incarcerated has increased. Some prisons already have social workers and psychologists who can be engaged in training students. The need for mental health services is great, and where such services are not available, supports for training can be built in. Our educational role must start with collaboration. We must work with correctional institutions to help them better understand what we have to offer and, more important, what they need.

WELFARE SYSTEM

The dismantling of the current welfare system has become a reality. The changes mandated by federal legislation are in process. Reports about the fate of those who have left the welfare system are beginning to appear, although the accounting is still inadequate relative to the claims of the number of people who have disappeared from the welfare rolls. As reported recently in the *New York Times,* some of the touted success may be related to the fact that those first off are those easiest to employ successfully (DeParle, 1997). We now face a situation in which those about to lose benefits may be people whose lives are dominated by more intractable problems. Simply mandating that they find a job is not working or effective for many people who are more troubled and burdened, and not only because the number who will need jobs and the number of jobs that will be available do not match. As stories begin to surface about those whose circumstances, problems, trauma histories, and strengths are inadequate or insufficient, we are learning more about the dire consequences for people who, without major assistance and support, are not able to manage jobs.

Welfare-to-work programs work for some. If state welfare programs are serious about successfully moving more and more people into the work force, trained social workers ought to be involved. If job placement programs are to be at all effective for people currently about to leave the welfare system, child care, health care, job training, and clinical supports that prepare participants for existing job markets are necessary. Stable, meaningful participation in the work force and a move to economic self-sufficiency require a major shift for people who previously have not been actively employed. It requires building on people's strengths, managing their fears, and often, managing difficult lives. Social workers know how to help people with all of these tasks. Job training programs that attempt to initiate major life transitions ought to incorporate psychosocially oriented clinical services (Hartman, 1994). Social work may also have a contribution to make in helping work environments support employees who are new to the work force as well as in supporting the employers, who may sometimes have to make initial accommodations that are a stretch for them. Field internship opportunities for MSW students can be instituted in welfare-to-work programs, and schools of social work can become more proactively involved in the design of successful programs.

Conclusion

In contemporary practice, clinical services, both short- and long-term, may need to be integrated into other kinds of programs not specifically defined as clinical in nature but in which many problems in living come to the fore. Schools of social work have to become involved in program planning and structure in training for students. Public school systems, homeless programs, prisons, domestic violence programs, Head Start programs, AIDS programs, job and welfare programs, and so forth are all places where successful clinical work can occur. It may be necessary for schools of social work to assist in creating and sustaining small programs and agencies that build on a sense of community, offer multiple services, and empower mutual-aid relationships (Lightburn & Kemp, 1993). Placing students in such settings can provide opportunities for sustained and creative clinical work. For now, schools of social work have to take an active role in finding the financial resources to support faculty and student involvement in planning programs and in developing a new vision for training. This is not what many professional graduate schools ever envisioned. It is, however, what we must spend more of our time doing. We must rethink the context of clinical work and training, convince community organizations that schools of social work have something valuable to offer, and pursue the financial resources necessary to make training possible.

While we are doing all of this, we need to offer more to agencies that presently are willing to educate our students. We must be there both to help them train students and to assist them with problems that arise with students or within the agency programs themselves. Institutional support for the role of field liaison is essential if we are serious about meaningful partnering with agencies in field education. Conveying to agencies that the challenge belongs mutually to educational institutions and the world of practice is essential.

The message can be manifest in collaborative grant writing, effective feedback mechanisms, between practice settings and schools, forums for intellectual exchange, clear and responsive mechanisms for dealing with problematic students, collaborative research endeavors, and reliable support for supervision. The little existing research on fieldwork suggests that supervisors get little assistance in supervising. Schools can offer workshops and ongoing training to supervisors not only about supervision, but also on a wide array of professional issues. In New England, for example, all graduate schools of social work now pool their resources to sponsor workshops jointly that are open to supervisors from all the different systems.

While we productively look to the future, many students are voicing concern about what is currently available to them in their field training. Although disgruntled students are hardly a new phenomenon, in the present context their voices frequently take on a new urgency. Schools' levels of involvement in students' experiences frequently need to be intensified. Being available for problem solving more than ever can make the difference between a placement holding or folding. Even when effective problem solving has occurred, acknowledgment that a training site, although viable, may be less than optimal, may serve as necessary validation for some students. Validating legitimate concerns and being open to hearing dissatisfaction from students, who want to be as well prepared for the profession as students who previously were trained in a less burdened and more stable context, is the least that can be done. Students can then be engaged educationally in assessing the economic, political, and sociocultural factors that affect their training. Curricula must support the skills and information that enable students to understand the context in which they and their clients are functioning. As schools are challenged to think about innovative and creative practice, so can students be challenged as part of their educational journey.

Much of what is suggested here is a challenging undertaking. None of it provides a full measure of response in proportion to the problems we face. The ongoing crisis, however, does offer us another chance to think creatively, to reclaim and reshape much about the social work profession that has been historically successful, and to participate in creating new clinical and training opportunities that are more congruent with the complex needs of those whom we are committed to serve.

References

Adelman, H., & Taylor, L. (1997). Addressing barriers to learning: Beyond school-linked and full-service schools. *American Journal of Orthopsychiatry, 67,* 408–421.

Austin, D. (1997). The institutional development of social work education: The first 100 years and beyond. *Journal of Social Work Education, 33,* 599–611.

Bogo, M., Michalski, J., Raphael, D., & Roberts, T. (1995). Practice interests and self-identification among social work students: Changes over the course of graduate social work education. *Journal of Social Work Education, 31,* 228–246.

Budman, S., & Gurman, A. (1988). *Theory and practice of brief therapy.* New York: Guilford Press.

DeParle, J. (1997, November 20). Newest challenges for welfare: Helping the hard-core jobless. *New York Times,* pp. A1, A28.

Duncan, B., Hubble, M., & Miller, S. (1997). *Psychotherapy with "impossible" cases: The efficient treatment of therapy veterans.* New York: W. W. Norton.

Elias, E. (1994, June). *Forum on clinical interventions with the persistently mentally ill.* Forum held at Smith College School for Social Work, Northampton, MA.

Hartman, A. (1994). Winds of change. *Smith College Studies in Social Work, 64,* 211–220.

Hopps, J., Pinderhughes, E., & Shankar, R. (1995). *The power to care: Clinical practice effectiveness with overwhelmed clients.* New York: Free Press.

Lightburn, A., & Kemp, S. (1993). Urban family support: Empowering high-risk minority families in empowering families. In *Papers from the Seventh Annual Conference on Family-Based Services.* Riverdale, NY: National Association of Family-Based Services.

McDonald, L., Billingham, S., Conrad, T., Morgan, A., Nancy, O., & Payton, E. (1997). Families and schools together (FAST): Integrating community development with clinical strategies. *Families in Society, 78,* 140–155.

CHAPTER 43

The Impact of Managed Health Care Policy on Student Field Training

Deanna Brooks and Priscilla Riley

Managed care has altered the ways in which mental health, health, and substance abuse services are organized and delivered (Carson,1993; Cooper, 1993; Gorski,1993; Ray & Oss, 1993). Public–private and profit–nonprofit distinctions have blurred. Productivity and profit have become key motivating factors. Hospitalization has been reframed as stabilization of clients in crisis. Outpatient clinics now offer only brief or intermittent treatment or community-based home care and crisis services for patients with chronic illness. Private practice as an autonomous treatment context is disappearing. Emphasis on providing services at contained costs requires specialized practice skills, particularly rapid assessment, brief treatment, and the ability to document treatment outcomes. Practitioners have "shifted from a focus on relationships to a focus on tasks and outcomes" (Munson, 1996), and managed care accountability models do not emphasize supervision.

The rapid growth of managed care has had a dramatic impact on the social work profession, on most social work agencies, and on the training experiences of social work students (NASW, 1993; Strom & Gingerich, 1993). For several years Massachusetts agencies have experienced cutbacks in an era of state downsizing, reduced funding for social services, and privatization (Bocage, Homonoff, & Riley, 1995; Leadholm & Kerzner, 1993; Motenko et al., 1995). Changes led to staff layoffs, increased demands for staff productivity, and decreased or eliminated training programs. In a 1992 survey, conducted by Simmons College faculty, on the impact of the fiscal crises on agencies and student training in the Boston area (Bocage et al., 1995), managed care was frequently noted by respondents to be a factor complicating the education of students in the field. Cutbacks reduced the number of agency social workers, thereby leading to less-experienced supervisors. Increasingly difficult client problems led to demands for more experienced students.

Throughout the 1990s each new managed health care policy has created more stress for agencies, more fee-for-service work, and further downsizing of social work departments, especially in medical systems. Medical and mental health social work

NOTE: Originally published as Brooks, D., & Riley, P. (1996). The impact of managed health care policy on student field training. *Smith College Studies in Social Work, 66,* 307–316. This chapter is also based on a paper presented at the Annual Program Meeting of the Council on Social Work Education, February 1996, Washington, DC. The project was supported by a grant from the Simmons College Fund for Research.

services in hospitals have been drastically reduced as treatment shifts from institution to community, and to treatment models that mandate a continuum of care. Social services are frequently merged with case management services and are often provided by paraprofessional or nurses to cut costs (Brooks & Sankar, 1997). School-based, aging, and child and family services agencies are increasingly affected as Medicaid and Medicare contracts are privatized. The number of training sites and the amount of supervision time are reduced further each year. Field instructors' stress levels, changing social work role expectations, and long-held assumptions about quality care for clients continue to be affected.

These health care policy changes have also had a major effect on social work career planning and development. Personal discussions with recent graduates indicate that social workers are faced with entering a job market when they are uncertain whether the knowledge, values, and skills acquired during the master's program will be effective or marketable. New graduates are increasingly entering complex, nontraditional social work jobs with limited or absent social work supervision because more administrative supervision is geared to managed care expectations. The erosion of clinical supervision limits professional development and the expansion of advanced practice skills for new workers.

Communication with field training directors throughout the country highlights the growing concern about managed care nationwide as social work departments shrink, training sites decrease, and managed care companies show minimal investment in training. Field education departments are developing or expanding a greater range of nontraditional training sites, although often at a cost as nontraditional agencies may not have MSW supervisors or may be less prepared for training students. Field faculty are increasingly called on to provide more support and supervision to both students and field instructors.

Students, faculty, and field instructors have all expressed concerns about the difficulty of educating students in the field practicum because of these agency pressures and decreased training opportunities. A descriptive study was developed to examine in greater detail the impact of managed care policies on social work agencies, students, and field instructors and on the clients they serve. The study also attempted to identify the skills needed for current practice demands and to provide guidelines for curriculum development and school–agency collaboration.

Method

To explore the impact of changing health care policies on field training experiences, a survey questionnaire was developed and given to 200 second-year graduate students at Simmons College School of Social Work in Boston during 1994 and 1995. The survey was mailed to 80 field instructors of second-year students in 1995. Students and field instructors were not matched. The questionnaire included self-report responses to about 60 items in addition to open-ended questions. Based on responses from the 1994 student group, the questionnaire was expanded for 1995 students. Students' questions varied slightly from field instructors' questions.

Respondents were asked use a five-point Likert-type scale to rate their perceptions of the impact of managed care on their agencies, their practices, and student training. Questions focused on assessing agency and field instructor stress levels and on understanding emerging value conflicts regarding quality care. Identifying and evaluating competence levels in practice skills needed for managed care was also attempted. A list of skills for effective managed care practice was compiled from a review of the literature (Bistline, Sheridan, & Winegar, 1991; Sabin, 1991; Strom & Gingerich, 1993; Winegar, 1992). Open-ended questions explored field instructors' coping strategies, and both students' and field instructors' impressions of the integration of the school's curriculum with current practice demands.

The response rate was 48 percent, or 38 completed questionnaires, from field instructors, and 42 percent, or 84 responses, from students. The respondents represented a range of practice settings in the Boston area including inpatient and outpatient health and mental health centers, substance abuse programs, family services agencies, college counseling centers, employee assistance programs, and child welfare and child guidance agencies. Because Simmons is a clinical program, 71 percent of the respondents were in child and adult health and mental health outpatient or community agencies; the remainder represented inpatient health or mental health settings. Field instructors had an average of five years of supervisory experience, with a range of one to 15 years, and several supervised more than one student.

Findings

The majority of students and field instructors (86 percent of field instructors and 82 percent of 1995 students) thought their agencies had been affected by managed care. Fewer 1994 students (68 percent) reported an impact. The lower 1994 figure may represent increased awareness of managed care issues by 1995 students and the greater number of agencies affected the following year. Fifty-six percent of both students and field instructors reported feeling they had limited or no training in the theory or skills required for managed care practice.

In response to questions about the impact of managed care on agency life, 92 percent of field instructors reported an increased stress level; 73 percent expressed decreased job satisfaction, and 70 percent claimed decreased job security. Fifty-four percent of field instructors reported an increase in job cutbacks or layoffs, and many experienced increased productivity demands and staff shifts to fee-for-service jobs. Time allotted for traditional in-service training had decreased, although many field instructors reported an increase in meetings on brief treatment or documentation requirements. Fewer students (60 percent) reported an awareness of increased stress, but most field instructors felt they had shielded students from some of the staff turmoil.

When field instructors were asked to evaluate the effect of managed care on their own practices, 74 percent perceived client services as decreased, 85 percent reported shorter lengths of treatment, 55 percent felt the quality of client care had been compromised, and 47 percent experienced an increase in levels of client problems or pathology. Seventy-four percent of field instructors believed they spent more of their time doing paperwork. Many field instructors noted an increase in home-based services (39 percent), although students were doing slightly more (41 percent) than staff.

Although 50 percent of field instructors reported that student training levels had remained the same, 41 percent noted a decrease in the number of students in their agencies. Time spent supervising students had remained relatively intact, but 30 percent of field instructors claimed they had less available time, mostly as a result of productivity demands because supervisory time is not reimbursable. Student caseloads were reported as decreased in only one-third of agencies; however, students were doing more free care (44 percent) or nonbillable (44 percent) work and were seeing more difficult client problems. Students' low reimbursement rate added to

TABLE **43-1**

Student Competency in Managed Care Practice Skills

PRACTICE SKILL	STUDENTS' PERCEPTION[a] 1994	STUDENTS' PERCEPTION[a] 1995	FIELD INSTRUCTORS' RATING
Rapid assessment of mental health problems	3.7	3.6	3.17*
Rapid assessment of substance abuse	3.0	2.85	2.72
Use of DSM/diagnostic assessment skills	3.47	3.76	3.08
Creating behavioral treatment plans	3.05	2.85	3.05
Brief, focused treatment skills	3.26	3.17	3.00
Crisis management skills	3.37	3.39	3.41
Case management skills	3.66	3.50	3.51
Understand health care system	3.39	3.61	3.46
Familiar with community resources	3.22	3.30	3.35
Document treatment outcomes	3.22	3.09	2.67*
Ability to advocate for client	3.72	3.54	3.44

NOTES: Students were asked to assess their levels of competence in the practice skills on a scale of 1 to 5 (1 = limited, 3 = moderate, 5 = thorough). Field instructors were asked to assess how much their students had learned about these practice skills, using the same scale.
[a]Numbers refer to mean scores.
*$p = .05$.

caseload problems, and in many agencies productivity demands required staff social workers to fill their caseloads first. Length of treatment was shorter for most clients, but managed care guidelines in Massachusetts often allowed more treatment time for client services supported by Medicaid; therefore, students frequently worked with longer-term clients who were on Medicaid or who received free care.

When asked to compare their current work to three years before, 48 percent of field instructors reported more use of cognitive–behavioral approaches, and 40 percent stated that they used more solution-focused approaches to treatment; however, both students and field instructors continued to use psychodynamic and family systems theories to inform their work. Field instructors (70 percent) reported spending more time teaching the administrative skills required for managed care practice, and 36 percent of field instructors noted increased time discussing ethical issues in client care. The questionnaire did not elicit specific details about value conflicts, but several supervisors mentioned concerns that managed health care did not offer effective treatment to clients with chronic illness or multiple problems, particularly due to restrictions in length of treatment.

Students evaluated their own progress in learning skills useful for practice in a managed care work world. The skills for effective managed care practice compiled from a review of the literature (Bistline et al., 1991; Sabin, 1991; Strom & Gingerich, 1993; Winegar, 1992) are included in Table 43-1. Students' perceived level of competence in these practice skills was compared to field instructors' ratings of their students' skill level (student and field instructor were not matched). Data analysis of student and field instructor ratings indicated close agreement. Students' self-ratings and instructors' ratings of students fell in the moderate range for most practice skills. In two skill areas, rapid assessment of mental health problems and documenting treatment outcomes, students rated themselves significantly higher than they were rated by field instructors.

Both students and field instructors were in agreement about which managed care practice skills needed more attention in the school of social work curriculum. Eighty-five percent of students felt they needed more substance abuse content; 83 percent desired more brief treatment skills; 78 percent requested more cognitive–behavioral techniques, and 59 percent wanted increased focus on diagnostic skills. About half the field instructors agreed with students, especially increasing brief treatment and cognitive behavioral content.

In 1994 Simmons School of Social Work added a second-year elective course in managed care that integrated policy and practice issues. A second section of the course was offered in 1995. In addition, a component of a required introductory course, called "The Organizational Context," exposed students to managed care issues. Many students felt the managed care elective was helpful and that it should be both required and offered earlier in the curriculum. They also asked for more linkage between policy issues and practice, including strategies for affecting practice change rather than just reacting to change. Other students requested practice cases that encouraged more short-term, behavioral interventions. Another group of students recognized "you can't do it all in two years!" Field instructors were pleased to see that the School of Social Work was concerned about new practice trends, but some instructors felt there was an overreaction to managed care issues and feared we would not continue to "Teach the basics! They're still important."

Coping Strategies

Field instructors were asked to identify coping strategies they had developed to increase their sense of competence or control during this period of rapid change. Examples of their responses to the open-ended question were grouped into the following four themes.

1. Managing time and goals differently

    Clearly stating that we can no longer provide indefinite open-ended treatment was difficult but necessary. It helped to feel more honest and ethical about what we can and can't provide.

    Expect to do less.

    Attitude change.

    Have more realistic expectations of what I can accomplish; prioritize responsibilities.

    Streamline paperwork expectations.

    Use a computer to help with forms.

    Better time management.

2. Collaborative efforts to educate and support each other

    Increased in-service training on short-term and cognitive–behavioral strategies.

    Collaborate; we're all in it together.

    Seek support and techniques from colleagues.

    Continued dialogue—keep informed—continual repetition of administrative changes.

Stop feeling defeated and controlled and join together in strategies to access treatment in spite of the obstacles.

Discussions of possible activist positions to take.

3. Strategies to figure out what managed care wants—learn what levels of care they will approve

   Learn the language of managed care.

   Learn to rewrite treatment plans in behavioral terms.

   Educate the client–consumer about insurance from the time of intake.

4. Reframing the changes as opportunities to increase knowledge

   Begin to validate other theoretical perspectives—more biological or cognitive–behavioral.

   Many clients do get better with short-term strategies; the work feels satisfying.

   Clinicians need better assessment skills, a wider range of interventions.

   Recognize that many managed care skills are valuable, especially problem-focused and cognitive–behavioral.

   Learn to advocate for clients to reduce the risk of compromised services.

Discussion

The results of the surveys confirmed the impression that managed health care policies have had a major impact on field agencies, field instructors, and student training in Massachusetts. The majority of field instructor respondents were experiencing stress, both about changing practice roles and interventions and about job security. Most students were protected from agency stress levels but felt their education had been affected by decreased supervision time and caseloads and the need to learn practice skills that were still new to their supervisors.

Schools of social work have usually relied on agencies to provide students with orientation and training on the intricacies of various health care and service delivery policies. With rapidly changing policies and diminishing time and resources, many agencies are unable to give adequate time for this important area. In other instances, supervision time is used for the administrative details of managed care, with the students shortchanged educationally because adequate attention cannot be given to issues such as developing detailed psychosocial assessments, understanding client diversity, processing interviews and the use of self, or integrating psychodynamic or family systems theories with practice.

Both students and field instructors looked to the School of Social Work to teach students policy and practice skills needed for managed health care services. They emphasized the need for more curriculum content on brief treatment, cognitive behavioral approaches, and skills for working with substance abuse. In addition, they targeted the need for new areas of knowledge and skills such as advocacy for clients within their managed care plan, competence in documenting problem-focused and behavioral treatment plans, and measuring treatment outcomes.

Although some agencies were still providing in-service training, field instructors clearly felt the need to upgrade their skills and engage in dialogues about changing practice trends. Although many of the respondents were trained during "easier times," the new cohort of field instructors, trained under managed care guidelines, often received limited clinical supervision or opportunities to develop advanced practice skills and felt less prepared to provide in-depth field instruction. Schools of social work have an opportunity to help field instructors and agencies by offering continuing education programs that focus on skill building, provide a conceptual framework for new interventions, and integrate social work values in practice.

Strategic Action Plan

As managed care continues to expand, social work educators need to move from the "denial stage" (Gorski, 1993) and evaluate its ongoing impact on the social work profession and on the training of social work students. Rapidly changing health care policies challenge us to keep up-to-date and to develop creative strategies for the future direction of social work roles, social work curricula, and field training. Social work educators need to make a commitment to change while maintaining the integrity and value base of the profession. Collaboration within the school and within the social work community is a first step.

In response to this study, the Simmons College School of Social Work faculty began multilevel efforts to learn from our students and our affiliated field agencies about current student training and practice issues. The survey findings were presented by the authors at a faculty meeting, which resulted in cross-sequence discussions to evaluate the curriculum and its conflicting demands. Faculty struggle with the dilemma of what can be removed from the curriculum to allow time for the managed care component of practice while preserving the foundation knowledge and value base of the social work profession.

Faculty from each sequence are working together to evaluate the current curriculum and recommendations from this study as well as similar recommendations from the joint CSWE–NASW (1996) Managed Care Project. Faculty goals include integrating existing agency documentation requirements with outcome measurement skills taught in research and practice classes. The aim is to increase students' capacity to evaluate their own practice skills and client outcomes. Content on social work practice in a managed care funding system continues to be a part of the curriculum. It is currently included in a required course to introduce new students to larger systems issues, "The Organizational Context." Two sections of a clinical issues seminar offered in the second year are focused on managed care. The seminars are opportunities for students to discuss and integrate practice, policy, and ethical issues in their work. Brief treatment and addictions courses are ongoing electives with a new elective on cognitive–behavioral skills offered this year. In addition, all faculty have been encouraged to incorporate a "managed care piece" in courses across the curriculum.

Focus groups consisting of local training directors, field instructors, and field faculty were organized by the Field Education Department to collaborate on mutual concerns related to educating students in a managed care world. Despite increased turmoil, agencies continue to express their commitment to training students and value the supervisory experience even though it increases workloads. Themes of the focus groups have included strategies for case finding and development of broader roles for interns within agencies. Sharing stories of agency stresses decreases the sense of isolation; provides support; and empowers training directors, field instructors, and field faculty in planning for change.

Agency field instructors and administrators were also invited to a full faculty meeting. The agenda focused on the current dilemmas and challenges in field training. Several issues were identified that have also been noted in the recent social work literature on managed care (Jarmon-Rohde, McFall, Kolar, & Strom, 1997; Newsome, 1996; Strom-Gottfried, 1997). One challenge is developing a range of writing skills. Demands for more rapid, problem-focused records require the ability to document current functioning levels and use DSM pathology models. Students were seen as losing the capability to develop more detailed psychosocial histories and the capacity to apply critical thinking skills to integrate strengths perspectives into assessments and treatment planning. Another challenge is the need to develop students' communication skills to use in advocacy, negotiation, and collaboration with multiple client systems. Integrating individual, psychodynamic techniques with broader case management practice skills was also discussed as both a dilemma and a challenge.

Implications for the Future

Since the survey was completed, the Massachusetts Medicaid contract has twice been given to new managed care companies. Managed Medicaid and Medicare continue to be hot political issues. New mergers and agency downsizing occur across the country every day. New trends include a shift from fee-for-service models to capitated payment models of managed care.

Massachusetts schools of social work have thus far been successful in maintaining Medicaid reimbursement for social work services provided by trainees, but each new contract and administrative change threatens to delete reimbursement; therefore, agencies and field departments are once again challenged to find creative solutions. If students are unable to work with Medicaid clients, many agencies will further reduce or eliminate the numbers of trainees. It would also be tragic to deprive students of opportunities to work with the vulnerable client populations social workers have historically served.

In a previous health care service conflict, Massachusetts deans, field directors, and NASW had been successful in advocating with the Massachusetts legislature and a prior managed care company for services provided by second-year social work trainees. Mindful of that accomplishment and the ongoing threat to student training by changes in managed care policies, field training directors and agency leaders, with the help of NASW, need to continue to work together to advocate for the training of professional social workers for managed care practice. We also need to collaborate to document, research, and articulate the valuable services provided by social workers.

Schools of social work will need to include more specialized clinical content on brief treatment and cognitive–behavioral interventions, as well as the broader range of case management skills needed for managed care practice. Schools also have a unique opportunity to develop continuing education programs to support and update the skills of field instructors. Field education departments will need to provide more supervision support to an increasing number of junior field instructors who have limited clinical supervision. The role of the faculty advisor–Field liaison will expand, much like the expanding case management roles of students and supervisors. There will be an increased need to negotiate student–agency problems, to advocate for training needs with administrators, to fill the gaps resulting from diminished supervision time, and to manage the ethical decision-making dilemma among a student's idealized role, client need, and limited resources.

In summary, social workers can and do provide unique services that managed care companies value, including knowledge of clinical case management for complex problems, home-based and family treatment, and the formal and informal resources and support networks in communities. Schools of social work and the social work profession need to document and articulate these skills to managed care companies and ensure that training prepares social workers for a place in the future health care delivery system.

References

Bistline, J., Sheridan, S., & Winegar, N. (1991). Five critical skills for mental health counselors in managed care. *Journal of Mental Health Counseling, 13,* 147–152.

Bocage, M., Homonoff, E., & Riley, P. (1995). Measuring the impact of the fiscal crisis on human service agencies and social work training. *Social Work, 40,* 701–705.

Brooks, D., & Sankar, S. (1997, March). *Social work case management: A new challenge in field education.* Paper presented at the Annual Program Meeting of the Council on Social Work Education, Chicago.

Carson, D. (1993, Fall). Managed care: A provider perspective. *New Directions for Mental Health Services, 59,* 81–88.

Cooper, M. (1993, November/December). A second look at managed care. *Addiction & Recovery,* pp. 7–10.

Council on Social Work Education & National Association of Social Workers. (1996, May). *Strategic action plan: Social work and managed care* [Draft]. Alexandria, VA: Council on Social Work Education.

Gorski, T. (1993, November/December). Managed care: A guide to survival. *Addiction & Recovery,* p. 6.

Jarmon-Rohde, L., McFall, J., Kolar, P., & Strom, G. (1997). The changing context of social work practice: Implications and recommendations for educators. *Journal of Social Work Education, 33,* 29–46.

Leadholm, B., & Kerzner, J. (1993, July/August). Implementing a system of public managed care: The Massachusetts experience. *Behavioral Healthcare Tomorrow,* pp. 36–38.

Motenko, A., Allen, E.A., Angelos, P., Block, L., DeVito, J., Duffy, A., Holton, L., Lambert, K., Parker, C., Ryan, J., Schraft, D., & Swindell, J. (1995). Privatization and cutbacks: Social work and client impressions of service delivery in Massachusetts. *Social Work, 40,* 456–463.

Munson, C. (1996). Autonomy, technology, managed care and clinical social work mental health services. *Smith College Studies in Social Work, 66,* 241–260.

National Association of Social Workers, Council on the Practice of Clinical Social Work. (1993). *The social work perspective on managed care for mental health and substance abuse treatment.* Washington, DC: Author.

Newsome, M. (1996). Preparing for a managed care environment. *Social Work Education Reporter, 44,* 1, 16.

Ray, C., & Oss, M. (1993, Fall). Community mental health and managed care. *New Directions for Mental Health Services, 59,* 89–98.

Sabin, J. (1991). Clinical skills for the 1990s: Six lessons from HMO practice. *Hospital and Community Psychiatry, 42,* 605–608.

Strom, K., & Gingerich, W. J. (1993). Educating students for the new market realities. *Journal of Social Work Education, 29,* 78–87.

Strom-Gottfried, K. (1997). The implications of managed care for social work education. *Journal of Social Work Education, 33,* 7–18.

Wilson, C. V. (1993, Fall). Substance abuse and managed care. *New Directions for Mental Health Services, 59,* 99–106.

Winegar, N. (1992). *The clinician's guide to managed mental health care.* New York: Basic Books.

CHAPTER 44

Managed Care and Merger Mania: Strategies for Preserving Clinical Social Work Education

Joshua Miller

This chapter will consider the impact of such changes in the delivery of clinical social work services as managed care, downsizing, and agency mergers on master's-level social work field education. Training directors at 15 mental health agencies that serve as clinical social work internship sites for the Smith College School for Social Work (SSW) in nine states were asked to respond to a survey about the impact of managed care on their student training programs. The results of this descriptive research will illustrate the substantial challenges confronting clinical field education. I also will describe some of the creative strategies being used by agencies to ensure the continuation of social work training programs and will make some suggestions for ways in which schools of social work and social work agencies can collaborate to maintain quality clinical social work education.

Challenges Confronting Social Work Field Education

Field education has been an essential aspect of social work training since the profession's inception. A core tenet of all schools preparing professional social workers is that there should be a substantial amount of time spent in a supervised apprenticeship located in an agency that provides services to clients. In graduate social work programs, students usually spend at least half of their academic training (a minimum of 900 hours per year) in a field placement (Council on Social Work Education, 1995). At SSW, interns spend 1,100 hours per year in field practicums. However, over the past decade field education, particularly clinical practice, has been seriously tested by a number of market-driven forces.

Three related developments in the delivery of clinical services to clients have had a major impact on social work field education: (1) managed care, (2) agency downsizing, and (3) agency mergers to form increasingly larger corporate entities.

MANAGED CARE

Managed care, in its various permutations, has constituted a move toward a reimbursement system for health and mental health services that offers capitated payments for services that meet a set of requirements established by the payer, typically a private insurance company or a state Medicaid program (see chapter 3). As a result, agency professionals have lost a great deal of the autonomy they previously enjoyed in setting the terms and conditions of client treatment (Munson, 1996). McArthur and Moore (1997) described the impact of this change on physicians: "When a corporation employing physicians seeks profit by selling their services, the physician–employees cease to act as free agents" (p. 986). Whatever the professional discipline of the provider, the third-party payer now sets strict requirements about who can be seen, under what conditions, to what ends, and for how long.

The move to managed care has particularly affected social work training in both outpatient and inpatient mental health programs and in medical settings. Managed care has emphasized the necessity of providing billable hours, typically in-person interviews for which the agency can bill a payer. The apotheosis of this trend (for now, at least) has been the shift to employing professionals on a fee-for-service basis—the agency avoids the cost of paying for employee benefits (Lipkin, 1997), and practitioners are paid only for the hours they spend with clients. One reason for this tendency is that competitive pricing pressures have reduced the level of insurance payments to agencies below the actual cost of providing services if practitioners receive employee benefits. The implications of these trends in social work training agencies are that fewer staff are available to provide social work education. Those who do have salaried jobs are under pressure to provide billable hours and have less time available for social work training.

AGENCY DOWNSIZING

In the highly competitive "marketplace" of health and mental health services, agencies have had to cut costs to remain competitive and able to operate under price restrictions imposed by the third-party payers. Geller (chapter 3) has described the transformation of mental health services delivery as akin to shifting from a cottage industry orientation to industrialization. Many mental health agencies now describe themselves as companies or corporations, rather than as agencies and present themselves with corporate-style names, management structures, and marketing strategies. Nonprofit mental health centers compete with for-profit corporations providing mental health services, and the boundary between the two has become increasingly blurred.

An underlying theme has been the need to cut costs if the agency (corporation) is to survive. Because direct client hours generate billable income, cost cutting often comes from reducing or eliminating nonbillable services which, therefore, become expendable. Layers of middle management have been excised, often including the managers who coordinated professional training programs. Entire training departments have been eliminated. In multidisciplinary settings such as hospitals, there has been a consolidation of professional services, often in favor of one profession at the expense of others. For example, in hospitals, social workers have often been ousted in favor of nurses who can deliver medical services and (it is assumed) also pick up social services responsibilities such as discharge planning.

Downsized agencies and departments often require workers to carry more tasks and responsibilities, with higher productivity requirements and greater stress (Lipkin, 1997; see also chapter 43). Such workers have less time and energy to provide field education. It is more difficult to serve as a proud professional role model for students in agencies in which employees are not treated with professional respect and in which training is devalued.

AGENCY MERGERS

Agencies have been merging with other agencies and taken over in both friendly and unfriendly acquisitions. A prevalent mantra is that an organization must be large to survive—it must have the capital, purchasing power, clout, diversity, and range of programming that larger systems offer. Agencies believe (with some justification) that by offering a full range of services, they are more attractive to managed care companies seeking to purchase services.

Mergers and takeovers have made it necessary for schools of social work to negotiate training agreements with much larger systems. Successful field internship programs are often the result of ongoing relationships forged through personal contact and understanding that develops over time between field personnel in schools of social work and training staff in agencies. These relationships result in successfully matching students with agencies, because personnel in field offices know the kind of experience they can expect an intern to have, agency staff, in turn, are familiar with the academic preparation an intern will bring to the placement. In larger systems, personal relationships matter less because there is a tendency toward bureaucratization and homogeneity and decision making about training programs becomes increasingly centralized and less contextualized.

Mergers that take place in the middle of placement years frequently disrupt ongoing educational experiences. When one agency is taken over by another agency, field offices and students often experience sudden changes in the nature of field placements, with markedly changed placement expectations. Such changes are often abruptly and unilaterally implemented by the new corporate entity.

All of the above trends also have led to a greater staff turnover, sometimes after a student is already placed. Schools of social work must work with new supervisors and training directors who are unknown to them. These changes diminish the predictability and consistency of field placements, problems which make successful matching of student and agency (never a scientific enterprise) even more difficult. Staff morale and identification with the agency also are often negatively affected by mergers and takeovers—another factor that can undermine supervisory effectiveness.

What Agencies Report about Their Ability to Provide Clinical Social Work Training

RESEARCH METHODOLOGY

A survey was mailed to the training directors at 18 mental health agencies in nine states that served as field sites for SSW internships. The impetus for the survey was developed in an ad hoc task force comprising NASW Massachusetts Chapter members and representatives from the state's graduate schools of social work. The task force was formed in response to a threatened change in the state's Medicaid reimbursement policy for social work interns placed in mental health settings (see chapter 43 for a description of the task force). All agencies that served as affiliated training sites for SSW (in 1996–97) were selected for inclusion in the survey if they were primarily an outpatient mental health program and were not located in Massachusetts. (Massachusetts agencies were not included because the task force that spawned the survey already had a great deal of data about the impact of managed care on Massachusetts mental health centers). Fifteen (83 percent) of the surveys were returned.

The goal of this research was to provide descriptions of the impact of managed care on graduate-level clinical social work internships. The survey (see Figure 44-1) was a qualitative instrument that asked respondents to describe

- the impact managed care was having on their agency's ability to educate students
- how Medicaid reimbursement worked for interns in their state
- what fiscally feasible strategies they were using to educate students.

FIGURE **44-1**

Survey of Training Directors

March 10, 1997

Dear Agency Training Director,

I am writing to you to ascertain what impact managed care has had on your ability to educate social workers in training. If you could briefly answer the following questions, I would appreciate it. (Please write on back if you need more space.)

1. Your name and your agency name.
2. Are the services provided by social work interns reimbursed by Medicaid when they see clients? (If there is a difference between first- and second-year students, please differentiate.)
3. If you do receive reimbursement, at what rate?
4. If you do not receive reimbursement, how are you able to afford to give interns cases?
5. Has your ability to give students cases changed over the past few years? (Explain.)
6. Have you developed any new strategies to ensure that students receive adequate caseloads? (Describe.)
7. Any other comments?

Thank you for taking the time to do this. I will be sharing the results with other schools of social work and NASW as we all work together to ensure that quality social work education survives.

Sincerely,

Joshua Miller, Director of Fieldwork

FINDINGS

Mental health agencies usually rely on combined reimbursement streams from private insurers or state-administered Medicaid programs to pay for the bulk of their services. Some agencies also receive contract funding that comes from federal, state, or county agencies for targeted programs—for example, those for children who have been exposed to violence. Foundation grants also are available for demonstration projects, but these are time limited and not viable as ongoing revenue sources. Some income is generated from fee-paying clients, but that is quite limited in typical community mental health agencies that serve low-income clients. So, the two most important sources of funding for community mental health agencies are private insurers and Medicaid.

Accordingly, agencies lose income when a social work intern who cannot be reimbursed sees a client who would normally be paid for by either Medicaid or an insurer. This is the situation with which community mental health agencies have been grappling across the nation. However, the survey responses indicated that there are variations among Medicaid programs in different states, that is, some states fully reimburse social work interns, some partially reimburse them, some reimburse only second-year interns, and some states do not reimburse interns at all. The same is true for private insurance policies: Some reimburse for intern services, and others do not.

This hodgepodge of reimbursement policies has forced all community mental health centers that serve as internship sites to develop policies and mechanisms that make the cost of student training manageable. The survey indicated that agencies make different decisions about how to respond to the varied reimbursement policies for student interns, depending on the nature of the Medicaid policies in their states as well as the agency culture and philosophy in regard to student training.

For example, some agencies do not assign to interns any clients who can be reimbursed by Medicaid or by private insurers; the agencies assign only clients not covered by either funding source—for example, fee-paying clients or uninsured indigent clients who are not reimbursable. Other agencies have tried to expand the client base for interns by creatively identifying niches in which students can treat clients without a significant loss of income for the agency. For example, they assign clients covered by private insurance companies that will reimburse for interns, or clients who have languished on waiting lists, or clients who need updated intakes. Agencies also assign interns as secondary workers (assistants) to clients seen by a reimbursable agency employee who is the "primary clinician." This is often done with families, in which the intern works with one family member or a subgroup, or with groups in which the intern serves as coleader with an agency employee. Agencies also have assigned interns to work in programs funded by contracts where reimbursement is not an issue.

Despite the different ways in which agencies have responded to the constraints of managed care and the challenges posed by downsizing and mergers, the survey identified certain common themes, some of which are of serious concern.

- *The client pool for assignment to interns has been limited.* All agencies have had to re-examine which clients they can afford to assign to interns, thus shrinking the pool of available clients. One common result is that student caseloads have been much slower to develop, diminishing the depth and richness of internships.
- *Interns are being assigned more challenging cases.* Agencies report that managed care has caused them almost exclusively to serve clients who have conditions

that qualify them for third-party reimbursement. This situation has resulted in clinic caseloads dominated by clients with complex presenting problems, many of whom have histories of severe trauma. Although mental health agencies have always served such clients, there used to be a greater ability also to serve clients with less-severe problems. In the absence of these "lighter" cases, interns are being assigned more difficult and risky clients.

- *Interns are receiving less support.* Fewer staff are available for training and supervision, and those available have less time to devote to such activities. This trend, combined with interns being assigned more challenging cases, has led to a situation in which one respondent lamented, "Interns are being treated less like students and more like unpaid staff members."
- *Agencies are cutting back on internship slots.* A number of agencies reported that, because there are fewer cases available for interns and less staff time available for supervision and training, they have reduced the number of available internship slots.
- *Agencies are less willing to take first-year interns.* Because of less available supervision and training time and more complex cases, field offices in social work schools have found that mental health agencies are reluctant to take first-year interns. This finding was reported in the survey and also has been a topic of discussion by fieldwork coordinators who are members of the New England Consortium of Graduate Schools of Social Work. It is particularly true in states like Massachusetts, where only second-year students are reimbursed by Medicaid for seeing mental health clients.
- *There are diminished opportunities for long-term work.* Respondents reported that funders require solution-focused, goal-oriented work that can be completed in a limited number of sessions, typically fewer than 10. As a result, interns may have little or no exposure to long-term work with clients or to work that goes beyond addressing specific functional impairments defined in DSM-IV categories. This is consistent both with Brooks and Riley's findings (chapter 43) and with Donner's observations (chapter 42).

Discussion

Although some observers have argued that social workers should not be flocking to work in mental health settings (Specht & Courtney, 1994), many social workers do work in such organizations, and since the 1970s they have outnumbered both psychologists and psychiatrists in those settings (Ginsberg, 1995). Social workers have provided high-quality, low-cost mental health services. Many clients have benefited from social workers with excellent clinical skills and a working knowledge of social systems and social welfare policies. Social workers, perhaps more than any other mental health professionals, use a broad knowledge base that integrates psychological understanding with social consciousness. The profession's emphasis on the person-in-environment paradigm has equipped social workers with the capability to work with a wide range of clients and to use multiple modalities and a variety of interventions that address different levels and dimensions of the client's psychological and social worlds. Clients benefit from having social workers in mental health settings.

The future for social workers in such settings can only be ensured by collaborative efforts between social work schools and social workers in mental health agencies—efforts that address the problems and concerns raised in this chapter. If social work hopes to continue to have a professional presence in the delivery of mental health services, social work schools have to place students in mental health agencies. If social workers are phased out of mental health settings, one potential consequence is that the profession will be downsized (leading to diminished enrollments or even closure of schools of social work). Conversely, mental health agencies need to continue serving as social work training sites if the supply of clinical social workers competent to work in mental health settings is to be replenished. Social workers in agencies and social work schools are in this situation together and need one another to survive.

Based on this survey and my experience as director of fieldwork at SSW from 1994 to 1997, I have two modest recommendations for how schools of social work and social workers who practice in mental health agencies can respond to threats to clinical internships. They involve cooperative training and collective advocacy.

COOPERATIVE TRAINING

One of the disadvantages of managed care and merger mania is that nonprofit establishments have taken on the personas of for-profit corporate entities. With that has come a shift to values that emphasize competition and survival at the expense of rival agencies. Although free-market capitalism appears to have achieved hegemony in the political economy, social work has a value base, a code of ethics, and a tradition that have stressed cooperation and collaboration. That code is often at odds with today's prevailing ideology. Social work's commitment to the social well-being of the collectivity can serve as a counterpoint to the unfettered reverence of the marketplace.

Mental health agencies standing alone are faltering in their ability to train future social workers despite, in some cases, heroic efforts by staff. Rather than viewing other mental health and social services agencies as competitors, it could be fruitful to embrace them as training collaborators. Training consortia can be formed among similar agencies (for example, mental health centers) and also can be created among different types of agencies (for example, mental health clinics, schools, hospitals, college counseling centers, family services organizations, and child welfare agencies). Consortia also can be formed among private and public agencies, such as state departments of social services and mental health. Although individual agencies can no longer offer a full spectrum of training opportunities, consortia would have the ability to do so.

Multifaceted student (and staff) seminars could be offered through such consortia, thus offering trainings that would be richer and more diverse than trainings mounted by a single agency. Secondary rotations could be developed among different agencies to respond to the shortage of suitable cases for student assignment that some agencies are encountering. Secondary supervisors also could be assigned to interns, enhancing their exposure to professional role models. The formation of training consortia also might have a secondary consequence, fostering greater cooperation and teamwork among agencies participating in the consortia. These suggestions may sound formidable when agencies are engaged in a struggle for survival, but they would make it possible for social workers and other professionals to implement programs that reflect professional norms and values rather than mirroring the code of competitive free enterprise.

Schools of social work can help to foster such consortia through their field departments. Schools can help write proposals for grants that provide multiagency funding to support such programs. Faculty and field liaisons could provide consultation and offer direct teaching on behalf of training consortia. Continuing education credits could be offered to agency personnel. Schools also could work with agencies to design research instruments that would evaluate how successful such programs are, to demonstrate the value of internships both for clients and for developing competent future professionals. Schools of social work also should redesign curricula and continuing education programs better to meet the needs of students and practitioners in the field. Such curricula would respond to the realities of mental health practice today while affirming the humanistic and collective values that have characterized the profession.

Interdisciplinary collaboration should be encouraged. Other professions also are suffering from the consequences of managed care and merger mania, and clients benefit from interdisciplinary cooperation and teamwork. Social workers should not only design collaborative social work training ventures but also should reach out to other professionals to develop interdisciplinary programs, both within agencies and through collaboration among professional schools. Such collaborations should include disciplinary training but also might stimulate more interdisciplinary supervision. Although every profession, understandably, feels it is important for its members to supervise its professionals in training, an expansion of interdisciplinary secondary supervision would be beneficial to all.

Ultimately, many administrators are concerned with the quality of the services their agencies deliver (as well as the cost), not the profession that is providing them. The superintendent for a school district that served as a field site for social work interns once remarked to me that he could not care less whether services were delivered by social workers, psychologists, family therapists, or other professionals. What mattered to him was the quality of services, access to those services, and the ability of professionals to move beyond professional parochialism and competitiveness to work collaboratively with each other on behalf of children and families. Such professional cooperation and collaboration could be further enhanced by strengthening interdisciplinary training programs.

COLLECTIVE ADVOCACY

Both schools of social work and social workers in mental health settings have a vested interest in continuing social work training programs. Working in concert they can be more effective in advocating and lobbying for the conditions necessary to support training as part of a long-term strategy on behalf of consumers. Local chapters of NASW can help pull together advocacy groups of social work educators and social work practitioners to lobby on behalf of training programs.

Advocacy will involve government lobbying efforts at the federal and state levels as well as with federal and state agencies that regulate and oversee Medicaid programs. It also will involve working together with consumers to challenge restrictive policies that limit reimbursement by private insurers for professionals in training.

Social work training, like medical programs, uses professional internships. That educational practice expands units of service but requires funding. Pressure should be applied to funders to include training costs in requests for proposals. Agencies need to band together to demand training funds that reflect the value of training to the quality of care over time. They also should treat agencies that "lowball" training costs to gain contracts much as unionized workers have traditionally treated scabs.

This battle is not one that social workers should fight alone. Other professionals, including psychologists, nurses, and doctors, also have a vested interest in supporting training programs. Social workers should encourage their national organizations to band together with the national organizations of other professions to advocate for standards that include support for professional training.

Conclusion

Managed care and merger mania are disrupting the life cycle of professional social work training in mental health settings. They undermine the development of the profession and ultimately the well-being of clients. Ironically, clinical social work training is thriving in settings that do not depend on capitated payments and rely primarily on contract funding rather than third-party reimbursements (for example, schools, prisons, women's shelters, homeless programs, child welfare departments, and family services agencies). Some of this change has been positive. Social workers are returning to traditional settings that the profession had forsaken in favor of mental health settings perceived as more prestigious.

However, there is also a risk in that trend. Capitation can easily move beyond health and mental health services. Any service can be capitated, and in the cathedral of the free market, where the reigning political economy is profit driven, the lure of cost cutting invites more managed care (see chapter 10). And, as I argued earlier, social workers provide many important services to clients and make important contributions to the field of mental health.

Accordingly, I suggest that social workers confront this modern challenge not by retreating into the past but by drawing on values and traditions that have sustained the profession and are still relevant today. I advocate for collaboration among mental health and social services agencies, among agencies and schools of social work, among social workers and consumers, and among social workers and other professionals. Such collaboration should aim to enact cooperative programs that expand and preserve professional training and to support policies that recognize professional training as a critical component of delivering mental health services.

Social philosopher Richard Rorty (1996), in an essay imagining that he was looking back at the present from the year 2096, wrote that the market-driven inequalities of the late 20th century were viewed as an incomprehensible abomination, much as our generation views slavery. In 2096, he anticipated, an ethic of fraternity will replace selfish individualism, but not before "decades of despair and horror were required to impress Americans with lessons that now seem blindingly obvious" (p. 156).

Perhaps it will eventually appear blindingly obvious that acceding to the short-term profit taking and unbridled competition of managed care and merger mania is a mistake. For now, we can at least work together on behalf of quality services for consumers, which include viable training programs for social workers and other professionals and are based on the principles of fraternity and collaboration.

References

Council on Social Work Education. (1995). Curriculum policy statement. In R. L. Edwards (Ed.-in-Chief), *Encyclopedia of social work* (19th ed., Vol. 3, p. 2653). Washington, DC: NASW Press.

Ginsberg, L. (1995). *Social work almanac* (2nd ed.). Washington, DC: NASW Press.

Lipkin, H. (1997). Social work in crisis. *Focus, 24*(10), 1, 8.

McArthur, J. H., & Moore, F. D. (1997). The two cultures and the health care revolution: Commerce and professionalism in medical care. *JAMA, 277,* 985–989.

Munson, C. E. (1996). Autonomy and managed care in clinical social work practice. *Smith College Studies in Social Work, 66,* 241–260.

Rorty, R. (1996, September 29). Fraternity reigns: The case for a society based not on rights but on unselfishness. *New York Times Magazine,* pp. 155–158.

Specht, H., & Courtney, J. (1994). *Unfaithful angels: How social work has abandoned its mission.* New York: Free Press.

PART SEVEN

Research

CHAPTER 45

Trends in the Evaluation of Managed Mental Health Care

H. Stephen Leff and Lawrence S. Woocher

The past 10 years have witnessed dramatic growth in the prevalence and variety of managed care arrangements overseeing the provision of mental health services. Once largely a feature of the private sector and private insurance, managed care has more recently been expanding in public-sector programs, particularly Medicaid. As this expansion into the public sector and into systems serving the most vulnerable populations continues and accelerates, there is a great need for knowledge about how managed care works and about the potential impact it may have on consumer satisfaction and outcomes, service use and cost, provider satisfaction, and family burden. Yet, the rate of knowledge generation has not kept pace with the rate of system change. Policymakers and system stakeholders are relying heavily on evaluation studies that are currently underway to expand the knowledge base on the effects of managed care.

This chapter describes work currently in progress by the Evaluation Center@ HSRI (Human Services Research Institute)[1] to develop a database and related materials for tracking evaluations of public managed behavioral health care.[2] We expect that this database will be a dynamic one with studies being added as new evaluations are initiated. The database will be made available to clinicians, policy makers, regulators, service recipients, evaluators, and other stakeholders who have an interest in how these studies are being conducted and in what will and will not be learned from them. In developing the database, we have been influenced by the work of Hurley, Freund, and Paul (1993), who assessed the earliest evaluations of Medicaid managed care.

At this point, we have not reviewed all the evaluations in process. However, we have reviewed a purposive sample, selected through discussions with evaluators,

NOTE: Originally published as Leff, H. S., & Woocher, L. S. (1998). Trends in the evaluation of managed mental health care. *Harvard Review of Psychiatry, 5,* 344–347.

[1]The Evaluation Center@HSRI is a technical assistance center for the evaluation of adult mental health systems change funded by a cooperative agreement with the Center for Mental Health Services in the Substance Abuse and Mental Health Services Administration.

[2]We are also reviewing completed managed care evaluations. However, that review will not be described here. As a related activity, we have initiated an Internet discussion group on the topic of evaluations of managed behavioral health care called MBHEVAL. For more information, call Michael Carter at HSRI, 617-876-0426, ext. 312.

health services researchers, and federal officials, to illustrate important trends in evaluation designs and content. Our goal in this review has been to develop a template for the database. To date, we have formulated a template that includes the funding sources and purposes of the evaluations, the characteristics of the plans compared, the population under study, the major study domains and instruments, and the evaluation designs. These attributes speak to what will be learned, the degree of certainty and generalizability of the knowledge, those questions that will remain unanswered, and the timeline for the production of this knowledge. Below, we present the template that we have developed and describe the initial group of evaluations we have reviewed.

Funding Sources and Purposes of Evaluations Being Conducted

The evaluations of managed care currently being conducted can be classified by funding source and purpose. The major categories are

- State-initiated and -funded projects conducted because of a Health Care Financing Administration (HCFA) requirement linked to a Medicaid waiver. Waivers release states from having to adhere to certain Medicaid regulations that would interfere with aspects of managed care, such as the assignment of people to plans.
- Federal agency–initiated and –funded evaluations that are announced in requests for proposals or applications and can take the form of grants, cooperative agreements, or contracts. Studies funded by grants give investigators more control over evaluation questions, design, and methods than do contracts, which often specify these aspects of the evaluation. Cooperative agreements fall between grants and contracts in the discretion they give to evaluators.
- Investigator-initiated studies, in which investigators obtain funding from federal agency or foundation research programs not specific to managed care to evaluate a Medicaid managed care plan. In those studies, which can complement or enhance a state-initiated evaluation, researchers are able to select their own research questions, designs, and methods.

Our analysis includes the following evaluations:

- An evaluation of ICare, a health maintenance organization (HMO) for people with disabilities in Milwaukee County, Wisconsin, conducted by the HSRI. This evaluation is an example of a state-initiated study and is being conducted under a contract with the State of Wisconsin.
- An evaluation of the Oregon Health Plan conducted by Health Economics Research under contract to HCFA, an example of a federally initiated study.[3]
- A coordinated evaluation of managed care in five sites around the nation (Philadelphia, Hawaii, Oregon, Florida, and Virginia) funded through

[3]Although this evaluation is examining all health care services covered under the Oregon Health Plan, we limit our analysis to Phase II of the evaluation, which focuses on people with disabilities.

cooperative agreements by the Substance Abuse and Mental Health Services Administration (SAMHSA), another example of a federal initiative.[4]

- A federally initiated evaluation of five states (Tennessee, Hawaii, Oklahoma, Kentucky, and Rhode Island) operating managed care programs under 1115 waivers, conducted by Mathematica Policy Research, Inc., under contract to HCFA, with additional funds provided by SAMHSA to address mental health and substance abuse issues.
- An investigator-initiated evaluation of Colorado's Medicaid managed care system conducted by the Institute for Mental Health Services Research of the University of California at Berkeley through a grant from the National Institute of Mental Health (NIMH).

Taken together, these evaluations cover more than a dozen separate managed care plans.

Characteristics of Plans Compared

Reviewing our sample of evaluations suggests that one major consideration for researchers evaluating managed care is how to define managed care. The term "managed care" is commonly used to describe a wide variety of organizational or financial arrangements designed to reduce cost and improve coordination of care.

Four areas of plan difference earmarked as important to the evaluation of managed care in the evaluations reviewed are

1. the manner and degree to which plans integrate physical and mental health services
2. the way in which risk is distributed
3. the breadth of covered services
4. the developmental stage of plans.

With respect to the integration of services, mental health services can be provided by a single organization also delivering physical health care (that is, integrated), by a subcontractor to that organization, or by a different organization entirely (that is, carved out). In some plans risk is borne by only a managed care organization and not by subcontractors or individual providers. In others, the risk is shared with subcontractors, and in still others it is shared with providers as well. Managed care plans also differ in the types and amounts of mental health services they cover. Plans may vary widely, particularly with respect to responsibility for providing psychosocial services such as rehabilitation and residential services. Finally, managed care plans can differ in their stage of development or maturity. Some plans under study may be the first organization to hold a managed care contract at their site; others may follow a previous managed care contractor. Each condition may carry unique challenges in several areas, such as development or maintenance of the provider network, adopting or establishing clinical practice guidelines, and building relationships with other state agencies. Additionally, some plans may be only

[4]The SAMHSA study includes a total of 21 sites, five in each of four target populations: adults with severe mental illness, adults with chemical dependency, children with severe emotional disorders, and adolescents with substance use problems. We limit our analysis to the sites studying adults with severe mental illness.

starting operations, whereas others may be in the second or even third year of operations. In each of these areas, evaluators are struggling to conceptualize and measure important differences.

Nevertheless, in the evaluations we have reviewed to date, the overwhelming majority focus on a comparison of managed care versus traditional fee-for-service systems rather than comparisons of different forms of managed care. Moreover, the majority of evaluations center on program models that "carve out" mental health services and do not distribute risk to providers. Only a small number of studies (the evaluations in Florida, Oregon, Virginia, and Wisconsin) include plans that integrate physical health and mental health care (Wisconsin's program integrates physical and mental health care but carves out the population of people with disabilities). And only two (Oregon and Virginia) distribute risk to subcontractors or individual providers. In nearly all cases, the evaluations examine first-generation managed care systems, most of which are relatively mature, having been operating for at least two years. We hope that future evaluations of managed care will study a greater variety of plan models to inform policymakers about the relative merits of different options. However, cross-site evaluations, particularly ones designed with common protocols and data collection procedures, such as the multisite evaluations funded by HCFA and SAMHSA, do hold promise for comparing programs with different characteristics, if appropriate adjustments can be made for differences in enrollees and contextual factors.

Major Study Domains and Instruments

Our review suggests that evaluators of managed care are in consensus on the key domains to be studied. All evaluations will analyze service use, cost, consumer satisfaction, and outcomes. Most studies also are examining service quality as separate from outcomes. The SAMHSA-funded multisite study did not require reporting on service quality, but the sites do have plans to work to establish a common strategy for examining issues of quality of care. There is also considerable, although somewhat less, consensus on the outcomes instruments being used (Sederer & Dickey, 1996). All or nearly all of the evaluations are using the Medical Outcomes Study Short-Form Health Survey (Ware & Sherbourne, 1992), a brief measure of mental and physical health status. Other common instruments are the Quality of Life Interview (Lehman, 1988); the Addiction Severity Index (McLellan, Luborsky, Woody, & O'Brien, 1980) and the CAGE (Mayfield, McLeod, & Hall, 1974), to measure substance abuse; and the Mental Health Statistical Improvement Program Task Force's (1996) Consumer-Oriented Mental Health Report Card to measure satisfaction and empowerment. Those instruments collectively suggest a focus on consumer self-report measures rather than clinician ratings and interviewer ratings based on clinical interviews. The emphasis on evaluation from the consumers' perspective has been fostered by the growing consumer movement in mental health (McLean, 1995) and the widespread adoption of Total Quality Management strategies exemplified by the principle of "customer-mindedness" (Gustafson & Hundt, 1995).

Evaluation Design Characteristics

A number of research design factors limit the generalizability of evaluation findings. Because managed care implementation is most often driven by policy and administrative concerns rather than scientific ones, decision makers may see random assignment or even comparison groups as more of a programmatic complication than an evaluation necessity. This has left evaluators and researchers in the less-than-ideal situation of comparing managed care populations with populations that are either excluded from the managed care system or in different geographic areas. In most cases, however, data necessary for risk adjustment are available, and evaluators can, in theory, adjust for some differences in the demographic and clinical characteristics of the populations. However, it remains to be seen how convincing those adjustments will be.

The other major obstacle facing researchers designing evaluations is the lack of pre-managed care data, thus forcing inferences to be drawn from two or more measurements that occur post-implementation. This is particularly true for analysis of client-level outcomes data. Only two of the studies we reviewed—Colorado and Wisconsin—were able to collect data from clients both before and after they enrolled in managed care. For information regarding service use and cost, evaluators are typically able to turn to archival Medicaid claims data for a pre–managed care measurement. In this case, conversely, the difficulty is more associated with the lack of high quality and complete encounter data once managed care has been implemented. This was cited as a problem in early studies of Medicaid managed care (Hurley et al., 1993) and continues to be a concern for evaluators. This type of data problem is most often associated with start-up programs.

A related design issue is the duration of follow-up periods. Most evaluations collect follow-up data a relatively short time after the initial data collection. Often, this timing is in response to limited resources, but it can also be a response to the fact that control groups are scheduled to be maintained outside of managed care for only a short time. The SAMHSA-funded studies and the Wisconsin evaluation all conduct client follow-up data collection six months after the initial measurement. Other studies follow consumers for as long as two years. However, considering the episodic nature of severe mental disorders, one might question whether these follow-up periods are adequate. If one hypothesizes, for example, that the way in which managed care will make its impact is through more limited hospitalization and shorter lengths of stay, a research design would want to capture a sufficient number of people who would at some point during the study become acutely ill and require hospitalization or some other intensive treatment. Even a two-year follow-up may not be enough time with sample sizes on the order of 200 to 300 people per group. Because of this issue, two of the five sites in the SAMHSA study have chosen to oversample people who become hospitalized during the study period. Nevertheless, the relatively short follow-up periods pose another limitation on the knowledge that will be gained from the studies of managed care currently underway.

Conclusion

Policymakers grappling with decisions about managed mental health care have a pressing need for knowledge about its effects. Through federal and state initiatives and those of field investigators, studies addressing this need are currently planned or underway, with additional evaluations on the horizon. Although there will not be randomized experiments, many studies will approximate quasi-experiments. The current set of evaluations will generate substantial knowledge on how managed mental health care compares with traditional fee-for-service systems in terms of service use and cost and on consumer outcomes, including health status, symptomatology, functioning, quality of life, and satisfaction. Most studies currently underway will not compare different types of managed care—an additional pressing policy need. However, if adjustments for differences in enrollees and contextual factors can be made, multisite comparisons may produce information comparing managed care plans with each other.

Because most studies will not be completed until the fall of 1999, it seems likely that the reports that policymakers require will not be readily available until after the millennium. The information summarized here, which represents work in progress, is presented to stimulate additional evaluations of managed care that address some questions that will be unanswered or inadequately answered by the current studies. Although it would be ideal to have greater knowledge sooner, current efforts to evaluate managed mental health care are an improvement over the pioneering evaluations of managed physical health care described by Hurley et al. (1993) which, on the whole, were less methodologically rigorous, less timely, and gave less attention to cross-site synthesis.

References

Gustafson, D. H., & Hundt, A. S. (1995). Findings of innovation research applied to quality management principles for health care. *Health Care Management Review, 20*(2), 16–33.

Hurley, R. E., Freund, D. A., & Paul, J. E. (1993). *Managed care in Medicaid: Lessons for policy and program design.* Ann Arbor, MI: Health Administration Press.

Lehman, A. (1988). A quality of life interview for the chronically mentally ill. *Evaluation and Program Planning, 11,* 51–62.

Mayfield, D., McLeod, G., & Hall, P. (1974). The CAGE questionnaire: Validation of a new alcoholism screening instrument. *American Journal of Psychiatry, 131,* 1121–1123.

McLean, A. (1995). Empowerment and the psychiatric consumer/ex-patient movement in the United States: Contradictions, crisis and change. *Social Science and Medicine, 40,* 1053–1071.

McLellan, A. T., Luborsky, L., Woody, G. E., & O'Brien, C. P. (1980). An improved diagnostic instrument for substance abuse patients: The Addiction Severity Index. *Journal of Nervous and Mental Disorders, 168,* 26–33.

Mental Health Statistics Improvement Program Task Force. (1996). *The MHSIP Consumer-Oriented Mental Health Report Card.* Rockville, MD: Center for Mental Health Services.

Sederer, L. I., & Dickey, B. (1996). *Outcomes assessment in clinical practice.* Baltimore: Williams & Wilkins.

Ware, J. E., & Sherbourne, C. D. (1992). The MOS 36-Item Short-Form Health Status Survey (SF-36). I. Conceptual framework and item selection. *Medical Care, 30,* M253–M265.

CHAPTER 46

Research Needs in Managed Behavioral Health Care

Nancy W. Veeder and Wilma Peebles-Wilkins

The current roles and job functions of social workers in managed care systems, as well as the blurring of social work roles with other disciplines, need further evaluation and assessment. Additionally, over the past decade, managed health and behavioral health care systems have evolved to such an extent that there is greater need for federal and state regulation and outcome data documenting the success of this approach to patient care. Cost-effectiveness and services delivery efficacy are the two primary goals of a managed care system. Research studies have primarily focused on the effectiveness of cost containment, models of managed care, characteristics of behavioral health care, case management services, service utilization patterns, the relationship between the employer and the managed care organization partnerships, resource allocation and access to care, pricing, and similar content. As efforts are made to understand the suitable roles for social workers in this evolving health care delivery system, there continues to be a need for expanded knowledge about patient care outcomes.

This chapter will examine the research needed to assess the achievement of the two primary goals of cost-effectiveness and services delivery efficacy in relation to managed behavioral health care outcomes. Background and current issues in managed behavioral health care will be discussed as they relate to the State of Massachusetts and to our efforts at better preparing social workers for practice in this growing system of care.

Managed Behavioral Health Care Defined

Definitions for managed health and behavioral health care are varied, representing both diverse and evolving models of care. A recent review of the history and research on Medicaid and managed care described *managed care* as a "broad array of health care financing and delivery arrangements" (Rowland, Rosenbaum, Simon, & Chait, 1995b, p. x). Corcoran and Vandiver (1996) defined *managed care* as the "administration or oversight of health and mental health services by someone other than the clinician and the client" (p. 1), thus getting to the core of the professional autonomy issues surrounding this system of patient care.

NOTE: This chapter is a modification of the original version prepared for the National Institute of Mental Health in collaboration with Cassandra Clay, Iris Cohen, Jennifer Coplon, Carolyn Dillon, Scott Miyake Geron, and Gail Steketee.

Other similar definitions addressing the traditional professional role are characterized by Goodman, Brown, and Dietz (1992) and Alperin and Phillips (1997), who described a system of "patient care that is determined by external review procedures rather than exclusively by the practitioner" (p. 5). Winegar and Bistline (1994) described "systems and technologies aimed at organizing and managing both the clinical and financial services to a given population of consumers" (p. 17).

Still other definitions include descriptions of primary mechanisms of financing such as capitation, pricing, care management, and utilization review (Austed & Hoyt, 1992; Feldman, 1991; Hutchins, 1996). One important point agreed to by all is that managed care systems are prepaid insurance systems.

For purposes of this chapter, the definition by Winegar (1992) is the most useful: "managed mental health care has as its focus the marshaling and coordinating of the appropriate clinical and financial resources necessary for each client's care. Essentially, managed care clients' needs are matched to appropriate treatment resources, and then the delivery and outcome of these resources are monitored" (p. 8). Cost containment and the results of services delivery, the two primary goals of managed behavioral health care as noted earlier, are captured in the Winegar definition. Cost-effectiveness and services delivery efficacy serve as the organizing framework for this chapter as managed behavioral health care issues are further examined.

Issues in Managed Behavioral Health Care

This section is an overview of managed behavioral health care issues, recognizing that many similar issues have first emerged in managed health care in general. A discussion of the related categories follows within which research needs will be examined.

There are significant challenges in determining the effects of managed care on such indicators as cost, access, and outcomes. The difficulties stem from the wide range of managed care configurations currently available, such as multiple models of health maintenance organizations (HMOs) and preferred provider organizations (PPOs), the many variations of prepayment or capitation used, and the rapid development of new organizational and financing arrangements in managed care. The complexity in organizations and financing mechanisms makes both comparison and generalization difficult.

Managed behavioral health care coverage differs from health care costs coverage in general and, although many health care plans provide some mental health coverage, patient care is a more complex issue. Mechanic (1993) described the historic inequities and economic turmoil associated with mental health care and noted that "mental health benefits may seem difficult to manage within the context of health insurance reform because they require that policymakers confront the complexity of relations between acute and long-term care, between medical and social services, and between services provided by physicians and those offered by other health care professionals" (p. 349). Health coverage such as HMOs, PPOs, and point-of-service (POS) plans—the major variants of managed care—provide some mental health coverage, but they tend to be restrictive. For example, chronic mental illness is not covered in many plans. Mechanic (1993) also noted the limited coverage of both inpatient and outpatient care—30 to 45 inpatient days and 20 to 30 outpatient visits—and the fact that copayments, deductibles, capitation, and so on must be factored into the equation. The services available within the majority of managed care plans are seen by most mental health professionals as too limited for people with severe and persistent mental illness (Mechanic, Schlesinger, & McAlpine, 1995).

Feldman (1991) asserted that managed mental health may be, at best, an oxymoron and at worst, an exercise in futility. "At its best, managed mental health can improve quality, reduce inappropriate utilization, control costs and protect mental health and substance abuse benefits from a society that has not infrequently been inclined to reduce them" (p. xv). Acknowledging also the value of protecting people from unnecessarily using up their benefits, Feldman went on to say that at its worst, "managed mental health can fall victim to greed, deprive people of services they really need, truncate the role of mental health providers and successfully cut costs by damaging the quality of the clinician/patient relationship so central to the success of the therapeutic process" (p. xv). Lay audiences have been repeatedly exposed to anecdotal accounts in the media about the shortcomings of both managed health and behavioral health care.

In an article in the *New York Times,* Toner (1996) observed that "Louise" was well off not to have to deal with the "billion-dollar bureaucracy" about which she was so concerned during the Clintons' aborted health care reform efforts. Louise's greater peace of mind notwithstanding, the advent—indeed the total takeover—of health and behavioral health care services delivery by managed care has given rise to hotly debated positive and negative positions.

The sifting and weighting of factors for or against managed care are the functions of research. Issues in managed behavioral health care include the following: regulation, costs, access, services rationing, care-giving ethics, professional autonomy and education, and quality of services delivered. These categories provide the framework for the discussion of research needs later in this chapter.

REGULATION

Since the Health Maintenance Act of 1973, health and behavioral health care across the country have become increasingly "privatized," managed in a context termed "corporate welfare" and perceived as a for-profit venture (Cornelius, 1994; Freeman & Trabin, 1994). This "privatization" has made federal and state government regulation of managed care practices extremely difficult.

A bipartisan battle over the regulation of health benefits and managed care corporate practices was predicted for 1997 by U.S. Representative John Dingell of Michigan, the senior Democrat on the House Commerce Committee, which has jurisdiction over many managed care issues. For example, managed care companies have been forced to address problems raised by both consumers and lawmakers in the matter of postpartum reimbursable length of stay (managed care originally set six hours' hospital stay; a federal law now mandates 48-hour maternity stays) and length of time permitted for a woman in the hospital after a mastectomy (managed care companies originally set only outpatient payment for such procedures; when legislation was about to be introduced, managed care companies allowed mastectomies to be performed in the hospital). Not only does there appear to be a disregard for the physical aspects of major procedures such as childbirth and mastectomies, but an almost total disregard for potential behavioral health complications is also evident.

Another managed care practice due for regulation at the federal level is that of writing contracts with provider physicians that prevent them from recommending treatments not covered in the managed care health plan ("Battle over Managed Care Rules Expected to Intensify," 1996). Legislation that will set new rules for mental health coverage and make it more difficult for insurers to deny coverage to people based on pre-existing medical conditions is also planned for the near future. In almost every instance, external threats of legislation or sanctions and actual lawsuits in several states have strongly motivated managed care companies to regulate themselves.

There is growing concern in other areas as well, such as the "proprietariness" of treatment protocols and computerized patient information, which will be discussed in subsequent sections of this chapter. In the words of Bill Gradison, president of the Health Insurance Association of America, "the big, somewhat underreported health care story of 1996 is that the Congress, in a bipartisan manner, has moved into regulating health insurance, which they have not done before" (quoted in Toner, 1996, p. 3). To emphasize the seriousness of the lack of regulation issue as it pertains to managed health and behavioral health care, a presidential panel was appointed to recommend ways to protect consumers in this new and fiercely competitive health marketplace.

COSTS

Health economist Uwe Reinhardt has said, "Someone had to say to doctors and patients, you cannot have all these resources all the time" (quoted in Toner, 1996, p. 1). Managed care is a response to the failure of one of the major goals of health care—reasonable costs. The American public has two other major goals in relation to the health care system: (1) universal health insurance, so that health care is available and accessible when needed and (2) patients' freedom to choose doctors and other health care professionals, coupled with the equally important doctors' independence to choose appropriate treatment (Samuelson, 1996, p. 13).

Managed care thus far has seemed to stem from cost increases. Between 1965 and 1989, health spending rose 8 percent of gross domestic product; in 1996, employers' health care premiums rose less than 1 percent, whereas in 1991 the increase was 11.5 percent. In short, managed care's "triumph over 'fee-for-service' medicine has been stunning" (Samuelson, 1996, p. 13). This result has come about largely through managed care's providing both insurance and health care simultaneously.

Cost-effective procedures used by managed health and behavioral health care systems may include elimination of costly elective procedures; capitation; prospective utilization reviews to determine treatment necessity; diminution of medication waste; de-emphasis on research funding; more efficient and effective treatments for increasingly parsimonious cost; resources allocation for prevention; and privatization of Medicaid and other formerly not-for-profit and publicly funded categories and institutions such as hospitals, the penal system, and child welfare services.

Supporters of managed care also point to improvements in health care and cost containment by means of preventive care emphasis and elimination of waste. For example, proponents argue, there are more immunizations and more screenings for breast cancer. There is far more early detection and outright prevention of disease. It also has been argued that poor people and people of color have been provided greater access to primary care.

Opponents generally criticize managed care for giving the public less than it needs. Opponents also maintain that restrictions in service may be good for profits, but they are bad for patients. Detractors also question such cost containment policies as any or all of the following: services monies being diverted to administrative costs (Christensen, 1995), lack of access to services by the most at-risk populations, services rationing (so-called "profit versus people") (Borenstein, 1990; Kane, 1992), and a shift in control of finances from the provider–clinician to the corporation. Additionally, state Medicaid "carve-outs" for defined populations and services raise issues about alternative systems of care for those excluded (see Bachman, Burwell, Abers, Herz, & Jackson, 1997).

ACCESS

With the exception of primary care, as noted earlier, access to health and behavioral health services, particularly by known "at-risk" groups, is perceived as a major problem in managed care systems. In addition to expensive pre-existing health and behavioral health conditions for which managed care companies would prefer to deny access, there is public outcry about the actual or potential neglect of poor people. This particular issue has come to a head with a variety of recent public hospital acquisitions and mergers by private health care corporations ("Future of a Medical Center," 1996; "Questions about a Hospital Deal," 1996; "Selling of a Hospital," 1996). This issue interacts with both the costs and regulation factors in that there are currently no regulations that mandate the private corporations to serve the poor, a large part of whom were previously served by public hospitals and Medicaid. With the privatization of Medicaid and demographic changes in states such as Massachusetts, there is greater concern about culture- and language-related accessibility as well.

SERVICE RATIONING

"Whether applied to mental or physical health, all forms of managed care represent attempts to limit the use of services" (Iglehart, 1996, p. 131). Because universal insurance and unlimited choice by both consumer and physician would make costs explode, "controlling costs requires rationing, either by income or bureaucracy (governmental or private). Some people or medical services have to be excluded" (Samuelson, 1996, p. 13). This variable interacts with the access variable.

A major rationing issue is whether

> as Medicaid, too, turns increasingly to managed care, for-profit companies will be challenged to achieve their bottom-line objectives and still provide adequate care for the many poor beneficiaries who suffer from severe and persistent mental illness. . . . A crucial question is whether people with chronic mental illness in the United States will receive an adequate share of the available Medicaid funding when managed care becomes the chief method of rationing. (Iglehart, 1996, p. 135)

CARE-GIVING ETHICS

Ethical issues are numerous, particularly those professional ethical issues that appear to be at variance with many of the philosophies and operations of managed care systems. Not surprisingly, the largest body of descriptive issues-oriented literature in managed care exists in relation to ethics (Chervenak & McCullough, 1995; Christensen, 1995; Emanuel, 1995; Holleman, Edwards, & Matson, 1994; Howe,

1995; Jecker & Pearlman, 1992; Morreim, 1995; Pellegrino, 1995; Phillips, 1997; Sabin, 1994a; Sulmasy, 1995; Zoloth-Dorfman & Rubin, 1995). These ethical issues relate to denial of service, premature termination of services, confidentiality, lack of outcome data, and so on.

Additional ethical issues raised have to do with personal and financial self-interest versus the best interests of the client (Backlar, 1996; Doner, 1995; Emanuel & Dubler, 1995; Geraty, Hendren, & Flaa, 1992; Hall, 1994; NASW, 1996; Rodwin, 1995; Rosner, 1995; Sabin, 1994b). Other ethical issues include who has the right to disseminate which types of information, under which circumstances, and to whom. Issues related to information dissemination are the ownership of client assessment, diagnostic, and ongoing treatment data (is it the professional provider or the managed care company?) and the compiling and sharing of client information with inappropriate third parties, frequently without client knowledge or permission (Davidson & Davidson, 1996; Gostin et al., 1993; Koppel, 1996; Scarf, 1996; Weimer, 1990).

A major ethical area focuses on diagnostic categories and their appropriate initial application and subsequent use in therapeutic interventions. Assessment and diagnostic catch-22s, such as "overdiagnosing" for purposes of managed care reimbursement, have come under fire, as has the practice of "overdiagnosis" using the DSM-IV classifications of pathology when, in fact, brief treatment lengths permitted by managed care necessitate client competencies and strengths assessments (Stern, 1993). Other ethical issues raised include lack of interest in serving people who are poor and severely mentally ill (chapter 2); the necessity for informed consent and the proper nature of consumer freedom of choice (Koppel, 1996); and statutory appeal provisions and sanctions available for inadequate, poor, or damaging treatment outcomes (NASW, 1996).

Finally, Olsen (1995) cautioned about the ethical concerns regarding the nature of outcome data in the field of mental health. He reviewed ethical cautions specific to six types of outcome measurements (utilization, clinical report, patient reports, objective measures of diagnostic entities, objective measures of functioning, and multifactor research) and discussed the difficulties in defining good outcomes for mental health interventions. He also advocated for process measures rather than strictly outcome measures as better fulfilling obligations to generations of the future.

PROFESSIONAL AUTONOMY AND EDUCATION

Another trend, in part a direct result of managed care, is the steady drift away from emphasis on professionalism to increased focus on meeting the goals of the organization.

> Perhaps most offensive to mental health professionals is the challenge to professional accountability that is the essence of managed care. . . .This assertion of corporate responsibility overrides, or at the very least inserts an unsought second opinion into the relationship with the patient. Clinicians in all the mental health professions resent this intrusion, pointing to its cost, its inconvenience, and the subjective, even capricious, nature of the decisions made by case managers, who may have considerably less training than the professionals with whom they interact. (Shore & Beigel, 1996, p. 117)

This shift in focus has led to loss of clinical and professional autonomy and, perhaps most important, to loss of consumer choice in many if not most respects (Munson, 1996; Sederer & Mirin, 1994). Weimer (1990) succinctly observed, "while psychiatrists were prominent in [managed care's] early development, cost pressure forced higher-paid practitioners out of clinical and administrative positions. That's occurring already in 'big business' psychiatry, with predictable deterioration in clinical sophistication. Reducing clinicians to bureaucratic service workers degrades the system" (p. 1055).

Professional social work, in particular, must educate and re-educate its practitioners for practice in managed care. It must not remain true that "the field of social work has left itself vulnerable to having its services defined as merely medical-like interventions, and therefore evaluated as either medically unnecessary or non-efficacious from a medical perspective" (Cornelius, 1994, p. 60).

Several professional competencies need to be developed specifically for practice in managed care environments: culturally competent practice, namely, tailoring services in ethnoculturally appropriate venues, languages, and services delivery packages; client problem assessment with emphasis on strengths and a life model of human development, rather than pathology-based assessment models; interventions designed for prevention, not simply for amelioration; development of uniquely social work–oriented intervention protocols (what the profession of nursing calls "critical pathways" or "care paths"; they are ubiquitous in both nursing and medicine); brief psychological and social interventions; client advocacy; interdisciplinary collaboration; and outcome research. Training and retraining should be focused specifically on services delivery to seriously mentally ill populations (Lefley, Bernheim, & Goldman, 1989).

Additional competencies should include interdisciplinary collaboration and other collaborative relationships, including those with clients, policymakers, and legislators; consumer participation; advanced case management (Billig & Levinson, 1989); group work; community building, to include community practice and knowledge about community self-sufficiency (Weil, 1996); joint micro–macro assignments and field training opportunities; coalition building; prevention; physical health and its impact on emotional well-being; management for change (strategic management); information technology; marketing; managing in public, nonprofit, and for-profit organizations (Billig & Levinson, 1989; Edwards, Cooke, & Reid, 1996; Freeman 1996; Goplerud, 1995; Johnson & Rubin, 1983; McNutt, 1995; Strom & Gingrich, 1993; Weil, 1996); and advocacy, particularly in relation to the severely mentally ill and substance-abusing populations (Cornelius, 1994).

One of the major criteria for autonomous practice is the generation of the profession's own knowledge base. Social work falls short in this regard. One of the major stated tenets of managed care systems is that outcomes be assessed in terms of two major outcome criteria—cost-efficiency and services delivery effectiveness. There is a need continuously and adequately to document the effectiveness of the more traditional approaches to patient care. Social work must, therefore, instill in its practitioners a commitment to encourage and conduct research. For example, several authors have noted that research is needed "in problems or issues in combating severe long-term mental illness and a commitment to link training and research with community agencies and systems that provide services for the severely mentally ill" (Lefley, Bernheim, & Goldman, 1989, p. 462; see also Cornelius, 1994; Kamerman, 1996). A commitment must be made to evaluate every aspect of managed care, from services delivered and their outcomes, to administrative issues, to ethical concerns, to policies generated and implemented, to protocol proprietorship and other legal and statutory issues, and to the comparative viability of managed care approaches to behavioral health care.

SERVICE QUALITY

Some tentative evidence exists that short-term cognitive interventions work well for clients with diagnoses of depression, for example. However, because existing studies take small samples and do not have control or comparison samples of either long-term treatment or no treatment at all, managed behavioral health care is still faced with this dilemma.

Despite the growth of managed care for mental health and substance abuse services, "there are few reliable data to address issues concerned with the quality of care provided under such programs" (Mechanic, Schlesinger, & McAlpine, 1995, p. 20). The paucity of knowledge in the area of managed behavioral health care "stems in part from a failure of past research to address the complexity and diversity of managed care arrangements" (p. 19).

There are currently no such cumulative clinical research studies. In reviewing Anders' (1996) *Health Against Wealth: HMOs and the Breakdown of Medical Trust,* Samuelson (1996) noted, "mass clinical studies don't yet show that managed care has systematically eroded quality" (p. 13). This means, of course, that there are also not extant studies of a controlled clinical nature which show that managed care systems have improved the quality of care. Proponents of managed care systems argue that consumer satisfaction, the main outcome measure of interest to managed care companies, is actually quite high. It is said that consumers like the access to a more affordable product, which also has low out-of-pocket costs, more comprehensive benefits, and more emphasis on prevention. It is asserted that even Medicare recipients, who do have a choice, are increasingly choosing managed care plans (Toner, 1996).

SUMMARY

In summary, the many issues in the burgeoning managed behavioral health systems that have been briefly addressed here provide a fertile framework for research. Samuelson (1996) pointed out that "managed care's full effects aren't yet clear, because the system is evolving. But the idea that crass commercialism is corrupting medicine is less beguiling than it seems. Open-ended spending was also corrupting medicine and—just as important—hijacking the nation's social priorities" (p. 13). A major point to keep in mind is that the health care system exists in a fluid, sometimes even volatile, political and ideological social context. If nothing else, that makes designing and implementing research all the more complex and the research findings frequently politically "loaded." Research needs in managed behavioral health care, with particular reference to the Massachusetts experience, will be discussed in the following sections.

Existing Research in Managed Behavioral Health Care

MASSACHUSETTS MANAGED BEHAVIORAL HEALTH CARE EXPERIENCE: HISTORY, CURRENT PRACTICE, AND RESEARCH

Managed care companies view Medicaid as the next large market opportunity. Massachusetts was the first state to introduce "a state-wide managed-care plan for mental health services with its Medicaid program" (Iglehart, 1996, p. 134; see also Leadholm & Kerzner, 1995; Minkoff, 1994). In July 1992, the state enrolled

375,000 beneficiaries with and without disabilities in a Medicaid managed care program. Recently in Massachusetts there have been several takeovers of hospitals formerly serving large populations of poor people by private, for-profit health care corporations, causing great public and professional consternation. Massachusetts has experienced all the issues attendant to managed behavioral health care systems outlined in previous sections of this chapter.

Several early research efforts have been undertaken in the state to address the performance of managed behavioral health care implementation in Massachusetts. The evaluation of the state's managed care Medicaid program, mandated and underwritten by the Health Care Financing Administration, was conducted by researchers at Brandeis University, Florence Heller School for Advanced Studies in Social Welfare (Callahan, Shepard, Beinecke, Larson, & Cavanaugh, 1995). That study found that mental health expenditures were reduced by $47 million, or 22 percent of levels predicted without managed care. In addition, no overall decreases in access to care or quality of care were found. Reduced lengths-of-stay, lower prices, and fewer inpatient admissions were the major factors. However, for children and adolescents, readmission rates increased slightly, and providers for that group were less satisfied than they were before managed care was adopted. Provider dissatisfaction may have resulted from less costly types of 24-hour care being substituted for inpatient hospital care. These findings were thought to give some support for the usefulness of a managed care program for mental health and substance abuse services and for its applicability to high-risk populations.

Subsequent studies of the Massachusetts Medicaid Mental Health/Substance Abuse Program (Beinecke & Lockhart, 1996; Beinecke & Perlman, 1996) expanded findings from the Callahan and colleagues (1995) study. Providers reported improvement in access to care, appropriate utilization, and quality; 90 percent of clients were either moderately or severely ill, and client severity of illness continued to increase; the average length of hospital stay was 11 days and decreased slightly each subsequent year; on average, 13 percent of clients were readmitted within 30 days, and readmission rates were fairly stable; 87 percent of clients received appropriate aftercare planning, and aftercare planning had improved; the managed care company's clinical review decisions continued to be rated highly; and over half of the providers felt that the changes in services delivery had been helpful to clients, whereas one-quarter of providers believed that they had not been helpful.

One qualitative study of social work and client impressions of privatization and cutbacks in services delivery from September 1991 to May 1992 in nine Massachusetts social services organizations found the following: increased demands on social workers for higher productivity levels and more documentation; deterioration in collaborative work environments; an inability to meet treatment goals; more severe client conditions on entering and leaving the system; and increased demands for inappropriate services delivery—in short, original gains that had been made by expanded community services were now being reversed by systems beset by too many cuts (Motenko et al., 1995).

In a survey of fiscal crises conducted across 200 student social worker training site agencies, Bocage, Homonoff, and Riley (1995) found that the impact of budget cuts, largely resulting from cost-cutting managed care approaches, was severe. More than half of the responding agencies reported a reduction in supervisory staff over the past year and an increased reliance on less experienced staff for intern supervision. Even when not directly affected, agencies reported being indirectly affected by lack of resources in other agencies.

CASE MANAGEMENT IN BEHAVIORAL HEALTH RESEARCH

The majority of empirical studies in managed behavioral health care are in relation to case management as a major services delivery mode (see Mechanic, Schlesinger, & McAlpine, 1995, for a review of what they term "high-cost case management"). Like managed care, case management has many definitions and models. Case management in a variety of its forms has been examined as an intervention mode with a range of target populations, especially people with chronic mental illness. However, in a methodological review of more than 30 studies of case management, Chamberlain and Rapp (1991) found "a paucity of outcome research on case management . . . and an added lack of comparability of those studies reviewed in terms of intervention, purpose, subjects and outcomes" (pp. 184–185).

A study comparing two case management strategies found little difference between them (Sands & Cnaan, 1994), and a comprehensive descriptive study of the state of case management programs by the Center for Psychiatric Rehabilitation, Boston University, found that, despite perceived ambiguity of case management, in practice there are consistencies that point to an "ideal type" of case management (Ellison, Rogers, Sciarappa, Cohen, & Forbess, 1995).

Case management is frequently used to coordinate a care plan and services for patients in a capitated managed care system. According to Quinlivan et al. (1995), clients who received intensive case management had fewer inpatient days and lower costs for mental health services. However, such intensive case management is costly and may not necessarily be desired by companies that prefer not to encourage follow-up services and referrals (Durham, 1994).

Other studies of outcomes of case management with people who have serious mental illness, including those who are homeless, have produced mixed but largely positive results (Biegel, Tracy, & Corvo, 1994; Borland, McRae, & Lycan, 1989; Dietzen & Bond, 1993; Dixon, Friedman, & Lehman, 1993; Goering, Wasylenki, Farkas, Lancee, & Ballantyne, 1988; Grella & Grusky, 1989; Harris & Bergman, 1988; Intagliata & Baker, 1983; Korr & Cloninger, 1991; Rife, First, Greenlee, Miller, & Feichter, 1991; Rubin, 1992).

OUTCOME STUDIES OF MANAGED BEHAVIORAL HEALTH CARE: COST-EFFECTIVENESS

In addition to the Massachusetts Medicaid study reported above, which did find cost savings subsequent to the initiation of a managed care system for Medicaid clients (Callahan et al., 1995), several other studies have addressed the cost issue including reviews of the effect of managed care on costs or outcomes (Miller & Luft, 1994). HMOs, compared with traditional fee-for-service reimbursement, are thought to have lower hospitalization rates but greater use of outpatient services; it is unclear whether the outpatient costs offset the lowered impatient costs (Bodenheimer & Grumbach, 1995). Fiscally speaking, it is significant to note that premiums for managed care plans have been rising at the same rate as those for indemnity plans.

A review by the Kaiser Commission on the Future of Medicaid of the research literature that assesses 20 years of Medicaid managed care experience with low-income families (mostly women and children enrolled in Aid to Families with Dependent Children) took four areas for examination: (1) effect of Medicaid managed care on access to care, (2) effect on health care costs, (3) effect on the quality of care and patient satisfaction, and (4) whether the special populations were served (Rowland et al., 1995a). Medicaid managed care had mixed results on access to care, primarily shifting the type and site of care. The use of specialists and emergency rooms declined, but managed care had little effect on the number of doctor visits, use of preventive services, or inpatient hospital care.

The studies reviewed also indicated difficulty in attributing cost savings directly as a result of managed care becoming the major provider in Medicaid. For example, some programs did obtain savings, but others showed higher costs. Another frequent confounding factor was low managed care provider payment levels. Other observers have noted concerns: "While most observers considered access and capacity in Medicaid managed care to be good, there was some concern about the future, particularly in light of reduced payment rates to HMOs" (Holahan, Bovbjerg, Evans, Wiener, & Flanagan, 1997, p. 42).

These dichotomous findings and concerns have implications for Medicaid managed care for people with mental illness, even though the studies were for managed care for the general Medicaid population, particularly because the authors predicted "continued growth in managed care by states under Medicaid as well as by private health insurers to improve service delivery and stabilize costs" (Rowland et al., 1995b, p. 6). In fact, there is growing evidence that some state authorities have already contracted with managed behavioral health care vendors to provide services to the public sector (Essock & Goldman, 1995; Holahan et al., 1997).

People with severe mental illness are a group of clients that health plans have tried to avoid enrolling because of the high cost of their care (Schlesinger & Mechanic, 1993). It also should be kept in mind that managed care systems can avoid high-risk patients by not contracting with providers known for specializing in high-risk conditions (Luft, 1996).

Dickey and Azeni (1992) compared a prior-approved managed care program to a concurrent review managed model. They found that although concurrent review showed limited effectiveness, prior approval showed none. The authors pointed out that pressures by insurers and corporations to limit lengths of stay may be countered by pressures to fill beds, particularly in specialized programs such as treatment of eating disorders and substance abuse.

A study comparing an experimental fixed-prepayment system (case-based reimbursement) for patients requiring psychiatric hospital care and a regular payment system found that costs for those in the experimental group were lower per patient and per admission and that cumulative costs for patients in the program were not calculated. Treatment outcomes and patients' satisfaction with hospital care were comparable for the two groups (Sederer et al., 1992).

A study of Wisconsin's community support programs and services for people with severe mental illness, which are paid for by managed Medicaid, found that amounts of medication and psychotherapy appeared less than adequate, especially for clients with the most severe and persistent mental illness. Case management for an hour per week appeared to be "effective and sufficient" for clients with chronic mental illness who were established rather than new. The high proportion of clients with severe mental illness who were not covered suggested a problem with client access to benefits. A further disturbing finding was that payments for community-based services were smaller than payments for inpatient stays for this group (Hollingsworth, 1994).

SERVICES DELIVERY EFFICACY

Numerous studies of the prevalence of chronic and severe mental illness, several by race and class, have been reported (Adler, Boyce, Chesney, Folkman, & Syme, 1993; Bruce, Takeuchi, & Leaf, 1991; Dohrenwend et al., 1992; Kessler & Neighbors, 1986). A few studies have also addressed services needs of the mentally ill population (Dorwart & Hoover, 1994; Morse, Calsyn, Allen, & Kenny, 1994). These needs fall generally in the categories of cost-effectiveness; services relevance, accessibility, and availability; and services delivery efficacy.

Several outcome studies of managed behavioral health care have been reported. For example, Douglass and Torres (1994) examined an innovative managed care program designed to deliver health care services to poor people while reducing excessive emergency room and inpatient care. The following variables were examined: differences in off-program utilization, use of clinical services, hospitalization, and patient satisfaction. Findings indicated that patients responded favorably to the program; however, off-program utilization was substantial, and emergency room and inpatient care were not significantly reduced. The authors concluded that "how such a program is managed and administered, and a provider's degree of motivation, govern the extent to which it succeeds in reducing health care costs and increasing patient satisfaction" (p. 83).

A study of rehabilitative day treatment compared with supported employment for people with severe mental disorders found that eliminating day treatment and replacing it with a supported employment program could improve integration into competitive jobs in the community (Drake et al., 1994). A national survey of home health and behavioral health care organizations' need to understand about managed care organizations' perspectives found that both home health care and managed care need to better understand each others' strengths: "Communication with managed care companies must improve. New and more effective measures of clinical outcomes and patient satisfaction must be developed and used" (p. 24).

In a Swiss study of differences between those who chose managed care and those who chose indemnity health insurance plans, it was found that joiners of the managed care system had significantly lower mental health status but not somatic health status. Therefore, "people who join managed care organizations may have substantial uncovered needs for psychiatric care. Minimum mandatory benefits for mental health care may be an effective countermeasure to unequitable self-selection" (Perneger, Allaz, Etter, & Rougemont, 1995, p. 1020).

A study of predictors of outpatient mental health care utilization by primary care patients in an HMO found that a high level of mental health services were purchased outside of the HMO. Even when the illness was severe, the demand for services was reduced because of increased copayment rates. Equity and clinical need were determined to be essential considerations in cost-containment measures.

Two outcome studies of interventions with mentally ill populations were undertaken, each of which took a fairly large sample. Thompson (1985) found that characteristics associated with treatment outcome among 519 clients with mental illness in a partial hospitalization program included previous state hospitalizations, age at admission to hospital, age of onset of mental illness, intelligence, and parental history of mental illness. A second study (Wells et al., 1993) evaluated quality of care outcomes associated with the implementation of the Medicare Prospective Payment System (managed care funded) among 2,746 depressed elderly patients in 297 acute care general medical hospitals. The study found that after implementation of the

Medicare system (prior to managed care auspices), the quality of care for the depressed elderly patients improved, and there were no marked increases in adverse clinical outcomes. However, after implementation, the quality of patient care was moderate at best, and more than one-third of the sample had unacceptable clinical status at the time of discharge.

In an early survey of 1,471 adults with chronic mental disabilities in community support systems, sponsored by the National Institute of Mental Health, the authors concluded that

> [presaging many of the current issues] the problem of chronically mentally ill people remains a major mental health and social welfare challenge. The magnitude of the problem is sure to grow. . . .the prevalence of chronic mental disorder and disability is certain to increase as the large cohort of young acute and chronic patients age. Only an unlikely technological fix could reverse this trend. . . . With support, adequate financing, and imagination, the chronically mentally ill could enjoy a reversal of a century of neglect. (Tessler, Bernstein, Rosen, & Goldman, 1982, p. 211)

FUTURE RESEARCH NEEDS IN MANAGED BEHAVIORAL HEALTH CARE

In general, research questions should flow from the regulation, cost, access, rationing, practice, ethical, and educational issues outlined above. A range of research methodologies has been suggested, from controlled clinical trials using an experimental or quasi-experimental format to more process- and outcome-oriented qualitative study approaches. Mechanic, Schlesinger, and McAlpine (1995) suggested that "the heterogeneity of managed care is perhaps the strongest reason for extensive process evaluations" (p. 49).

It is good to keep in mind a caveat in relation to strictly "scientific" experimental research designs, namely, that "efficacy research (employing highly sophisticated experimental designs in controlled clinical trials) has been notoriously unable to provide busy clinicians with the research findings that might add value to their practice by indicating which treatments are actually effective under naturalistic, real-world conditions" (Freeman & Trabin, 1994, p. 23).

It is clear that the most viable future research in managed behavioral health care will include both quantitative and qualitative approaches and will address cost-effectiveness and services delivery efficacy issues simultaneously in the research design and implementation. Following are some suggested future research areas and questions.

Cost-Effectiveness

- Is managed care cost-effective? With whom? With which treatments and for what duration? Services provided by which professional or nonprofessional?
- How do various payment approaches affect the provision of care?
- How do for-profit and not-for-profit delivery systems compare on cost-effectiveness indicators?
- How do for-profit and not-for-profit delivery systems compare in relation to actual and proportional expenditures on services versus administration?

- How do immediate versus long-term costs–benefits of managed care systems compare?

Services Delivery Efficacy

Needs Assessments

- Define, describe, and calibrate services needed and demanded by specific target groups.
- Determine what professional competencies are needed for behavioral health care practice.
- Determine what services are needed by culturally diverse populations and which services are available to meet those diverse needs.

Development Needs for Assessment, Diagnostic, and Outcome (Including Follow-up) Measurement Instruments

- initial protocols (care pathways) and goals as outcome evaluation benchmarks (Balassone, 1991; Dorwart, 1990)
- other outcome tool development (Harvard–Pilgrim Mental Health Patient Assessment Tool)
- case recording for quality assurance (Corcoran & Gingrich, 1994)
- culturally sensitive assessment, diagnostic, and intervention protocols.

Access and Rationing

- Which groups do and do not have access to behavioral health care services? Why?
- For whom and under which circumstances are services rationed?
- Is there market research to target underserved groups and increase access and utilization?
- Are managed care systems available and responsive to culturally diverse populations?

Services Delivery Outcome Evaluations

- measuring benefits and outcomes effectiveness of managed behavioral health interventions (Hargreaves & Shumway, 1989; Kane, Bartlett, & Porthoff, 1995; McCarthy, Gelber, & Dugger, 1993; Mirin & Namerow, 1991; Monkman, 1991)
- comparison of for-profit and not-for-profit delivery systems on services delivery efficacy indicators
- determination if people with chronic mental illness receive an adequate share of Medicaid funding when managed care becomes the chief mechanism of funding in the formerly public sector
- comparisons of how various lower-cost treatments are affecting patient mental health and other quality-of-life factors
- comparisons of different professionals delivering different services
- assessments of effectiveness of interdisciplinary teams versus solo interventions
- effects of managed care policies

- effects of managed behavioral health care on families of people with mental illness
- short-term versus longer-term interventions with people with more chronic mental illness
- intensive treatment versus periodic interventions; missed therapeutic sessions versus spaced sessions for various types of problems
- relationship of diagnosis to outcomes of brief and longer interventions
- comparison of service outcomes between two groups of mental health consumers, one in a managed behavioral health plan and the other group not in a managed care plan (outcomes in relation to such factors as readmissions, functional levels, maintenance in the community)
- follow-up studies to determine goal attainment maintenance as well as consumer satisfaction (consumer satisfaction does not necessarily covary with desirable clinical outcome)
- determination if treatment outcomes are different for various cultural groups and that utilization patterns vary according to cultural variables
- determination if treatment outcomes are improving or declining as a result of use of nonphysician providers in companies' networks
- provider decision making (Gottlieb, 1989).

Professional Autonomy and Education

- social workers who are taking leadership roles in defining, developing, and studying managed care operations
- advanced case management versus less-skilled interventions outcomes
- viability of community-building
- viability of preventive interventions
- strength/competency approaches to assessment and intervention versus psychodynamic approaches
- social work practitioner as part of the treatment team
- in interprofessional collaboration situations, ownership of the treatment planning process. Who prevails when there is disagreement? Who controls the review or consultation process?
- a stifling of the development of new drugs and other clinical improvements for people with mental illness.

Conclusion

Much work remains to be done to document the efficacy of patient outcomes in a behavioral health system driven by cost containment. Access to quality patient care for people who are poor, who have a primary language other than English, or who have chronic and persistent mental health problems remains a concern for services delivery under managed behavioral health care. Mechanic (1993) reminded us that our judgment about the effectiveness of managed behavioral health care must address "the problems of those with serious and persistent disabling illness, who depend on the health system for their functioning, perhaps even for their lives" (p. 363).

The full implications of issues such as professional autonomy, alterations of the traditional professional–patient relationship, and patient choice need further study. Shore and Beigel (1996) observed that

> The challenges to all mental health professionals are to prepare themselves to assume responsibility for population-based practice without losing concern for the care of individual patients and to strike a balance between individual professional responsibility and corporate accountability. . . . The challenges to the definition of illness, professional ethics, the allocation of professional resources, and professional accountability brought by the emergence of managed behavioral health care . . . must be resolved by professionals and managed behavioral health care companies working together to craft new forms of professional practice. (p. 118)

The available knowledge base about managed behavioral health care must be expanded.

Outcome studies that extend beyond a focus on cost containment and which better document services delivery efficacy are essential. For example, many studies show an increase in outpatient usage and suggest that outpatient care is more cost effective than inpatient care; however, the full meaning of this trend in terms of both quality of patient care and cost-related factors is yet to be determined. "It is only when we develop a more complete picture of the process by which managed care affects outcomes that its potential for achieving efficiency while protecting or enhancing quality can be fully realized" (Mechanic, Schlesinger, & McAlpine, 1995, p. 50). These challenges must be met with the assistance of empirical data so that the best of the past is reformulated into the best of current and future managed behavioral health care services delivery packages that will maximally combine cost-effectiveness and services delivery efficacy. The profession of social work is faced with the challenge of re-examining and redefining its role in the context of this empirical data.

References

Adler, N. E., Boyce, T., Chesney, M. A., Folkman, S., & Syme, L. (1993). Socioeconomic inequalities in health. *JAMA, 269,* 3140–3145.

Alperin, R. M., & Phillips, D. G. (1997). *The impact of managed care on the practice of psychotherapy. Innovation, implementation, and controversy.* New York: Brunner/Mazel.

Austed, M. F., & Hoyt, C. S. (1992). The managed care movement and the future of psychotherapy. *Psychotherapy, 29,* 109–113.

Bachman, S., & Burwell, B., Abers, L. A., Herz, L., & Jackson, B. (1997). *Medicaid carve-outs: Policy and programmatic considerations.* Princeton, NJ: Center for Health Care Strategies.

Backlar, P. (1996). Managed mental health care: Conflicts of interest in the provider/client relationship. *Community Mental Health Journal, 32,* 101–106.

Balassone, M. L. (1991). A research methodology for the development of risk assessment tools in social work practice. *Social Work Research & Abstracts, 27*(2), 16–23.

Battle over managed care rules expected to intensify. (1996, November 24). *Boston Sunday Globe,* p. 12.

Beinecke, R. H., & Lockhart A. (1996). *A provider assessment of the Massachusetts managed mental health/substance abuse program: Year four.* Boston: Suffolk University, Department of Public Management.

Beinecke, R. H., & Perlman, S. (1996). *Providers' assessment of the MHMA mental health/substance abuse program outpatient treatment protocols.* Boston: Mental Health Corporation of Massachusetts.

Biegel, D. E., Tracy, E. M., & Corvo, K. N. (1994). Strengthening social networks: Intervention strategies for mental health case managers. *Health & Social Work, 19,* 206–216.

Billig, N. S., & Levinson, C. (1989). Social work students as case managers: A model of service delivery and training. *Hospital and Community Psychiatry, 40,* 411–413.

Bocage, M. D., Homonoff, E. E., & Riley, P. M. (1995). Measuring the impact of the fiscal crisis on human services agencies and social work training. *Social Work, 40,* 701–705.

Bodenheimer, T. S., & Grumbach, K. (1995). *Understanding health policy. A clinical approach.* Norwalk, CT: Appleton & Lange.

Borenstein, D. B. (1990). Managed care: A means of rationing psychiatric treatment. *Hospital and Community Psychiatry, 41,* 1095–1098.

Borland, A., McRae, J., & Lycan, C. (1989). Outcomes of five years of continuous case management. *Hospital and Community Psychiatry, 40,* 369–376.

Bruce, M., Takeuchi, D. T., & Leaf, P. J. (1991). Poverty and psychiatric status. *Archives of General Psychiatry, 48,* 470–474.

Callahan, J. J., Shepard, D. S., Beinecke, R. H., Larson, M. J., & Cavanaugh, D. (1995). Mental health/substance abuse treatment in managed care: The Massachusetts Medicaid experience. *Health Affairs, 14,* 173–184.

Chamberlain, R., & Rapp, C. (1991). A decade of case management: A methodological review of outcome research. *Community Mental Health Journal, 27,* 171–188.

Chervenak, F. A., & McCullough, L. B. (1995). The threat of the new managed practice of medicine to patients' autonomy. *Journal of Clinical Ethics, 6,* 320–323.

Christensen, K. T. (1995). Ethically important distinctions among managed care organizations. *Journal of Law, Medicine & Ethics, 23,* 223–229.

Corcoran, K., & Gingrich, W. J. (1994). Practice evaluation in the context of managed care: Case-recording methods for quality assurance reviews. *Research on Social Work Practice, 4,* 326–337.

Corcoran, K., & Vandiver, V. (1996). *Maneuvering the maze of managed care: Skills for mental health practitioners.* New York: Free Press.

Cornelius, D. S. (1994). Managed care and social work: Constructing a context and a response. *Social Work in Health Care, 20,* 47–63.

Davidson, J. R., & Davidson, T. (1996). Confidentiality and managed care: Ethical and legal concerns. *Health & Social Work, 21,* 208–215.

Dickey, B., & Azeni, H. (1992). Impact of managed care on mental health services. *Health Affairs, 11,* 197–204.

Dietzen, L. L., & Bond, G. R. (1993). Relationship between case manager contact and outcome for frequently hospitalized psychiatric clients. *Hospital and Community Psychiatry, 44,* 839–843.

Dixon, L., Friedman, N., & Lehman, A. (1993). Compliance of homeless mentally ill persons with assertive community treatment. *Hospital and Community Psychiatry, 44,* 581–583.

Dohrenwend, B. P., Levav, I., Shrout, P. E., Schwartz, S., Naveh, G., Link, B., Skodol, A. E., & Stueve, A. (1992). Socioeconomic status and psychiatric disorders: The causation–selection issue. *Science, 255,* 946–952.

Doner, K. S. (1995). Managed care: Ethical issues. *JAMA, 274,* 609.

Dorwart, R. A. (1990). Managed mental health care: Myths and realities in the 1990s. *Hospital and Community Psychiatry, 41,* 1087–1091.

Dorwart, R. A., & Hoover, C. W. (1994). A national study of transitional hospital services in mental health. *American Journal of Public Health, 84,* 1229–1234.

Douglass, R. L., & Torres, R. E. (1994). Evaluation of a managed care program for the non-Medicaid urban poor. *Journal of Health Care for the Poor and Underserved, 5,* 83–98.

Drake, R. E., Becker, D. R., Biesanz, J. C., Torrey, W. C., McHugo, G. J., & Wyzik, P. F. (1994). Rehabilitative day treatment vs. supported employment: I. Vocational outcomes. *Community Mental Health Journal, 30,* 519–532.

Durham, M. L. (1994). Healthcare's greatest challenge: Providing services for people with severe mental illness in managed care. *Behavioral Sciences and Law, 12,* 331–349.

Edwards, R. L., Cooke, P. W., & Reid, P. N. (1996). Social work management in an era of diminishing federal responsibility. *Social Work, 41,* 468–479.

Ellison, M. L., Rogers, E. S., Sciarappa, K., Cohen, M., & Forbess, R. (1995). Characteristics of mental health case management: Results of a national survey. *Journal of Mental Health Administration, 22,* 101–112.

Emanuel, E. J. (1995). Medical ethics in the era of managed care: The need for institutional structures instead of principles for individual cases. *Journal of Clinical Ethics, 6,* 335–338.

Emanuel, E. J., & Dubler, N. N. (1995). Managed care: Ethical issues. *JAMA, 274,* 610.

Essock, S. M., & Goldman, H. H. (1995). States' embrace of managed mental health care. *Health Affairs, 14,* 34–44.

Feldman, S. (1991). *Managed mental health services.* Springfield, IL: Charles C Thomas.

Freeman, E. M. (1996). Welfare reforms and services for children and families: Setting a new practice, research, and policy agenda. *Social Work, 41,* 521–532.

Freeman, M. A., & Trabin, T. (1994). Managed behavioral healthcare: History, models, key issues, and future course. *Behavioral Health Alliance,* p. 23.

The future of a medical center [Editorial]. (1996, November 11). *Boston Globe,* p. A12.

Geraty, R. D., Hendren, R. L., & Flaa, C. (1992). Ethical perspectives on managed care as it relates to child and adolescent psychiatry. *Journal of the American Academy of Child and Adolescent Psychiatry, 31,* 398–402.

Goering, P. N., Wasylenki, D. A., Farkas, M., Lancee, W. J., & Ballantyne, R. (1988). What difference does case management make? *Hospital and Community Psychiatry, 39,* 272–276.

Goodman, M., Brown, J., & Dietz, P. (1992). *Managing managed care.* Washington, DC: American Psychiatric Press.

Goplerud, E. N. (1995). Why prevention is important for managed behavioral healthcare. *American College of Mental Health Administration Newsletter, 15*(2), 1–2.

Gostin, L. O., Turek-Brezina, J., Powers, M., Kozloff, R., Faden, R., & Steinauer, D. D. (1993). Privacy and security of personal information in a new health care system. *JAMA, 270,* 2487–2493.

Gottlieb, G. L. (1989). Diversity, uncertainty, and variations in practice: The behaviors and clinical decisionmaking of mental health care providers. In C. A. Taube, D. Mechanic, & A. A. Hohmann (Eds.), *The future of mental health services research* (pp. 225–251). Rockville, MD: U.S. Department of Health and Human Services.

Grella, C. E., & Grusky, O. (1989). Families of the seriously mentally ill and their satisfaction with services. *Hospital and Community Psychiatry, 40,* 831–835.

Hall, R. C. (1994). Legal precedents affecting managed care. The physician's responsibilities to patients. *Psychosomatics, 35,* 105–117.

Hargreaves, W. A., & Shumway, M. (1989). Effectiveness of services for the severely mentally ill. In C. A. Taube, D. Mechanic, & A. A. Hohmann (Eds.), *The future of mental health services research* (pp. 253–283). Rockville, MD: U.S. Department of Health and Human Services.

Harris, M., & Bergman, H. (1988). Misconceptions about use of case management services by the chronic mentally ill: A utilization analysis. *Hospital and Community Psychiatry, 39,* 1276–1280.

Holahan, J., Bovbjerg, R., Evans, A., Wiener, J., & Flanagan, S. (1997). *Health policy for low-income people in Massachusetts.* Washington, DC: Urban Institute.

Holleman, W. L., Edwards, D. C., & Matson, C. C. (1994). Obligations of physicians to patients and third-party payers. *Journal of Clinical Ethics, 5,* 113–120.

Hollingsworth, E. J. (1994). Managed care plan performance since 1980: A literature analysis. *JAMA, 271,* 1512–1519.

Howe, E. G. (1995). Managed care: "New moves." Moral uncertainty, and a radical attitude. *Journal of Clinical Ethics, 6,* 290–305.

Hutchins, J. (1996). Managing managed care for families. *Empowering Families, 5*(2), 6–7.

Iglehart, J. K. (1996). Health policy report. Managed care and mental health. *New England Journal of Medicine, 334,* 131–135.

Intagliata, J., & Baker, F. (1983). Factors affecting case management services for the chronically mentally ill. *Administration in Mental Health, 11,* 75–91.

Jecker, N. S., & Pearlman, R. A. (1992). An ethical framework for rationing health care. *Journal of Medicine and Philosophy, 17,* 79–96.

Kamerman, S. B. (1996). The new politics of child and family policies. *Social Work, 41,* 453–465.

Kane, R. L., Bartlett, J., & Porthoff, S. (1995). Building an empirically based outcomes information system for managed mental health care. *Psychiatric Services, 46,* 459–461.

Kane, R. A. (1992). Case management. Ethical pitfalls on the road to high-quality managed care. In S. M. Rose (Ed.), *Case management and social work practice* (pp. 219–228). New York: Longman.

Kessler, R. C., & Neighbors, H. W. (1986). A new perspective on the relationship among race, social class, and psychological distress. *Journal of Health and Social Behavior, 27,* 107–115.

Koppel, T. (1996, November 8). Mental health care privacy and managed care [Transcript]. *Nightline,* pp. 1–5.

Korr, W. S., & Cloninger, L. (1991). Assessing models of case management: An empirical approach. *Journal of Social Service Research, 14,* 129–146.

Leadholm, B. A., & Kerzner, J. P. (1995). Public managed care: Comprehensive community support in Massachusetts. *Administration and Policy in Mental Health, 22,* 543–552.

Lefley, H. P., Bernheim, K. F., & Goldman, C. R. (1989). National forum addresses need to enhance training in treating the seriously mentally ill. *Hospital and Community Psychiatry, 40,* 460–470.

Luft, H. S. (1996). Modifying managed competition to address cost and quality. *Health Affairs, 15,* 23–38.

McCarthy, P. R., Gelber, S., & Dugger, D. (1993). Outcome measurement to outcome management: The critical step. *Administration and Policy in Mental Health, 21,* 59–68.

McNutt, J. G. (1995). The macro practice curriculum in graduate social work education: Results of a national study. *Administration in Social Work, 19*(3), 59–74.

Mechanic, D. (1993). Mental health services in the context of health insurance reform. *Milbank Quarterly, 71,* 349–364.

Mechanic, D., Schlesinger, M., & McAlpine, D. D. (1995). Management of mental health and substance abuse services: State of the art and early results. *Milbank Quarterly, 73,* 19–55.

Miller, R. H., & Luft, H. S. (1994). Managed care plan performance since 1980: A literature analysis. *JAMA, 271,* 1512–1519.

Minkoff, K. (1994). Community mental health in the nineties: Public sector managed care. *Community Mental Health Journal, 30,* 317–321.

Mirin, S. M., & Namerow, M. J. (1991). Why study treatment outcome? *Hospital and Community Psychiatry, 42,* 1007–1013.

Monkman, M. M. (1991). Outcome objectives in social work practice: Person and environment. *Social Work, 36,* 253–258.

Morreim, E. H. (1995). Lifestyles of the risky and infamous. From managed care to managed lives. *Hastings Center Report, 25*(6), 5–12.

Morse, G. A., Calsyn, R. J., Allen, G., & Kenny, D. A. (1994). Helping homeless mentally ill people: What variables mediate and moderate program effects? *American Journal of Community Psychology, 22,* 661–683.

Motenko, A. K., Allen, E. A., Angelos, P., Block, L., DeVito, J. A., Duffy, A., Holton, L., Lambert, K., Parker, C., Ryan, J., Schraft, D., & Swindell, J. A. (1995). Privatization and cutbacks: Social work and client impressions of service delivery in Massachusetts. *Social Work, 40,* 456–463.

Munson, C. E. (1996). Autonomy and managed care in clinical social work practice. *Smith College Studies in Social Work, 66,* 241–260.

National Association of Social Workers. (1996). *NASW code of ethics.* Washington, DC: Author.

Olsen, D. P. (1995). Ethical cautions in the use of outcomes for resource allocation in the managed care environment of mental health. *Archives of Psychiatric Nursing, 9*(4), 173–178.

Pellegrino, E. D. (1995). Interests, obligations, and justice: Some notes toward an ethic of managed care. *Journal of Clinical Ethics, 6,* 312–317.

Perneger, T. V., Allaz, A-F., Etter, J-F., & Rougemont, A. (1995). Mental health and choice between managed care and indemnity health insurance. *American Journal of Psychiatry, 152,* 1020–1025.

Phillips, D. G. (1997). Legal and ethical issues in the era of managed care. In R. M. Alperin & D. G. Phillips (Eds.), *The impact of managed care on the practice of psychotherapy: Innovation, implementation, and controversy* (pp. 171–184). New York: Brunner/Mazel.

Questions about a hospital deal [Editorial]. (1996, November 29). *New York Times,* p. 22.

Quinlivan, R., Hough, R., Crowell, A., Beach, C., Hofstetter, R., & Kenworth, K. (1995). Service utilization and costs of care for severely mentally ill clients in an intensive case management program. *Psychiatric Services, 46,* 365–371.

Rife, J. C., First, R. J., Greenlee, R. W., Miller, L. D., & Feichter, M. (1991). Case management with homeless mentally ill people. *Health & Social Work, 16,* 58–67.

Rodwin, M. A. (1995). Conflicts in managed care. *New England Journal of Medicine, 332,* 604–607.

Rosner, F. (1995). Managed care: Ethical issues. *JAMA, 274,* 609–610.

Rowland D., Rosenbaum, S., Simon, L., & Chait, E. (1995a). *Medicaid and managed care: Lessons from the literature. A Report of the Kaiser Commission on the Future of Medicaid.* Washington, DC: Kaiser Commission on the Future of Medicaid.

Rowland, D., Rosenbaum, S., Simon, L., & Chait, E. (1995b). Medicaid and managed care: Lessons from the literature [Review]. *News and Issues.* National Center for Children in Poverty (NCCP), 6.

Rubin, A. (1992). Is case management effective for people with serious mental illness? *Health & Social Work, 17,* 138–150.

Sabin, J. E. (1994a). A credo for ethical managed care in mental health practice. *Hospital and Community Psychiatry, 45,* 859–860, 869.

Sabin, J. E. (1994b). Caring about patients and caring about money: The American Psychiatric Association code of ethics meets managed care. *Behavioral Sciences and the Law, 12,* 317–330.

Samuelson, R. J. (1996, November 24). Mismanaged care. Review of G. Anders, *Health against wealth: HMOs and the breakdown of medical trust. New York Times,* p. 13.

Sands, R. G., & Cnaan, R. A. (1994). Two modes of case management: Assessing their impact. *Community and Mental Health Journal, 30,* 441–457.

Scarf, M. (1996, June 16). Keeping secrets. *New York Times Magazine,* pp. 38–41.

Schlesinger, M., & Mechanic, D. (1993). Challenges for managed competition from chronic illness. *Health Affairs* (Suppl.), 123–137.

Sederer, L. I., Eisen, S. V., Dill, D., Grob, M. C., Gougeon, M. L., & Mirin, S. M. (1992). Case-based reimbursement for psychiatric hospital care. *Hospital and Community Psychiatry, 43,* 1120–1126.

Sederer, L. I., & Mirin, S. M. (1994). The impact of managed care on clinical practice. *Psychiatric Quarterly, 65,* 177–188.

The selling of a hospital [Editorial]. (1996, November 21). *Boston Globe,* p. A22.

Shore, M. F., & Beigel, A. (1996). The challenges posed by managed behavioral health care. *New England Journal of Medicine, 334,* 116–118.

Simon, G. E., Von Korff, M., & Durham, M. L. (1994). Predictors of outpatient mental health utilization by primary care patients in a health maintenance organization. *American Journal of Psychiatry, 151,* 908–913.

Stern, S. (1993). Managed care, brief therapy, and therapeutic integrity. *Psychotherapy, 30,* 162–175.

Strom, K., & Gingrich, W. J. (1993). Educating students for the new market realities. *Journal of Social Work Education, 29,* 78–87.

Sulmasy, D. P. (1995). Managed care and the new medical paternalism. *Journal of Clinical Ethics, 6,* 324–326.

Tessler, R. C., Bernstein, A. G., Rosen, B. M., & Golman, H. H. (1982). The chronically mentally ill in community support systems. *Hospital and Community Psychiatry, 33,* 208–211.

Thompson, C. M. (1985). Characteristics associated with outcome in a community mental health partial hospitalization program. *Community Mental Health Journal, 21,* 179–188.

Toner, R. (1996, November 24). Harry and Louise were right, sort of. *New York Times,* section 4, pp. 1, 3.

Weil, M. O. (1996). Community building: Building community practice. *Social Work, 41,* 481–499.

Weimer, S. R. (1990). Taking issue: The benefits and drawbacks of managed care. *Hospital and Community Psychiatry, 41,* 1055.

Wells, K. B., Rogers, W. H., Davis, L. M., Kahn, K., Norquist, G., Keeler, E., Kosecoff, J., & Brook, R. H. (1993). After implementation of the Medicare prospective payment system. *American Journal of Psychiatry, 150,* 1799–1805.

Winegar, N. (1992). *The clinician's guide to managed mental health care.* New York: Haworth Press.

Winegar, N., & Bistline, J. (1994). *Marketing mental health services to managed care.* New York: Haworth Press.

Zoloth-Dorfman, L., & Rubin, S. (1995). The patient as commodity: Managed care and the question of ethics. *Journal of Clinical Ethics, 6,* 339–357.

Epilogue: Inhumane versus Humane Managed Care

Albert R. Roberts

Dean Anita Lightburn and Professor Gerald Schamess have compiled and edited a state-of-the-art sourcebook on the current policies, controversies, clinical knowledge, case studies, and research strategies on managed care practices. Lightburn and Schamess have vast experience in developing curriculum and training programs for clinical social workers, health care administrators, and future social workers. Sixty-two of the nation's leading experts have made important contributions to this book. This magnum opus is the most comprehensive in scope, well-written, and timely volume published to date on managed care. It provides the necessary information, guidelines, and blueprints for maximizing opportunities for humane managed care as we enter the 21st century. This long-awaited volume will help all social workers and other human services professionals better understand and advocate for humane managed care in both public and private sectors. Lightburn and Schamess are to be congratulated on completing this innovative book project. It surpasses my high expectations.

Until recently, the overriding purpose of managed care has been to keep spiraling costs under control through profit-driven corporate principles and values. Managed care policies, systems, and practices were originally developed with a preventive orientation for all healthy people to stay healthy. Unfortunately, in many states, managed care systems have ignored the health care needs of the chronically ill, chronically mentally ill, and developmentally disabled populations. This encyclopedic volume, in accord with the social work profession's strong voice and concern for humane health and mental health care for all people in need, provides the organizational models, agency perspectives, ethical challenges, legal concerns, changing practice perspectives, professional education strategies, and research guideposts to optimize the delivery of health and behavioral health care services.It examines the dangers inherent in cost shifting, corporate takeovers, and mergers.

This outstanding book was completed in response to the National Association of Social Workers' (NASW's) fervent commitment to social justice and humane care through building consensus, forming coalitions, and advocating for oppressed and vulnerable populations. The focus of the book includes a calling for quality care for all individuals and families at risk. This book provides avenues for maximizing health care services and corrective action in communities where oppressed groups are being denied services.

Managed care has resulted in revolutionary changes in the organization, accessibility, and delivery of health and mental health services in the United States. It has been estimated that by the beginning of the 21st century almost 90 percent of health insurance plans will mandate that their subscribers receive health and mental health care through a managed care network. Many practitioners are scrambling to find a place for themselves in this new era of managed care. Some practitioners—frustrated by the burdensome managed care procedures and regulations and the lower payment rates—have left practice altogether. Others have joined managed care networks because they were experiencing a dwindling clientele, with more of their consumers informing them that their new health benefits program permitted service delivery only from the XYZ health maintenance organization (HMO). Still other practitioners have tried to organize their own managed care networks with the goal of having a say in the way the organization reduces costs and improves the quality of care.

HMOs and preferred provider organizations (PPOs) were originally developed with the goal of bringing affordable and accessible health care to the public, but few authorities realized how complex and profit-oriented these organizations would become. The original HMOs (for example, Kaiser Permanente Health Plan) were nonprofit organizations, and they focused primarily on preventing illness and coordinating care for those who were ill. Unfortunately, what began as a humane and efficient system of health care delivery evolved into a highly competitive, big-business, profit-making enterprise, wherein the interests of the shareholders took precedence over the interest in providing medically appropriate health and mental health services.

The enrollees of the early HMO plans were primarily young and middle-aged (under age 65)—and healthy—working people. But as time went on, the HMOs' target populations expanded to serve Medicaid and Medicare beneficiaries, as well as people with chronic illness and disabilities. And these newer populations typically have health care needs that are much more complex and costly than the groups that HMOs originally intended to serve. This has resulted in a greater need for specialists, expensive diagnostic procedures, and higher hospital costs.

Patients and practitioners alike are furious when they hear about chief executive officers (CEOs) of managed care organizations annually receiving compensation packages in excess of $10 million while at the same time the HMO dictates an enrollee be denied access to an advanced diagnostic tool such as a magnetic resonance image (MRI) examination, or a woman who has had a mastectomy be discharged from the hospital before her physician believes she is ready to go home.

The proliferation of managed care companies throughout the United States will have a significant effect on every professional social worker. As we approach the beginning of the 21st century, each social worker must define her or his own role vis-à-vis managed care. Will social workers choose to work within managed care systems and promulgate the rules and regulations that govern that system of care? Or will they remain apart from the managed care system and serve as advocates for consumers, advising them of their rights to file grievances and appeals against the system, if they have been denied medically necessary services?

Humane Managed Care? will make a significant contribution toward increasing our understanding of the issues, controversies, and innovative practices in today's managed care environment. The challenges and opportunities before us have been thoroughly discussed in this volume. Because the overwhelming majority of health and mental health professionals completed graduate school prior to the expansion of managed care, they lack many of the administrative and practice skills necessary to prosper economically in the managed care environment. However, most social workers were educated and trained with the ideals and ethics of our profession's founders: Jane Addams, Dorothea Dix, Ida Cannon, Bertha Capen Reynolds, Mary Richmond, and Harriet Bartlett. Therefore, our advocacy, social action, and coalition-building skills and sensitivity to vulnerable populations will help us meet the challenge in the tradition of our founders (from the Charity Organization Movement and the Progressive Era)—to facilitate humane care in health, mental health, and child care settings.

This book is a major first step in information sharing necessary to persuade our clinical colleagues about the critical importance of the latest opportunities and managed care strategies for all people, regardless of their income levels or pre-existing medical and mental disorders. The next important step should be the planning and publication of a special issue of *Social Work* on humane managed care. Simultaneous planning efforts should be made for a national conference on humane managed care, jointly convened by NASW, the American Nursing Association, and the American Psychiatric Association. Finally, legislative and lobbying efforts need to gain momentum in the important next few years as we enter the new millennium. NASW, the Clinical Social Work Federation, the National Council of Community Mental Health Centers, and the Society of Hospital Social Workers need to unite in support of consumer-protection legislation for managed care consumers. All social workers should support NASW's political action committee, PACE, both in helping draft and in lobbying for new legislation needed to remove barriers to quality health care for people with chronic mental illness, serious physical illness, and developmental disabilities. Furthermore, we should be advocating for federal and state legislation that will mandate such new opportunities for social change and social work practice as revising and negotiating state Medicaid laws and contracts, providing clinical case management, and developing multidisciplinary teams in community clinics.

Managed care—a humane goal, or an albatross? Within communities throughout the United States, there has been much discussion of and growing media attention to the negative and devastating irreversible effects of denying necessary medical procedures to people in the early stages of a chronic or terminal illness (such as cancer). As social workers we all believe in human dignity and the individual's ability to change and improve their health and environment. The "albatross" would be dismissing the challenge, focusing only on self-interest, and giving up the hope that people (for example, hospital administrators, HMO medical directors, legislators, CEOs) can and do change. The albatross would be to give up by changing careers, or by staying neutral and allowing big business and major corporations to dictate to and disenfranchise nondominant cultural and racial groups and people with chronic illnesses and developmental disabilities. As client advocates, educators, group members, change agents, community organizers, clinical practitioners, and legislative advocates, we have the ability and power to join together in transforming inhumane and narrow care to humane care for all citizens in need.

Index

G

H

I

J

K

L

M

N

U

V

W–Y

About the Editors

Gerald Schamess, MSS, is professor of social work at Smith College School for Social Work, Northampton, Massachusetts, and editor of the *Smith College Studies in Social Work.* He has published widely on treatment process and group treatment for children and adolescents, and has practiced clinically since 1958.

Anita Lightburn, MSS, MEd, EdD, is dean and Elizabeth Marting Truehaft Professor at Smith College School for Social Work and a member of the Academy of Practice. She has taught clinical social work practice for 25 years and is an author and consultant. Before assuming the deanship in 1994, she was a practicing clinician and an associate professor at Columbia University School of Social Work, New York. Recent research includes family support for at-risk families and knowledge development to support work with traumatized children and families.

About the Contributors

Gunnar Almgren, PhD, is an assistant professor at the School of Social Work at the University of Washington and former director of the social work department at the University of Washington Medical Center. His research throughout the past several years has concerned the linkages among race, ethnicity, social class, and health outcomes.

Richard H. Beinecke, DPA, ACSW, is an assistant professor, department of public management, Suffolk University, Boston.

Candyce S. Berger, MSW, PhD, is the director of social work and patient care services at the University of Michigan Hospitals and Health Center and is an associate professor and assistant dean at the University of Michigan School of Social Work. She is past-president of the Society for Social Work Administrators in Health Care.

Cindy Brach, MS, is a health policy researcher at the Agency for Health Care Policy and Research's Center for Organization and Delivery Studies, where she conducts research on managed care. She received her master's degree in public policy from the University of California, Berkeley, and is presently a doctoral candidate there.

Amy Braverman, MSW, is a clinical social worker in the psychiatric emergency services of a northeastern university teaching hospital. She is a graduate of the Smith College School for Social Work.

Deanna Brooks, MSW, LICSW, is a clinical associate professor and the associate director of field education at Simmons College School of Social Work, Boston. She also lectures at Boston College School of Social Work.

James J. Callahan, MSW, PhD, is a research professor and the director of the National Institute of Mental Health Training Program in Mental Health Services Research at the Heller School, Brandeis University, Waltham, Massachusetts.

Jay Callahan, PhD, is an assistant professor at the Jane Addams College of Social Work, University of Illinois at Chicago. He has been active in the American Association of Suicidology and on the Northern Illinois Critical Incident Stress Management Team and also maintains a private practice. His research interests are traumatic stress, crisis intervention, and suicidology.

Alfred Carter, MD, is in the full-time private practice of psychiatry in Springfield, Massachusetts, and is a member of the Steering Committee for the Health New England Mental Health/Substance Abuse Program. He is also a clinical instructor in psychiatry at Tufts University School of Medicine.

Doreen Cavanaugh, PhD, is a research associate at the Institute for Health Policy of the Heller School. She was formerly a regional director in the Office of Children in Massachusetts.

Jeanette R. Davidson, PhD, ACSW, is an associate professor and chair of direct practice at the University of Oklahoma School of Social Work. She was formerly an associate professor at Columbia University School of Social Work. Her research and writing include interracial marriage, cultural diversity in social work education, and legal or ethical issues concerning managed care.

Kay Davidson, DSW, is dean and professor at the University of Connecticut School of Social Work. Before taking that position, she was a faculty member in the schools of social work at both Hunter College and Columbia University. She is active in the Society of Social Work Leaders in Health Care.

Tim Davidson, PhD, is an associate professor in the department of human relations at the University of Oklahoma. Since 1973 he has worked alternately in public mental health, private practice, and as an adjunct professor. His experience is in outpatient, inpatient, residential, and day programs.

King Davis, PhD, is a professor of public mental health policy and planning at the Virginia Commonwealth University School of Social Work, Richmond. He is a former commissioner of the Virginia Department of Mental Health, Mental Retardation, and Substance Abuse Services.

Susan Donner, PhD, is a clinical social worker and associate dean of the Smith College School for Social Work, Northampton, Massachusetts. She was director of fieldwork there for almost 10 years. Her areas of interest are field education, self-psychology, administration, diversity, and the relationship between meditation and clinical insight.

Matthew P. Dumont, MD, is a psychiatrist at Westborough State Hospital in Massachusetts. For 16 years he directed a community mental health clinic in Chelsea, Massachusetts. His book *Treating the Poor* describes his experience of being laid off from that directorship during a privatization and budget-cutting campaign implemented by the state's Department of Mental Health.

Carol Edelstein, MSW, is a poet and fiction writer who supports her writing life through an independent psychotherapy practice and through her work as a clinical supervisor in a community mental health center.

Joyce Edward, CSW, BCD, is cofounder and the first cochair of the National Coalition of Mental Health Professionals and Consumers. She is a part-time member of the faculty at the Smith College School of Social Work, Northampton, Massachusetts and coeditor of *Fostering Healing and Growth,* published in 1996 by Jason Aronson.

Eileen Elias, MEd, is a senior policy analyst for the Substance Abuse and Mental Health Services Administration, Center for Mental Health Services. She served as Commissioner of Mental Health for the Commonwealth of Massachusetts from 1991 to 1996 and is recognized for helping create responsive and accountable systems from fragmented services by working closely with key stakeholders at national, state, local, and provider levels.

Suzanne Gelber, PhD, is executive vice president and chief marketing officer at Managed Health Network, San Rafael, California. She is a member of the advisory boards of *Managed Behavioral Health News*, the Florida Mental Health Institute in Tampa, and six national managed care research projects.

Jeffrey L. Geller, MD, MPH, is professor of psychiatry at the University of Massachusetts Medical School, the director of public-sector psychiatry at the University of Massachusetts Medical Center, and the central Massachusetts area medical director for the Massachusetts Department of Mental Health. He is active in the American Psychiatric Association, serving on the editorial board, as book review editor, and as

First Person Account column editor for *Psychiatric Services.* He teaches the mental health policy course at the Smith College School for Social Work.

Maury Goodman, MPA, is a research associate in the department of public management at Suffolk University, Boston.

Sidney H. Grossberg, MSW, PhD, BCD, is the executive director of Counseling Associates, Inc., Southfield, Michigan, and a member of the continuing education faculty, Smith College School for Social Work, Northampton, Massachusetts. He is a Distinguished Practitioner, National Academy of Practice in Social Work, and a member of the board of directors, American Board of Examiners in Clinical Social Work.

Stephen R. Hall, PhD, is the executive director of The Resource Exchange, a Colorado community-centered board serving people with developmental disabilities. His current interests are in transforming a large human services organization into neighborhood locations with allegiance to and support from neighbors rather than government.

Eva Havas, MSW, PhD, is assistant dean for part-time programs and a clinical associate professor of social work at the Boston University School of Social Work. With 20 years of social work practice experiences, she has publications and conference presentations focused on social policy, families, and health care delivery.

Joel Kanter, MSW, LCSW, has been a practicing social worker since graduating from Smith College School for Social Work in 1974. He is senior case manager at the Mount Vernon Center for Community Mental Health in Fairfax, Virginia, and is in private practice. His many publications focus on the community care of people with severe mental illnesses.

Patricia Kelley, PhD, LISW, BCD, is a professor in and the director of the School of Social Work, University of Iowa, Iowa City. She also practices part-time as an independent clinical social worker in Cedar Rapids. Her teaching and scholarship are in the area of clinical practice with families.

Mary Jo Larson, PhD, is a senior research scientist at the New England Research Institutes.

H. Stephen Leff, PhD, is senior vice president at the Human Services Research Institute (HSRI), Cambridge, Massachusetts, and an assistant professor of psychology at the Harvard Medical School. He is principal investigator and director of the Evaluation Center@HSRI, a program funded by the Center for Mental Health Services to provide technical assistance nationally for evaluating adult mental health systems change.

Benjamin Liptzin, MD, is chair of the department of psychiatry at Baystate Health System in Springfield, Massachusetts, and is professor and deputy chair of psychiatry at the Tufts University School of Medicine.

Amy Lockhart, BA, is a research associate in the department of public management, Suffolk University, Boston.

Sue Matorin, MS, ACSW, is the program director of the Cornell Psychiatry Intensive Managed Care program. She is also an adjunct associate professor at the Columbia University School of Social Work, where she serves as vice chair of the school's advisory council. She is on the executive committee of the NASW New York City Chapter.

Joshua Miller, MSW, PhD, is an associate professor and chair of the social policy sequence at Smith College School for Social Work, Northampton, Massachusetts. Formerly, he held the position of director of fieldwork there. He has worked as a caseworker, group worker, family therapist, community organizer, and agency director and is presently engaged in research and publication about the intersection of family, community, and social policy.

Terry Mizrahi, MSW, PhD, is a professor at the Hunter College School of Social Work of the City University of New York. There she chairs the social health field of practice and directs the Education Center for Community Organizing. She also cochairs the Health Care Policy and Practice Network of the NASW New York City Chapter.

Carlton E. Munson, MSW, PhD, is a professor and the doctoral program director at the University of Maryland School of Social Work, Baltimore. He has held faculty appointments at Catholic University of America, Washington, DC; the University of Houston; and Fordham University at Lincoln Center, New York. He is the founding editor of *The Clinical Supervisor,* an interdisciplinary journal devoted to supervision research.

Roberta Myers, MSW, BCD, is the program chair of the clinical certificate program in theory and practice through the Washington State Society for Clinical Social Work and Family Services, Seattle. She maintains a private psychotherapy practice in Bellevue, Washington. Her training includes completion of the Psychoanalytic Psychotherapy Program at the Seattle Institute for Psychoanalysis.

Marc Navon, LICSW, is the director of the behavioral health program at Neighborhood Health Plan, an affiliate of Harvard Pilgrim Health Care, Boston. He previously served as director of utilization management for the Massachusetts Department of Mental Health.

Wilma Peebles-Wilkins, PhD, ACSW, is dean and a professor at Boston University School of Social Work. Before her appointment at Boston University, she was director of the undergraduate social work program and associate head of the department of sociology, anthropology, and social work at North Carolina State University, Raleigh.

Michael S. Perlman, MD, has been in the full-time private practice of psychiatry in Northampton, Massachusetts, since 1976. His major clinical interests include approaches to treatment-resistant mood disorders, especially psychotherapy with patients who have bipolar disorder, and paradoxical and dialectical approaches to apparently irreconcilable conflicts.

Janet D. Perloff, PhD, is an associate professor in the School of Social Welfare and the School of Public Health at the University of Albany, State University of New York. She has research interests in the delivery of health services to low-income and other disadvantaged populations and has published widely on the effect of Medicaid on access to maternal and child health care.

Elizabeth V. Phillips, MSW, PhD, is president of the Clinical Social Work Federation. She conducts a private practice in New Haven, Connecticut, having been a clinical professor at the Yale University School of Medicine Department of Psychiatry. She is a founding member of the Clinical Social Work Guild–Office and Professional Employees Union International–AFL/CIO.

Jay M. Pomerantz, MD, is in full-time private psychiatric practice in Longmeadow, Massachusetts. He has served as a Peace Corps staff physician in Panama and later as Peace Corps medical director for Latin America. He is on the clinical faculty of Tufts Medical School and is a lecturer on psychiatry at Harvard Medical School.

Frederic G. Reamer, PhD, is a professor in the graduate program of the School of Social Work, Rhode Island College, Providence. His research, teaching, and social work practice have focused on the areas of criminal justice, affordable housing, social policy, and professional ethics. He served as the chair of the NASW committee that drafted the *NASW Code of Ethics.*

Cheryl Resnick, DSW, is an assistant professor of social work and the coordinator of gerontology at Georgian Court College in Lakewood, New Jersey. She received her graduate degree from Yeshiva University and has 20 years of experience in health care.

Priscilla Riley, MSW, LICSW, is an associate professor and the director of field education at Simmons College School of Social Work, Boston. She cochairs the North American Network of Field Educators and Directors.

Albert R. Roberts, PhD, is a professor of social work and criminal justice at the School of Social Work, Rutgers University, Piscataway, New Jersey. He is the editor-in-chief of the journal *Crisis Intervention and Time-Limited Treatment.* He has authored more than 130 scholarly publications, including 20 books.

Gary Rosenberg, PhD, is the Edith J. Baerwald professor of community medicine (social work) and senior vice president at the Mount Sinai Medical Center. He serves as editor-in-chief of *Social Work in Health Care,* and has written and published extensively. Having received a number of awards, he is a recipient of the Ida M. Cannon Award of the Society for Hospital Social Work Directors as well as the society's past-president.

Suzanne Sankar, MSW, LICSW, is an assistant professor in the field education department of Simmons College School of Social Work, Boston. She is the former coordinator of the Mystic Clinic of the Somerville Mental Health Center, Somerville, Massachusetts.

Leslie Scallet, JD, is a vice president of The Lewin Group, Fairfax, Virginia, specializing in mental health and substance abuse. She is recognized nationally as an expert in managed behavioral health care, mental health policy, development and dissemination of policy information, health care reform, legislative advocacy, and client rights.

Phebe Sessions, MSW, PhD, is an associate professor and chair of the social work practice sequence at Smith College School for Social Work, Northampton, Massachusetts. Her research and scholarly interests have focused on clinical practice in low-income communities and understanding the relevance of philosophical issues for social work practice.

Donald S. Shepard, PhD, is a research professor at the Heller School, Brandeis University, Waltham, and an adjunct lecturer at the Harvard School of Public Health.

Madeline Silva, RN, CCM, is a utilization and case management liaison for Health Cost Consultants and an independent consultant in the field of managed care. At the time of this writing, she was manager of case management at Blue Cross/Blue Shield of the National Capital Area.

Alan B. Siskind, MSW, PhD, is executive vice president of the Jewish Board of Family and Children's Services, New York, vice president of the Coalition of Voluntary Mental Health Agencies, and the first vice chair of the Human Services Council of New York. He also serves as an adjunct professor at Columbia University School of Social Work.

Ellen Gelhaus Tighe, MSW, LCSW, at the time of writing, was a social worker in the Maternal Infant Care Program at Metropolitan Nashville General Hospital.

Alisa Trugerman, PhD, works with United Behavioral Health, New York, overseeing the network and interfacing with accounts throughout the northeastern United States. She has several years of experience in the provision of psychological services to children, adolescents, and families in school and outpatient settings and has served as assistant director of the marital–family program for a large group practice in Connecticut.

Rita Vandivort-Warren, ACSW, has more than 15 years' experience in mental health and health administration, policy, and program development. She has served on the national board of directors for NASW and since 1989 has been working in NASW's national office, crafting the association's response on social work policy and practice in a number of areas, including mental health, managed care, and Medicaid.

Nancy W. Veeder, MSW, MBA, PhD, is an associate professor at Boston College Graduate School of Social Work, where she teaches research and management. She has been engaged in health and mental health services delivery research in the United States, Jamaica, West Indies, and Mauritius, Indian Ocean.

Darleen Vernon, MPH, PhD, manages the Healthy Options (Medicaid) program for Regence Blue Shield and oversees all aspects of that company's contract compliance with Washington State's Medical Assistance Administration. Her career has included community- and hospital-based assignments with the U.S. Army and 10 years with Walter Reed Army Institute of Research.

Susan E. Weimer, MSW, PhD, is an assistant professor of social work at West Texas A&M University, Canyon. Her clinical practice experience includes two years at Bellevue Hospital's Psychiatric Emergency Service, New York, and more than 10 years at the Child Guidance Center of Southern Connecticut, Stamford.

Lawrence S. Woocher, BS, is a project manager at the Human Services Research Institute (HSRI), Cambridge, Massachusetts. He manages the Evaluation Center@HSRI, a program supported by the Center for Mental Health Services to provide technical assistance in the evaluation of adult mental health systems change. He also manages a study of community placements for long-term residents of New Jersey's state psychiatric hospitals.

Humane Managed Care?

Cover design by **The Watermark Design Office**

Book design and composition by **Christine Cotting, UpperCase Publication Services**

Printed by **Boyd Printing Company**

RESOURCES FROM NASW PRESS TO HELP YOU THRIVE IN AN ERA OF MANAGED CARE

Humane Managed Care? *Gerald Schamess and Anita Lightburn, Editors.* This state-of-the-art volume looks at one of today's most complex challenges of social workers in managed care. With *Humane Managed Care?* you'll get an excellent grounding in major facts and issues and practical knowledge of real-life situations—everything you need to work critically and proactively in this environment.

ISBN: 0-87101-294-4. Item #2944. $29.95

Outcomes Measurement in the Human Services: ***Cross-Cutting Issues and Methods,*** *Edward J. Mullen and Jennifer L. Magnabosco, Editors.* This is the first-ever handbook to cover outcomes measurement for the human services profession. You will benefit from a wide range of expert thinking on outcomes measurement in mental and behavioral health and child and family services. Essential reading for practitioners dealing with managed care requirements and an important text for preparing new practitioners.

ISBN: 0-87101-275-8. Item #2758. $36.95

Managed Care Resource Guides, *Vivian H. Jackson, Editor.* These two guidebooks are designed to help social work practitioners thrive in a managed care environment—in agency settings or in private practice. The *Guides* are packed with practical information on the nuances and requirements of managed care.

Agency Settings: ISBN: 0-87101-245-6, Item #2456, $50.00
Private Practice: ISBN: 0-87101-247-2, Item #2472, $50.00

Handbook of Solution-Focused Brief Therapy, *Scott D. Miller, Mark A. Hubble, and Barry L. Duncan, Editors. Available from the NASW Press by special arrangement with the publisher, Jossey-Bass.* This comprehensive edited collection offers mental health practitioners a much-needed resource for applying solution-focused brief therapy techniques. The *Handbook* is a definitive guide for succeeding in an era of managed care.

ISBN: 0-7879-0217-9. Item #2179. $39.95

Prudent Practice: ***A Guide for Managing Malpractice Risk,*** *by Mary Kay Houston-Vega and Elane M. Nuehring with Elisabeth R. Daguio.* Social workers and other human services professionals face a heightened risk of malpractice suits in today's litigious society. This book provides practitioners a complete practice guide to increasing competence and managing the risk of malpractice. Included in the book and on disk are 25 sample forms and 5 sample fact sheets to distribute to clients.

ISBN: 0-87101-267-7. Item #2677, Windows disk. Item #2677A, Macintosh. $42.95

(Order form on reverse side)

ORDER FORM

	Title	Item #	Price	Total
__	Humane Managed Care?	2944	$29.95	________
__	Outcomes Measurement in the Human Services	2758	$36.95	________
__	Managed Care Resource Guides			
	Agency Settings	2456	$50.00	________
	Private Practice	2472	$50.00	________
__	Handbook of Solution-Focused Brief Therapy	2179	$39.95	________
__	Prudent Practice (Word for Windows disk)	2677	$42.95	________
__	Prudent Practice (Macintosh disk)	2677A	$42.95	________
			Subtotal	________
		+ 10% postage and handling		________
			Total	________

❐ I've enclosed my check or money order for $ ____________.

❐ Please charge my ❐ NASW Visa* ❐ Other Visa ❐ MasterCard

Credit Card Number ________________ Expiration Date ________________

Signature ________________________________

**Use of this card generates funds in support of the social work profession.*

Name ________________________________

Address ________________________________

City ________________ State/Province ________________

Country ________________ Zip ________________

Phone ________________ E-mail ________________

NASW Member # (if applicable) ________________________

(Please make checks payable to NASW Press. Prices are subject to change.)

NASW PRESS
P. O. Box 431
Annapolis JCT, MD 20701
USA

Credit card orders call
1-800-227-3590
(In the Metro Wash., DC, area, call 301-317-8688)
Or fax your order to 301-206-7989
Or order online at http://www.naswpress.org

Visit our Web site at http://www.naswpress.org. HMCBI98